Color Atlas of Human Gross and Microscopic Pathology

Gamal Dawood

Color Atlas of Human Gross and Microscopic Pathology

Second Edition

Springer

Gamal Dawood
Al-Azhar Faculty of Medicine
Cairo, Egypt

ISBN 978-3-031-76009-9 ISBN 978-3-031-76007-5 (eBook)
https://doi.org/10.1007/978-3-031-76007-5

This Springer imprint is published by the registered company Springer Nature Switzerland AG
The registered company address is: Gewerbestrasse 11, 6330 Cham, Switzerland

This Atlas is dedicated to:

The esteemed community of pathologists

Their keen eyes, unwavering commitment, and tireless pursuit of knowledge are the bedrock of accurate diagnoses to save countless lives. I am deeply honored to contribute to this noble field.

With profound gratitude to my family

My wife Professor Mariam Abu-Shady,

My brother Mostafa,

and the cherished memory of my late brother Atef.

Their unlimited love, support, and encouragement have been the foundation upon which this achievement stands.

Foreword

It is said that a picture is worth a thousand words. I can say that in this atlas, each picture is worth a million words—such is the quality of the images in this atlas. Pathology is a visual science—no words can accurately depict the lesions, gross and micro. Hence, this atlas by Prof. Gamal Dawood fills an important role in pathology education. "The Color Atlas of Human Gross Pathology, 2nd Edition," represents the culmination of 30 years of dedicated work in pathology by the author. This completely revised edition builds upon the success of the first edition.

Featuring over 1400 high-resolution color photographs and comprehensive explanations, this revised edition provides an unparalleled understanding of various pathological conditions across all body systems. It serves as an essential visual reference for students, residents, and practicing pathologists, offering detailed insights into both macroscopic and microscopic features of major diseases. The description of each lesion is so precise that one can reproduce it with paper and pencil. I would urge the students to draw sketches of gross and microscopic features in their laboratory notebooks.

Along with myriads of pathology educators around the world, I am grateful to Prof. Gamal Dawood for producing this labor of love.

Vinay Kumar

Biologic Sciences Division
and The Pritzker School of Medicine
University of Chicago
Chicago, IL, USA

Preface to the Second Edition

The second edition of the Color Atlas of Human Gross Pathology builds upon the success of the first edition, offering an even more comprehensive and visually stunning resource for both medical professionals and those fascinated by the intricate workings of the human body.

This atlas goes beyond traditional textbooks, utilizing the power of high-quality color photographs to bridge the gap between theory and practice. This edition boasts a significant increase in the number of images, from 421 in the first edition to over 1450 in this one showcasing a wider spectrum of diseased tissues and organs in exquisite detail. Each photograph has been meticulously chosen to showcase the macroscopic appearance of diseased tissues and organs with exceptional clarity. Furthermore, the quality of the existing images has been significantly improved, ensuring the most accurate and detailed representation of pathology available.

The first edition covered a vast amount of material, but the second edition took it a step further by including a brand-new chapter dedicated entirely to **"Diseases of the Ocular System."** This addition ensures complete coverage of all major body systems, providing a truly comprehensive reference point for understanding pathology throughout the human organism.

This atlas goes beyond simply presenting the macroscopic picture. Each image is accompanied by insightful text that explains the underlying pathology, its causes, and its clinical implications. However, the journey does not stop there. This edition delves deeper by incorporating microscopic images alongside the gross images. This dual approach allows you to not only see the macroscopic changes in diseased tissues but also understand the cellular and histological changes that underlie these alterations. This fosters a deeper understanding of the disease process and bridges the gap between clinical observation and a more in-depth pathological understanding.

The second edition further enhances its value by introducing a new section titled **"Ancillary Tools."** This section delves into the realm of immunohistochemistry and molecular/cytogenetic analysis, providing crucial information on positive immunohistochemical stains and molecular and cytogenetic profiles of specific diseases. This additional layer of information equips the reader with the most up-to-date tools for accurate diagnosis.

This edition introduces a new feature—**"Pearls."** These sections highlight critical information and key differentiating points between similar diseases. This invaluable addition helps to refine diagnostic skills and ensures a more nuanced understanding of the pathological landscape.

The organization of diseases within each chapter has been meticulously reviewed and improved. This edition presents diseases in a more systematic manner, facilitating a deeper comprehension of each disease category.

Whether you are a medical student embarking on your journey of learning, a seasoned physician refining your diagnostic skills, or simply an individual with a passion for human health, this atlas is a valuable asset on your path to knowledge. It serves as a visual companion, guiding you through the fascinating world of pathology and empowering you to recognize, diagnose, and ultimately contribute to the treatment of a wide range of medical conditions. We invite you to embark on this visual journey and delve deeper into the captivating world of human pathology.

Cairo, Egypt — Gamal Dawood

Acknowledgments

I would like to express my deepest gratitude to Dr. Ahmed Rabie, Assistant Professor of Pathology in the Department of Pathology at Al-Azhar Faculty of Medicine, Damietta Branch, Egypt. His contribution to the second edition of the Color Atlas of Gross Pathology has been invaluable.

Dr. Rabie's generous donation of the immunostained slides was instrumental in significantly clarifying some important lesions within the atlas. These slides have played a crucial role in enhancing the educational value of the atlas and will undoubtedly benefit countless readers in their pursuit of a deeper understanding of pathology.

I am truly humbled by Dr. Rabie's support and unwavering commitment to advancing our collective knowledge of pathological lesions. His dedication to the field is truly inspiring.

Book Description

Color Atlas of Human Gross Pathology, 2nd Edition, is an essential resource for both medical professionals and enthusiasts alike. This comprehensive reference book combines vivid imagery with detailed explanations to help individuals understand and identify various pathological conditions in the human body.

Within its pages, you will find about 1500 high-quality color photographs showcasing the macroscopic appearance covering a wide range of human disease entities. The images of the first edition were developed, and its quality has increased. Also, a new collection of high-quality images was added to increase the total number of photos from 421 in the first edition to over 1450 in this second edition. Also, a new chapter of "Diseases of the Ocular System" was added to complete the coverage of all body systems. So, both the quantity and quality of the photos are increased. Each image is accompanied by concise, informative text that explains the pathology, its causes, and its clinical implications.

The atlas does not stop at the gross pathology, though. It goes a step further by providing microscopic images that reveal the cellular and histological changes associated with each condition. This dual approach, linking macroscopic and microscopic features, is incredibly valuable in bridging the gap between clinical observation and in-depth understanding. Under "Ancillary Tools," the microscopic features are supplemented with mentioning the positive immunohistochemical stains and molecular/cytogenetic descriptions of the particular condition.

Also, a new addition under the title "Pearls" was highlighted to insert new information and differentiating points between certain diseases.

The diseases in each chapter were arranged in a more systematic way to facilitate the process of understanding the disease category.

Whether you are a medical student, a practicing physician, or simply someone passionate about the intricacies of human health, this color atlas is a valuable tool for honing your knowledge and sharpening your diagnostic skills. It is a visual journey through the world of pathology, making it easier to recognize, diagnose, and ultimately treat a wide range of medical conditions.

Contents

About the Author

Gamal Dawood a distinguished leader in the field of pathology, brings a wealth of experience and expertise to this atlas.

Professor Emeritus at the prestigious Al-Azhar Faculty of Medicine, Dr. Dawood's career spans over 40 years. His journey began in 1983 as a pathology tutor, culminating in a Ph.D. in Pathology in 1991 and a professorship in 2005.

He further enriched his knowledge through international experience, having served in universities across Libya and Saudi Arabia.

Since 1985, Dr. Dawood has honed his skills as a surgical pathologist, with a keen interest in dermatopathology. This unique combination allows him to curate an exceptional collection of complex and rare cases presented in this atlas.

His leadership extends beyond academia. He served as the Head of the Pathology Department at Al-Azhar Faculty of Medicine for 5 years (2013–2018).

Notably, Dr. Dawood is the Founder and Chairman of the Egyptian Society of Dermatopathology (ESDP), a testament to his dedication to advancing the field.

His remarkable contributions were recently recognized in the 2024 Power List of The Pathologist journal, where he was named one of the Top 100 most influential people in pathology and a Top 20 Hero of Pathology.

1 Diseases of the Cardiovascular System

1.1 Introduction

The circulatory system, including the heart and blood vessels, is vital for transporting nutrients and oxygen to organs and tissues. However, it is vulnerable to a variety of disorders and diseases that can alter its structure and function, affecting one specific component or the entire system.

Gross and microscopic examination of cardiac tissue at autopsy provides valuable insights into the underlying pathophysiological processes, guiding further investigations, treatment decisions, and research pursuits. Additionally, it helps to correlate clinical symptoms with the visible changes observed during autopsies or surgical interventions. This knowledge contributes to improved diagnostic accuracy, the development of effective treatment strategies, and a deeper understanding of cardiovascular pathology overall.

This chapter will cover the following topics:

1. Diseases of blood vessels
   (a) Atherosclerosis
   (b) Aneurysms
2. Cardiac Diseases
   (a) Ischemic heart disease
   (b) Valvular heart disease
   (c) Infective endocarditis
   (d) Hypertensive heart disease
   (e) Cardiomyopathy
   (f) Pericarditis

1.2 Diseases of Blood Vessels

1.2.1 Atherosclerosis

Atherosclerosis of Aorta

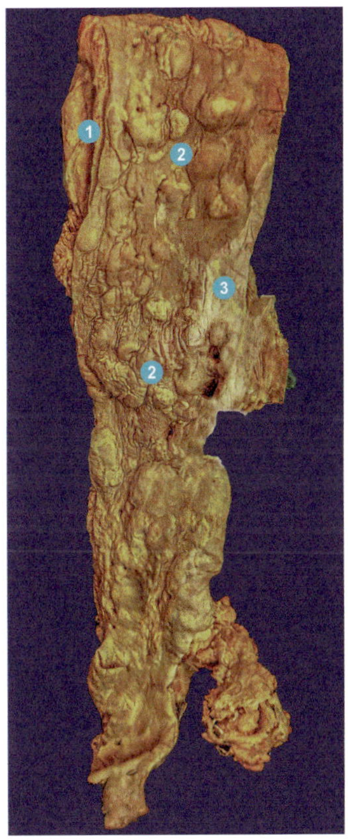

The aorta is displayed.

1. The wall of the aorta is thickened.
2. The intima shows multiple, yellow-white, raised atheromatous plaques and streaks causing longitudinal wrinkling.
3. Some atheromas are white and chalky due to calcification.

G. Dawood, *Color Atlas of Human Gross and Microscopic Pathology*, https://doi.org/10.1007/978-3-031-76007-5_1

Microscopic Picture of Atherosclerosis (a–c)

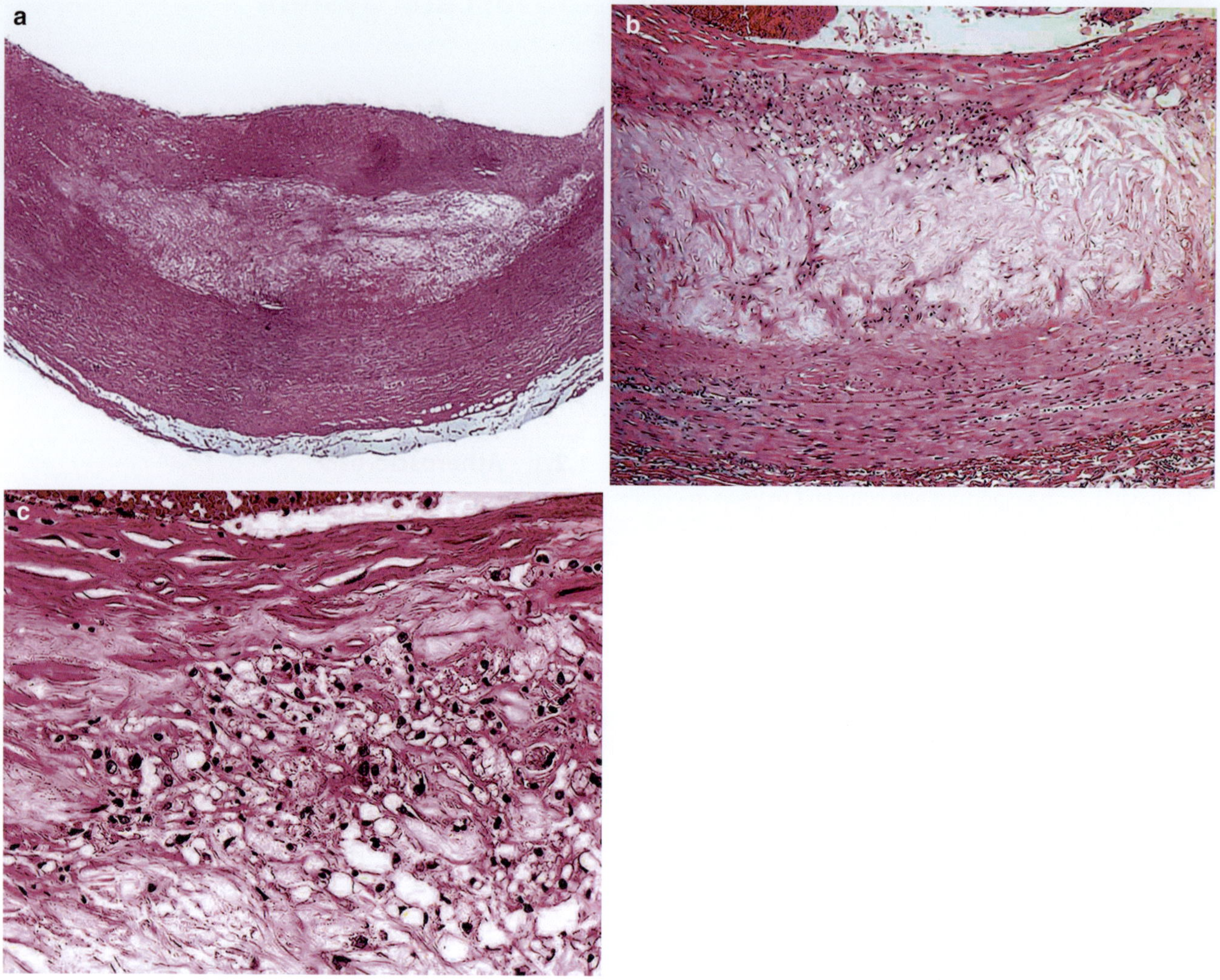

Sections show atheromatous plaque consists of a fibrinous cap and a necrotic core. The core contains lipids, dead cell debris, foam cells, fibrin, and other plasma proteins. It also includes macrophages, lymphocytes, smooth muscle cells, and areas of calcification (not shown in the sections).

Atherosclerotic Heart Disease

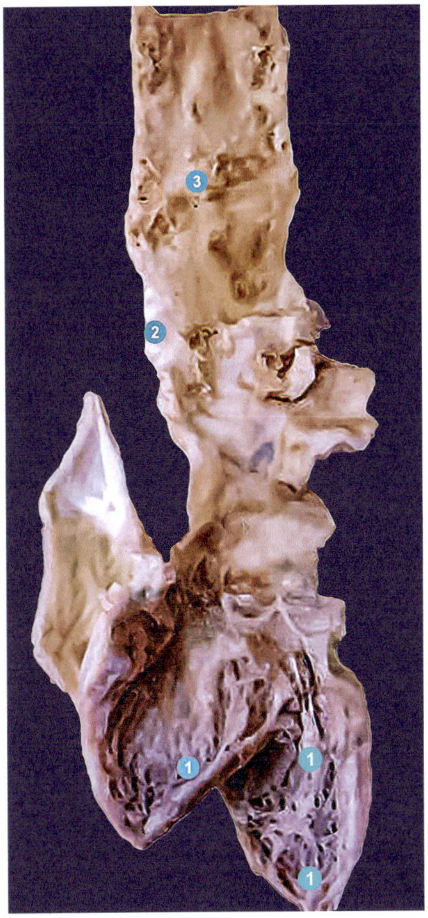

The opened heart and aorta are displayed.

1. The heart is small and shows focal fibrosis of the papillary muscle and wall of the left ventricle with a thinned-out apex due to chronic ischemia.
2. The wall of the aorta is thickened.
3. The intima shows multiple, yellow-white, raised atheromatous plaques and streaks causing longitudinal wrinkling. Some are white and chalky due to calcification.

Syphilitic Atherosclerotic Heart Disease

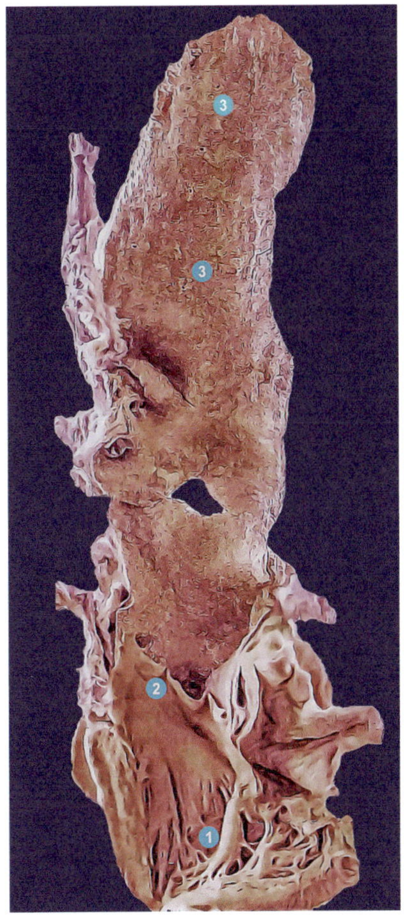

The specimen consists of an opened heart displaying its left ventricles, ascending aorta, and aortic cusps.

1. The heart is small and shows focal fibrosis of the papillary muscle and wall of the left ventricle.
2. The aortic valve cusps are rolled and thickened.
3. The aorta shows the characteristic irregular 'wood bark' appearance of the aortic intima. Atheromatous patches are seen around vascular openings.

Syphilitic Aortitis

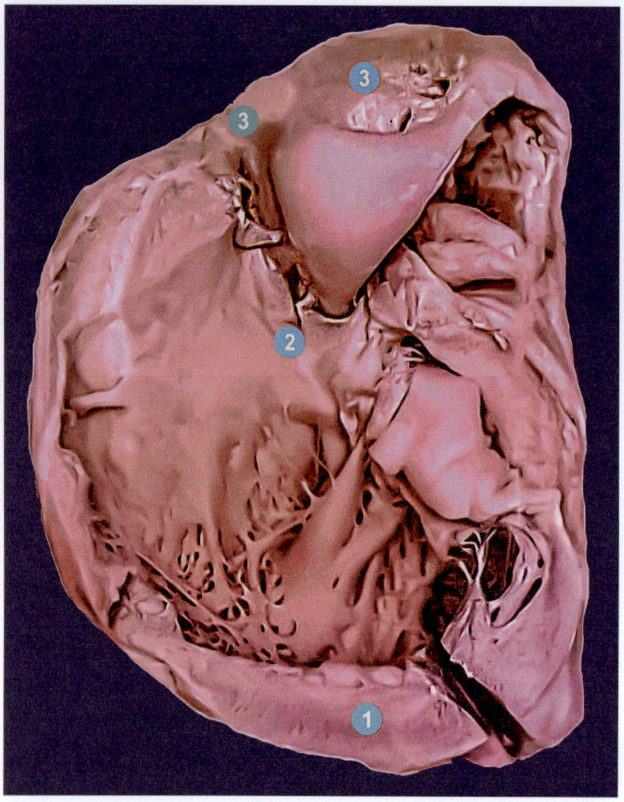

The specimen is an opened heart displaying the left ventricle, aortic cusps, and part of the aorta.

1. The left ventricle is hypertrophied and dilated.
2. The aortic cusps are thickened by white fibrous tissue.
3. The aorta shows ridges and yellow-white and raised atherosclerotic plaques around the roots of intercostal arteries.

Pearls

The appearance of syphilitic aortitis can vary depending on the stage of the disease and the individual's immune response. Gross pathology findings may also be influenced by coexisting conditions, such as atherosclerosis or other forms of vasculitis [1].

1.2.2 Aneurysms

Syphilitic Aneurysm of Aortic Arch with Laminated Thrombus

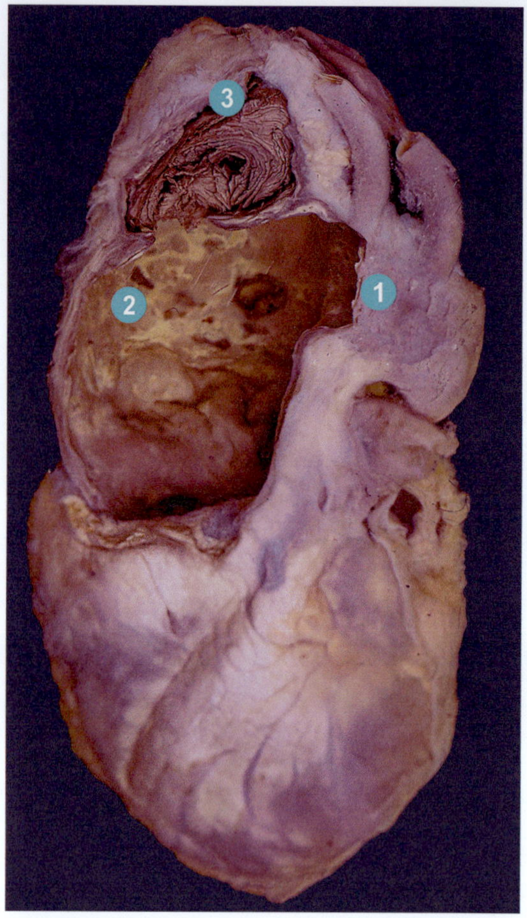

The specimen consists of a heart, ascending, and arch of the aorta.

1. The arch shows saccular aneurysmal dilatation.
2. The intima is brown blood-stained with the presence of thick, raised, irregular, yellow multiple atheromatous plaques.
3. The upper part of the aneurysm is filled with a laminated thrombus formed of alternating pale and dark layers, representing deposited platelets and RBCs, respectively.

Syphilitic Aneurysm of Aortic Arch

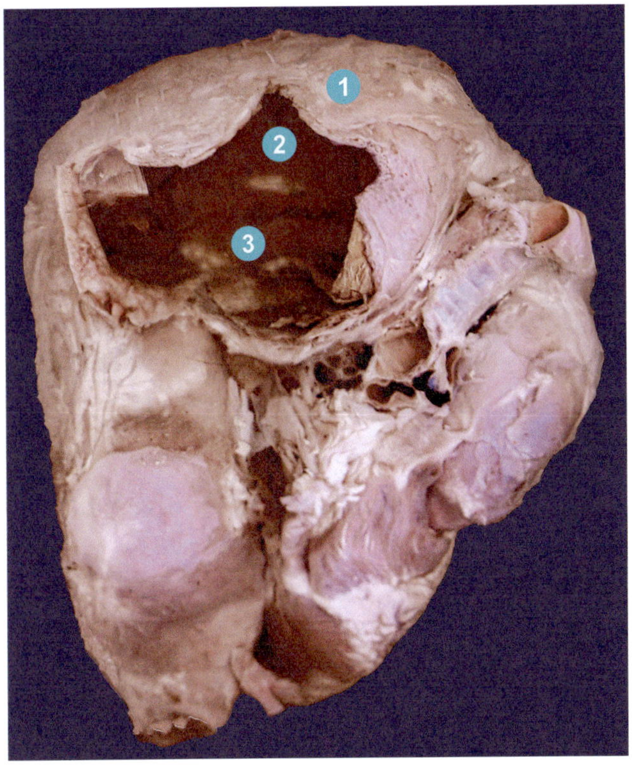

The specimen consists of a heart, ascending, arch, and descending aorta.

1. The arch shows saccular aneurysmal dilatation.
2. The intima is brown and blood-stained.
3. Thick, raised, irregular, yellow multiple atheromatous plaques.

Extra-parenchymal Renal Artery Aneurysm

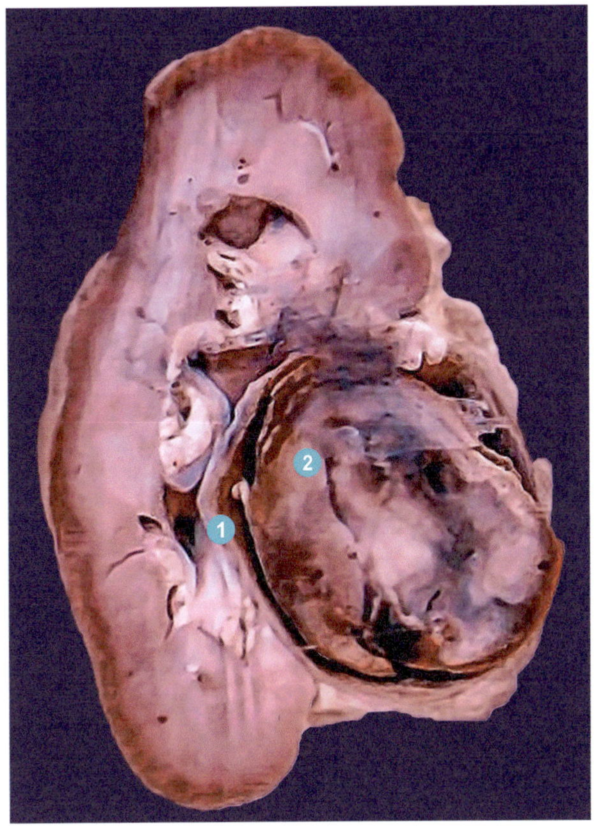

The specimen is left kidney sectioned longitudinally.

1. The renal artery shows aneurysmal dilatation outside the renal parenchyma.
2. The aneurysmal sac is filled with a large thrombus.

Ruptured Syphilitic Aneurysm of Aortic Arch

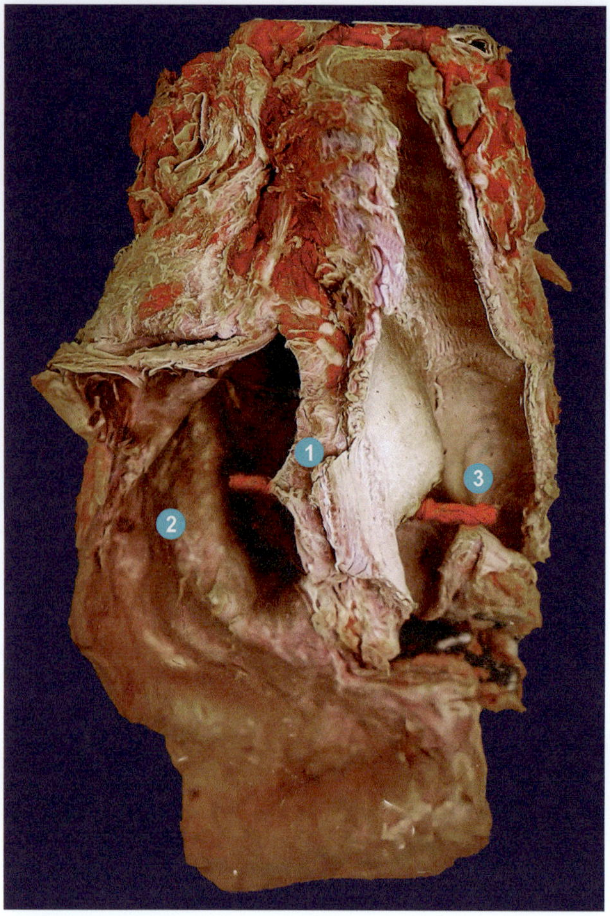

The specimen consists of a junction of the aortic arch and descending aorta and part of the trachea.

1. Aneurysmal dilatation of the aorta, which had ruptured into the bronchus with a fatal hemorrhage (the red rod points to the site of communication).
2. Atherosclerotic patches are seen in the aorta.
3. The bronchial mucosa is brown due to congestion.

1.3 Cardiac Diseases

1.3.1 Ischemic Heart Disease

Brown Atrophy of Heart

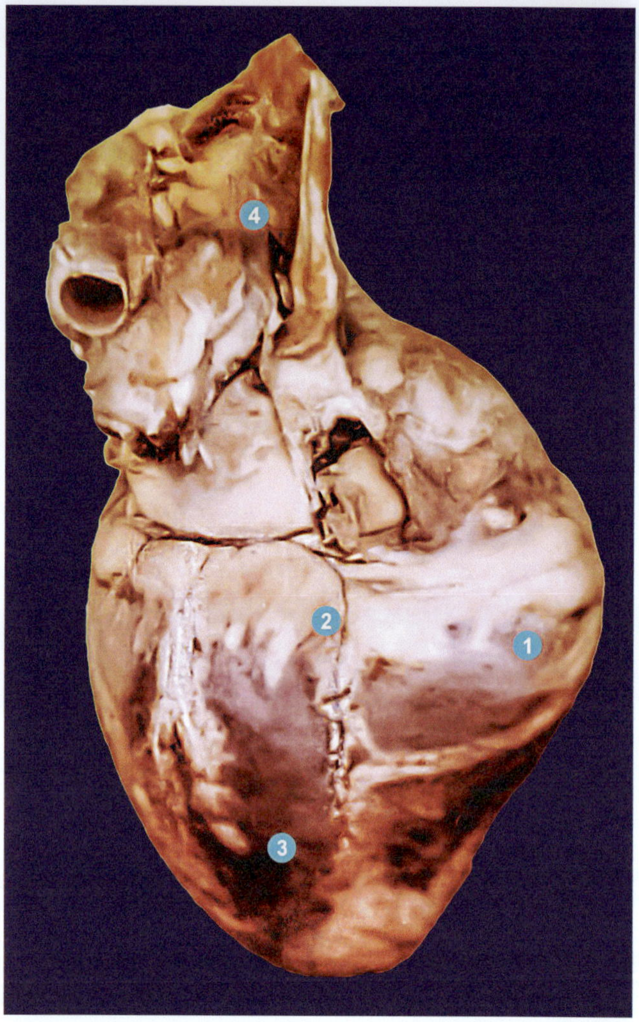

A human adult heart markedly reduced in size, obtained from an old patient with cancer esophagus, is mounted.

1. Pericardial fat is reduced or even disappears.
2. Coronary arteries are tortuous.
3. The myocardium is deep brown.
4. The root of the aorta shows atherosclerotic patches.

Microscopic Picture of Brown Atrophy of Heart (a)

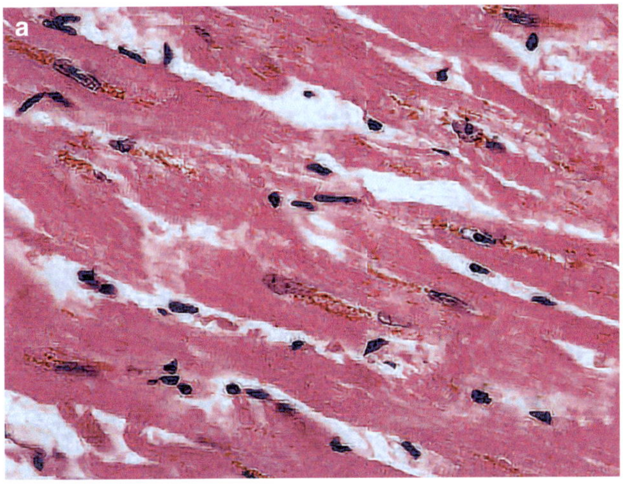

The section displays cardiac myocytes with yellow-brown lipofuscin pigment primarily around the nuclei.

Pearls

Brown atrophy of the heart is typically a secondary manifestation of an underlying systematic disease or cardiovascular disease, such as chronic congestive heart failure, pulmonary hypertension, or coronary artery disease. The brown discoloration and structural changes in the heart are primarily a result of chronic passive congestion and reduced blood flow within the myocardium with deposition of lipofuscin pigment [2].

Recent Myocardial Infarction (MI) and Recent Mural Thrombus (a)

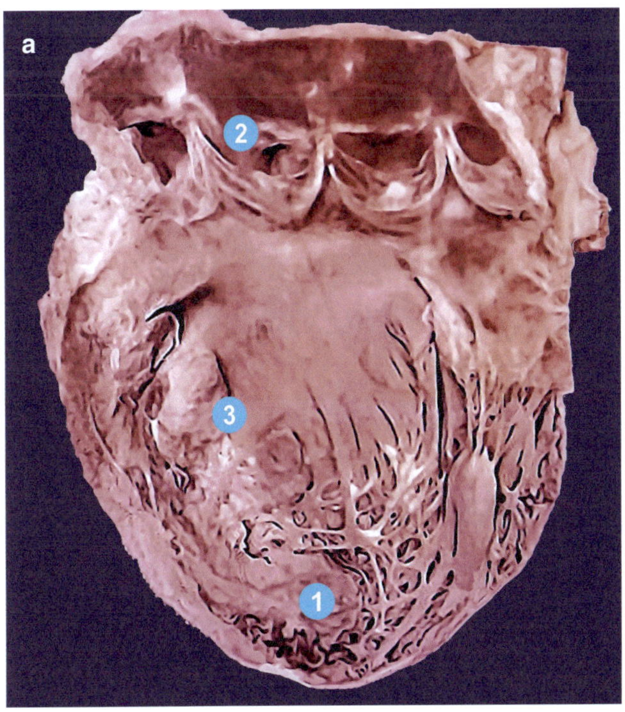

An adult heart is displayed. The specimen is formed of the interventricular septum with adjoining parts of both ventricles, with the root of the aorta and its cusps and coronary orifices attached to the upper part.

1. The wall of the left ventricle and the apex are opaque and covered on the endocardial surface by brown-red friable pieces of thrombus.
2. The coronary orifices are thrombosed.
3. Subendocardial edema

Microscopic Picture of Ischemic Myocardium (b)

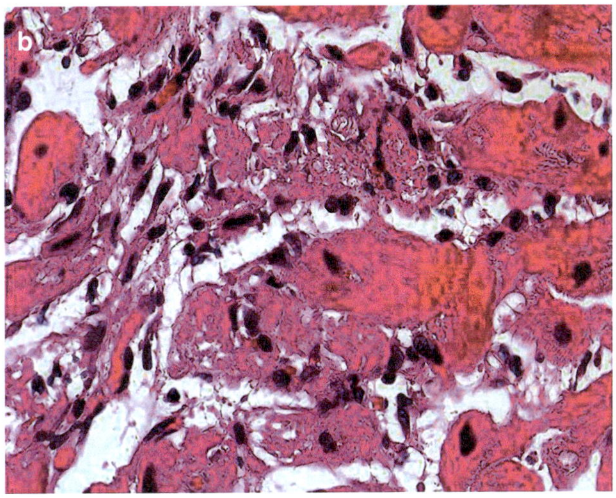

The section reveals cardiac myocytes with coagulative necrosis and contraction band necrosis. This is seen as dense pink bands within the myocytes due to sarcomere hypercontracture. This is accompanied by a slight inflammatory cellular infiltrate.

Microscopic Picture of Early Myocardial Infarction (c)

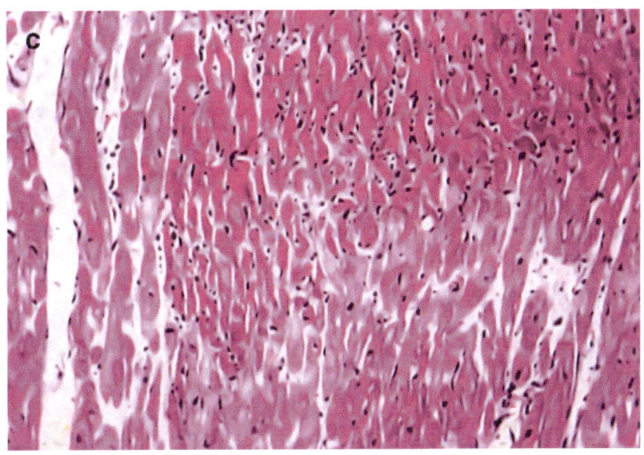

The section shows the earliest change in the form of hypereosinophilia (above) with an intense pink cytoplasm due to hyaline change. A sparse cellular infiltrate is observed.

Microscopic Picture of Recent Myocardial Infarction (d)

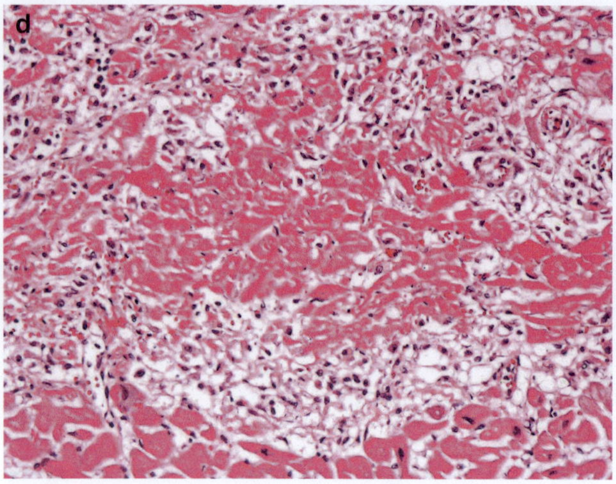

The section from an area of infarction shows a central zone of coagulative necrosis and a few inflammatory cells, fibroblasts (large vesicular nuclei), and damaged myocardial fibers with nuclear karyolysis.

Recent Myocardial Infarction (MI) and Recent Mural Thrombus with Chronic Ischemia

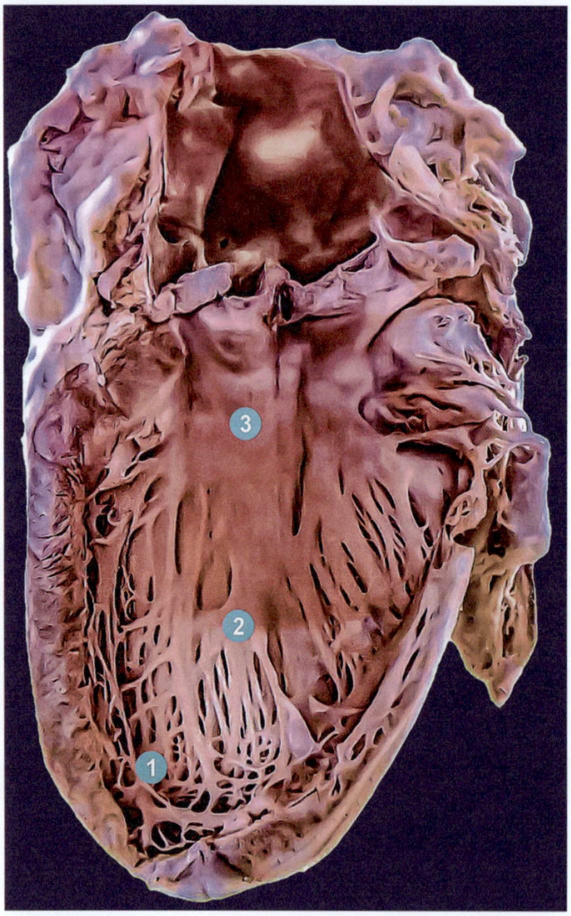

An adult heart is displayed. The specimen is formed of the interventricular septum with adjoining parts of both ventricles, with the root of the aorta and its cusps attached to the upper part.

1. The wall of the left ventricle and the apex are opaque and covered on the endocardial surface by brown-red friable pieces of thrombus.
2. The endocardium shows a focal white area of fibrosis, indicating chronic ischemia.
3. The ventricle is dilated.

Healed Myocardial Infarction (MI) with Mural Aneurysm

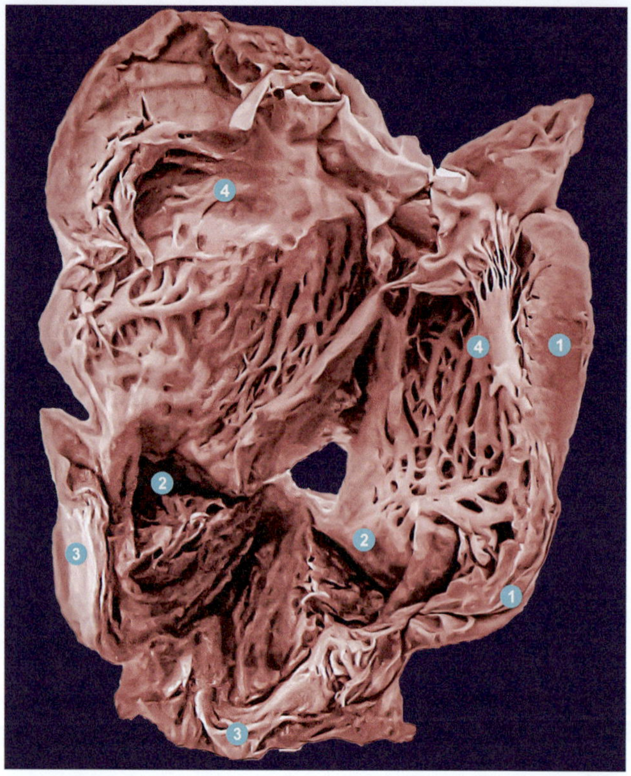

An adult heart is displayed and opened to show the left ventricle, aortic valve, and proximal aorta. The coronary arteries are not apparent in this dissection.

1. The left ventricular wall shows hypertrophy to a thickness and then thins at the apex to a few mm.
2. The apical endocardium has lost its normal pattern and appears somewhat smooth. This thin area forms an aneurysm that bulges towards the pericardium. The aneurysm is filled with a laminated thrombus.
3. The pericardium covering the aneurysm is thickened and white (indicating healed pericarditis).
4. The endocardium and papillary muscles are white due to fibrosis because of chronic ischemic heart disease.

Pearls

Healing, by fibrosis, commences about 3 weeks after acute infarction and is usually complete after 2 months. A study found that the protein YAP plays a critical role in the healing of MI because it is involved in regulating cell growth and proliferation. YAP could be a potential target for new therapies to promote healing after MI [3].

Another study found that a type of stem cell called epicardial adipose-derived stem cells (EAdSCs) can promote healing after MI. EAdSCs are located in the fatty tissue surrounding the heart, and the study found that they can migrate to the infarcted area and promote angiogenesis [4].

Cardiac aneurysms are made of scar tissue that has replaced previously infarcted myocardium. A protein called matrix metalloproteinase-9 (MMP-9) plays a role in the formation of myocardial aneurysm. MMP-9 is an enzyme that breaks down collagen, the main component of scar tissue [5]. However, the scar tissue does not contract normally, which predisposes to heart failure. Due to the altered blood flow in the aneurysm, a thrombus often forms on the wall (mural laminated thrombus).

Healed Myocardial Infarction (MI) with Mural Aneurysm

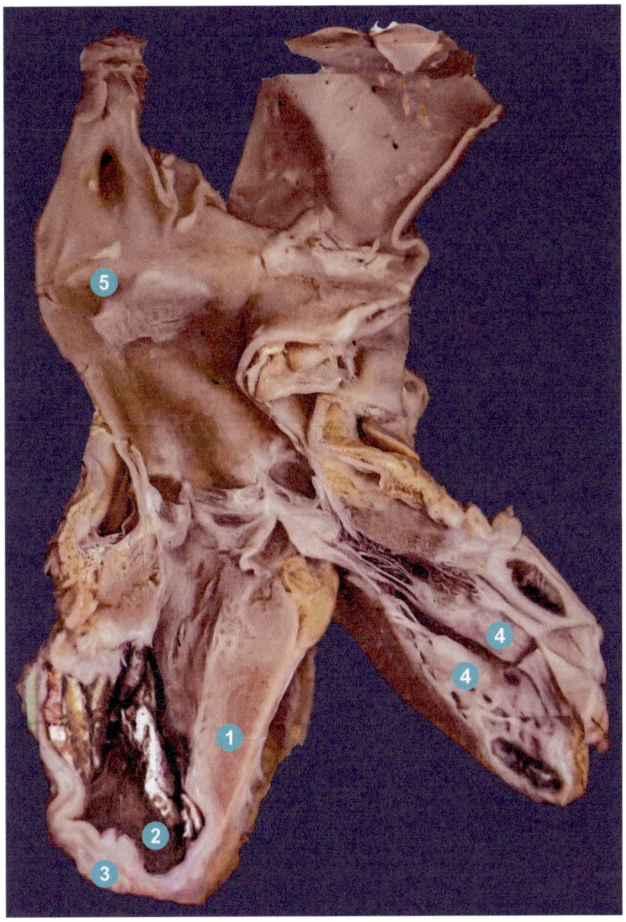

An adult heart is displayed and opened to show the left ventricle, aortic valve, and proximal aorta. The coronary arteries are not apparent in this dissection.

1. The left ventricular wall shows hypertrophy to a thickness and then thins at the apex to a few mm.
2. The apical endocardium has lost its normal pattern and appears somewhat smooth. This thin area forms the aneurysm, which bulges towards the pericardium and is filled with a laminated thrombus.
3. The pericardium covering the aneurysm is thickened and white (indicating healed pericarditis).
4. The endocardium and papillary muscles are white due to fibrosis because of chronic ischemic heart disease.
5. The aorta shows a yellow-white and raised atherosclerotic plaque.

Microscopic Picture of Myocardial Fibrosis (a, b)

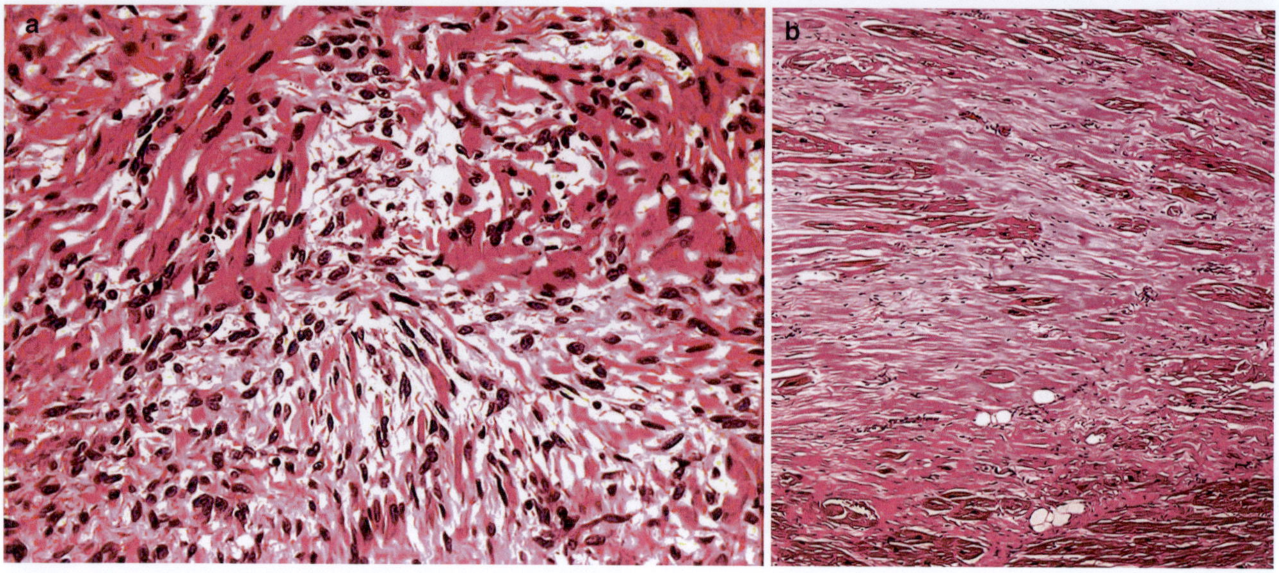

Sections show what is known as (replacement fibrosis) in which fibrous tissue replaces the dead cardiomyocytes with a disarray of the remaining cardiomyocytes. With time, an increase in collagen deposition occurs. In the maturation stage, the collagen fibers are dense and organized, and the scar tissue is less cellular.

Pearls

Replacement fibrosis occurs due to damage that results in the loss of heart muscle cells. Initially, fibrosis helps protect and maintain the heart's structure by adding connective tissue. However, if it becomes excessive, it can cause harmful scarring, further heart damage, and decreased heart function. Conditions like ischemic diseases, hypertension, and various cardiomyopathies involve fibrosis and changes in the extracellular matrix (ECM). As the heart becomes more damaged, it undergoes changes, such as enlargement of its chambers. Over time, the increasing burden on the heart enlarges the left ventricle and its cavity size. Since heart muscle cells don't naturally regenerate, the remaining ones enlarge to handle the extra load. This continuous process leads to more ECM changes, increased fibrosis, and eventually, heart failure [6].

1.3.2 Valvular Heart Disease

Mitral and Aortic Valve Stenosis (Rheumatic)

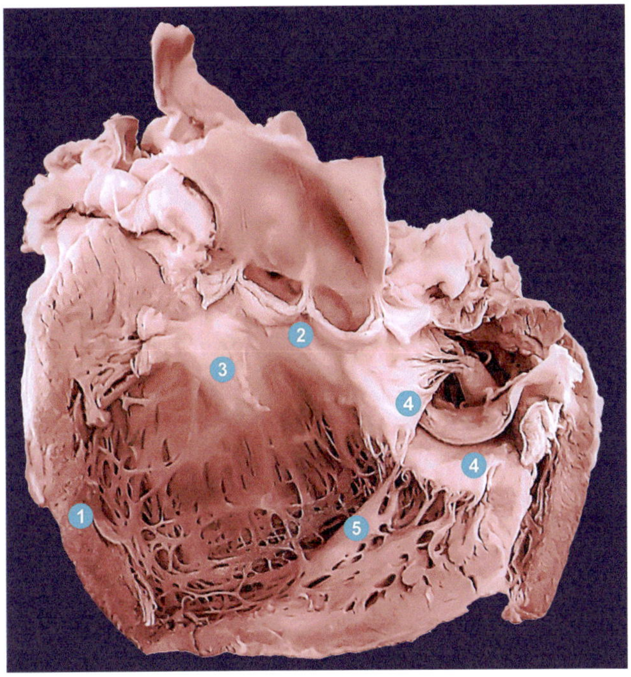

An opened heart displays its left and right ventricles, aorta and aortic cusps, and mitral valve. One of the papillary muscles was cut and turned up to display the mitral valve leaflet.

1. The heart is enlarged with dilatation and hypertrophy of the left ventricle.
2. The aortic cusps are thickened, fibrotic, and with rolled thick edges.
3. A white area of subendocardial fibrosis is seen at the root of the aorta.
4. The mitral valve shows thickened and fibrosed valve leaflets and cusps.
5. The papillary muscles are hypertrophied with fibrosis of chorda tendineae.

Mitral and Aortic Valve Stenosis (Rheumatic)

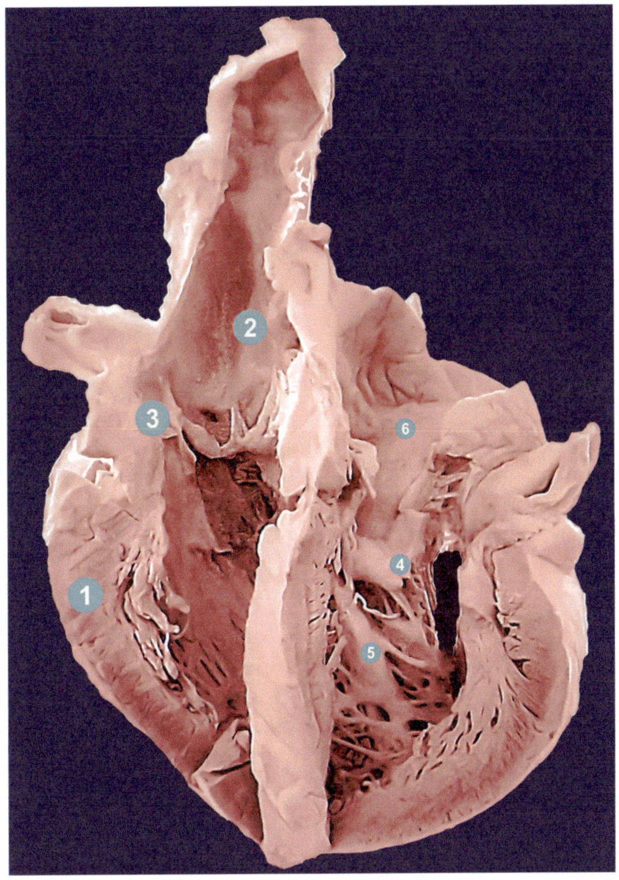

The specimen consists of an opened heart of a child displaying its left ventricle, aorta and aortic cusps, mitral valve, and left atrium.

1. The heart is enlarged with dilatation and hypertrophy of the left ventricle.
2. The root of the aorta shows yellow fatty streaks.
3. The aortic cusps are thickened and fibrosed and have rolled and thick edges.
4. The mitral valve shows thickened and fibrosed valve leaflets and cusps.

5. The papillary muscles are hypertrophied with fibrosis of chorda tendineae.
6. The left atrium shows diffuse subendocardial fibrosis.

Mitral and Aortic Stenosis

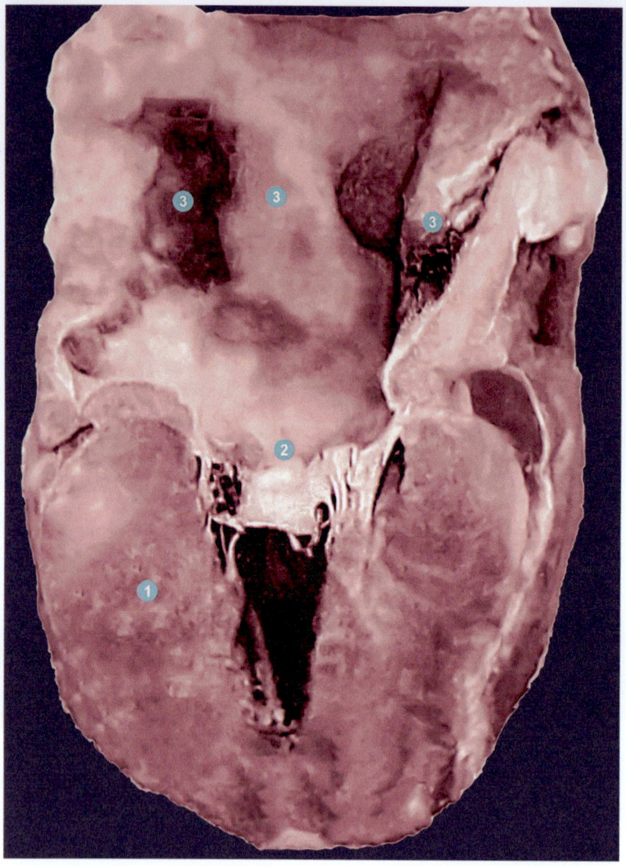

An adult heart is displayed and opened longitudinally.

1. Marked thickening of the wall of the left ventricle without dilatation (concentric hypertrophy), most probably due to aortic stenosis.
2. The mitral valve shows thickened, fibrosed cusps with stenosis of its orifice.
3. The left atrium is dilated and fibrosed with an ulcerated area covered with a thrombus on the left auricular appendage on the right side and another bigger thrombus on the left side of the atrium.

Aortic Stenosis (Rheumatic)

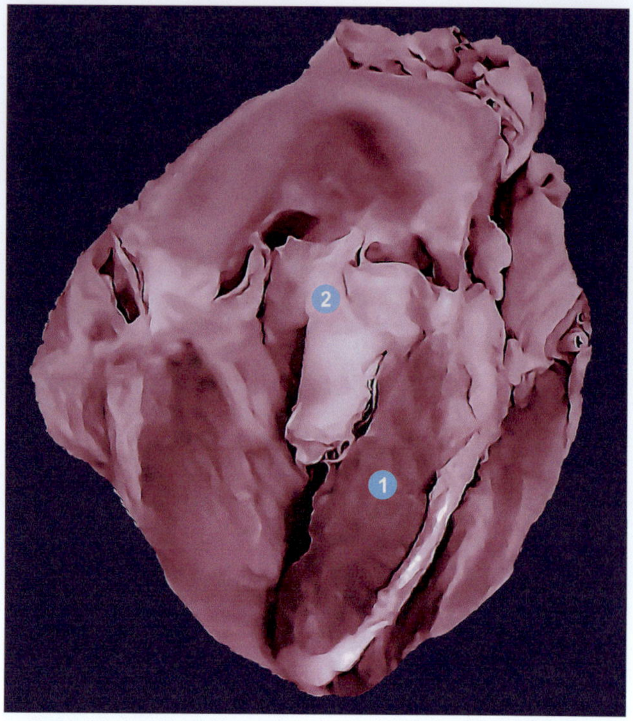

The mounted heart shows:

1. Marked thickening of the wall of the left ventricle without dilatation (concentric hypertrophy).
2. The aortic cusps show diffuse cuspal thickening that extends to their free edges and with commissural fusion, thickening in the basal half, fibrosis, and rolled thick edges. Aortic valve thickening of the cusps is typical aortic valve scarring.

Mitral Stenosis

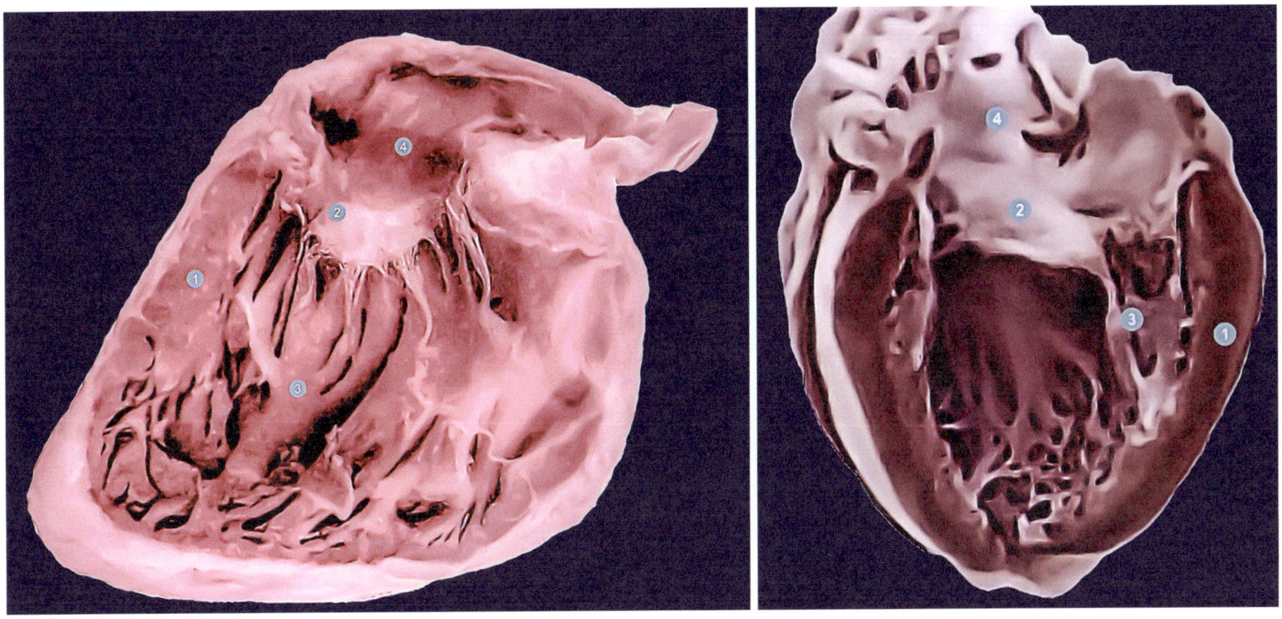

The specimen consists of an opened heart of a child displaying its left ventricle, mitral valve, and left atrium.

1. The heart is enlarged with dilatation and hypertrophy of the left ventricle.
2. The mitral valve shows thickened and fibrosed valve leaflets and cusps.
3. The papillary muscles are hypertrophied with fibrosis of chorda tendineae.
4. The left atrium shows diffuse subendocardial fibrosis.

Mitral Stenosis with Atrial Ball Thrombus

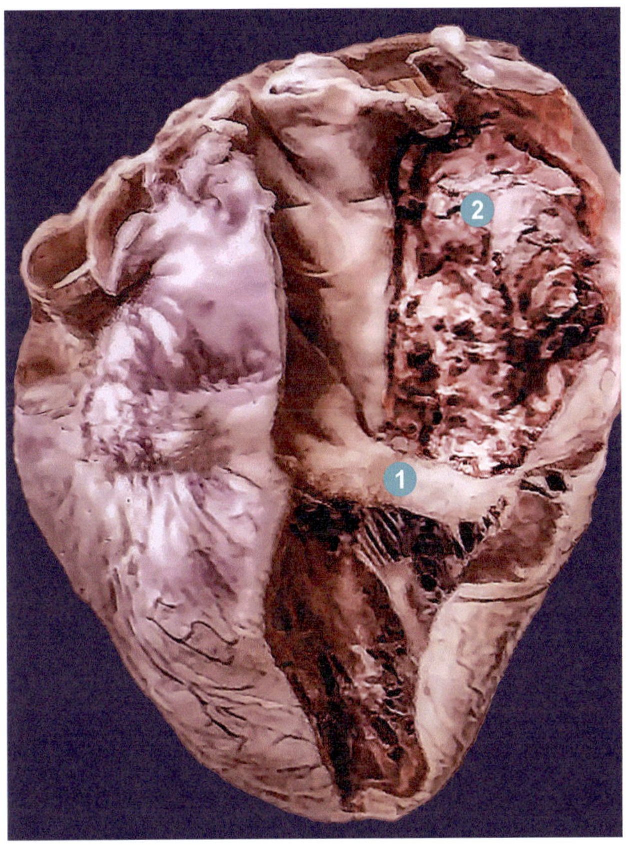

1. The mitral valve shows thickened fibrosed cusps with stenosis of its orifice.
2. The left atrium is dilated and fibrosed, with a large ball thrombus filling it. This is a complication of mitral stenosis and atrial fibrillation and a source of peripheral emboli.

1.3.3 Infective Endocarditis

Bacterial Endocarditis (a, b)

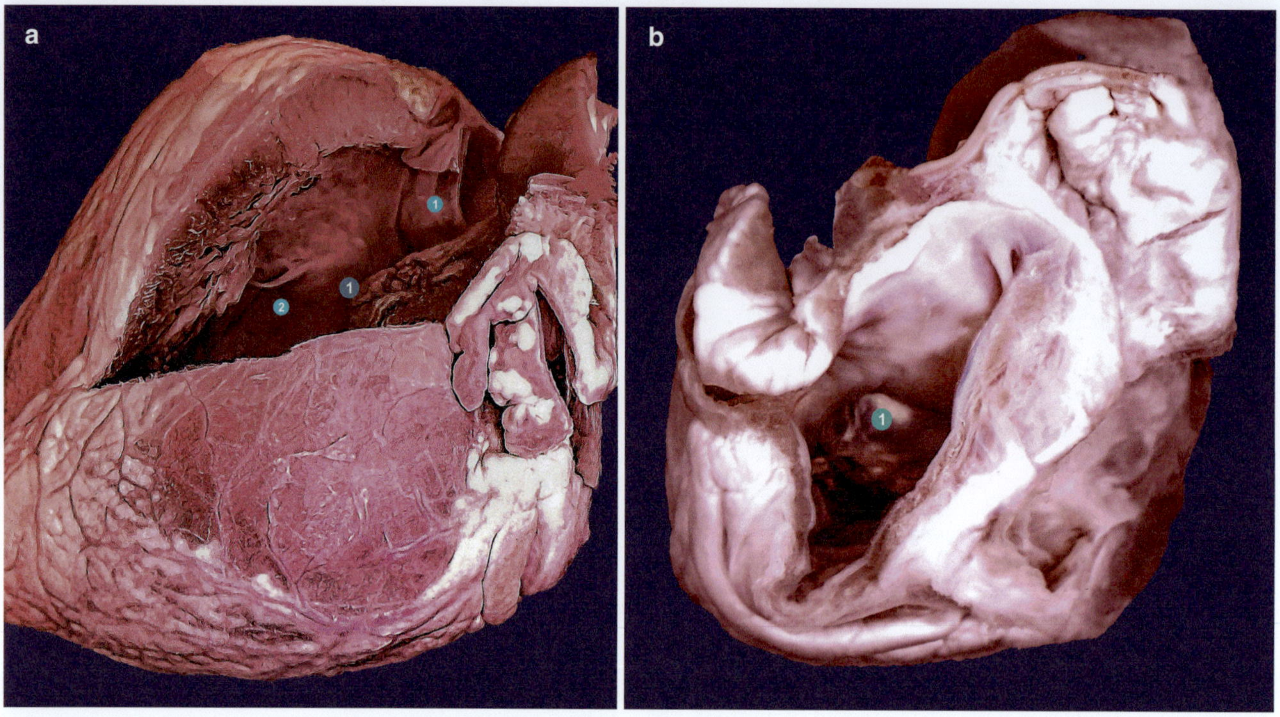

An adult heart with an open left ventricle is mounted.

1. A large polypoid, round, gray-brown vegetation is seen hanging from one of the normal-looking aortic cusps.
2. The left ventricle is dilated.

Mitral Stenosis and Bacterial Endocarditis

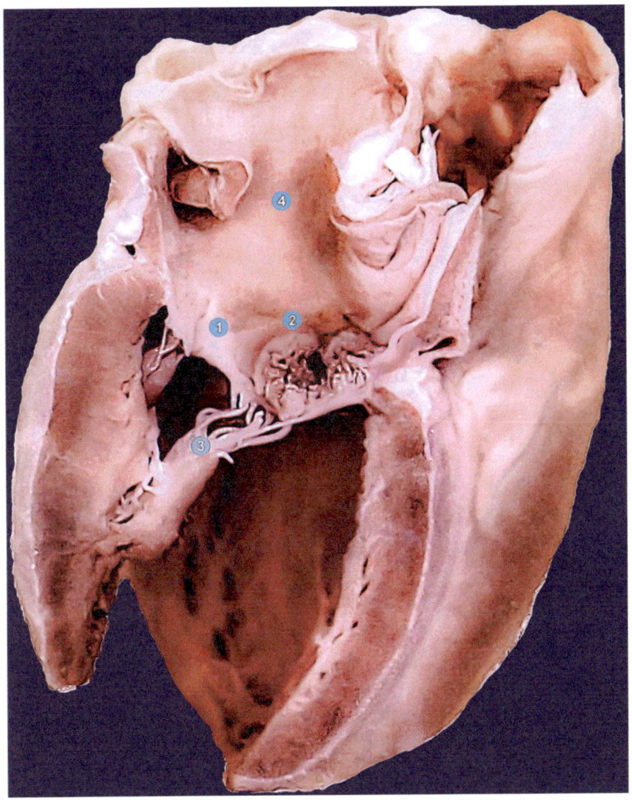

An opened heart displaying its left atrium, ventricle, and mitral valve.

1. Mitral valve cusps are markedly thickened and fused with stenosis of its orifice.
2. There is a circular area of superficial ulceration over the auricular surface of the mitral valve with some large brown vegetation.
3. The papillary muscles are thickened and hypertrophied with fibrosis of chorda tendinae.
4. The left atrium is dilated with fibrosis of the endocardium lining.

Mitral Stenosis and Bacterial Endocarditis

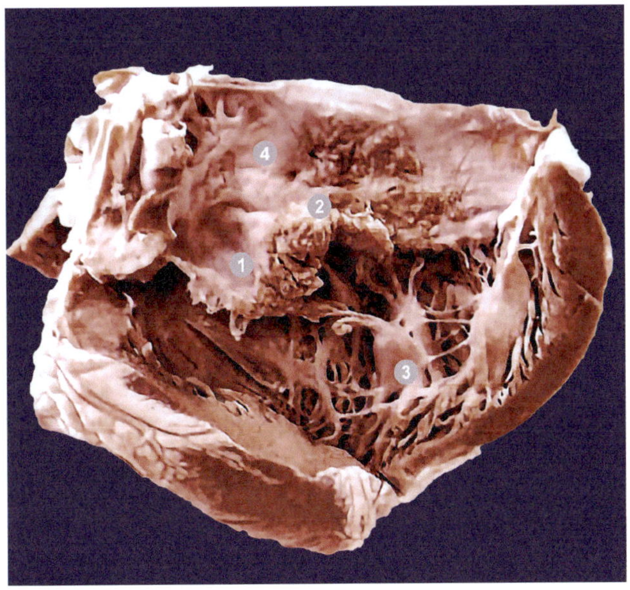

An opened heart displaying its left atrium, ventricle, and mitral valve.

1. Mitral valve cusps are markedly thickened and fused with stenosis of its orifice.
2. Yellow, irregular granular vegetations are seen attached to the atrial aspect of the mitral valve and extend into adjacent parts of the cusp or leaflets, chordae tendinea, and the endocardial surface of the left atrium.
3. The papillary muscles are thickened and hypertrophied.
4. The endocardium lining the left atrium is white fibrous. The left atrium is dilate.

Microscopic Picture of Bacterial Endocarditis (a, b)

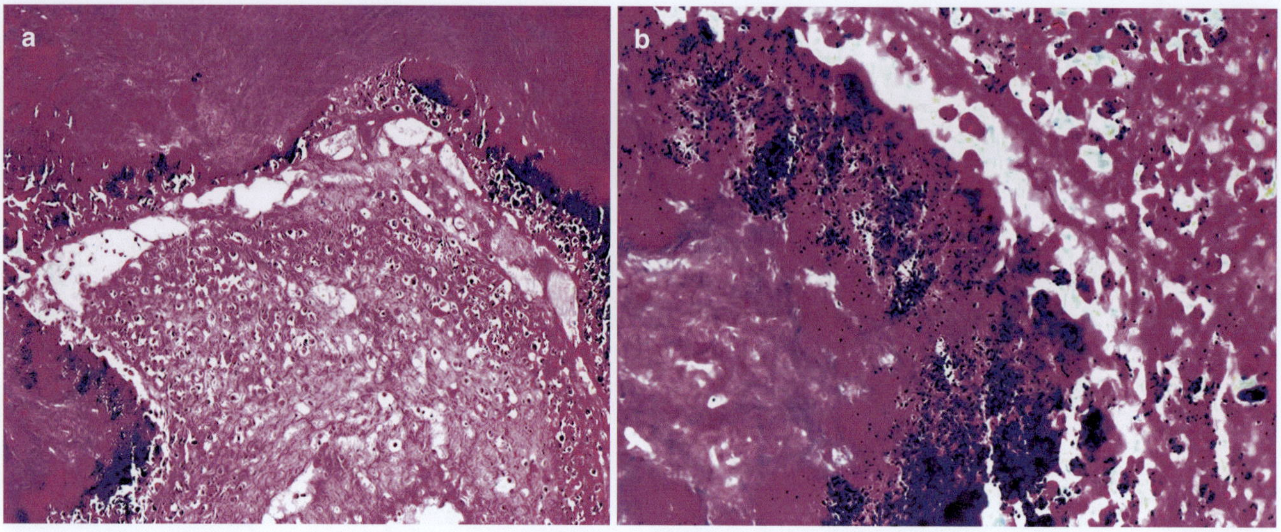

Sections show clumps of bacteria that can be seen superficially in the fibrin deposited on the valve leaflet. The dark coloration on hematoxylin and eosin stain may indicate the viability of bacteria.

1.3.4 Hypertensive Heart Disease

Hypertensive Heart Disease (a, b)

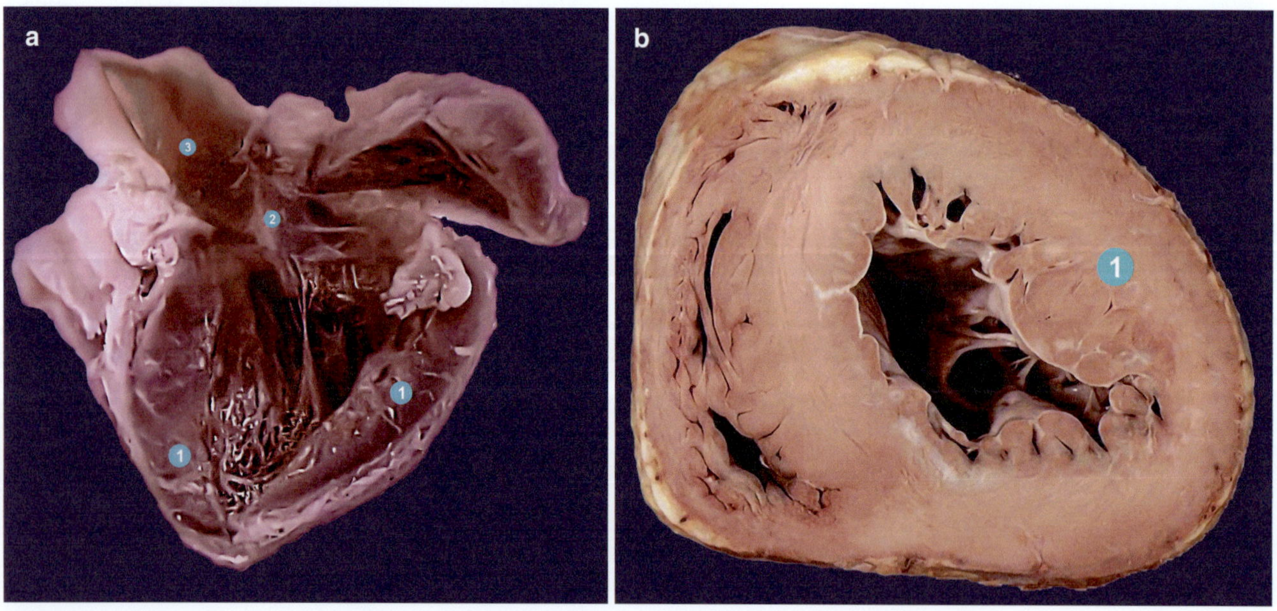

The specimen is an opened heart displaying the left ventricle, aortic cusps, and the proximal part of the aorta.

1. The wall of the left ventricle is hypertrophied with yellow discoloration due to fatty change, and fine white streaks of fibrosis in-between myocardial fibers. The transverse section (b) shows concentric hypertrophy of the wall of the left ventricle.
2. The aortic cusps are thin and translucent.
3. The root of the aorta shows atherosclerotic plaques.

Microscopic Picture of Hypertensive Heart Disease (c)

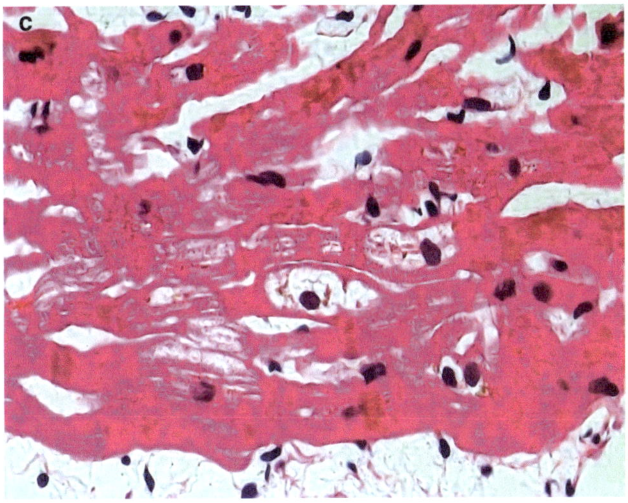

The section shows myocardial hypertrophy and contraction bands (typical of the left ventricular hypertrophy).

1.3.5 Cardiomyopathy

Hypertrophic Obstructive Cardiomyopathy (a, b)

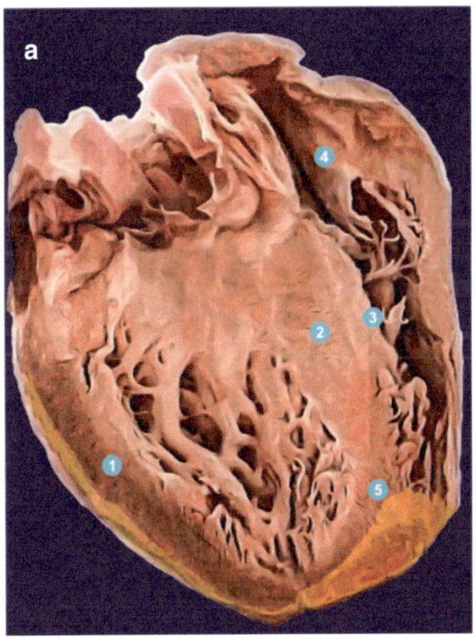

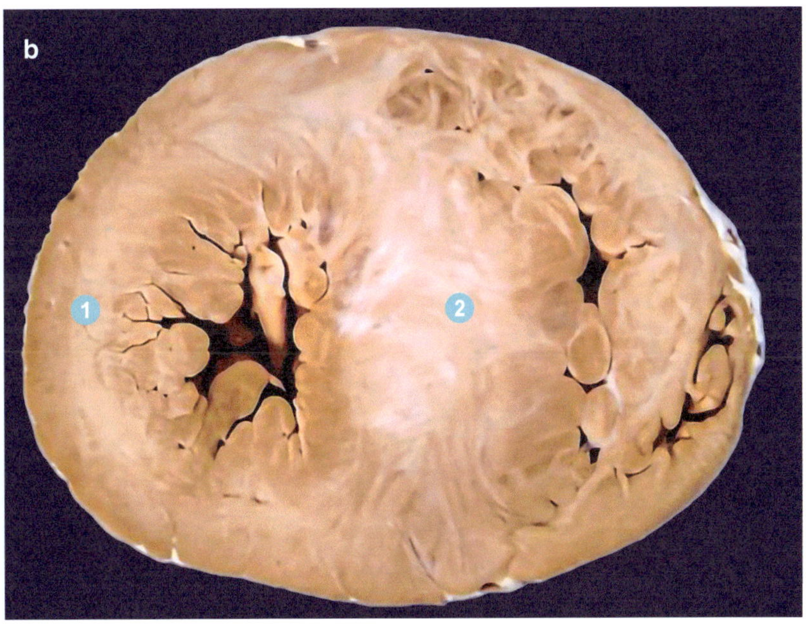

An adult heart is displayed and opened longitudinally.

1. There is thickening of the left ventricular wall.
2. Asymmetric hypertrophy of the interventricular septum, which bulges into the right ventricle (better shown in the transverse section in (b).
3. Papillary muscles are hypertrophied and displaced.
4. The mitral leaflet is enlarged and elongated.
5. Areas of fatty infiltration are seen in the ventricular wall.

Pearls

True cardiomyopathy is, by definition, any myocardial disease without an identifiable cause that appears noninflammatory. Hypertrophic cardiomyopathy is typified by asymmetrical left ventricular hypertrophy, especially of the septal wall. Most commonly, it is familial, and the mode of inheritance is autosomal dominant. Hypertrophic obstructive cardiomyopathy is a rare but important cause of unexpected sudden death [7].

Diagrammatic Representation of Hypertrophic Cardiomyopathy with Obstruction (c)

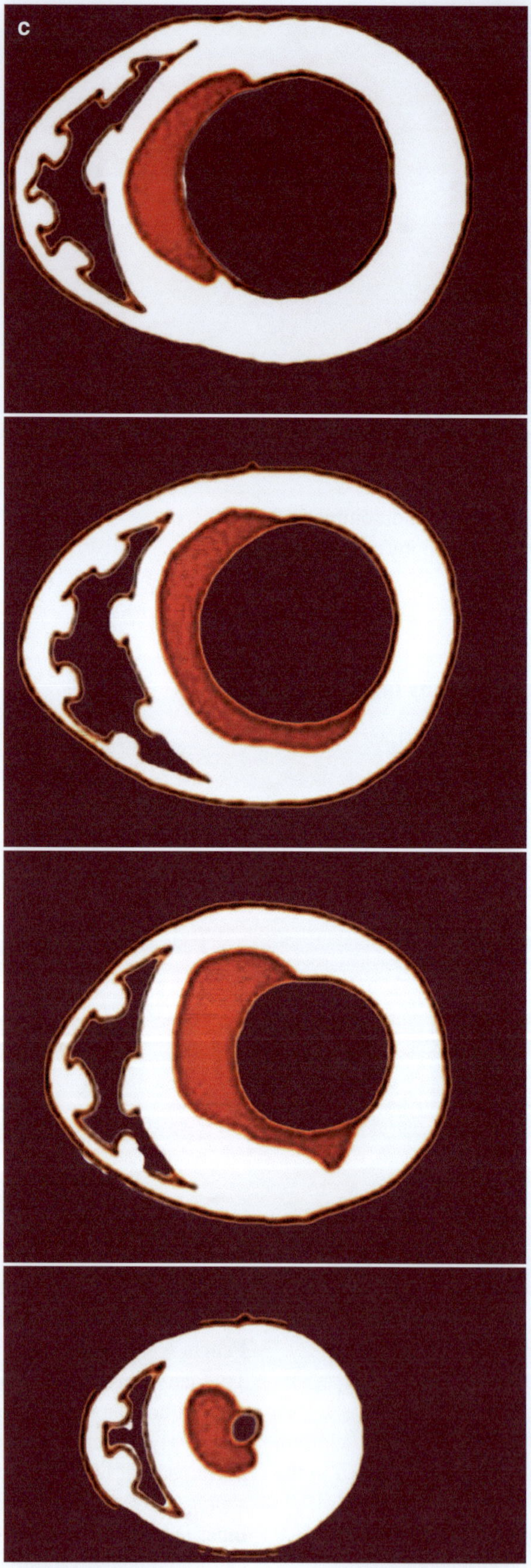

The abnormal fibers are principally confined to the asymmetrically thickened interventricular septum and extend for varying distances into the anterior and posterior left ventricular walls.

Microscopic Picture of Hypertrophic Obstructive Cardiomyopathy (d–f)

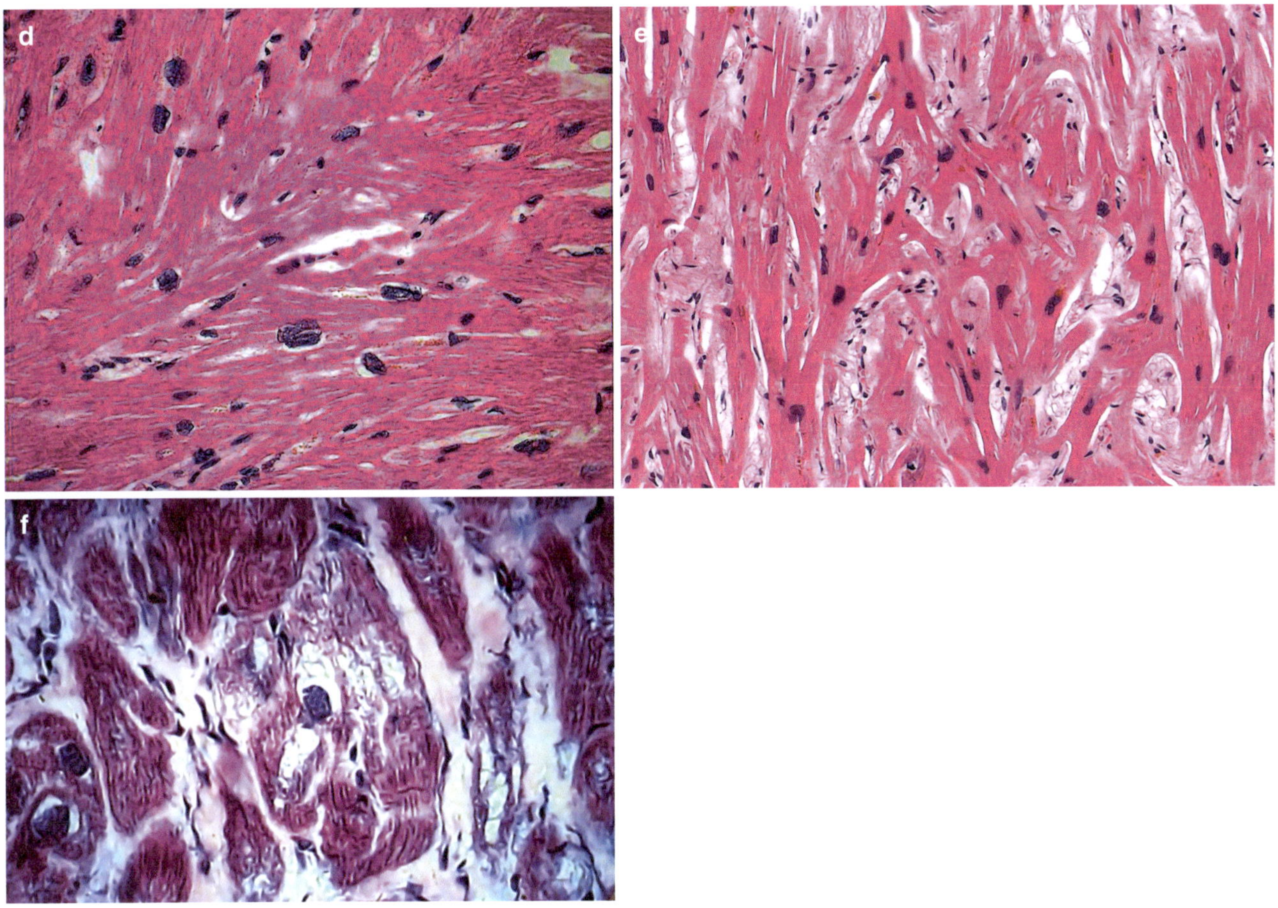

The section shows myocardial fibers in disarray, exemplified by short runs and severe hypertrophy of myocardial fibers separated by cellular connective tissue. (f) shows extremely hypertrophied myocardial fibers with bizarre nuclei (bottom left). The perinuclear halo is well illustrated in the center. Disintegrating myofibrils can be identified towards the top of the halo, giving a 'moth-eaten' appearance.

1.3.6 Pericarditis

Fibrinous Pericarditis (a, b)

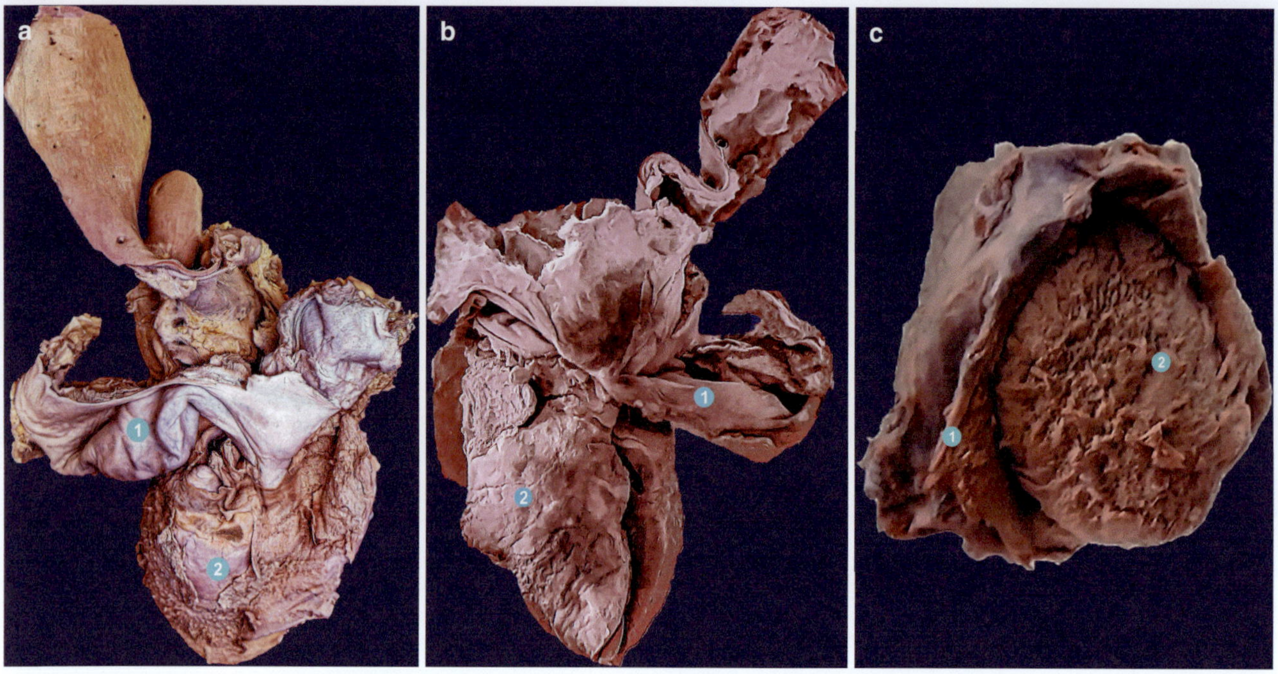

An adult heart is displayed.

1. The pericardial sac opened, and the parietal pericardium has been stretched out.
2. The visceral pericardium is covered by a thick, shaggy layer of fibrinous exudate, giving the "bread and butter" appearance.

Fibrinous Pericarditis (a, b)

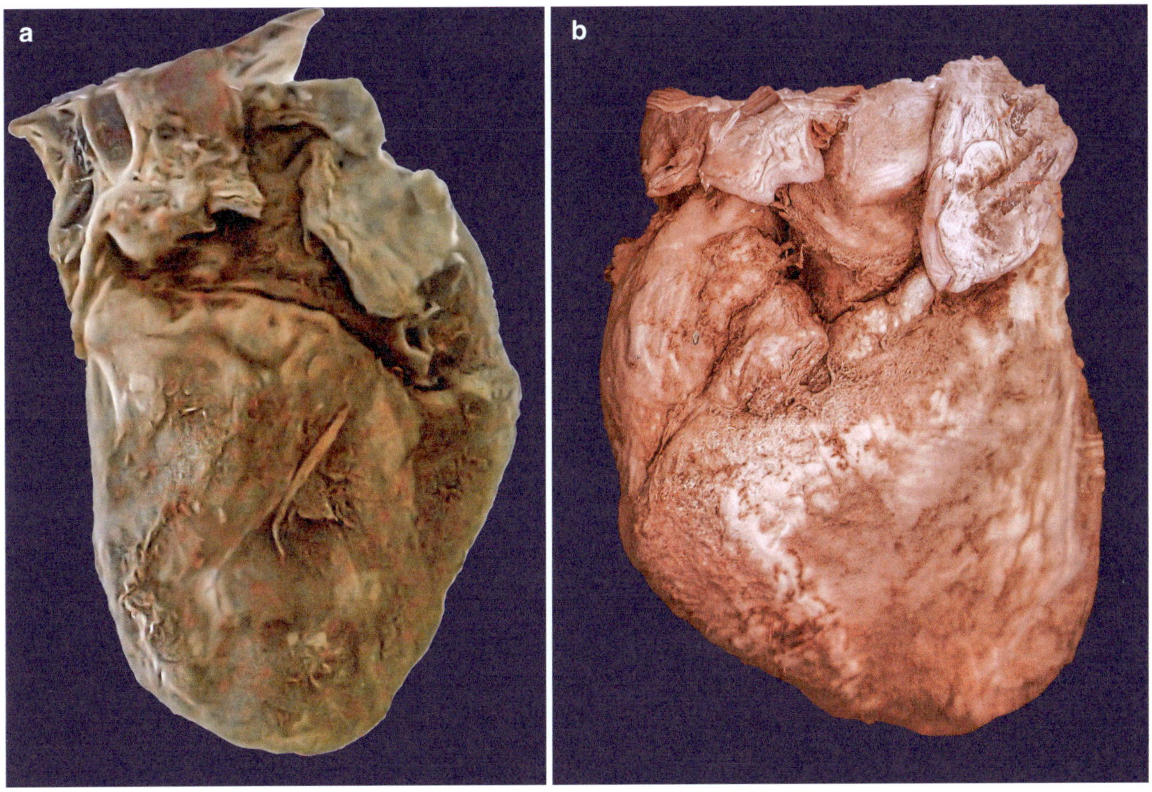

An adult heart is displayed. The visceral pericardium is covered by a brown, thick, shaggy layer of fibrinous exudate, giving the "bread and butter" appearance.

Microscopic Picture of Fibrinous Pericarditis (c)

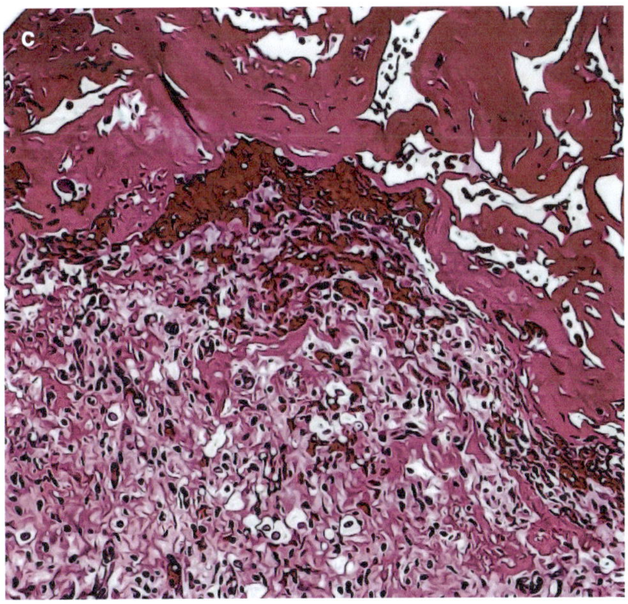

Sections show loosely arranged collagen fibers separated by edema, interstitial hemorrhage, and chronic inflammatory cells. The area is covered by eosinophilic fibrin.

Tuberculous Pericarditis

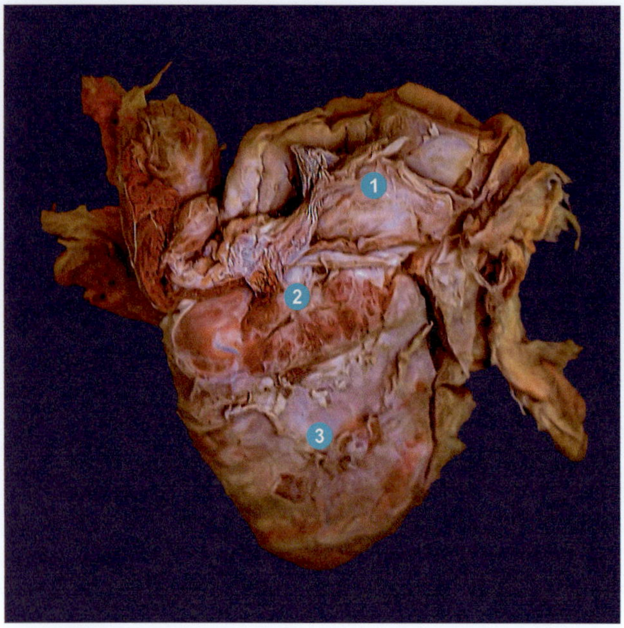

An adult heart with an open pericardial sac is displayed.

1. The parietal and the visceral pericardium are covered by a thick, shaggy layer of fibrinous exudate that extends up to the roots of great vessels.
2. Remains of marked inflammation and hemorrhage are seen at the roots of great vessels because this is the most dependent part during recumbency. The exudate was excessive and hemorrhagic. The inflammation was proved microscopically to be tuberculous.
3. There are some fibrous adhesions noted in the parietal pericardium, denoting healing in some areas.

Microscopic Picture of Tuberculous Pericarditis (a)

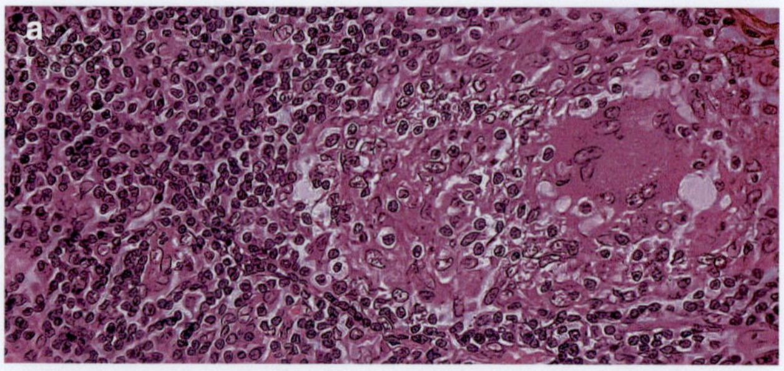

The section shows multiple tuberculous granulomas, formed of epithelioid cells, lymphocytes, and multinucleated Langhan's giant cells, seen at the surface of myocardial cells.

Healed Pericarditis

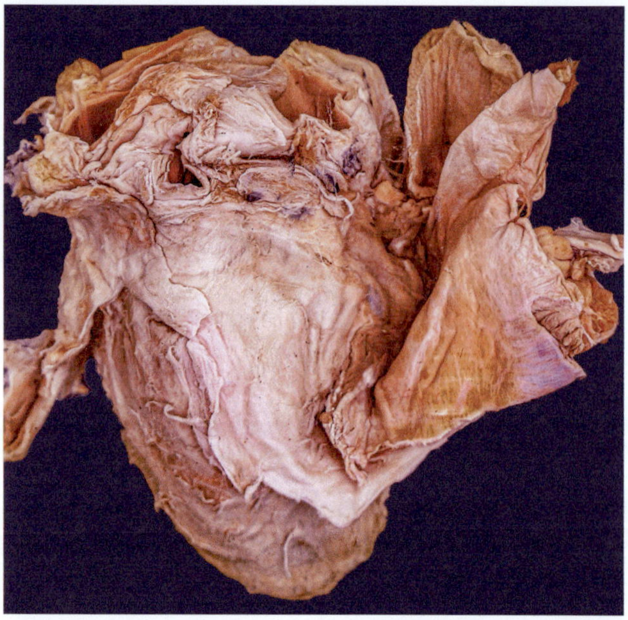

The heart is ensheathed by very thick white fibrous adhesions over the visceral and parietal pericardium and root of great vessels.

Constrictive (Adherent) Pericarditis

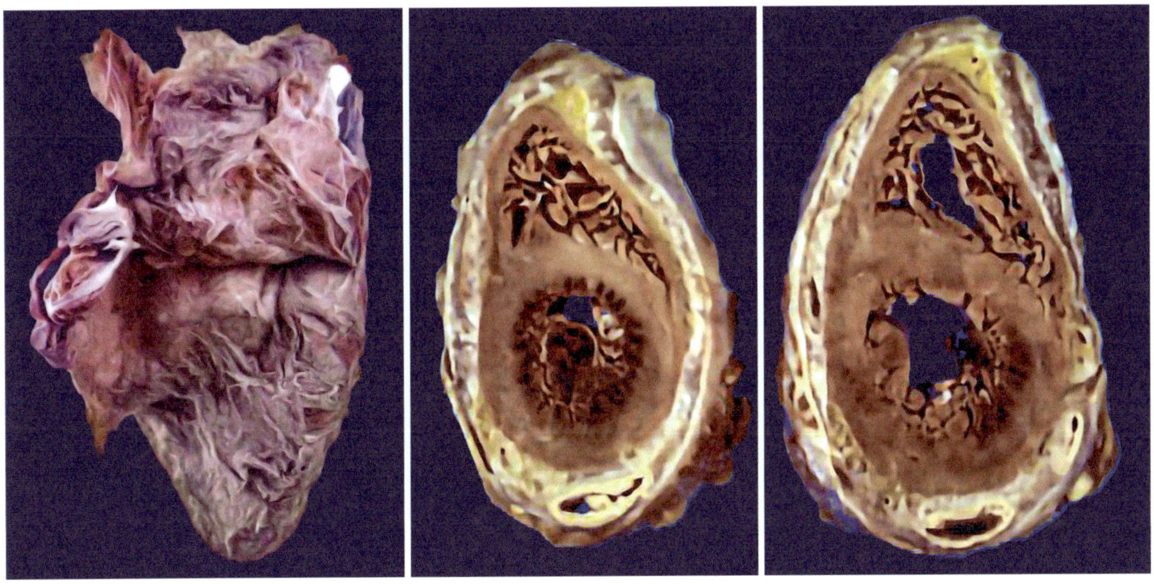

The heart is ensheathed by very thick white fibrous adhesions over the visceral and parietal pericardium and root of great vessels. This is the result of the healing of fibrinous pericarditis by fibrosis. The fibrous tissue was torn during the opening of the pericardial sac.

Constrictive (Adherent) Pericarditis

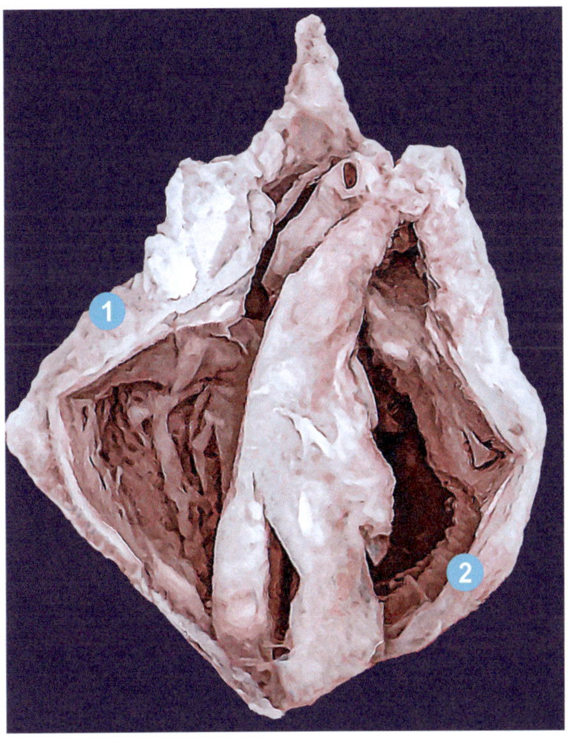

An adult heart is displayed.

1. The heart is ensheathed by very thick white fibrous adhesions over the visceral and parietal pericardium and root of great vessels.
2. The left and right ventricles are dilated and show moderate thickening of walls, indicating heart failure.

Pearls

Adhesive and constrictive pericarditis both involve pericardium inflammation but differ in causes and symptoms.

Adhesive Pericarditis

Origin: Result of acute pericarditis often due to infections, autoimmune conditions, or post-cardiac injury.

Pathophysiology: Involves fibrinous adhesions between pericardium layers, making them stick.

Symptoms: Includes chest pain and mild pericardial effusion. Doesn't usually impact cardiac function significantly.

Constrictive Pericarditis

Origin: Can arise from prior acute pericarditis, radiation therapy, tuberculosis, or unknown causes.

Pathophysiology: Chronic inflammation causes the pericardium to become thick and rigid, restricting heart movement.

Symptoms: Restricts the heart's filling ability, reducing cardiac output. Leads to exercise intolerance, swelling, fluid accumulation, and an enlarged liver.

While distinct, adhesive pericarditis can evolve into constrictive pericarditis with continued inflammation. Diagnosis involves patient assessment, imaging like echocardiography, and sometimes invasive evaluation.

It is important to note that while adhesive pericarditis and constrictive pericarditis are distinct entities, they are not mutually exclusive. In some cases, adhesive pericarditis can progress to constrictive pericarditis if there is ongoing inflammation and fibrotic changes in the pericardium. The clinical presentation, diagnostic evaluation, and management of these conditions are guided by a thorough assessment of the patient's history, physical examination, imaging studies (such as echocardiography and cardiac MRI), and sometimes invasive hemodynamic evaluation [8].

References

1. Girardi LN. (2017). Syphilitic aortitis: The bigger picture. The Journal of thoracic and cardiovascular surgery. 154 (2): e27-e28. https://doi.org/10.1016/j.jtcvs.04.052. Pubmed
2. Lee, H. J., Kim, S. W., Kim, S. H., Lee, C. H., & Kang, H. S. (2022). Lipofuscin accumulation is associated with increased autophagy in aging rat hearts. Aging Cell, 21(11), e13597. https://doi.org/10.1111/acel.13597. PMID: 35677386
3. Zheng A., Chen Q., Zheng L. (2022). The Hippo-YAP pathway in various cardiovascular diseases: Focusing on the inflammatory response. Front Immunol, 13: 971416. https://doi.org/10.3389/fimmu.2022.971416. PMCID: PMC9433876
4. Joo HJ, Kim J.H., Hong S.J. (2017). Adipose Tissue-Derived Stem Cells for Myocardial Regeneration. Korean Circ J. 47(2): 151–159. https://doi.org/10.4070/kcj.2016.0207. PMCID: PMC5378017
5. DeLeon-Pennell, K.Y., et al. (2017). Matrix Metalloproteinases in Myocardial Infarction and Heart Failure. Prog Mol Biol Transl Sci. 147: 75–100. https://doi.org/10.1016/bs.pmbts.2017.02.001. PMCID: PMC5576003.
6. Cho S., Paik D.T., Wu J.C. (2020). An extracellular matrix paradox in myocardial scar formation. Sig Transduct Target Ther. 5, 151. https://doi.org/10.1038/s41392-020-00270-z.
7. Borer J.S., et al. (2019). Atrial Fibrillation and Stroke in Patients with Hypertrophic Cardiomyopathy: Important New Insights. Thromb Haemost.: 119(3):355-357. doi: https://doi.org/10.1055/s--0039-1678724. PMID: 30759487.
8. Kisansa M. E., et al. (2018). Case of tuberculous pericarditis presenting as a giant pericardial adhesion and masquerading as a pericardial tumor SA J Radiol.: 22(1): 1359. https://doi.org/10.4102/sajr.v22i1.1359. PMCID: PMC6837817.

Diseases of Head and Neck

2

2.1 Introduction

The head and neck region is a complex anatomical area that comprises a variety of vital structures, including the brain, eyes, ears, nose, mouth, throat, and associated lymphatics.

In this chapter, we will discuss the gross and microscopic pathology of some head and neck lesions. Understanding the pathological features of these lesions is essential for accurate diagnosis, effective treatment, and appropriate follow-up.

Throughout this chapter, we will highlight the importance of a thorough examination as the foundation for accurate histopathological assessment and diagnosis. We will also emphasize the need for a systematic approach to gross examination as well as the value of correlating gross pathological findings with clinical history and radiological imaging.

The studied lesions will include the following:

1. Lesions in the Head Region
   (a) Nasopharyngeal carcinoma (NPC)
   (b) Carcinoma of the maxillary antrum
   (c) Ameloblastoma of maxilla
   (d) Papillary cystadenoma of parotid gland
2. Lesions in the Neck Region
   (a) Larynx
      - Syphilitic laryngitis
      - Intrinsic ulcerative carcinoma of the larynx
      - Extrinsic ulcerative carcinoma of the larynx
   (b) Thyroid Gland
      - Colloid nodular goiter
      - Primary thyrotoxic goiter
      - Thyroid carcinomas

2.2 Lesions in the Head Region

Nasopharyngeal Carcinoma (NPC)

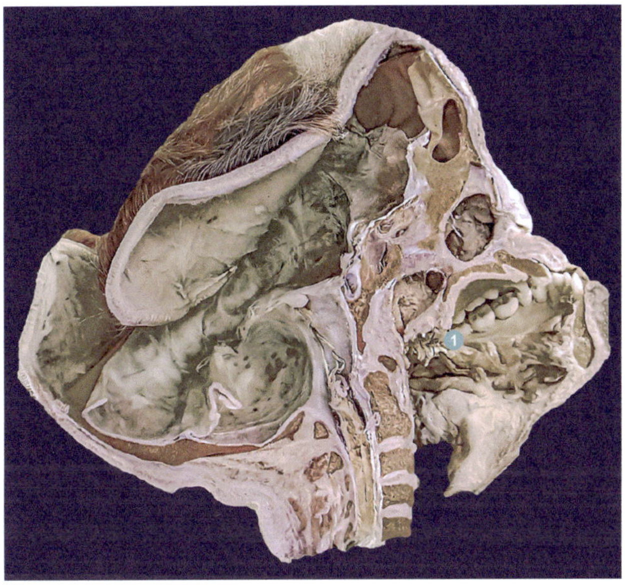

Head and neck bisected longitudinally are mounted.

1. Infiltrative, polypoid, gray-white tissue is seen at the nasopharyngeal recess (i.e., the fossa of Rosenmüller). Proved microscopically to be NPC.

G. Dawood, *Color Atlas of Human Gross and Microscopic Pathology*, https://doi.org/10.1007/978-3-031-76007-5_2

Microscopic Picture of Nasopharyngeal Carcinoma (NPC): Nonkeratinizing, undifferentiated subtype (a–d)

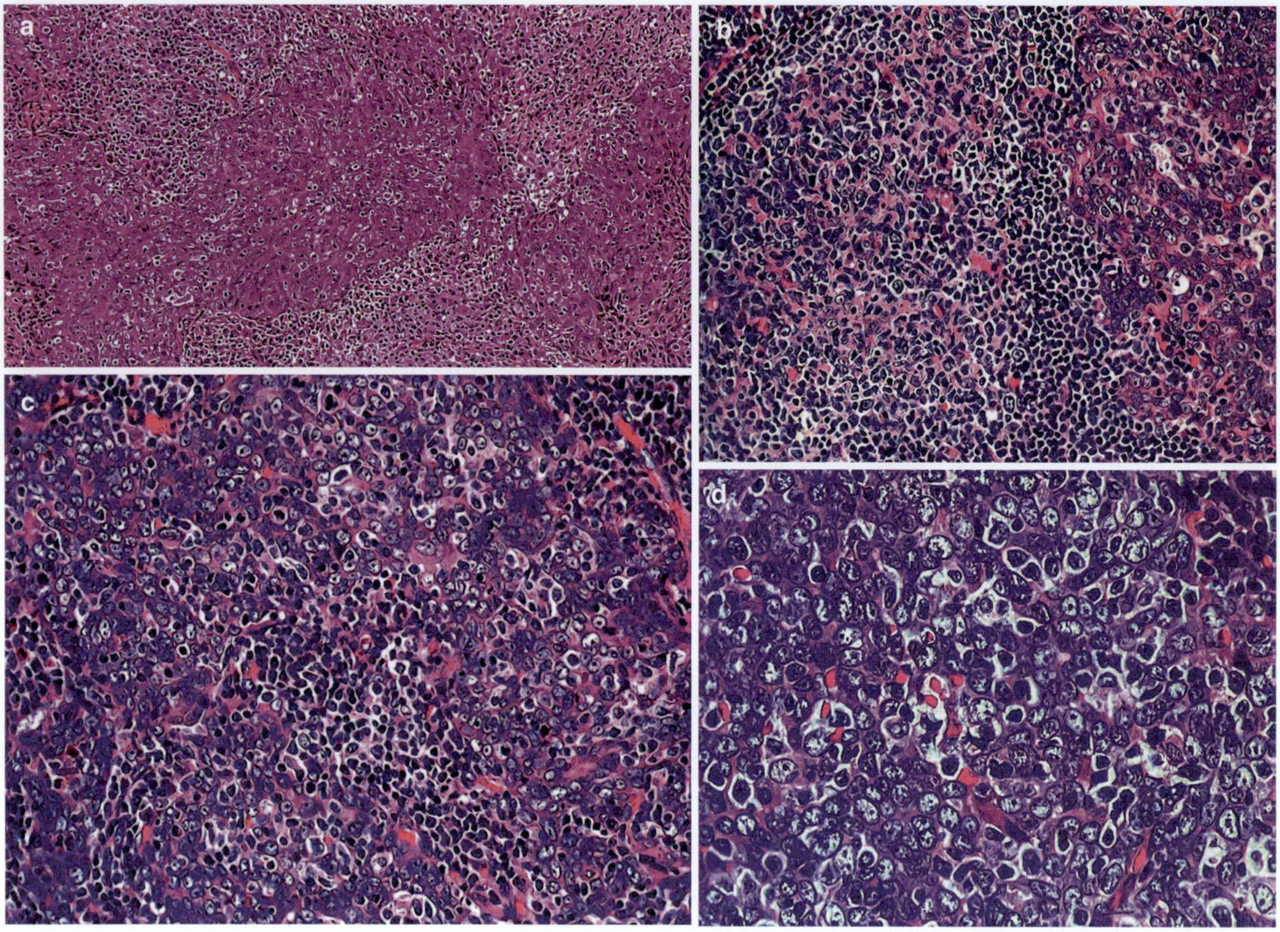

Sections show syncytial growth with oval or round vesicular nuclei and prominent nucleoli. There is a prominent inflammatory response in the adjacent stroma (Regaud pattern). Another part of the tumor presents the Schmincke pattern, where tumor cells spread out and mix with inflammatory cells without significant keratinization. Tumor cells have moderate eosinophilic to amphophilic cytoplasm, round nuclei, prominent eosinophilic nucleoli, and vesicular chromatin. Apoptosis and brisk mitotic activity are invariably present. Nonneoplastic lymphoplasmacytic infiltrate accompanies the tumor.

Ancillary Tools [1]

IHC:

Positive staining for pancytokeratin, high molecular weight CK, p63, and p40.

Molecular/cytogenetics Description:

Detection of Epstein-Barr virus (EBV) by PCR or ISH (EBER) was found in 75–100% of cases.

Carcinoma of Maxillary Antrum

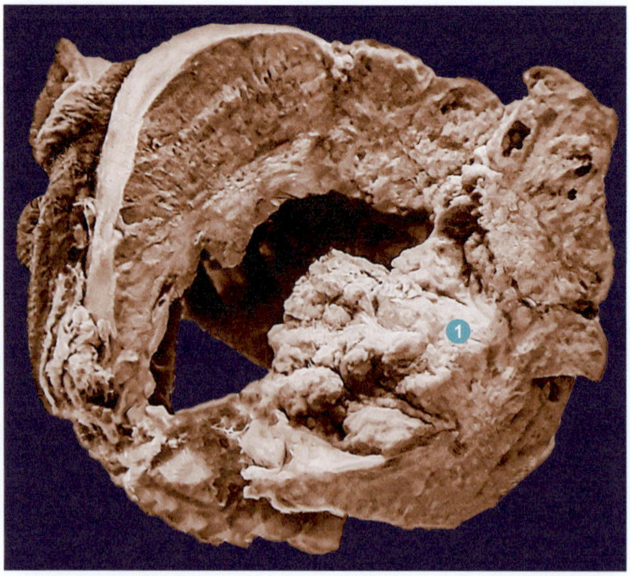

The left maxilla is mounted.

1. The bone is infiltrated by gray-white, fungating, firm, and crescentic mass arising from the lining of the maxillary antrum.

Microscopic Picture of Carcinoma of Maxillary Antrum (a)

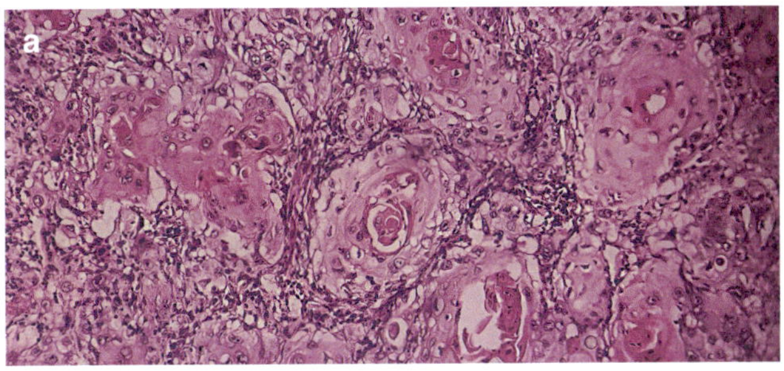

The tumor is a keratinizing squamous cell carcinoma arising from the squamous epithelium that lines the sinus.

Ancillary Tools [2]
IHC includes

Positive staining for AE1/AE3, CK5/6, CK7, CK903, p40, p63, and EMA.

Molecular/cytogenetics description:

p16 positive cases should be followed by high-risk HPV ISH or PCR for confirmation.

DEK::AFF2 fusion with RNA sequencing or DEK break apart FISH in DEK::AFF2 carcinoma

Pearls
The histopathology of carcinoma of the maxillary antrum is variable, but the most common type is squamous cell carcinoma. Other types include adenoid cystic carcinoma, adenocarcinoma, mucoepidermoid carcinoma, undifferentiated cancer, lymphoma, and occasionally malignant melanoma [3].

Ameloblastoma of Maxilla (a, b)

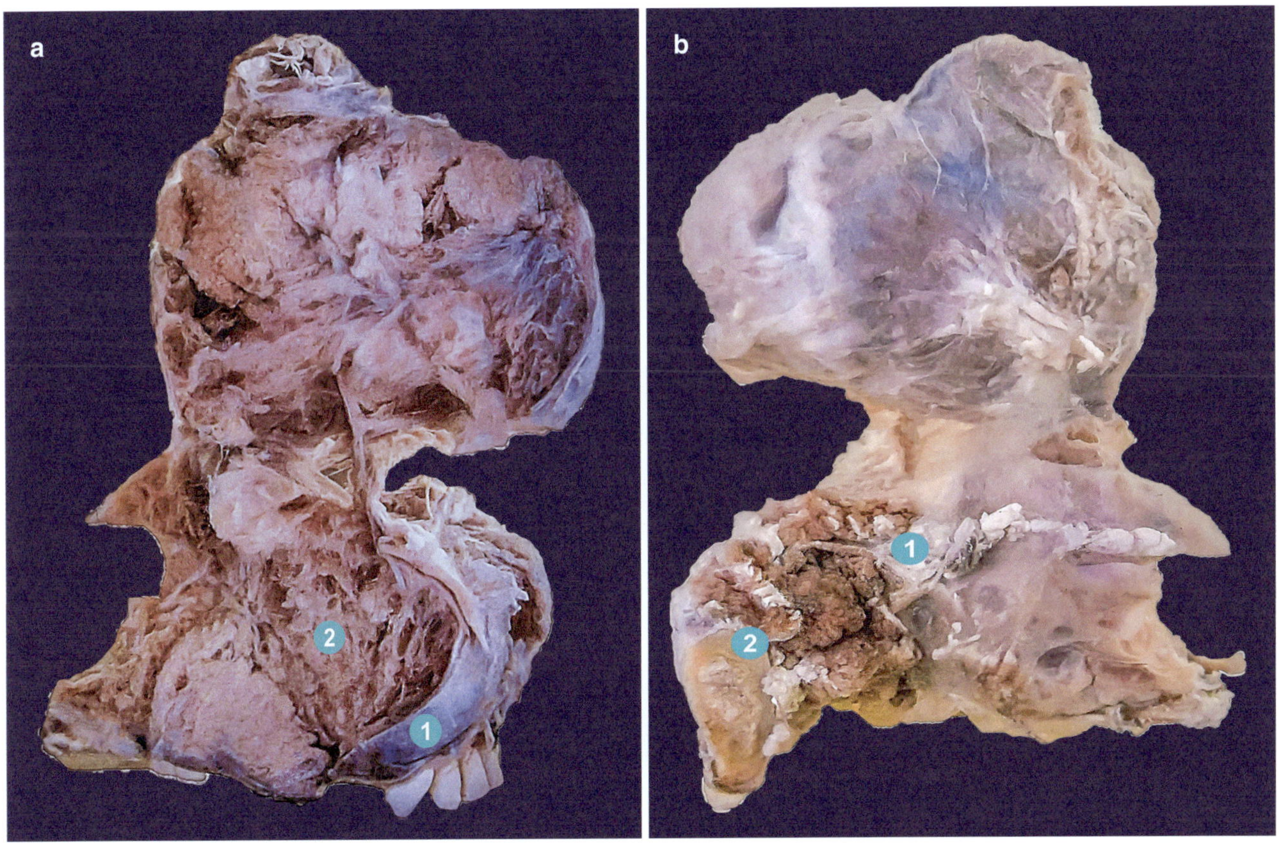

The left maxilla is mounted.

1. A tumor mass is seen originating above the teeth, which become irregular.
2. The tumor is gray-white, firm, partially cystic, and partially solid with complete infiltration of the maxilla.

Microscopic Picture of Ameloblastoma (Conventional Type) (c–i)

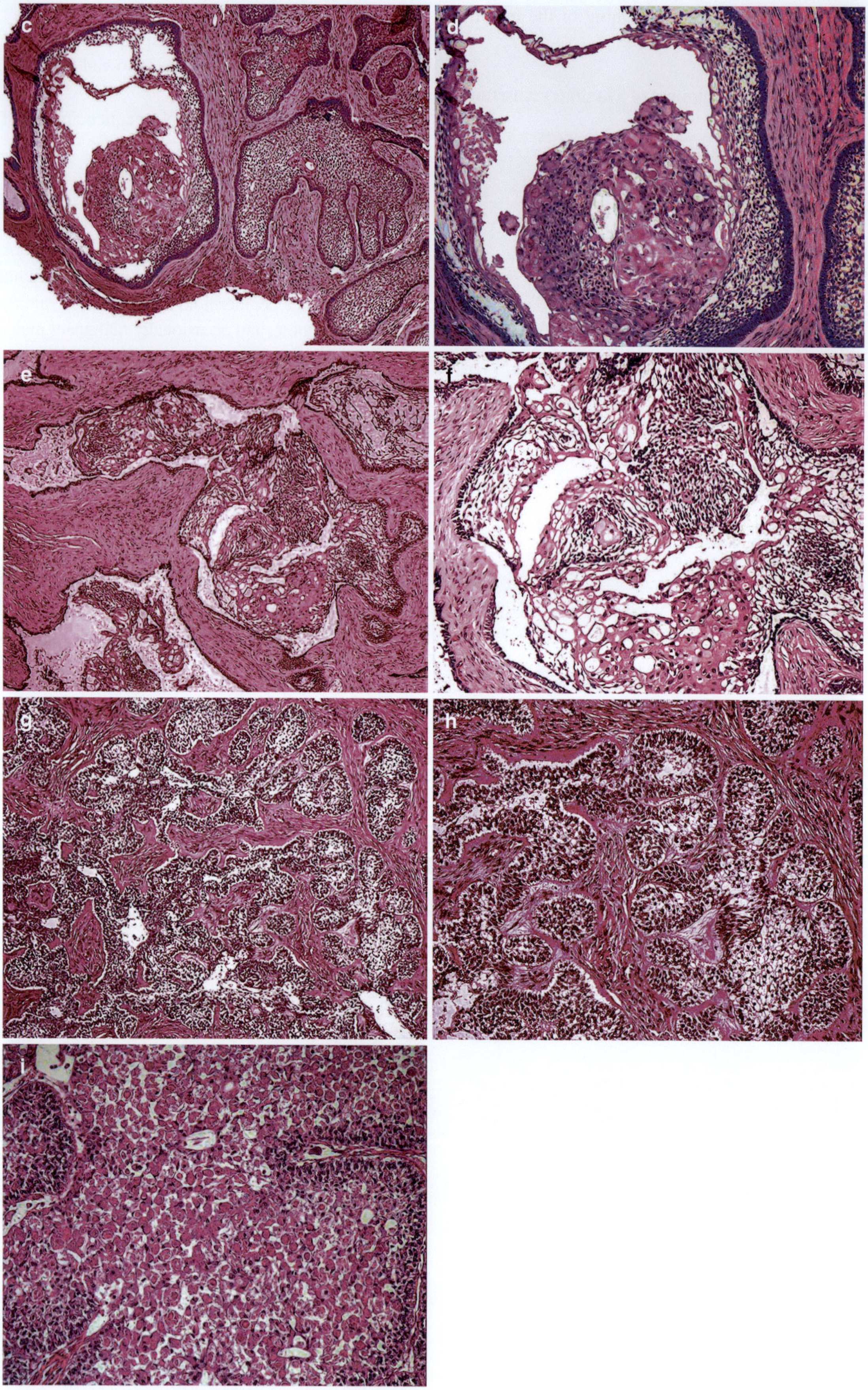

Sections show tumors consisting of variously shaped islands of odontogenic epithelium. These islands have outer columnar cells with nuclei facing away from the basement membrane and central cells that resemble the stellate reticulum of a developing tooth. These structures are surrounded by a dense collagen-rich stroma.

(c) Acanthotic pattern: in which areas of keratinization and cyst formation are seen in (c–f)
(d) Plexiform pattern: in which cords and sheets of anastomosing odontogenic epithelial cells; classic peripheral palisading and reverse polarity not always obvious (g, h)
(e) Granular Cell pattern: in which stellate reticulum-like cells have granular eosinophilic cytoplasm; less commonly involves cells at the periphery of nests (i)

Ancillary Tools [4]

IHC includes:

Positive staining for CK19 and CK14, CK5, CD56, calretinin, BRAF V600E (VE1), p63 and p40, FOXP1

Molecular/cytogenetics description:

Recurrent somatic and activating mutations in the mitogen-activated protein kinase (MAPK) pathway are present in ~80% of ameloblastomas identified in 2014 by 3 separate groups.

1. BRAF V600E (most common mutation; at least 60%)
2. RAS and FGFR2
3. Hedgehog signaling pathway; appears mutually exclusive from MAPK
4. In a recent study, 94% of the mandibular unicystic ameloblastomas revealed BRAF V600E mutations; in 1 BRAF wild-type mandibular tumor, an SMO p.L412F mutation was identified.

Pearls

Ameloblastomas display a wide variety of architectural patterns, including [5]:

1. Conventional type: its microscopic variants include follicular, plexiform, basal, acanthomatous, granular, and desmoplastic types. Follicular and plexiform patterns are the most common. Multiple patterns often coexist, and they have no clinical significance.
2. Unicystic type.
3. Extraosseous/peripheral type metastasizing ameloblastoma (rare).

Papillary Cystadenoma of the Parotid Gland (Warthin's tumor)

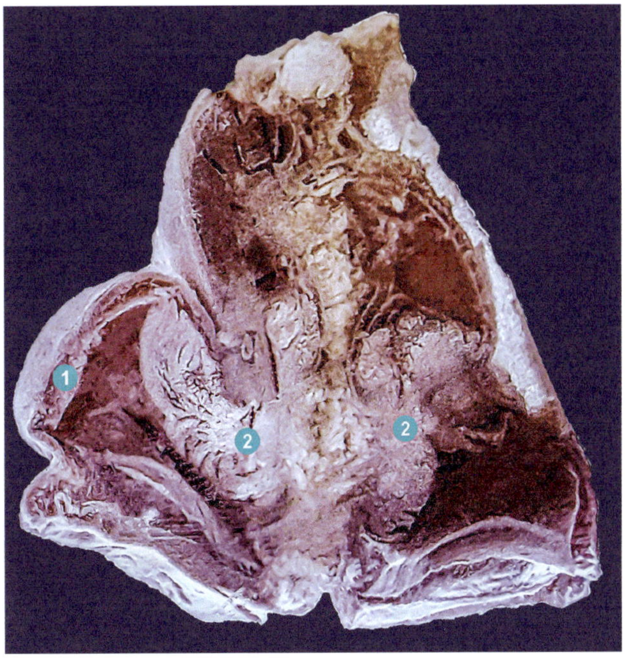

A tumor in the parotid gland is bisected longitudinally.

1. The cut section shows cystic, pink, well-defined, and encapsulated mass.
2. There are solid areas with fine branching papillary fronds and cystic brown areas that were filled with viscous brown fluid (machine motor oil).

Microscopic Picture of Papillary Cystadenoma Lymphomatosum (a–d)

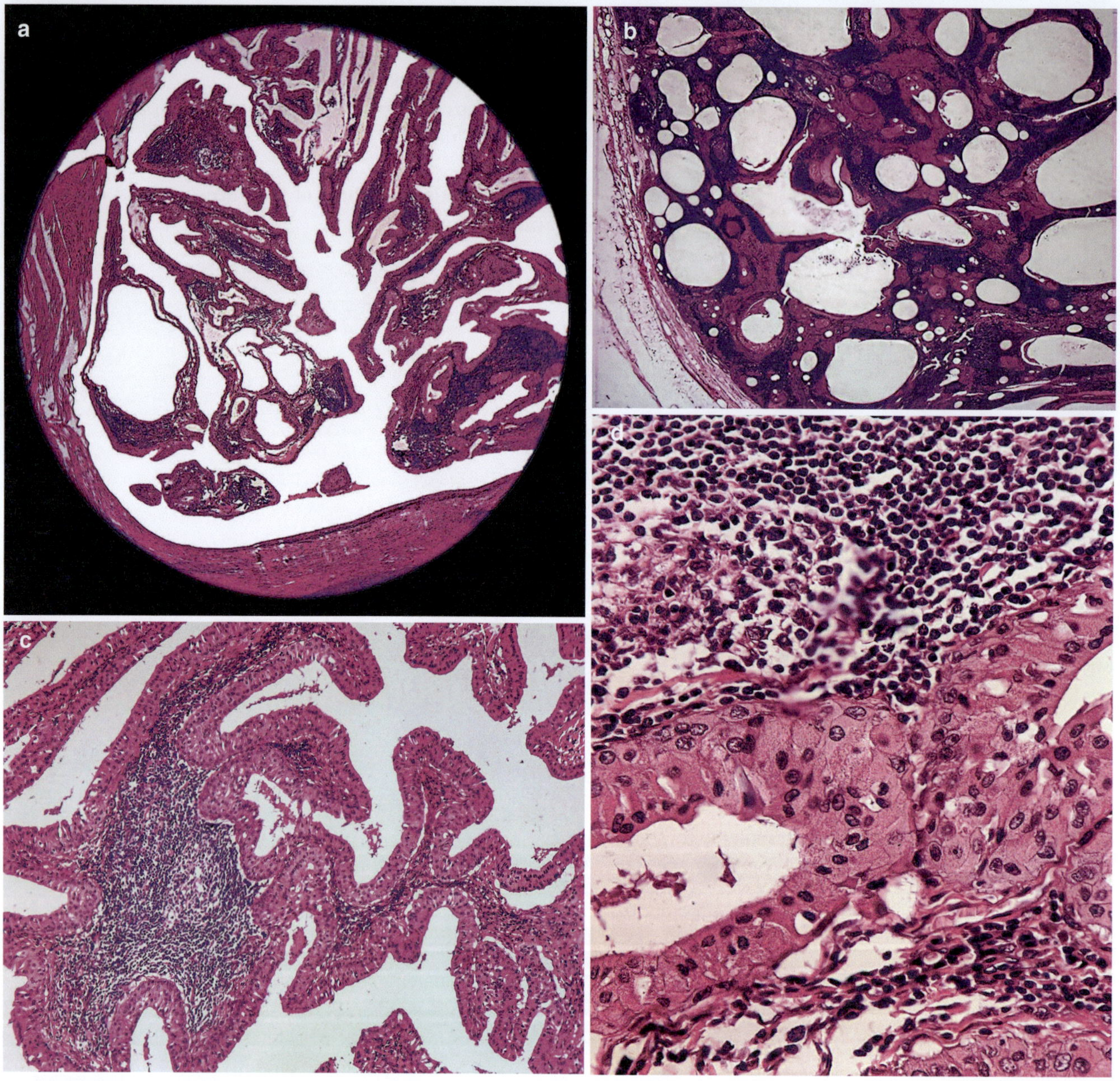

Sections of the tumor show papillary cystic structures, lined by bilayered oncocytic epithelium with brightly eosinophilic cytoplasm and round nucleus and surrounded by dense lymphocytic infiltrate with germinal center formation.

Ancillary Tools [6]

IHC includes:

Positive staining of all epithelial cells for pancytokeratin CK7, CK8/CK18, and EMA are positive in luminal (or inner) epithelial cells, while p63 and p40 show heterogeneous nuclear staining of the basal cells.

Lymphoid cells are positive for B cell markers (CD20) and T cell markers (CD3, CD4, CD8).

Molecular/cytogenetics description:

Absent MAML2 fusion.

2.3 Lesions in the Neck Region

2.3.1 Larynx

Syphilitic Gummatous Laryngitis

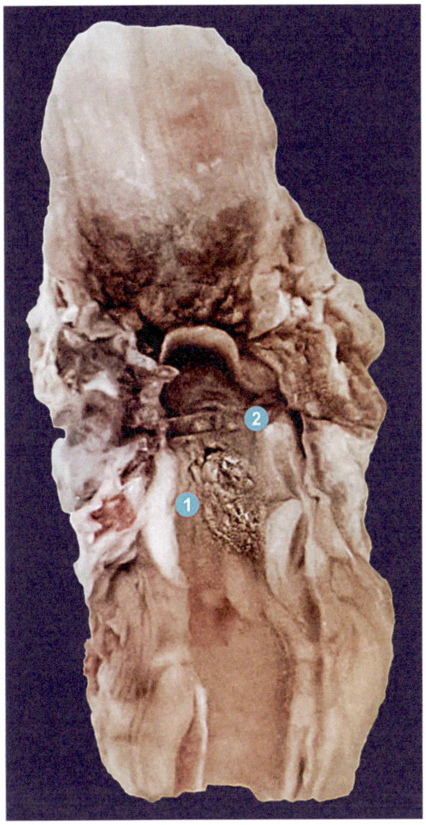

Tongue, larynx, and trachea are mounted.

1. The laryngeal mucosa appears irregularly puckered with small elevations and ulcerations.
2. Stenosis of laryngeal orifice.

Intrinsic Carcinoma of the Larynx

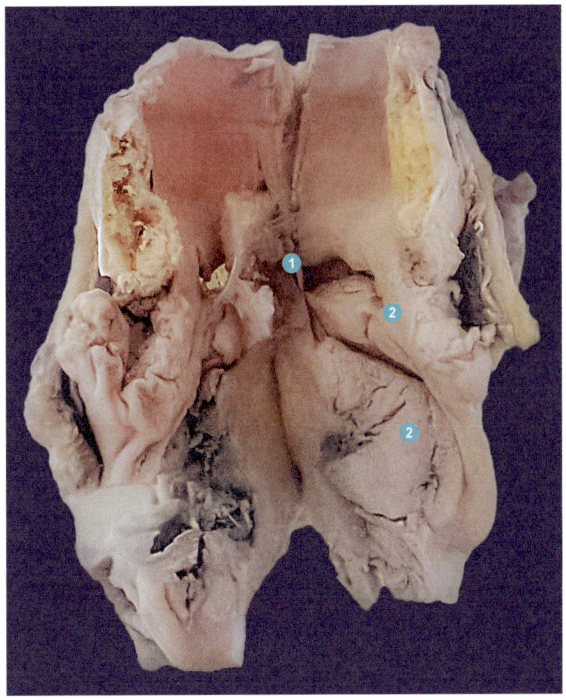

The larynx is mounted.

1. Both true and false vocal cords are infiltrated by malignant gray-white polypoid tumor mass with midline involvement.
2. The mass extends superiorly to involve the false vocal cord and inferiorly to involve the subglottic region.

Intrinsic Ulcerative Carcinoma of the Larynx

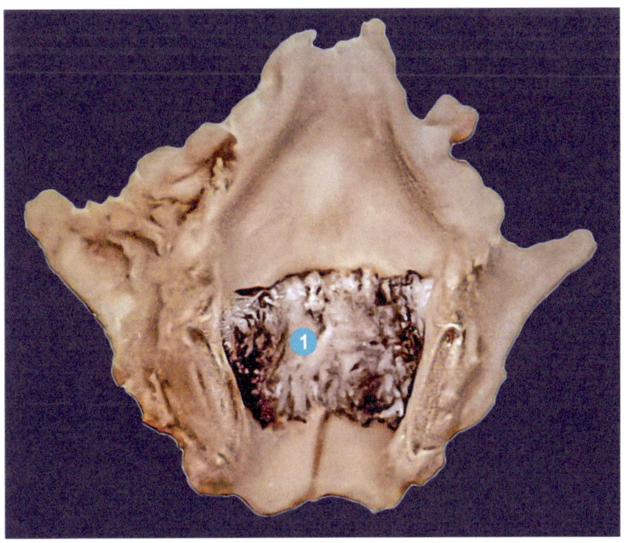

The larynx is mounted.

1. Both true and false vocal cords are infiltrated by an oval malignant tumor mass with raised edges. The ulcer extends superiorly to involve the false vocal cord.

Extrinsic (Supraglottic) Carcinoma of the Larynx

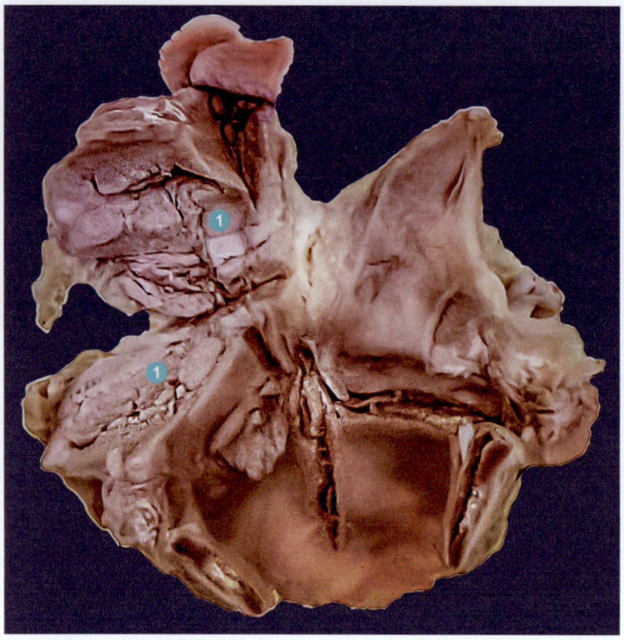

The larynx is mounted.

1. A large, pale gray, irregular mass is seen in the left supraglottic region infiltrating the surrounding structures and left vocal cord without midline involvement.

Glottic Laryngeal Carcinoma Extending into Subglottis

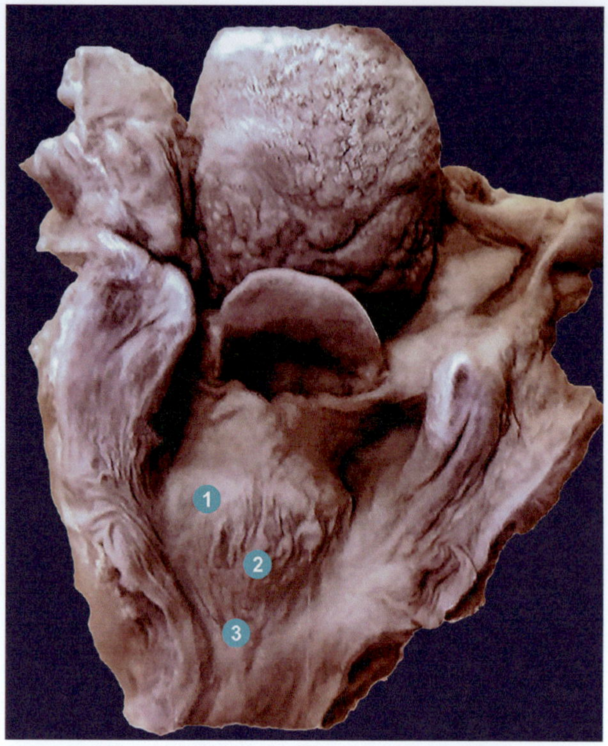

Tongue, larynx, and trachea are mounted.

1. A mass involves the left false vocal cord and extends down to the subglottis.
2. A submucosal nodule in the subglottis at the level of the cricoid cartilage.
3. Irregular and edematous subglottic mucosa covering the tumor with narrowing of the subglottic airway.

Microscopic Picture of Laryngeal Squamous Cell Carcinoma (a–c)

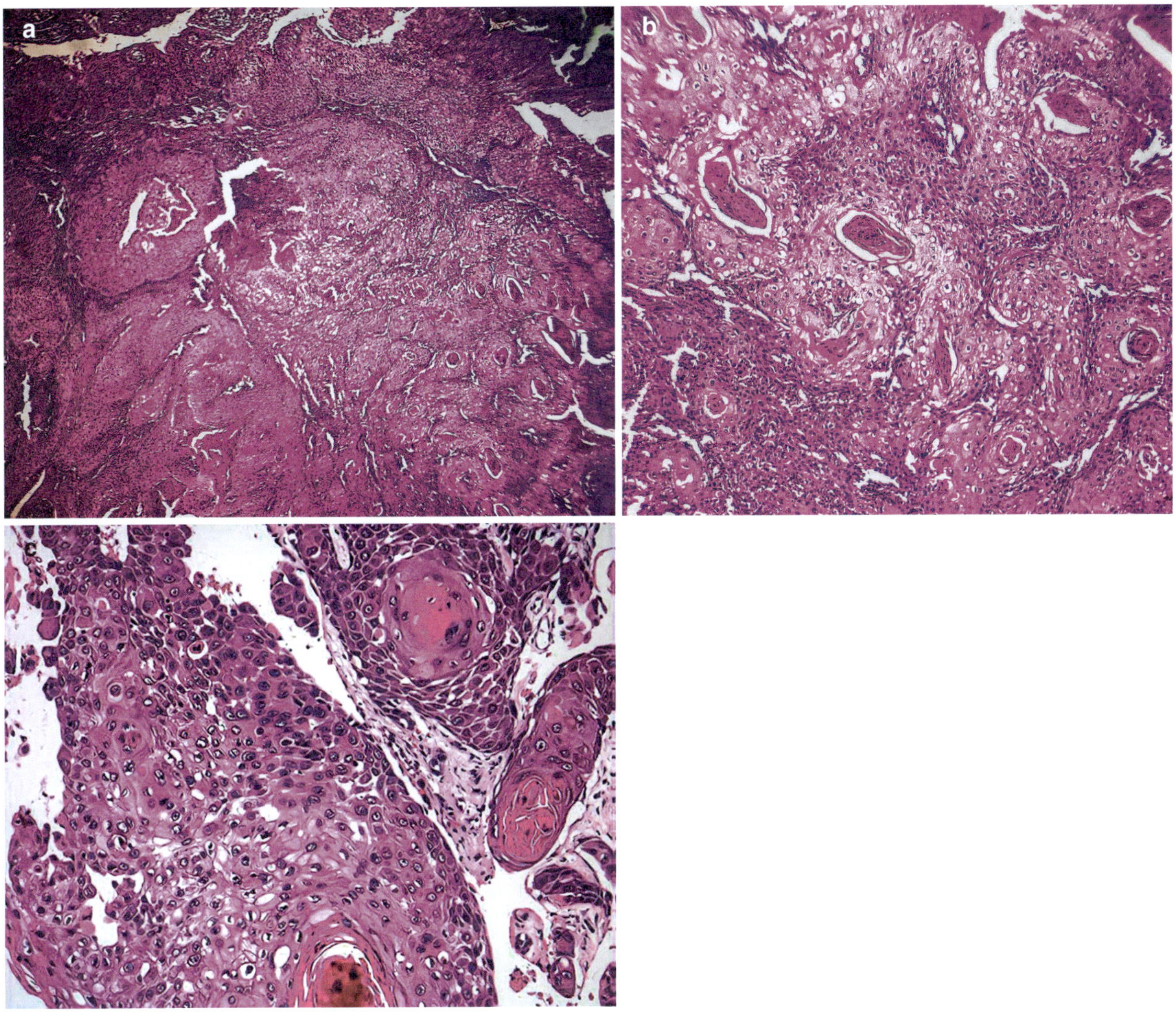

Sections show multiple nests formed of malignant squamous cells with central keratinization. The stroma is fibrous and infiltrated with chronic inflammatory cells.

Microscopic Picture of Laryngeal Mucoepidermoid Carcinoma (d–g)

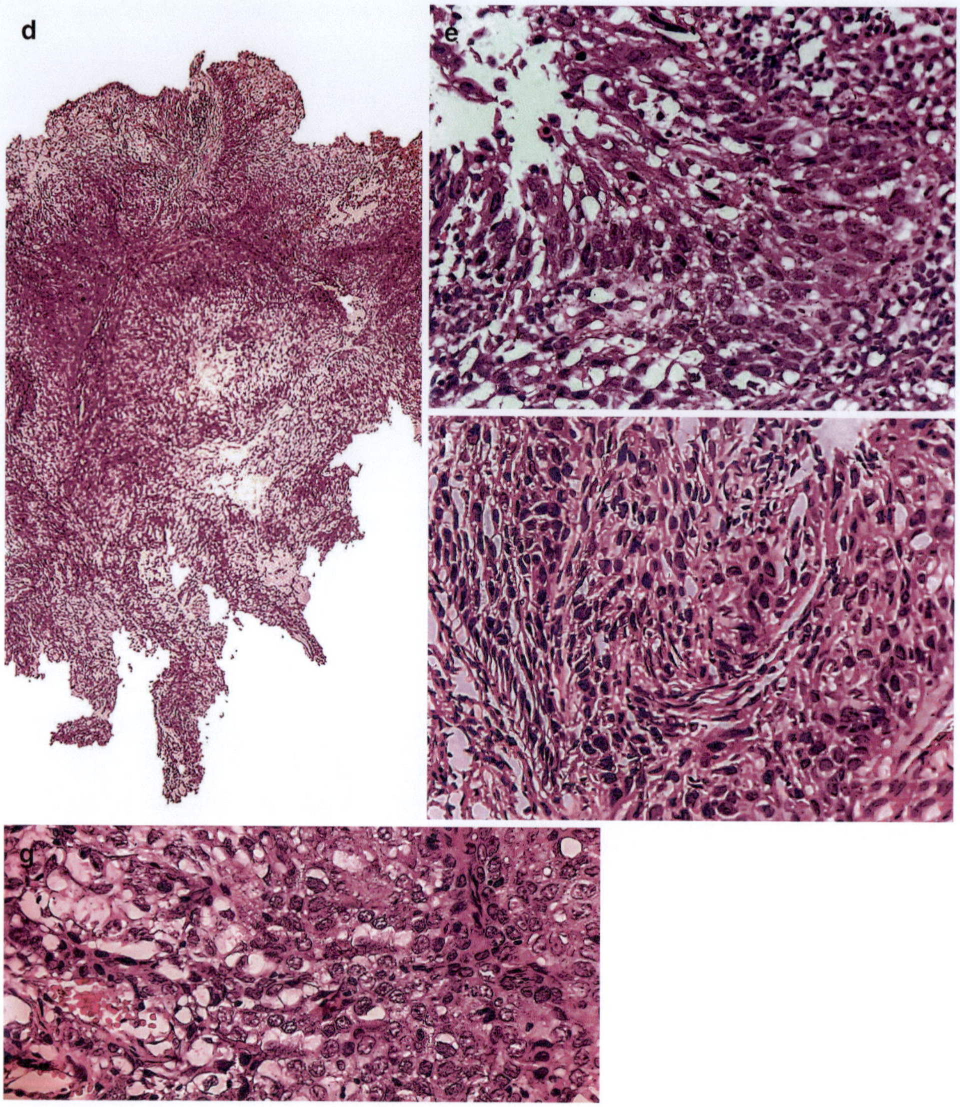

Sections show nests of tumor cells with both well-differentiated squamous cells, mucinous cells, and intermediate cells. Cytonuclear atypia was noted in the squamous component of the tumor.

Ancillary Tools

IHC includes [7]:

Positive staining for AE1, AE3, and p53 (50%, usually wild type).

Pearls

Primary cancers arising in the subglottic region are rare and are characterized by a long asymptomatic phase. More frequently, the subglottis is reached by tumors arising in the glottis or even the supraglottis through invasion of the paraglottic space. Involvement of the subglottis is associated with a relatively high frequency of stomal recurrences due to a peculiar lymphatic spread to the paratracheal nodes [8].

Pearls

Mucoepidermoid carcinoma is a common malignant neoplasm of the salivary glands. While quite common in the oral cavity, it is rare in the larynx. Laryngeal MECs affect the supraglottis (60%), followed by the glottis (30%) and the subglottis (10%). Because they tend to be developed submucosally, symptoms are usually mild, rendering early diagnosis difficult. In later stages, the manifestations are strongly related to the affected area. Supraglottic MECs generally cause dysphagia or even secondary otalgia, while glottic MECs appear with hoarseness or even stridor [9].

2.3.2 Thyroid Gland

Colloid Nodular Goiter

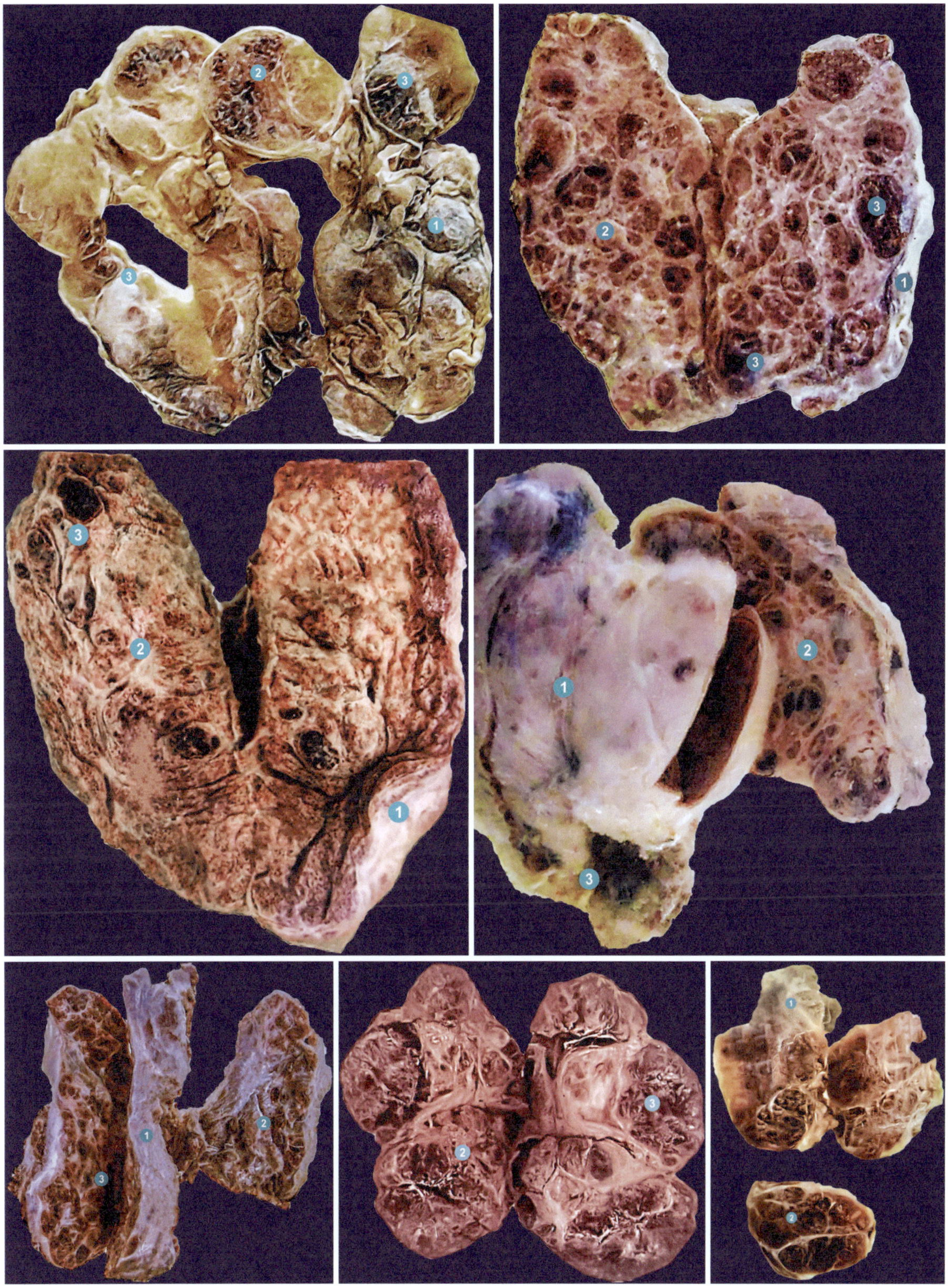

An enlarged thyroid is mounted.

1. It is irregular in shape, multinodular, and encapsulated.
2. The cut section is divided into loci by bands of fibrous tissue; the loci are variable in size and shape and filled with homogeneous gelatinous colloid.
3. Focal areas of hemorrhage, fibrosis, cyst formation, and calcification.

Microscopic Picture of Colloid Nodular Goiter (a, b)

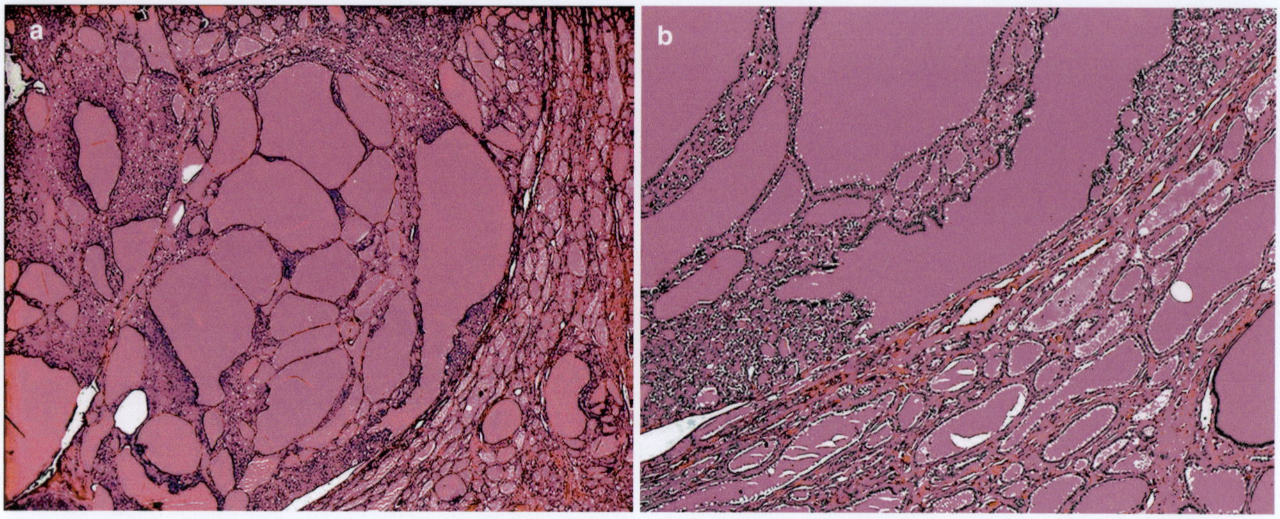

Sections show thyroid tissue divided into multiple nodules separated by bands of fibrous tissue. Each nodule is formed of thyroid follicles lined with cuboidal–flat epithelium and filled with dense, deeply eosinophilic colloid. Some follicles are cystically dilated, while others are hyperplastic.

Primary Thyrotoxic Goiter

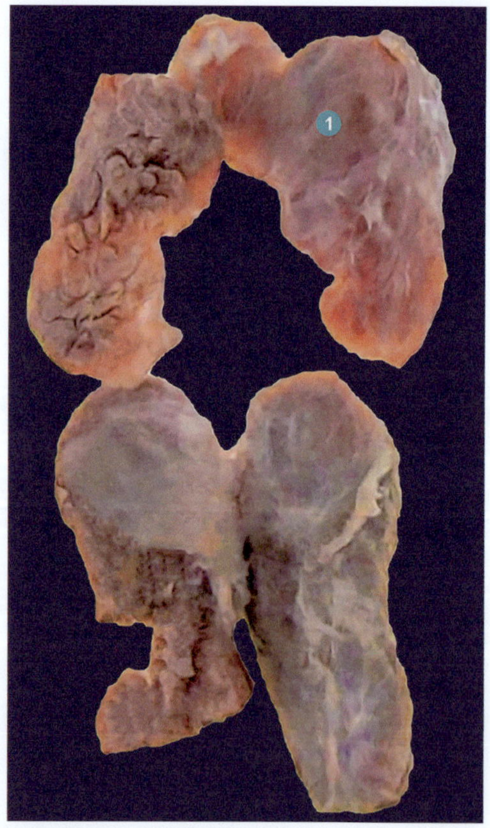

Two thyroid glands were removed from cases of thyrotoxicosis.

1. They are diffusely enlarged with fleshy cut sections and absent colloid.

Microscopic Picture of Thyrotoxic Goiter (a, b)

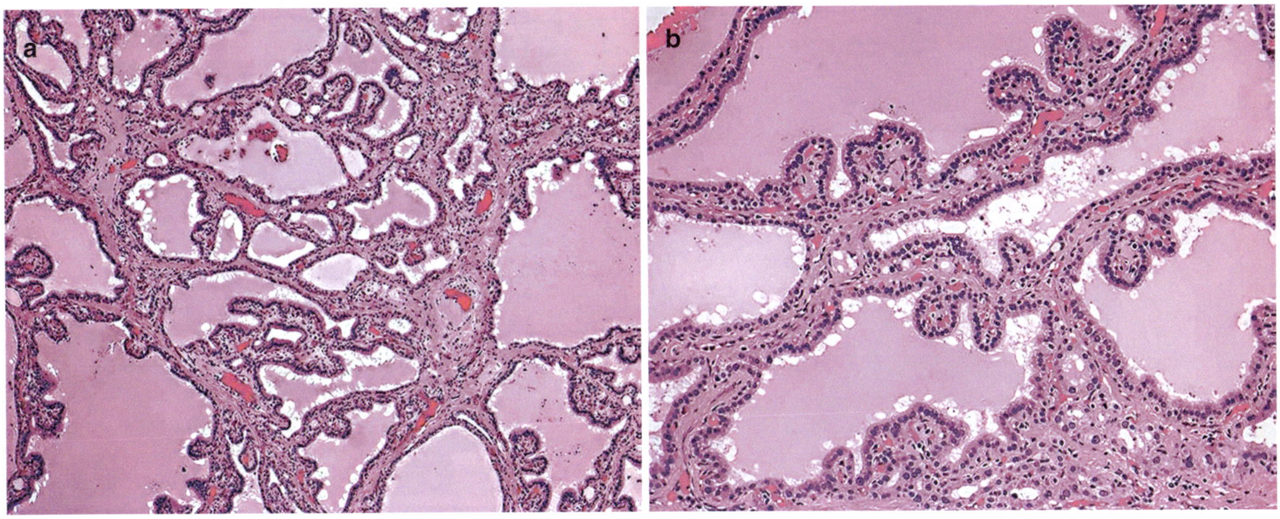

Sections show diffuse hyperplasia of thyroid follicles, which are variable in shape and lined with columnar epithelium thrown into papillae in areas. The follicles are filled with lightly eosinophilic colloid, which shows peripheral vacuolization. The stroma shows increased vascularity and lymphocytic inflammatory infiltrate.

Thyroid Carcinoma

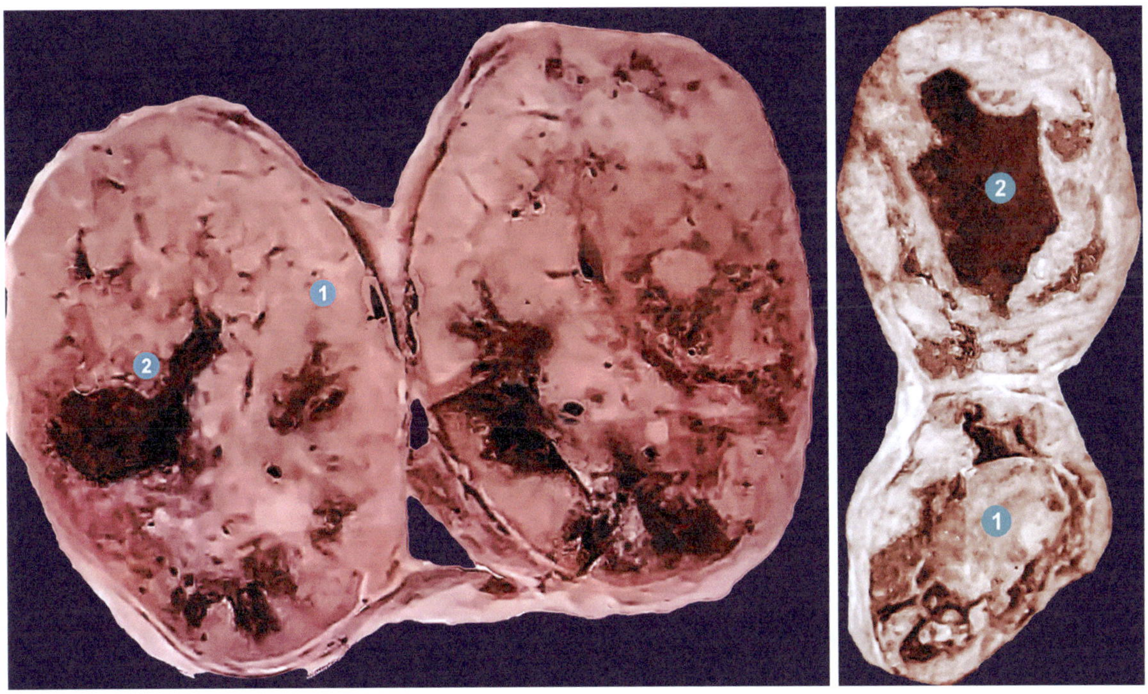

A partially encapsulated white-yellow mass was removed from the thyroid.

1. It has solid areas with focal areas of infiltration of the capsule.
2. Areas of hemorrhage and necrosis are seen.

Microscopic Picture of Papillary Thyroid Carcinoma (a–d)

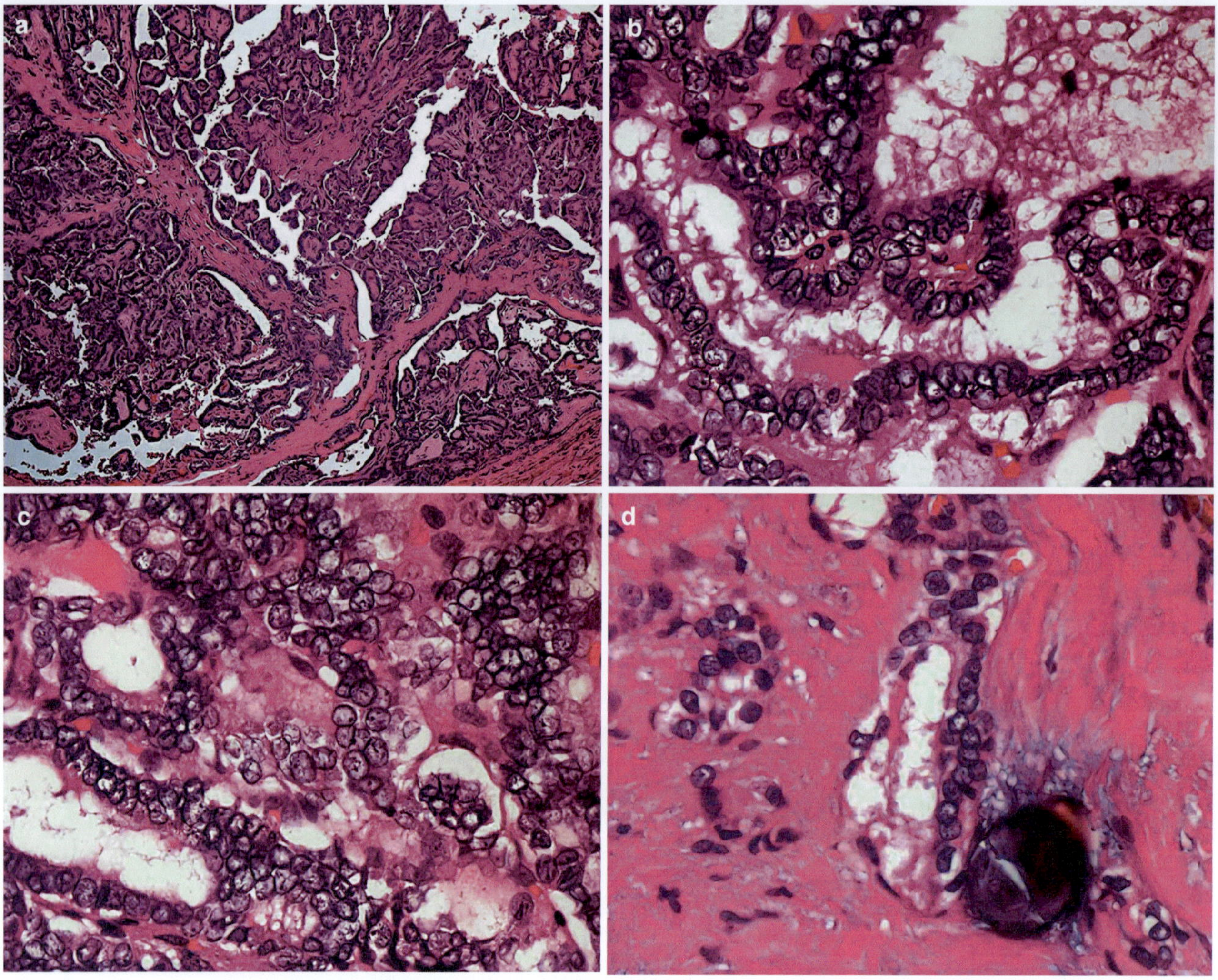

Thyroid tissue is infiltrated with complex, branching papillae with fibrovascular cores. The papillae are lined with columnar cells that have enlarged, oval, and overlapping round nuclei. The nuclear chromatin is clear or optically clear with margination, and the nuclei have a ground-glass appearance. Orphan Annie nuclei are also present. The nuclear membrane shows nuclear grooves and nuclear pseudoinclusions. Laminated microcalcification, known as psammoma body, is seen within the tumor. There is no capsular or vascular invasion.

Ancillary Tools

IHC of thyroid follicular cells includes [10]:

- Cytokeratin AE1/AE3, CK7, TTF1, thyroglobulin, and PAX8.

Variant-specific IHC includes:

- CDX2 for columnar cell variant (positive in 50% of cases)
- Beta catenin for cribriform morular variant showing abnormal nuclear accumulation
- Ki67 index is low (1–5%), and >10% is associated with aggressive histotype and higher recurrence risk.

Molecular and cytogenetic description [11]:

In 2014, The Cancer Genome Atlas (TCGA) published comprehensive genomic alterations. Key findings are [12]:

- BRAF is the most frequently mutated gene, occurring in 60% of cases

The most frequent mutation is BRAFV600E, which is associated with the classic variant and tall cell variant, as well as a low thyroid differentiation score (i.e., less differentiated).

BRAF is highly prevalent (80–90%) in PTC from coastal Asian countries with high iodine intake (Japan, Korea).

- RAS (HRAS, NRAS, and KRAS) occurs in 13%, in particular, follicular variant; RAS mutation is associated with a high thyroid differentiation score.
- Fusions involving BRAF, RET, PPARG, NTRK1, NTRK3, ALK, LTK, MET, FGFR2, or THADA are detected in 15%; among them, RET fusion is the most common, seen in 6%.

TERT promoter mutation is present in 10% and is often associated with aggressive histology, e.g., tall cell variant and poor prognosis.

Microscopic Picture of Follicular Thyroid Carcinoma (a–d)

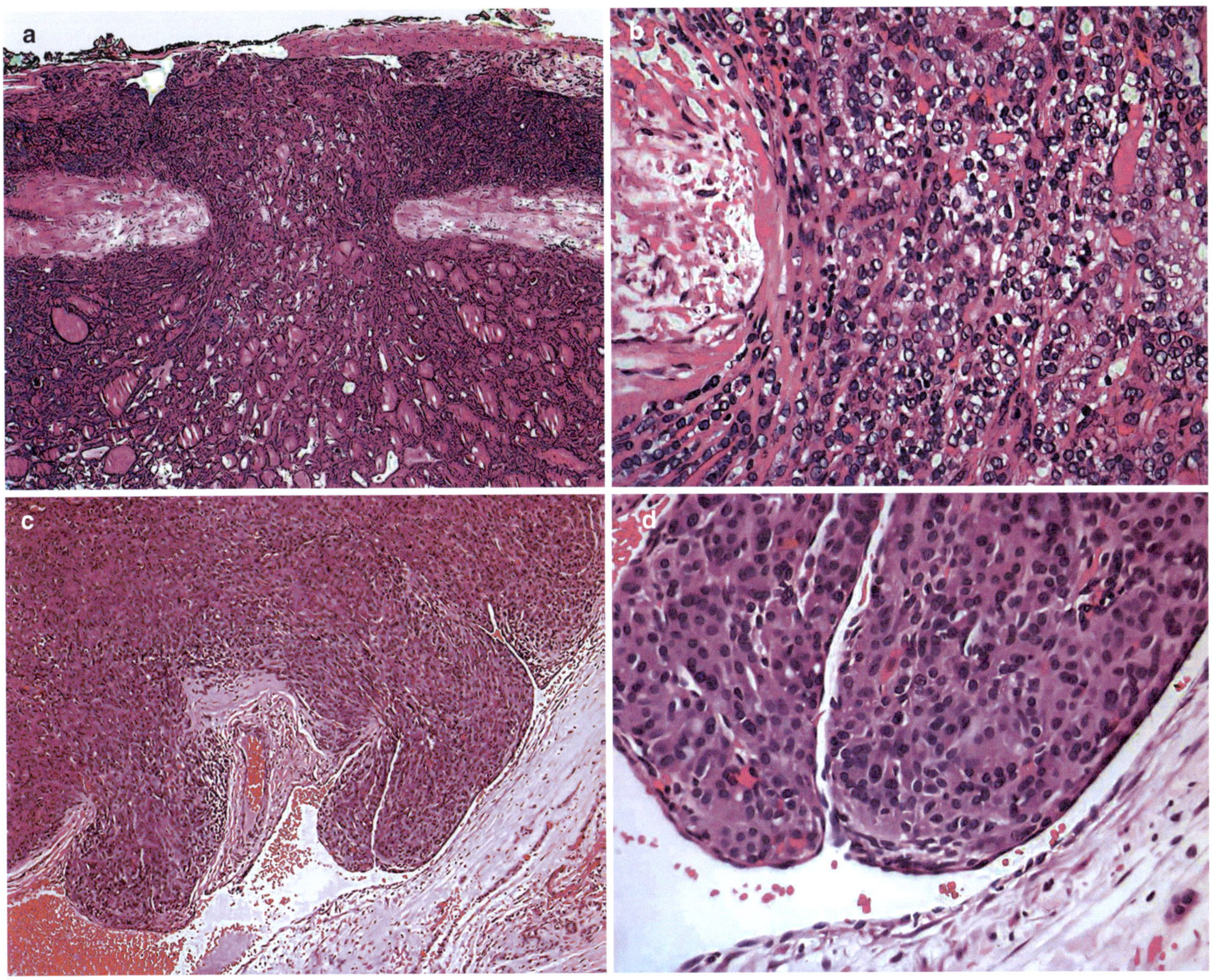

Sections show infiltration of the thyroid gland by closely packed follicular cells arranged in circular or oval patterns, forming follicles filled with colloid. These follicular cells exhibit a uniform appearance, resembling normal thyroid follicular cells. They possess round to oval nuclei with fine chromatin and prominent nucleoli. The cytoplasm is typically abundant and eosinophilic. Tumor cells infiltrate the thyroid gland capsule and extend into blood vessels, lymphatics, or adjacent structures.

Ancillary Tools [12]
IHC of thyroid follicular cells includes:

- Cytokeratin AE1/AE3, CK7, TTF1, thyroglobulin, and PAX8.

Molecular and cytogenetic description:

- Activated PI3K/AKT or RAS of the receptor tyrosine kinase signaling pathway
- NRAS and HRAS mutations in 49%, PAX8 and PPAR gamma rearrangements in 36%
- PI3CA and PTEN mutations in 5–10%

Tumors with rearrangement tend to be overtly invasive versus minimally invasive without this rearrangement.

Widely invasive carcinomas have a higher frequency of allelic loss than minimally invasive carcinomas.

Medullary Thyroid Carcinoma (a, b)

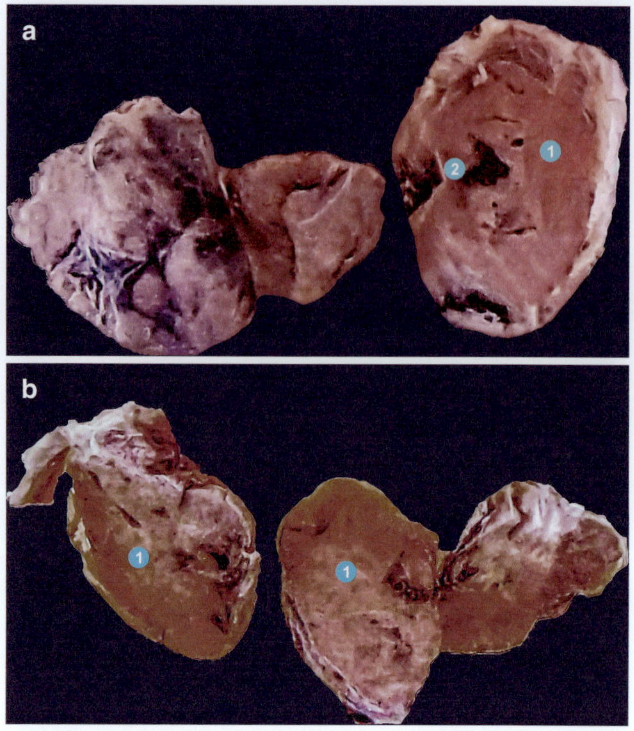

A sectioned thyroid gland is mounted.

1. The cut section shows a solid, firm, well-circumscribed, and unencapsulated mass. The cut surface is yellow tan.
2. Areas of hemorrhage and necrosis.

Microscopic Picture of Medullary Thyroid Carcinoma (c–l)

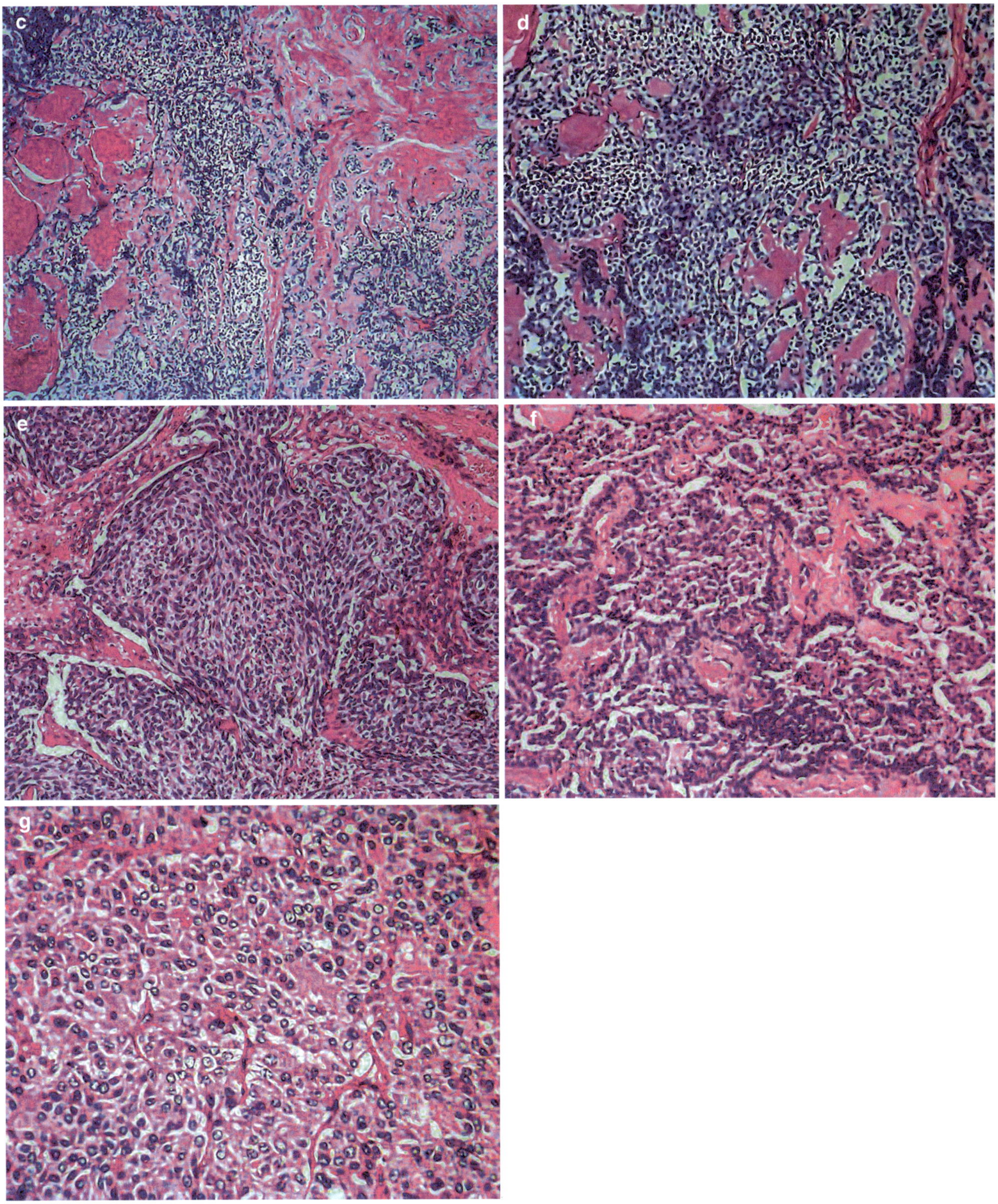

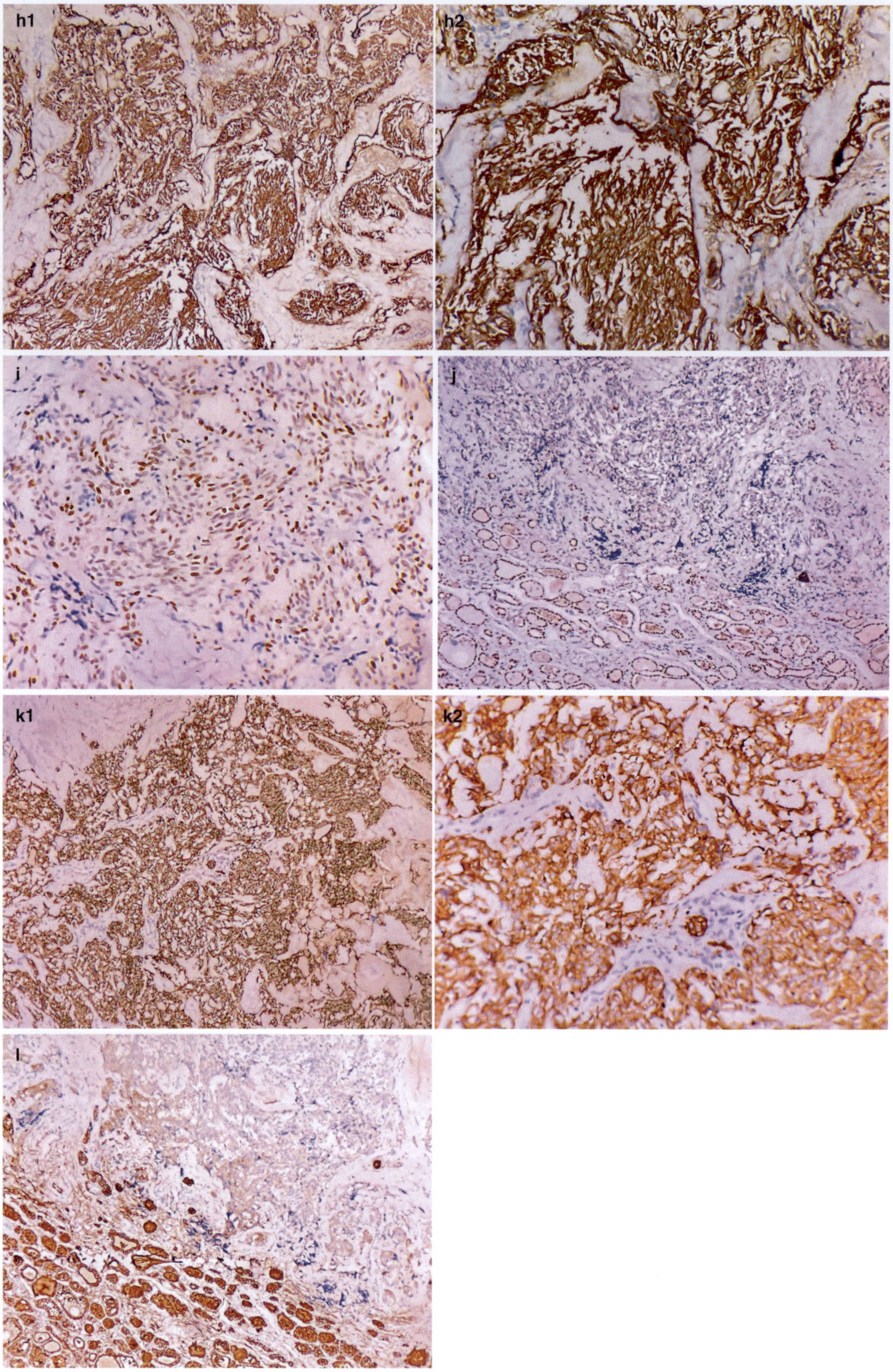

Sections show round, plasmacytoid, polygonal, or spindle cells (e) in nests, cords, or follicles (f), often mixtures of these cells. The tumor cells have round nuclei with finely stippled to coarsely clumped chromatin and indistinct nucleoli and eosinophilic to amphophilic granular cytoplasm. Generally low mitotic figures. Stroma has amyloid deposits from calcitonin and prominent vascularity with long cords of vessels.

Ancillary Tools

IHC [13]:

CEA (h1 and h2),

TTF1 (i) (weak to moderate),

PAX8 (j) (variable and weak)

Synaptophysin (k1 and k2)

Thyroglobulin (l) is negative in tumor cells but positive in entrapped thyroid follicles.

References

1. Petersson F. (2015). Nasopharyngeal carcinoma: a review. Semin Diagn. Pathol.32(1):54–73. https://doi.org/10.1053/j.semdp.2015.02.021. PMID: 25769204.
2. Tendron A. et al. (2022). Prognostic Analysis of HPV Status in Sinonasal Squamous Cell Carcinoma. Cancers (Basel). 14(8):1874. https://doi.org/10.3390/cancers14081874. PMID: 35454782.
3. Pérez-Sayáns M., et al. (2020) Clinicopathological features of 214 maxillary sinus pathologies. A ten-year single-center retrospective clinical study. Head Face Med.16: 24. doi: https://doi.org/10.1186/s13005-020-00239-x. PMCID: PMC7552481.
4. Nudell J. et al. (2014). Carcinoma ex-Schneiderian papilloma (malignant transformation): a clinicopathologic and immunophenotypic study of 20 cases combined with a comprehensive review of the literature. Head Neck Pathol. 8(3):269–86. doi: https://doi.org/10.1007/s12105-014-0527-7. PMID: 24519376.
5. El-Naggar AK. et al. (2022) WHO classification of head and neck tumors. International Agency for Research on Cancer; Lyon: Odontogenic and maxillofacial bone tumors; p. 205.
6. Kuzenko YV. et al. (2016): Pathogenesis of Warthin's tumor. Interv. Med. Appl. Sci. 8(2):41–48. doi: https://doi.org/10.1556/1646.8.2016.2.2. PMID: 28386459.
7. Chiesa F. et al. (2001). Surgical treatment of laryngeal carcinoma with subglottis involvement. Oncol Rep. 8(1):137–40. PMID: 11115585.
8. Joshi NP, et al. (2010). Unresectable basaloid squamous cell carcinoma of the trachea treated with concurrent chemoradiotherapy: a case report with review of literature. J Cancer Res.Ther. 6(3):321–3. doi: https://doi.org/10.4103/0973-1482.73341. PMID: 21119264.
9. Skliris JP. et al. (2023). A Case of Mucoepidermoid Carcinoma of the Larynx. Cureus. 15(1):e34455. doi: https://doi.org/10.7759/cureus.34455. PMID: 36874656; PMCID: PMC9980684.
10. Lam AK, Lee KT.(2022). Application of Immunohistochemistry in Papillary Thyroid Carcinoma. Methods Mol Biol. 2534:175–195. doi: https://doi.org/10.1007/978-1-0716-2505-7_13. PMID: 35670976.
11. Cancer Genome Atlas Research Network. (2014). Integrated genomic characterization of papillary thyroid carcinoma. Cell. 159(3):676–90. doi: https://doi.org/10.1016/j.cell.2014.09.050. PMID: 25417114.
12. Hunt JL. et al. (2003). A novel microdissection and genotyping of follicular-derived thyroid tumors to predict aggressiveness. Hum Pathol. 34(4):375–80. doi: https://doi.org/10.1053/hupa.2003.61. PMID: 12733119.
13. Rios A. et al. (2011). Histological and immunohistochemical profile of sporadic and familial medullary thyroid carcinoma. Endocrinología y Nutrición (English Edition). 58(10):521–528. doi: https://doi.org/10.1016/j.endoen.2011.07.005.

3 Diseases of Lungs

3.1 Introduction

The study of pathology of the lungs delves into the pathologic changes and abnormalities observed in the lungs, airways, and related structures. This branch of pathology encompasses a wide range of diseases, including congenital anomalies, infections, inflammatory disorders, neoplastic conditions, and occupational diseases, among others.

Understanding the gross and microscopic pathology of lungs is crucial for healthcare professionals, including pathologists, pulmonologists, thoracic surgeons, and radiologists, as it provides valuable insights into the underlying mechanisms and manifestations of respiratory diseases. By examining the pathologic features of diseased tissues and organs, clinicians can make accurate diagnoses, determine the severity of the condition, and plan appropriate treatment strategies.

The chapter will be organized in the following order:

1. Congenital Lung diseases:
   (a) Congenital Pulmonary bulla
2. Infectious Diseases:
   (a) Bacterial Pneumonia and Chronic Lung Abscess
   (b) Mycobacterial Disease and Tuberculosis
   (c) Parasitic Infection: Bilharziasis and Hydatid Cyst
3. Diseases of Cartilaginous and Non-Cartilaginous Airways
   (a) Bronchiectasis
   (b) Emphysema
4. Pulmonary Vascular Diseases
   (a) Pulmonary Infarction
   (b) Pulmonary Pyemic Abscesses
5. Neoplasms
   (a) Primary Malignant Tumors
      - Pulmonary Carcinomas
      - Malignant Mesothelioma
   (b) Metastatic Lung Disease

G. Dawood, *Color Atlas of Human Gross and Microscopic Pathology*, https://doi.org/10.1007/978-3-031-76007-5_3

3.2 Congenital Lung Diseases

Pulmonary Bulla (a, b)

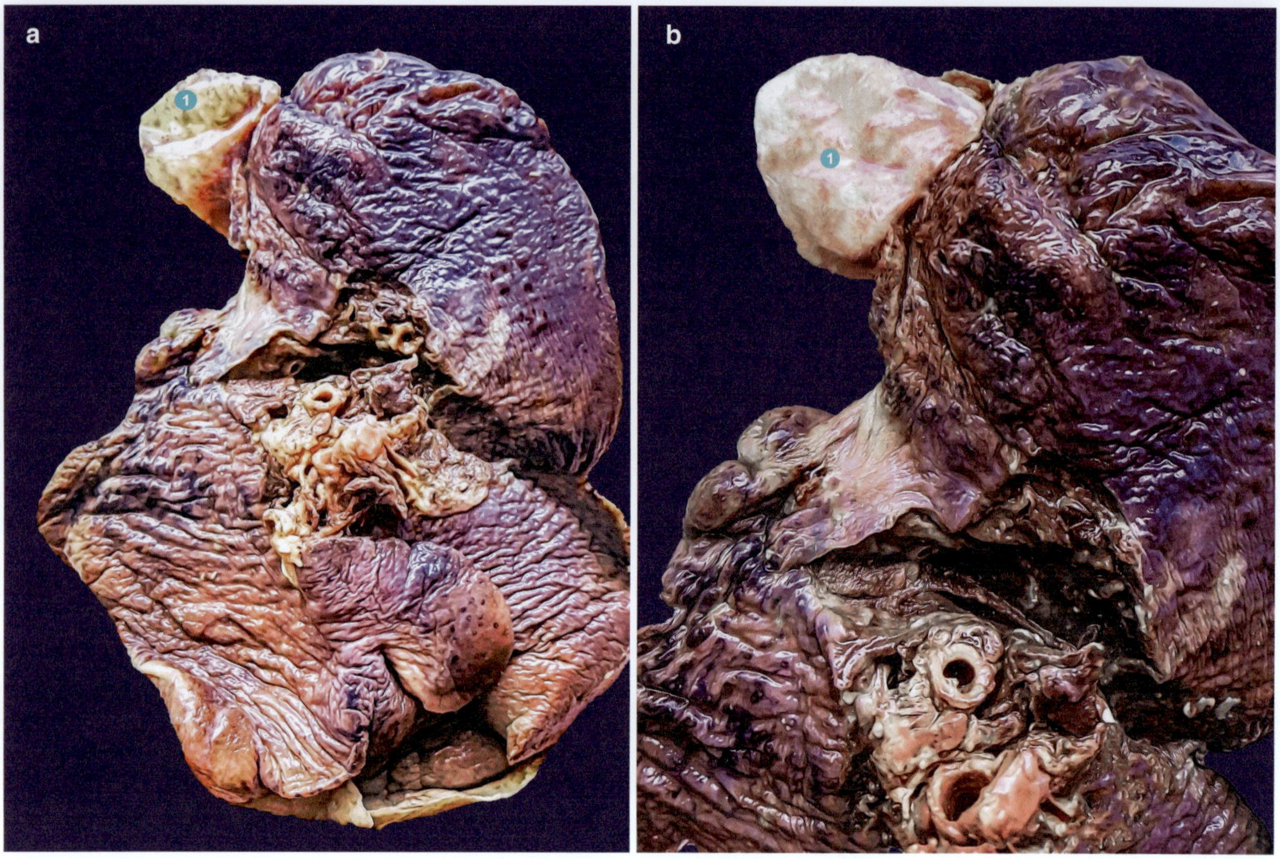

The lung is mounted.
The lung looks normal.

1. An air-filled cyst lined with a thin transparent membrane (visceral pleura) is seen at the apex.

Microscopic Picture of Pulmonary Bulla (c)

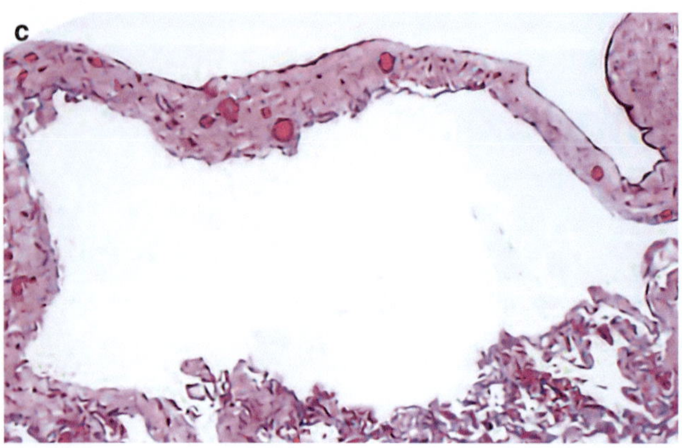

The section shows the periphery of the lung with a large dilated subpleural air space, lined by thin walls and surrounded by normal-looking air spaces. Focal fibrous pleural thickening is present. Neither inflammation nor interstitial fibrosis is seen.

Pearls

Pulmonary bulla can arise due to a variety of causes, including congenital abnormalities, underlying lung diseases, or trauma to the lung tissue [1].

3.3 Infectious Diseases

Lobar Pneumonia (Red and Gray Hepatization) (a, b)

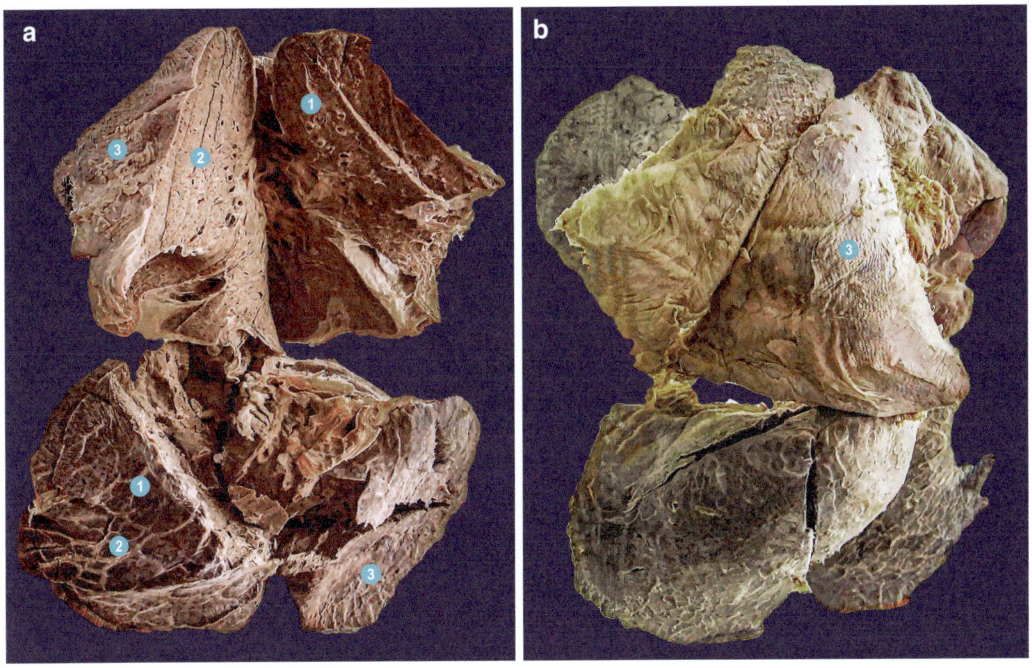

Two lungs bisected longitudinally are mounted.

1. Both are consolidated and firm.
2. The upper section is gray while the lower one is red.
3. Pleura is dull and lusterless.

Microscopic Picture of Lobar Pneumonia, Red Hepatization (c–e)

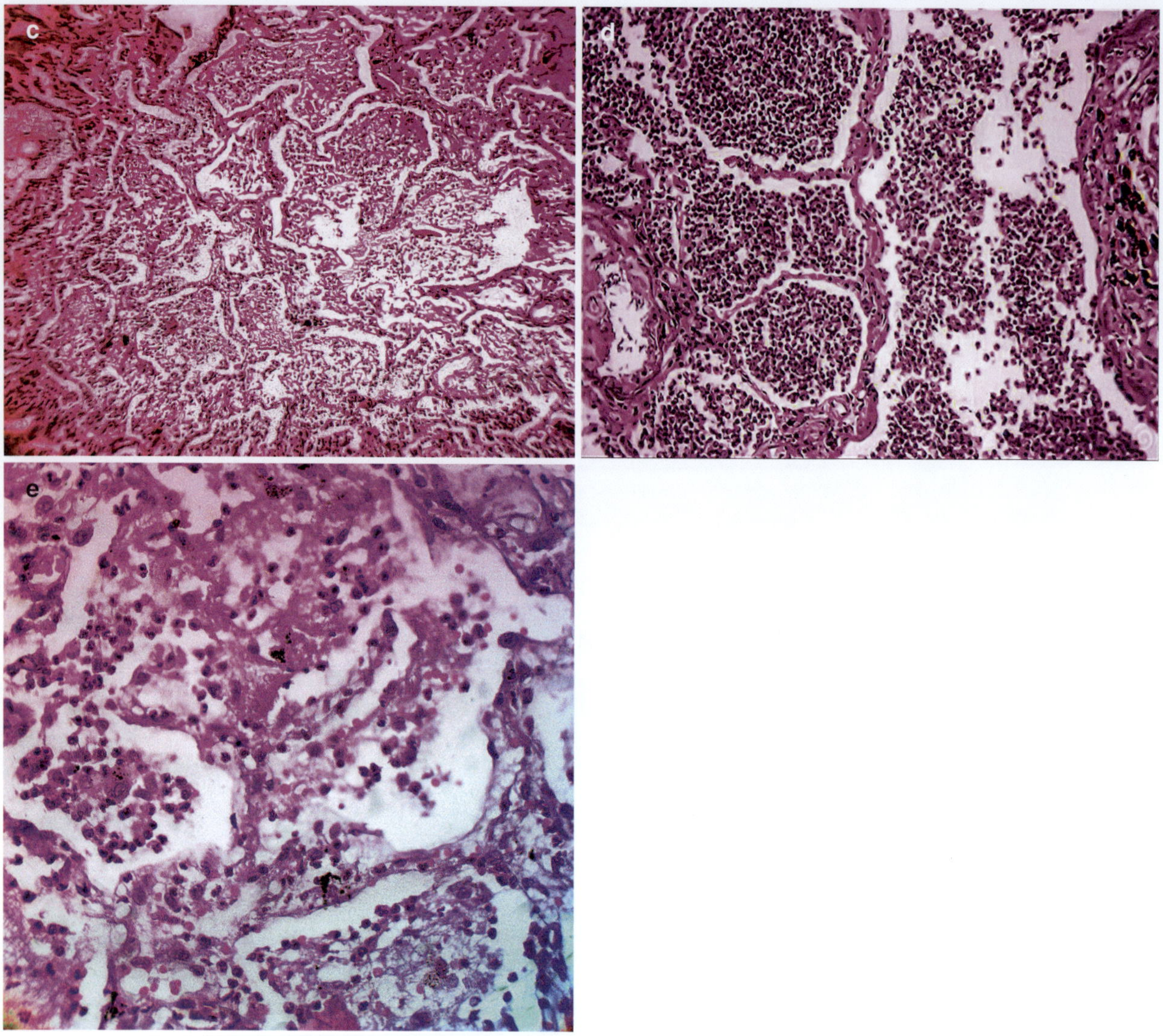

Sections show alveolar air spaces filled with an exudate formed of edema fluid and neutrophils admixed with fibrin. The exudate is so dense that it completely obliterates the air-spaces. The alveolar walls are thickened and congested.

Lobar Pneumonia (Gray Hepatization)

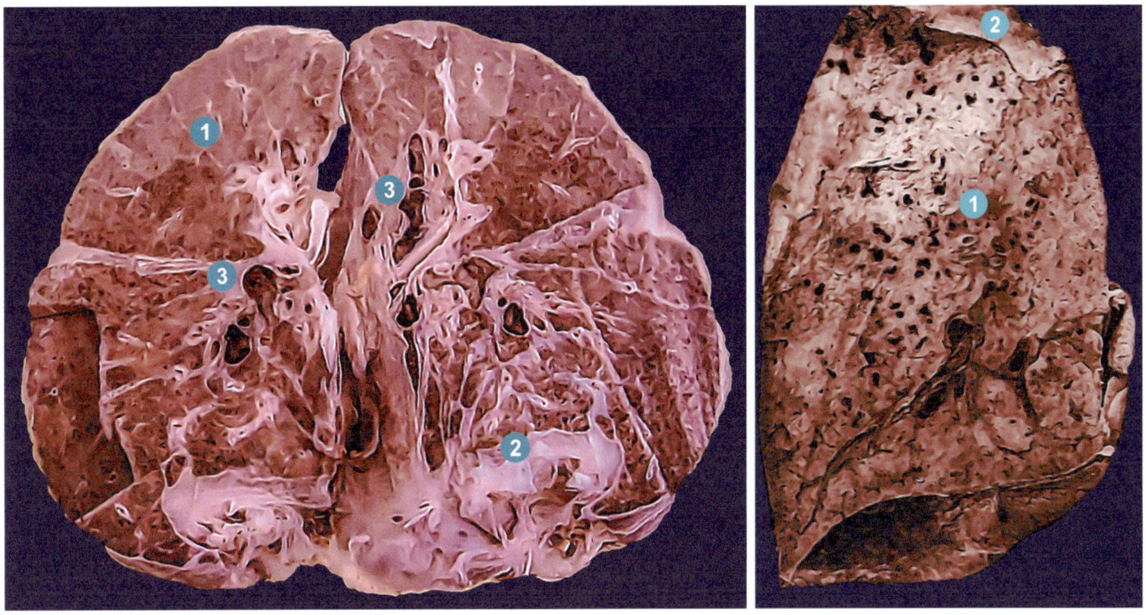

Lung bisected longitudinally is mounted.

1. The cut section is consolidated, firm, and gray-red.
2. Pleura is gray white and thickened.
3. Hilar lymph nodes are enlarged and anthracotic.

Microscopic Picture of Lobar Pneumonia, Gray Hepatization (a, b)

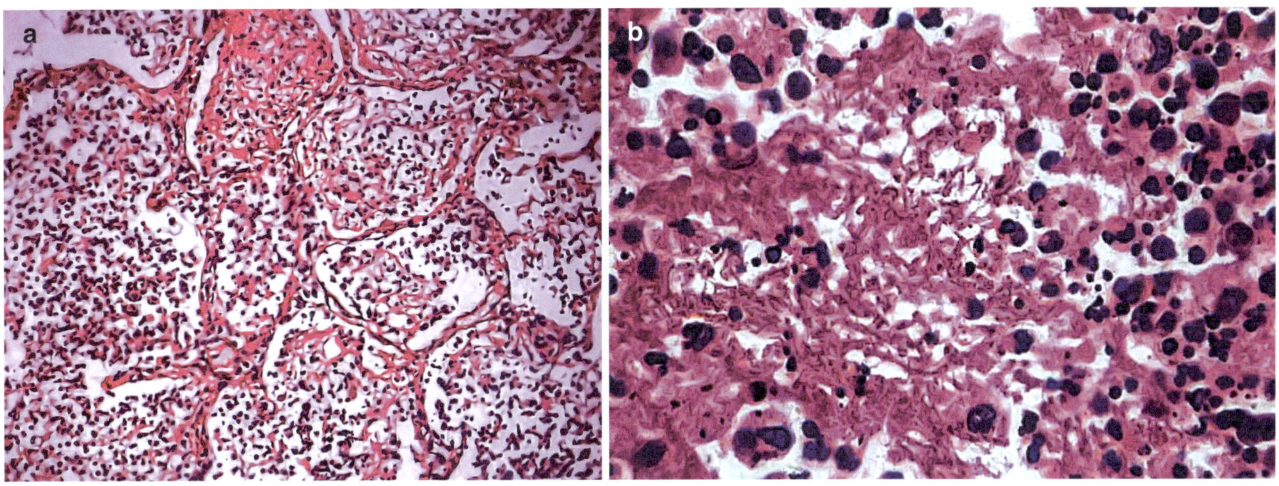

Sections show alveoli filled with exudate full of a lot of neutrophils, macrophages, fibrin, fluid exudate, and dead bacteria. The alveolar walls are thickened by edema.

Post-pneumonic Fibrosis (Organizing Pneumonia, "OP")

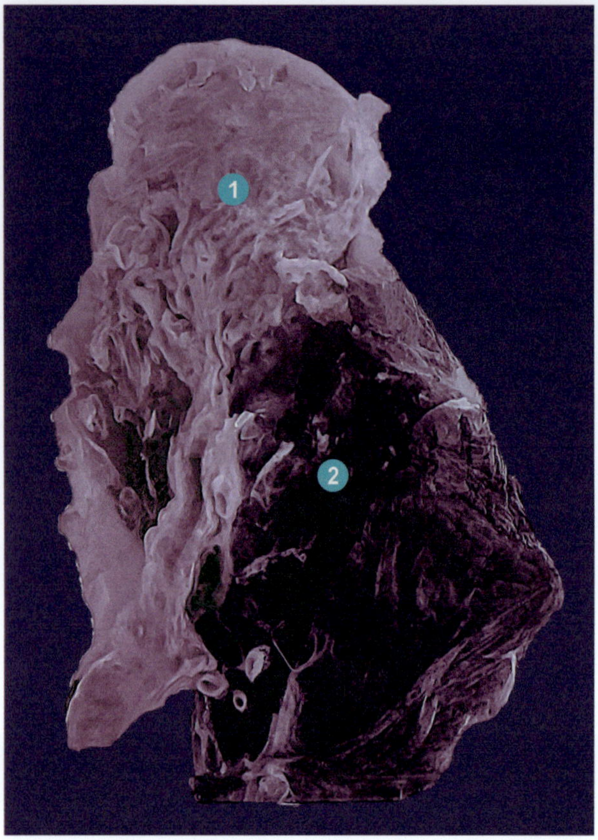

The lung is mounted.

1. The upper lobe is collapsed and turned into fibrous tissue covered with adherent dense white-gray pleura.
2. The rest of the lung is collapsed.

Microscopic Picture of Post-pneumonic Fibrosis (a, b)

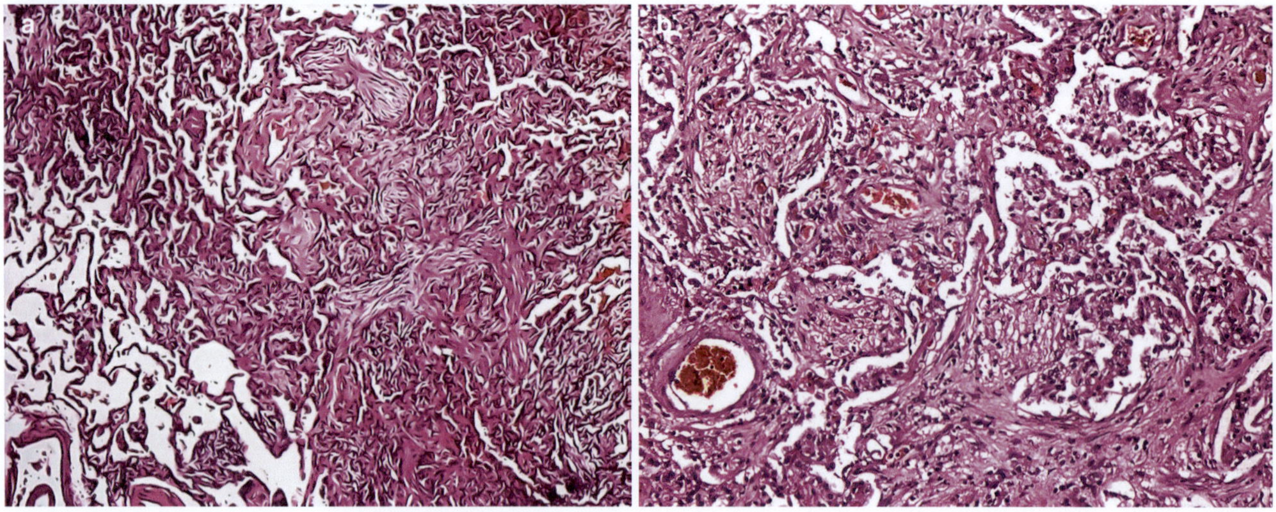

Sections show interstitial fibrosis, obliteration of alveoli by fibrous tissue, and increased lymphocytic infiltration and fibroblasts.

Bronchopneumonia

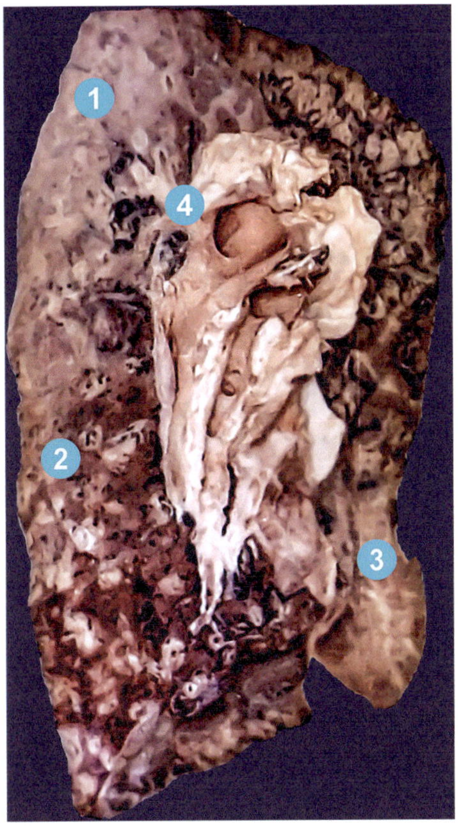

The lung is mounted.

1. The upper lobe is consolidated and yellow.
2. The lower lobe shows multiple, yellow, small foci separated by red lung tissue.
3. The lower part of the posterior border is pale and enlarged because of compensatory emphysema.
4. Hilar lymph nodes are slightly enlarged.

Microscopic Picture of Bronchopneumonia (a)

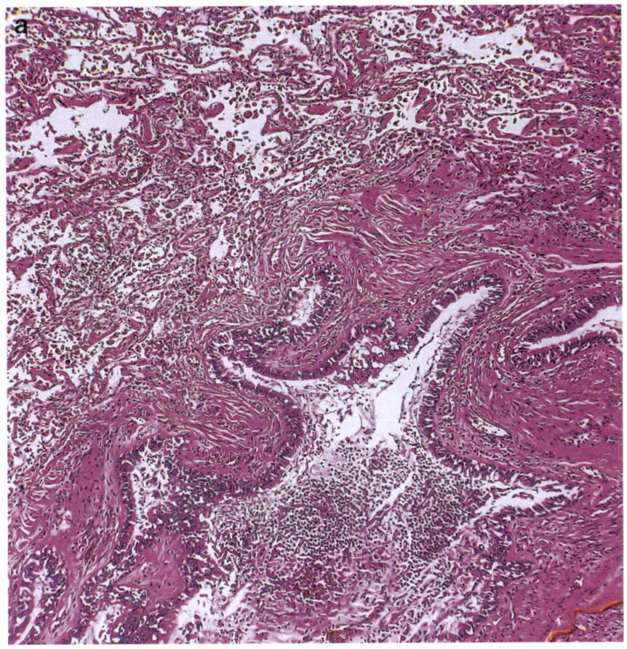

The section shows scattered areas of consolidation of the lung tissue around the bronchioles with evidence of bronchiolitis. The alveoli in these areas are filled with inflammatory cells, including neutrophils, lymphocytes, and macrophages, as well as fibrin. The walls of the alveoli are edematous, and some areas are necrotic.

Chronic Lung Abscess (a, b)

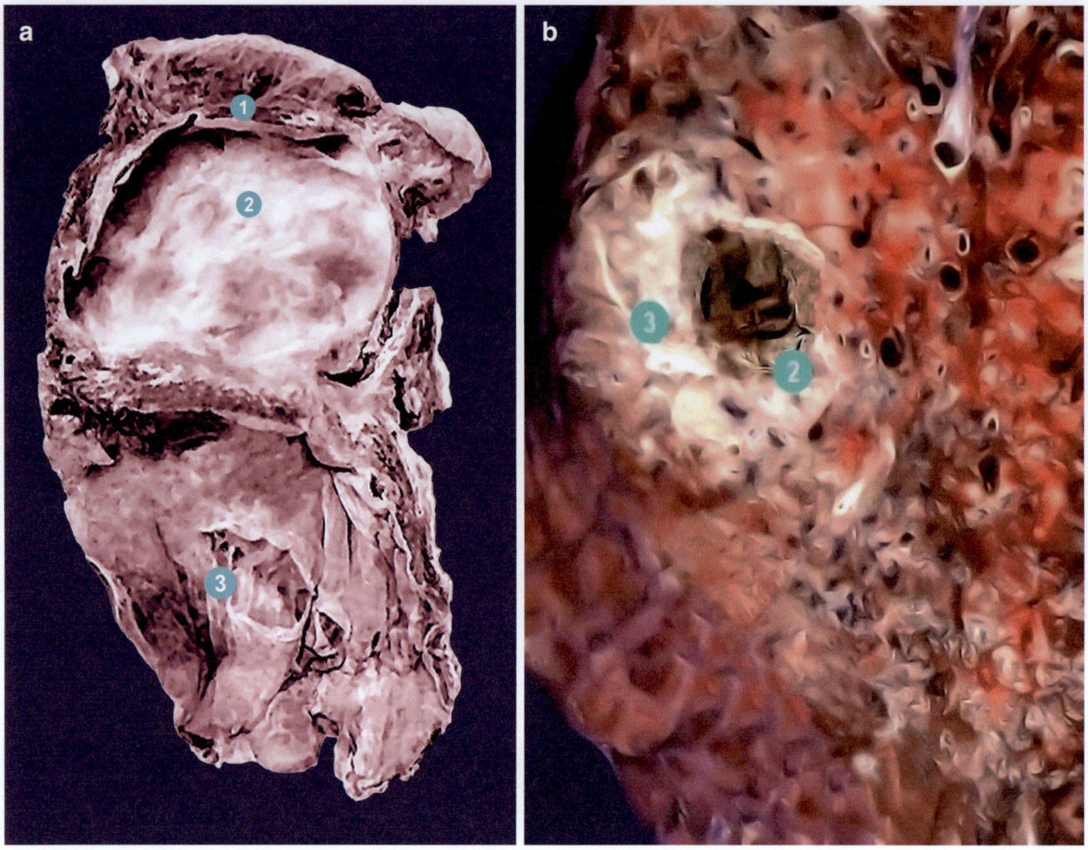

A sectioned lung is mounted.

1. The upper lobe is occupied by a cavity.
2. The cavity is lined with a well-defined, smooth, thick, and fibrous membrane.
3. The rest of the lung is atelectatic with areas of fibrosis.

Tuberculous Lymphadenitis of Tracheobronchial Lymph Nodes with Laryngitis and Tracheitis (a–c)

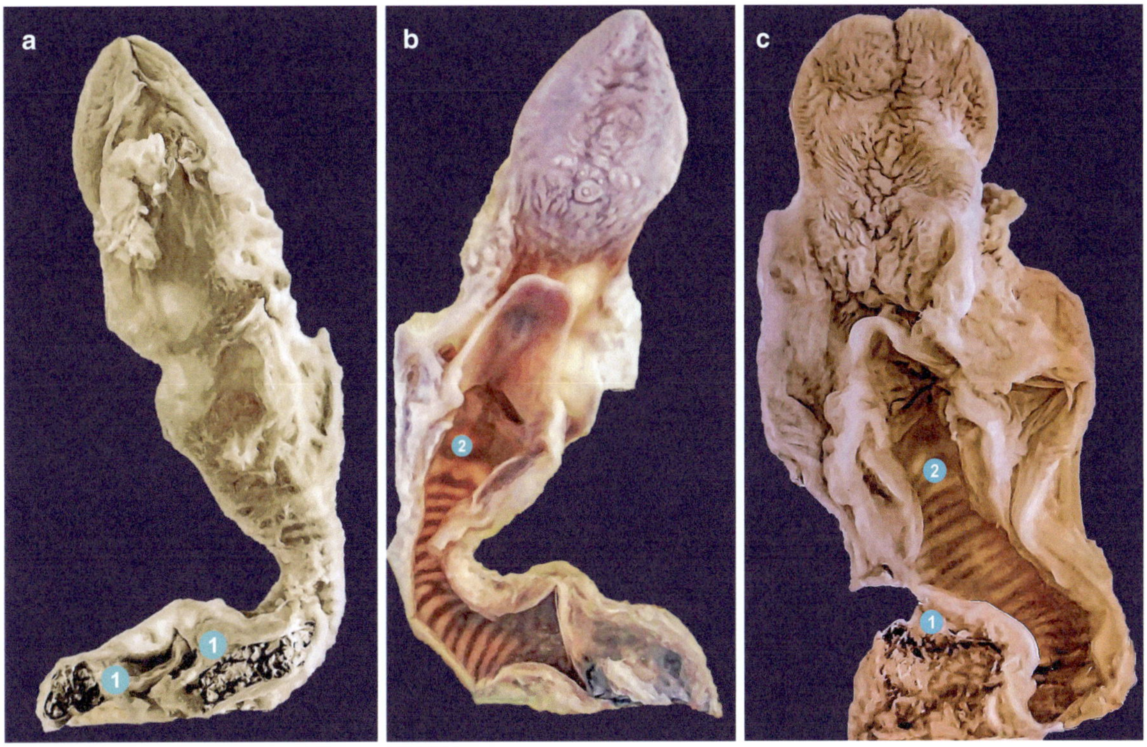

Tongue, larynx, and trachea are mounted with tracheobronchial lymph nodes.

1. The lymph nodes are enlarged, anthracotic, matted, and infiltrated with yellow foci of caseation.
2. The mucosa of the larynx and trachea is congested.

Primary Pulmonary Tuberculous Complex (a–c)

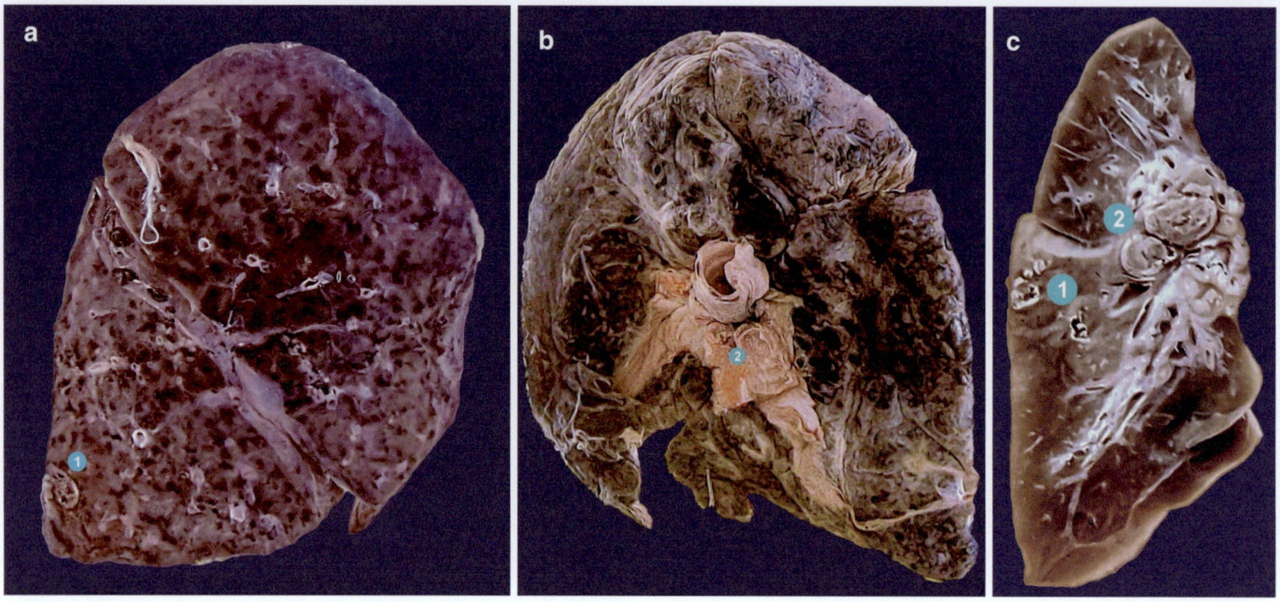

The lung is mounted.

1. The lung shows Ghon's focus: a round, well-circumscribed, subpleural, yellow area in the lower peripheral part of the inferior lobe.
2. The hilar lymph nodes are enlarged with a yellow caseating cut section.

Microscopic Picture of Tuberculous Lymphadenitis (d, e)

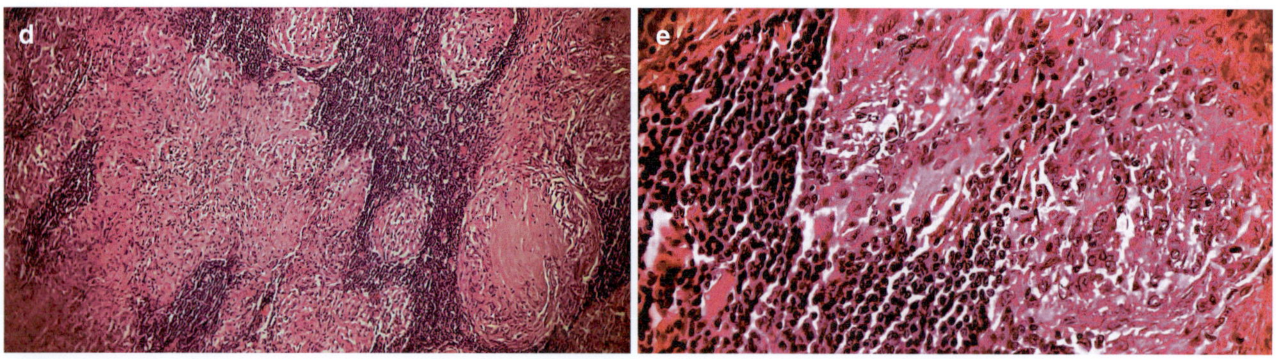

Sections show multiple tuberculoid granulomas in the lymph node. They are formed of epithelioid cells, histiocytes, Langhans giant cells, and lymphocytes with areas of caseation necrosis.

Chronic Fibrocaseous Pulmonary Tuberculosis (a, b)

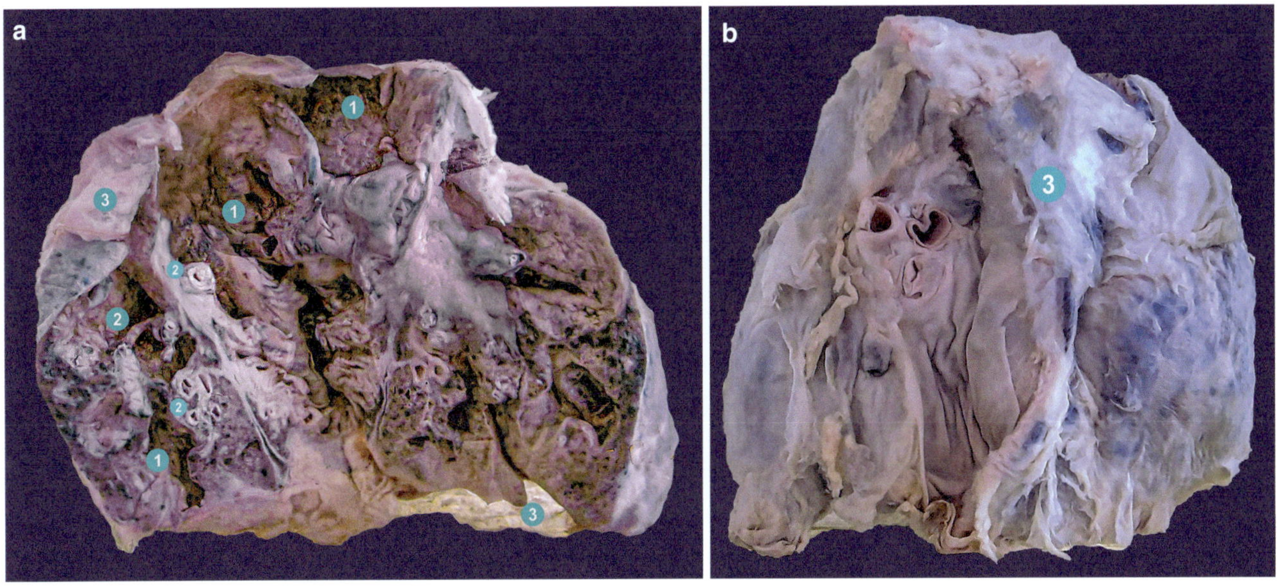

Lung bisected longitudinally is mounted.

1. The cut section shows multiple irregular cavities lined with smooth yellow fibrous tissue. The rest of the lung tissue shows atelectasis and yellow discoloration.
2. The cavities are traversed with fibrous cords representing obliterated and fibrosed blood vessels and bronchioles.
3. The pleura is thick, fibrous, and yellow.

Chronic Fibrocaseous Pulmonary Tuberculosis (a–c)

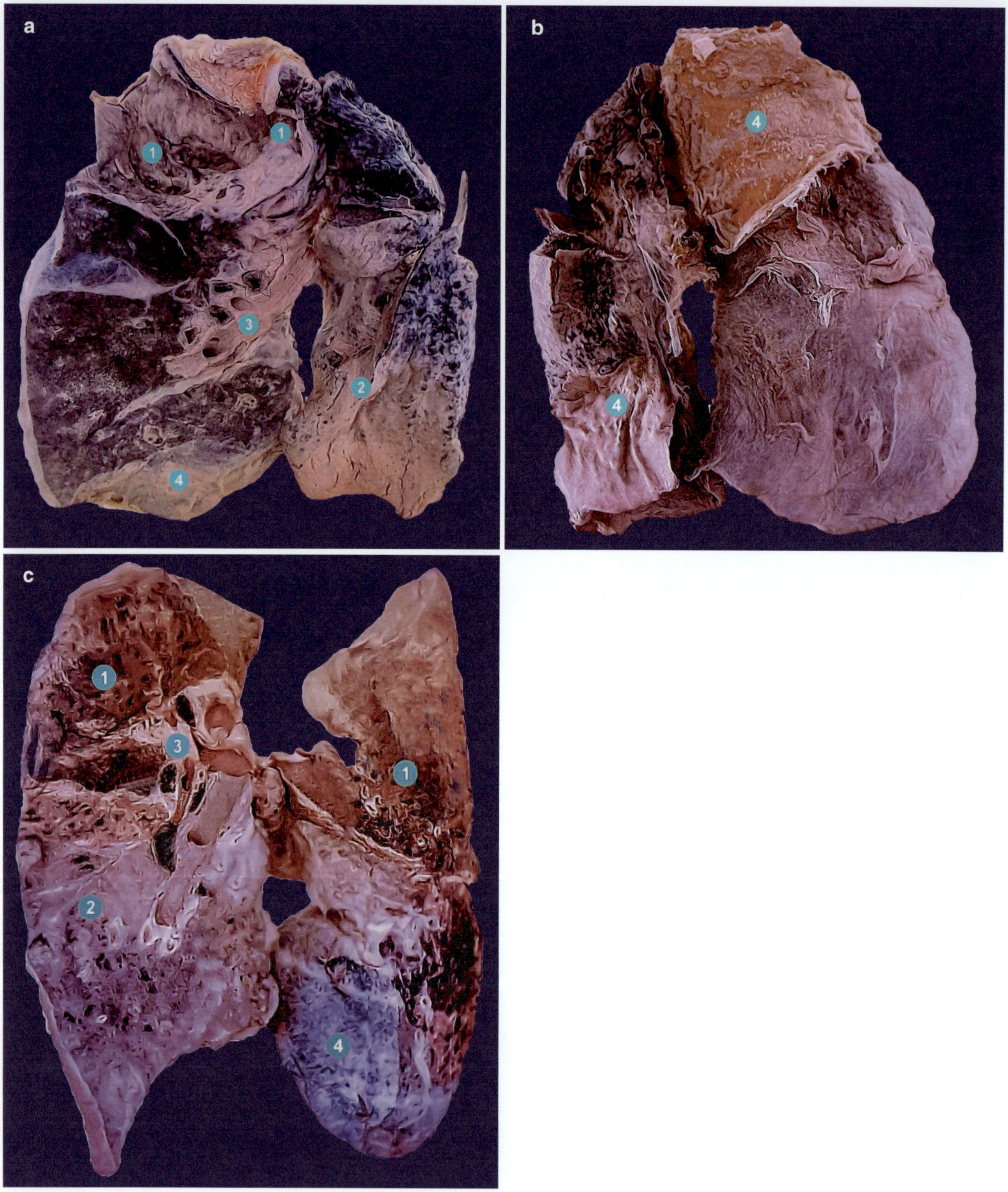

Two lungs are mounted.

1. The larger lung shows an apical, round, and large cavity lined with smooth yellow fibrous tissue and traversed with fibrous cords representing obliterated and fibrosed blood vessels and bronchioles.
2. The smaller lung shows fibrous yellow pleura and atelectasis.
3. Hilar lymph nodes are not enlarged but have a yellow caseating cut section.
4. The pleura is thick, fibrous, and yellow.

Miliary Tuberculosis (a, b)

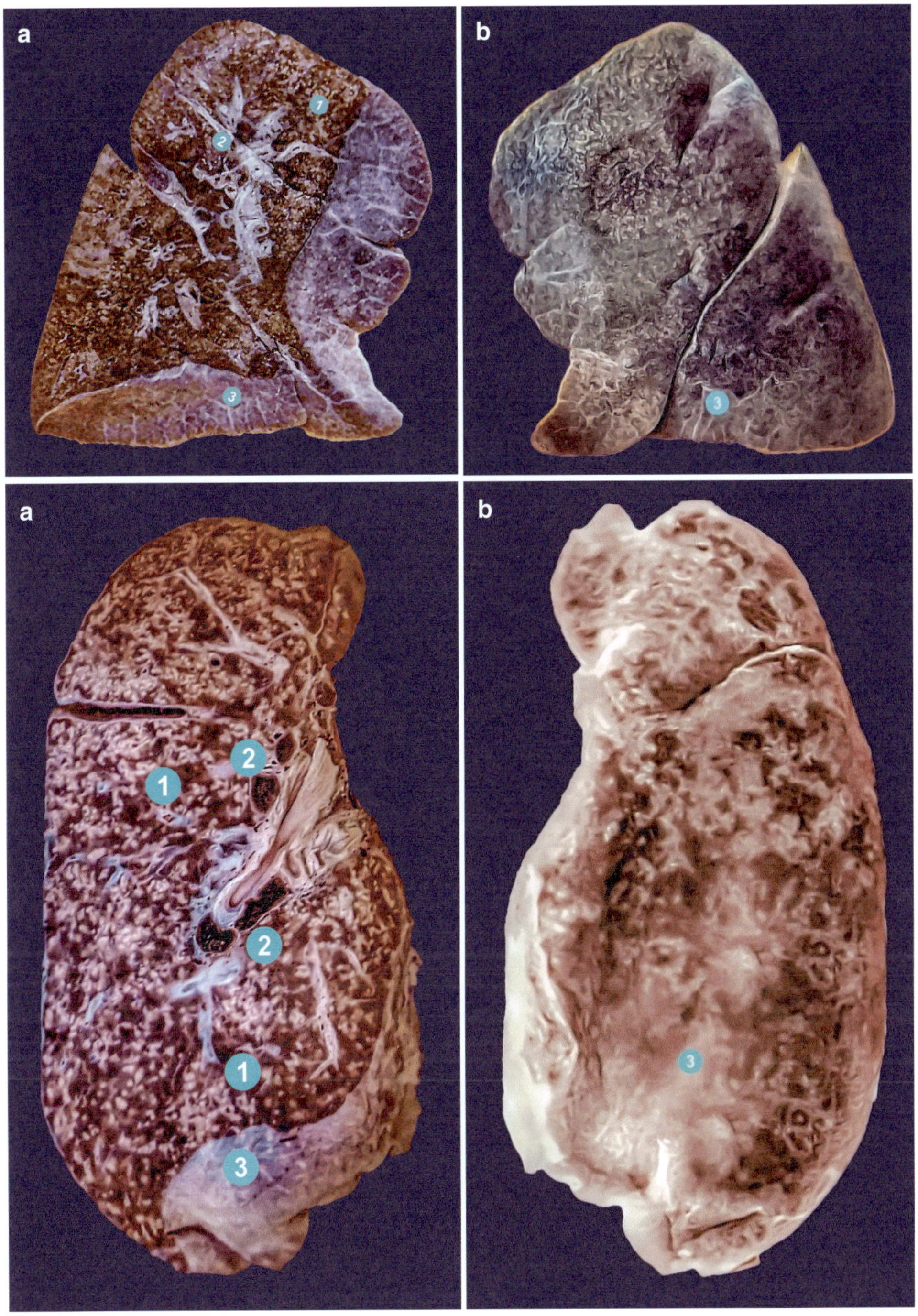

Normal-sized lung is mounted.

1. The lung is firm, red, and studded with multiple, small, yellow, subpleural nodules distributed uniformly, giving a mottled appearance. These nodules are typically 1–2 mm in diameter.
2. Tracheobronchial lymph nodes are large and anthracotic with focal caseation necrosis.
3. The pleura is thick, fibrous, and yellow.

Microscopic Picture of Miliary Tuberculosis (c–e)

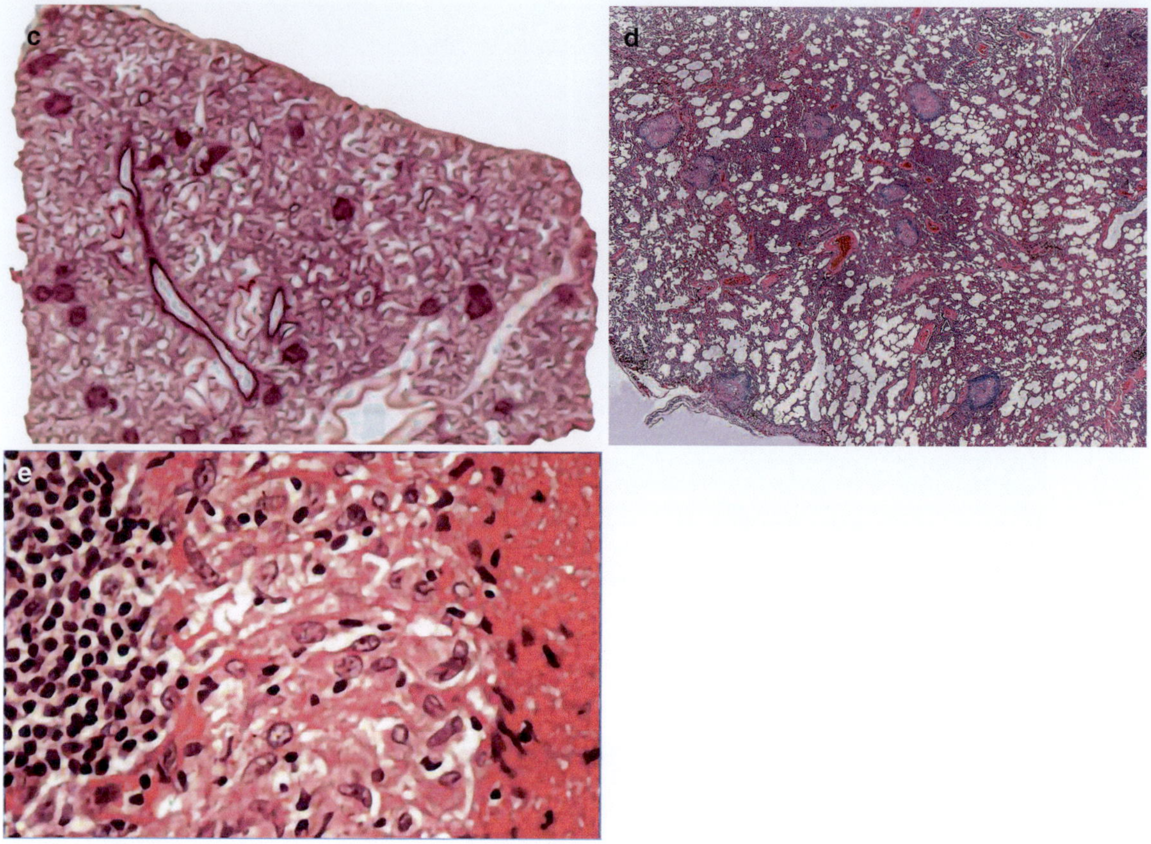

Sections show multiple scattered epithelioid granulomas (tuberculomas) formed of epithelioid cells, lymphocytes, and scattered Langhan's giant cells with the presence of caseous necrosis.

Miliary Tuberculosis

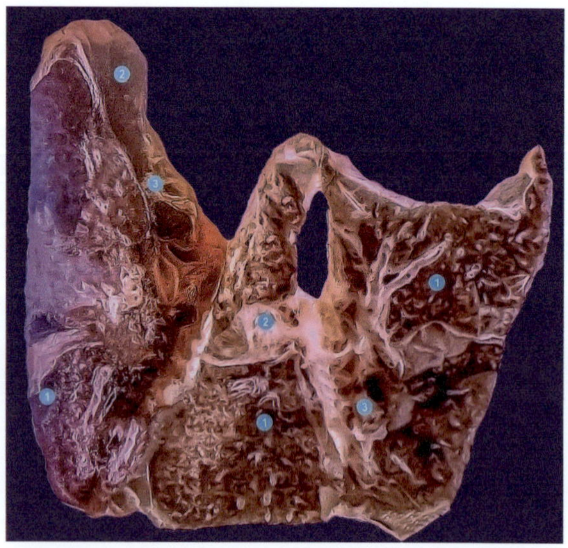

Three slices of lung tissue are mounted.

1. The lung is firm, red, and studded with multiple, small, yellow, subpleural nodules.
2. The pleura is thick fibrous and yellow.
3. Tracheobronchial lymph nodes are large and anthracotic with focal caseation necrosis.

Tuberculous Pneumonia with Early Cavitation

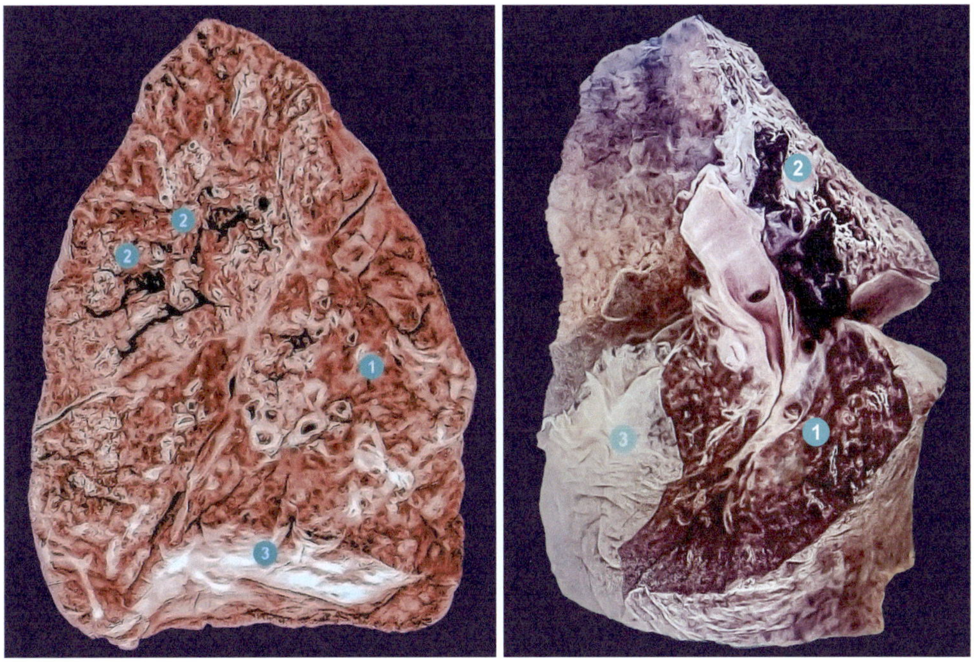

Lung bisected longitudinally is mounted.

1. The lung is consolidated and has sharp edges, a gray-yellow color (favoring the tuberculous nature of the lesion), with basal pink discoloration.
2. The upper lobe shows two small cavities with irregular walls.
3. Pleura is thick and fibrous.

Miliary Tuberculosis, Tuberculous Pneumonia with Early Cavitation

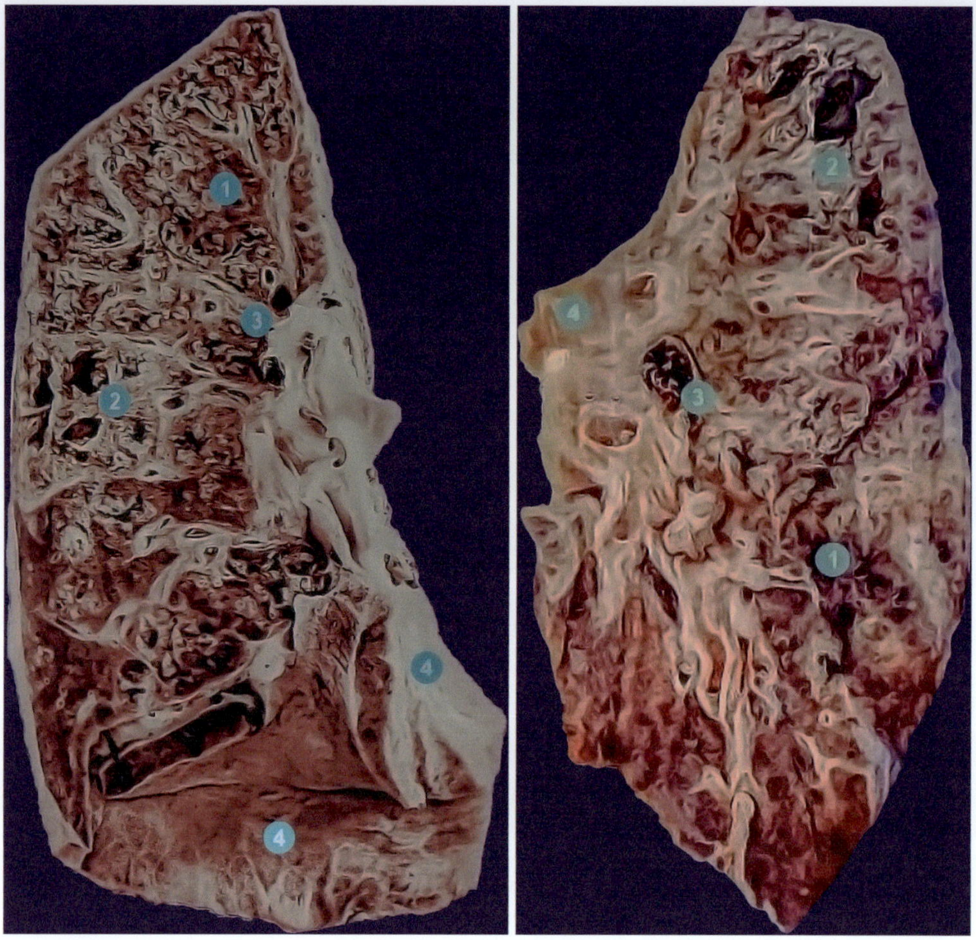

Lung bisected longitudinally is mounted.

1. The lung is firm, red, and studded with multiple, small, yellow, subpleural nodules.
2. The cut section of the upper lobe shows multiple irregular cavities with ragged walls.
3. Tracheobronchial lymph nodes are large and anthracotic with focal caseation necrosis.
4. The pleura is thick, fibrous, and yellow.

Miliary Tuberculosis, Tuberculous Pneumonia with Early and Chronic Cavitation

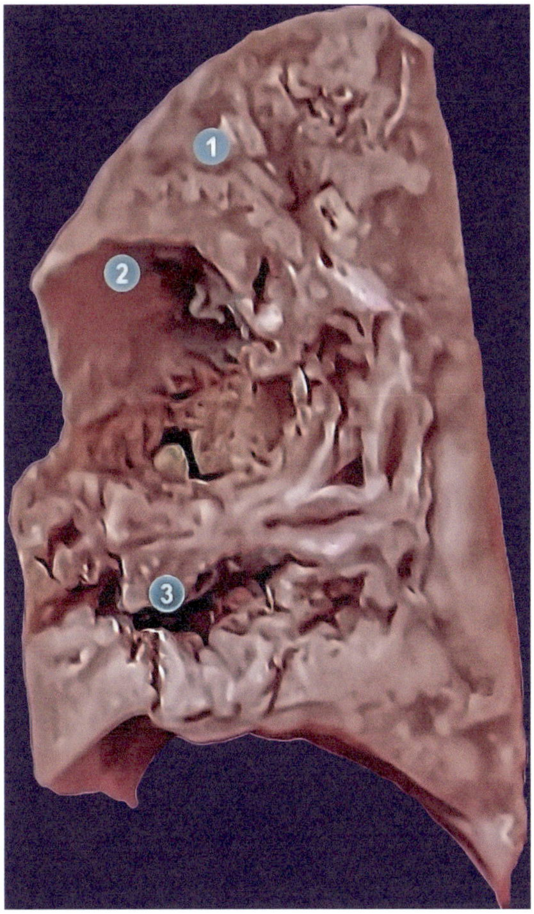

A lung is mounted.

1. The lung is firm, yellow-red, and studded with multiple, yellow, subpleural nodules.
2. A large cavity occupying most of the middle lobe of the lung is seen with a smooth inner lining. It is traversed by fibrosed cords, representing fibrosed bronchi and blood vessels.
3. Another smaller recent cavity is seen near the base of the lung with irregular walls.

Bilharziasis of the Lung

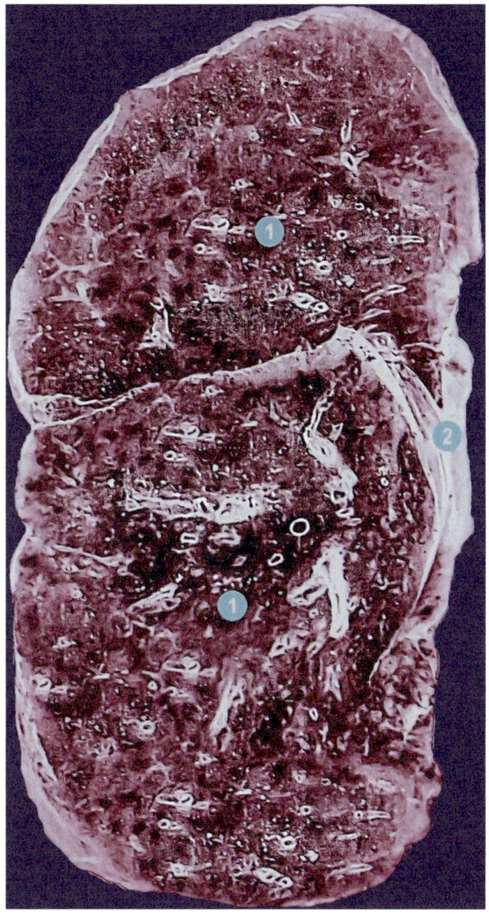

The lung is mounted.

1. The cut section shows multiple, small, pinhead-size, white lesions scattered all over the cut section. They don't show caseation.
2. Pleura is thickened.

Microscopic Picture of Pulmonary Bilharziasis (a)

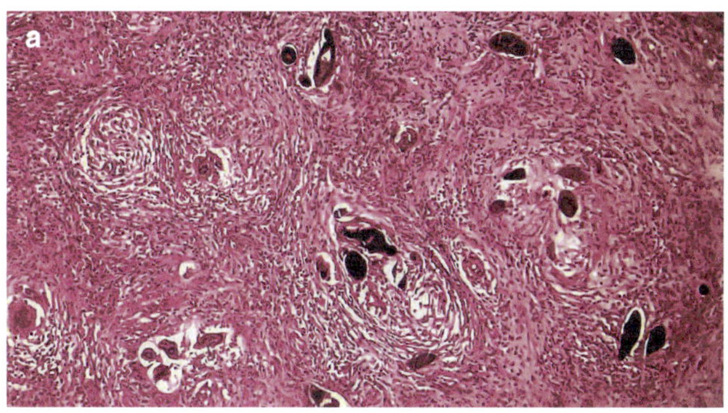

The section shows multiple calcified bilharzial ova surrounded by chronic inflammatory cells with areas of fibrosis.

Bilharzial Ayerza and Pulmonary Artery Aneurysm (a, b)

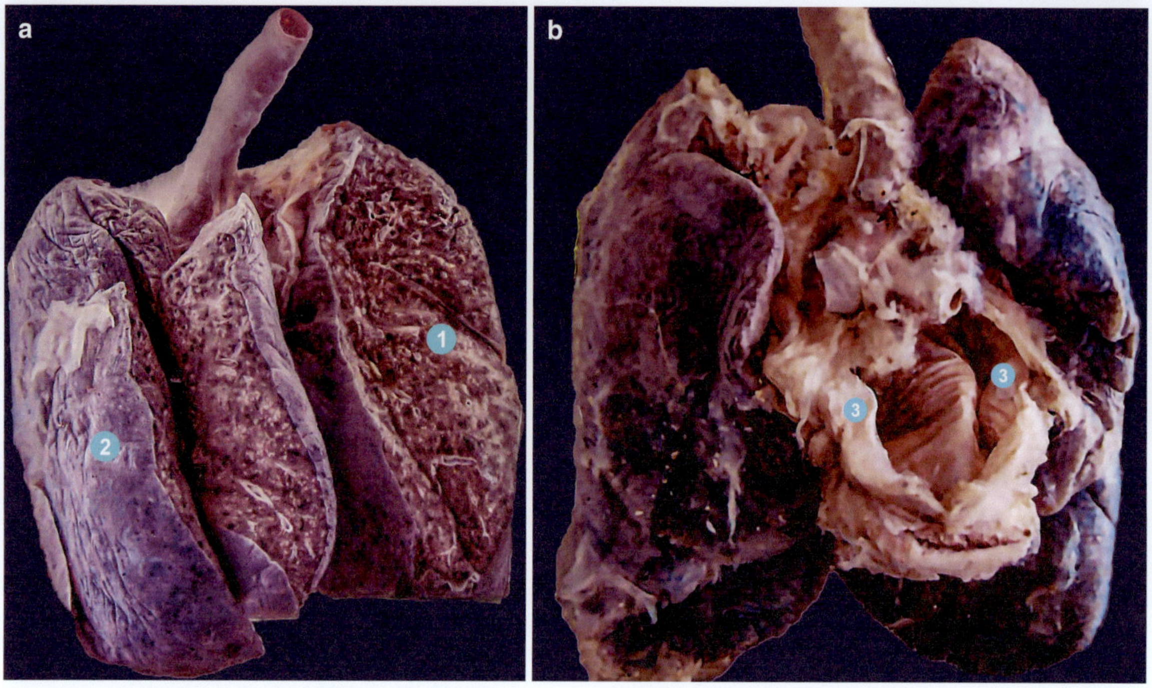

Lung is sliced into three slices with the trachea mounted.

1. The cut section is studded with multiple, small, white foci (bilharzial granulomas) (they are better felt than seen).
2. Pleura is thick and gray-white.
3. The pulmonary artery shows saccular dilatation and an atherosclerotic patch.v

Pulmonary Hydatid Cyst

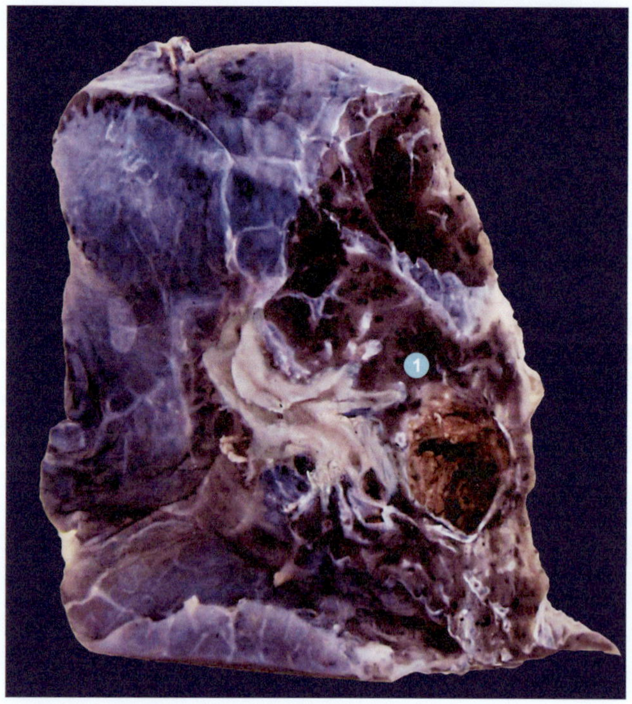

The lung is mounted.

1. A cystic, round cavity is seen occupying the lower lobe of the lung. The cavity is lined with a white membrane and surrounded by fibrous tissue.

Microscopic Picture of Pulmonary Hydatid Cyst (a)

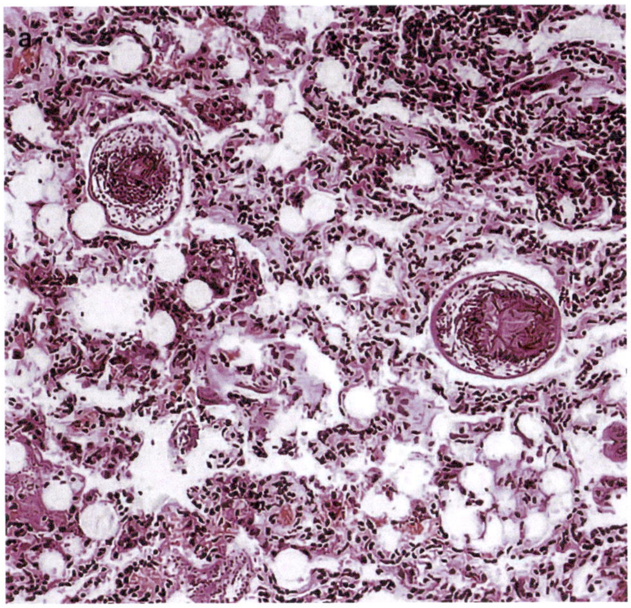

The section shows two scolices of *E. granulosus* seen among lung tissue with focal infiltration of lung parenchyma by chronic inflammatory cells.

3.4 Diseases of Cartilaginous and Non-cartilaginous Airways

Pediatric Bronchiectasis

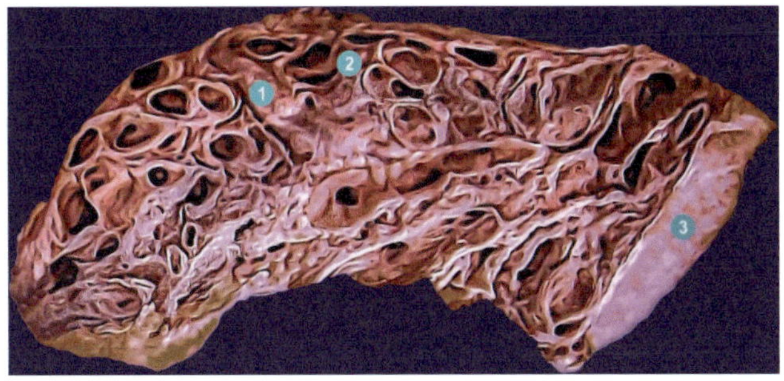

The lung of a child bisected longitudinally is mounted.

1. The lung is consolidated with a red-brown cut section.
2. Irregularly dilated bronchi lined with dirty yellow mucosa are seen.
3. Pleura is thick and gray-white.

Pearls

Bronchiectasis may result from multiple etiologies, including most commonly infection, congenital or genetic disorders, or idiopathic. A systematic review (12 studies involving 989 children) found that 63% had an underlying cause. Previous pneumonia (19%), primary immunodeficiency (17%), recurrent aspiration, including an inhaled foreign body (10%), and primary ciliary dyskinesia (7%) were implicated most commonly. It has been estimated that approximately 30% of cases of bronchiectasis are idiopathic [2].

Bronchiectasis

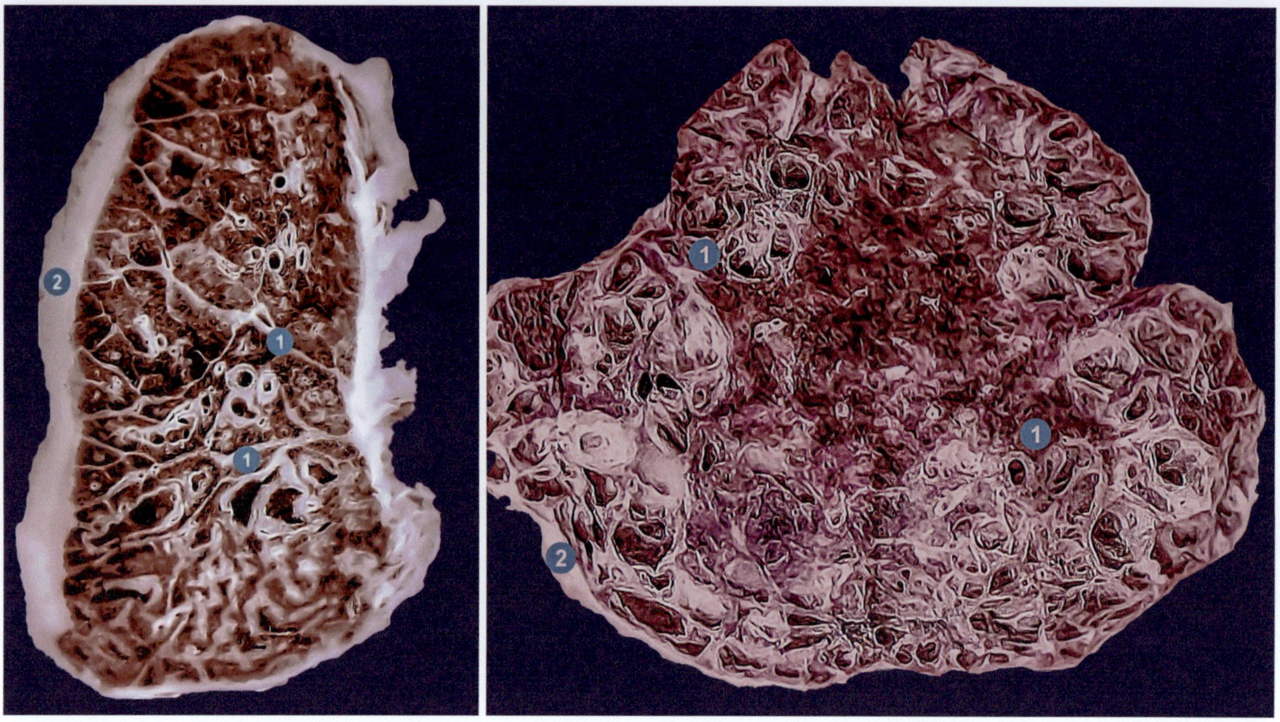

A slice of lung tissue is mounted.

1. The cut section is consolidated, firm, red-brown, and with irregular cystically dilated bronchi lined with a dirty yellow membrane.
2. Pleura is thick and gray-white.

Microscopic Picture of Bronchiectasis (a)

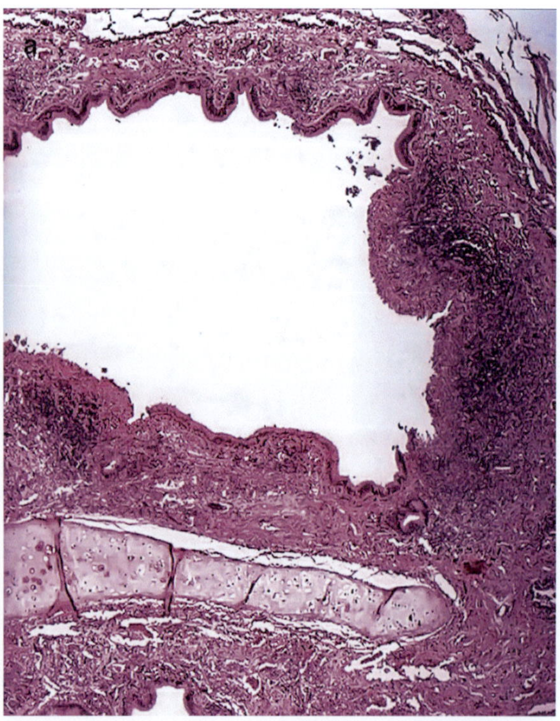

The section shows cystic dilatation and distortion of a bronchus, which is the most characteristic feature of bronchiectasis. Bronchial walls are thickened with inflammation of the bronchial mucosa and ulceration of the bronchial epithelium. The bronchial wall is infiltrated by inflammatory cells, including neutrophils, lymphocytes, which may be dense to form lymphoid follicles, and plasma cells. Granulation tissue formation and fibrosis are seen in the bronchial wall.

Emphysema with Atherosclerosis and Aneurysm of Pulmonary Artery (a, b)

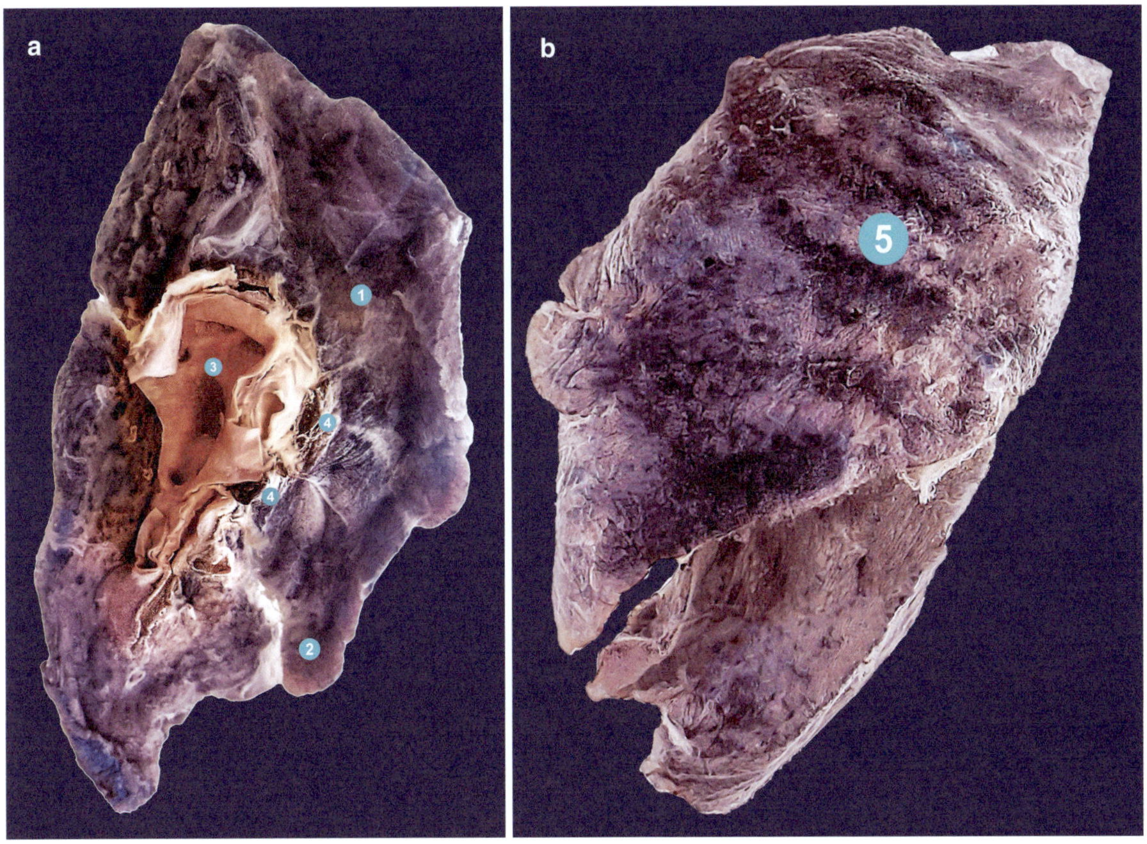

The lung is mounted.

1. The lung is voluminous and pale gray.
2. The anterior margin shows semitranslucent bulla.
3. The pulmonary artery is dilated and shows atherosclerotic plaques in the intima.
4. Tracheobronchial lymph nodes are large and anthracotic. Gray-white pleural adhesions are present.
5. Black stripes represent carbon particles deposited in septa.

Microscopic Picture of Emphysema (c, d)

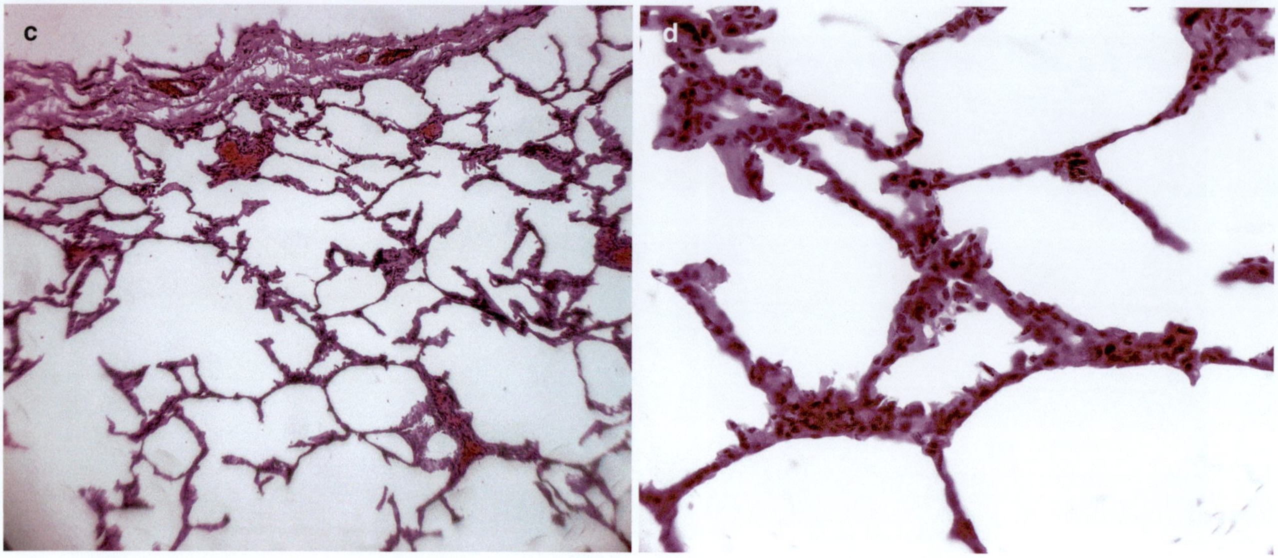

Sections show the destruction of alveolar walls with the formation of large air spaces. The remains of alveolar walls are seen as "spurs." Alveolar septa are thickened and fibrosed.

3.5 Pulmonary Vascular Diseases

Pulmonary Pyemic Abscesses (a, b)

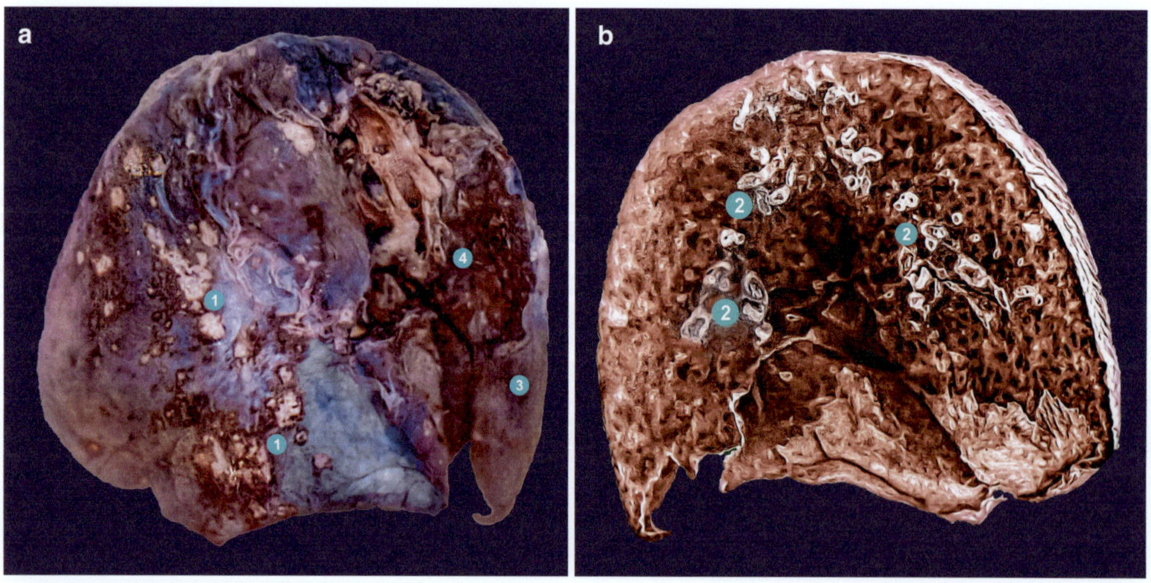

Lung bisected longitudinally is mounted.

1. The outer surface shows multiple small, yellow, depressed, subpleural pyemic abscesses surrounded by zones of congestion.
2. Small branches of the pulmonary artery are occluded with septic emboli.
3. The overlying pleura is thick and shows areas of congestion.
4. The lung is congested.

Pulmonary Infarction (a, b)

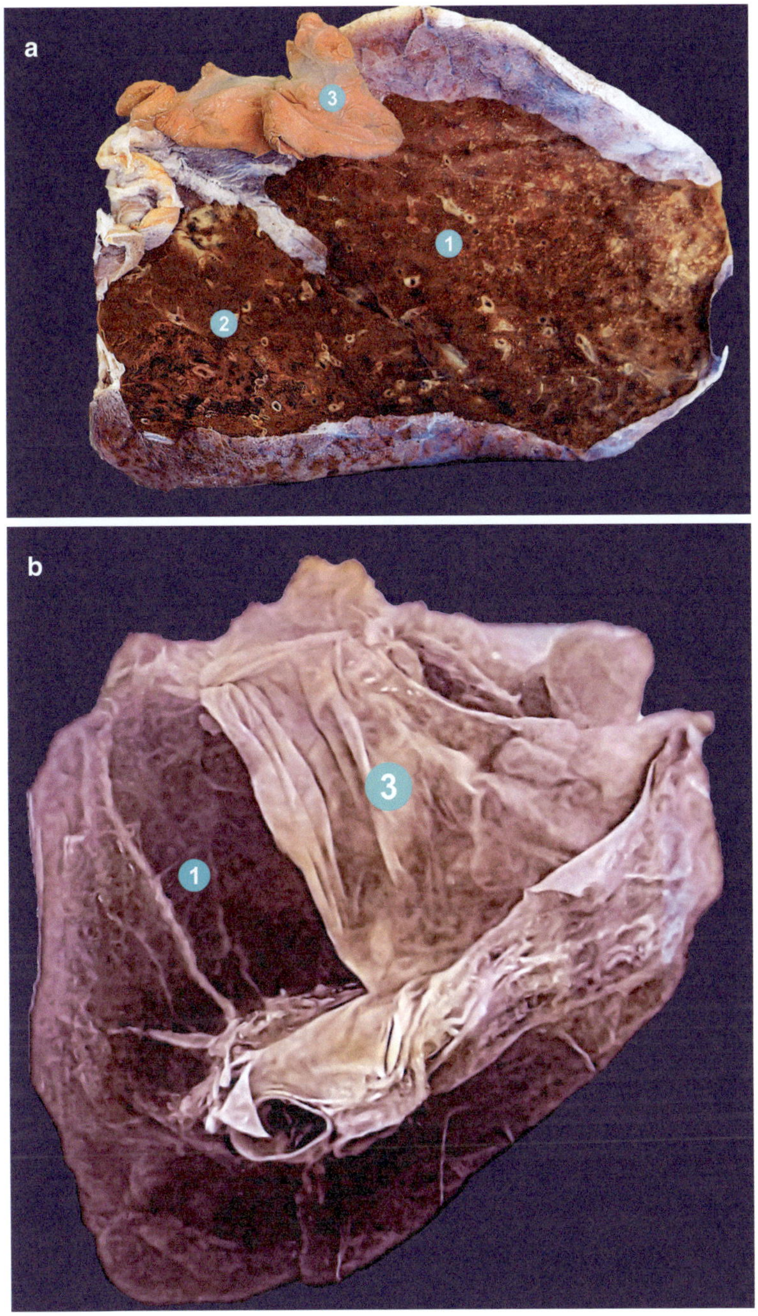

Lung bisected longitudinally is mounted.

1. The lung is red-brown, consolidated, and firm.
2. The cut section shows a darker triangular area with its base directed towards the surface.
3. Thickening of overlying pleura.

Microscopic Picture of Pulmonary Infarction (c–f)

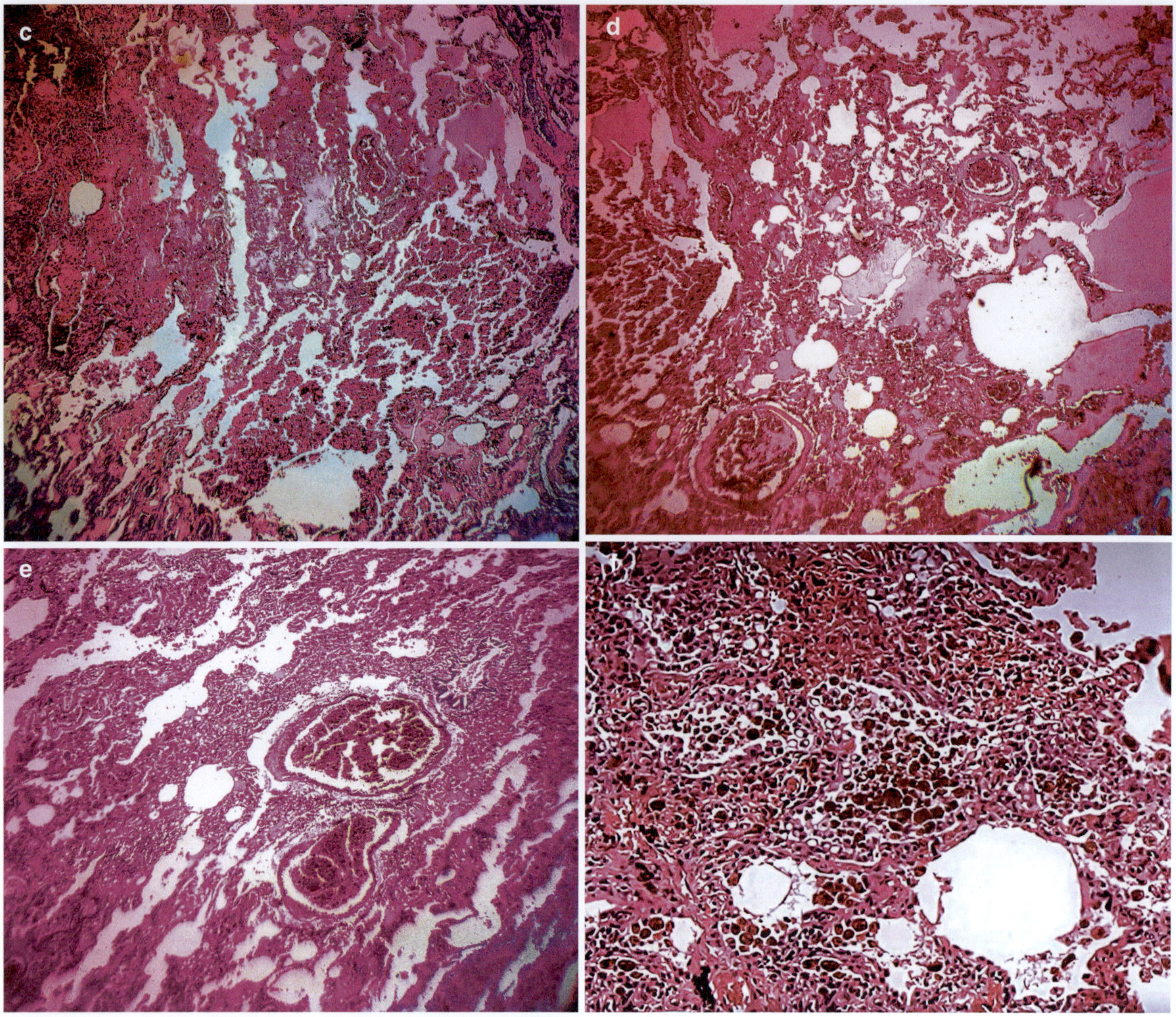

Sections show hemorrhagic necrosis in the lung parenchyma with the presence of thrombosed vessels and infiltration by inflammatory cells. The rest of the lung tissue shows evidence of chronic venous congestion. CVC of the lung is seen in the form of vascular congestion, alveolar congestion and edema, thickened alveolar septa, and the presence of siderophages (heart failure cells).

Pearls

During several prospective and retrospective studies, researchers have investigated the prevalence of pulmonary infarction (PI) in association with pulmonary embolism (PE), which is the most common etiology for the development of pulmonary infarction. The reported incidence of PI in the setting of PE is around 30%. Other disease states that can lead to pulmonary infarction include infection, malignancy, surgical iatrogenesis, amyloidosis, sickle cell disease, and vasculitis, among others. The early literature suggested that patients with underlying cardiac disease are at the greatest risk for developing a pulmonary infarction, as the hypothesis was thought to be due to poor collateral circulation, which in combination with pulmonary thromboembolism resulted in infarction. However, recent literature suggests the opposite is true. Specifically, younger patients without cardiopulmonary disease were found to be more likely to suffer a PI secondary to a PE. Experts hypothesized that longstanding local tissue hypoxia from chronic cardiopulmonary disease states led to the development of more robust bronchial vascular collateralization, which protected parenchyma from infarction [3].

3.6 Neoplasms

3.6.1 Primary Malignant Tumors

Bronchogenic Carcinoma (Central Type) (a, b)

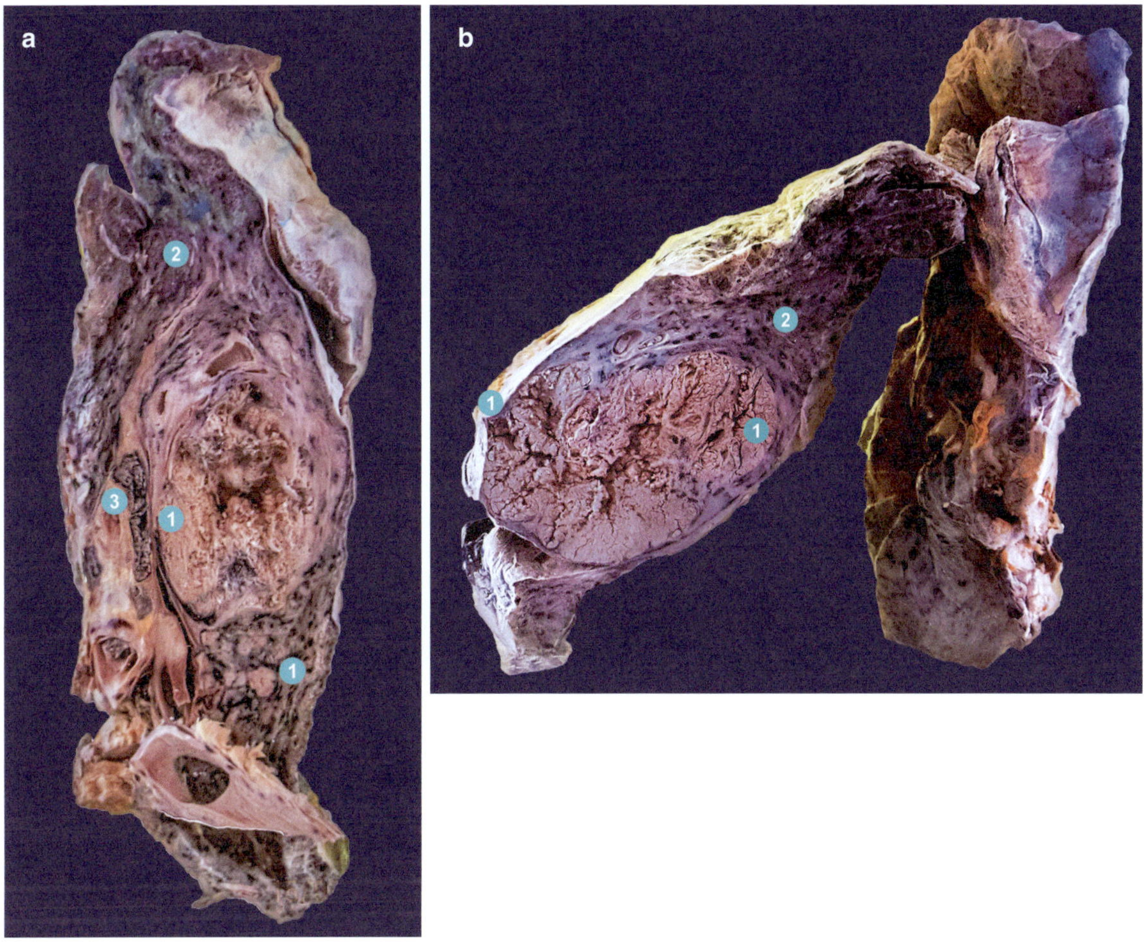

Lung bisected longitudinally is mounted.

1. The main bronchus is infiltrated and destroyed by irregular, white, necrotic tumor tissue, which also infiltrates the surrounding lung tissues and pleura.
2. The rest of the lung shows atelectasis.
3. The hilar lymph nodes are enlarged and infiltrated by tumor tissue.

Microscopic Picture of Bronchogenic Carcinoma (Small Cell Lung Carcinoma, SCLC) (c–k)

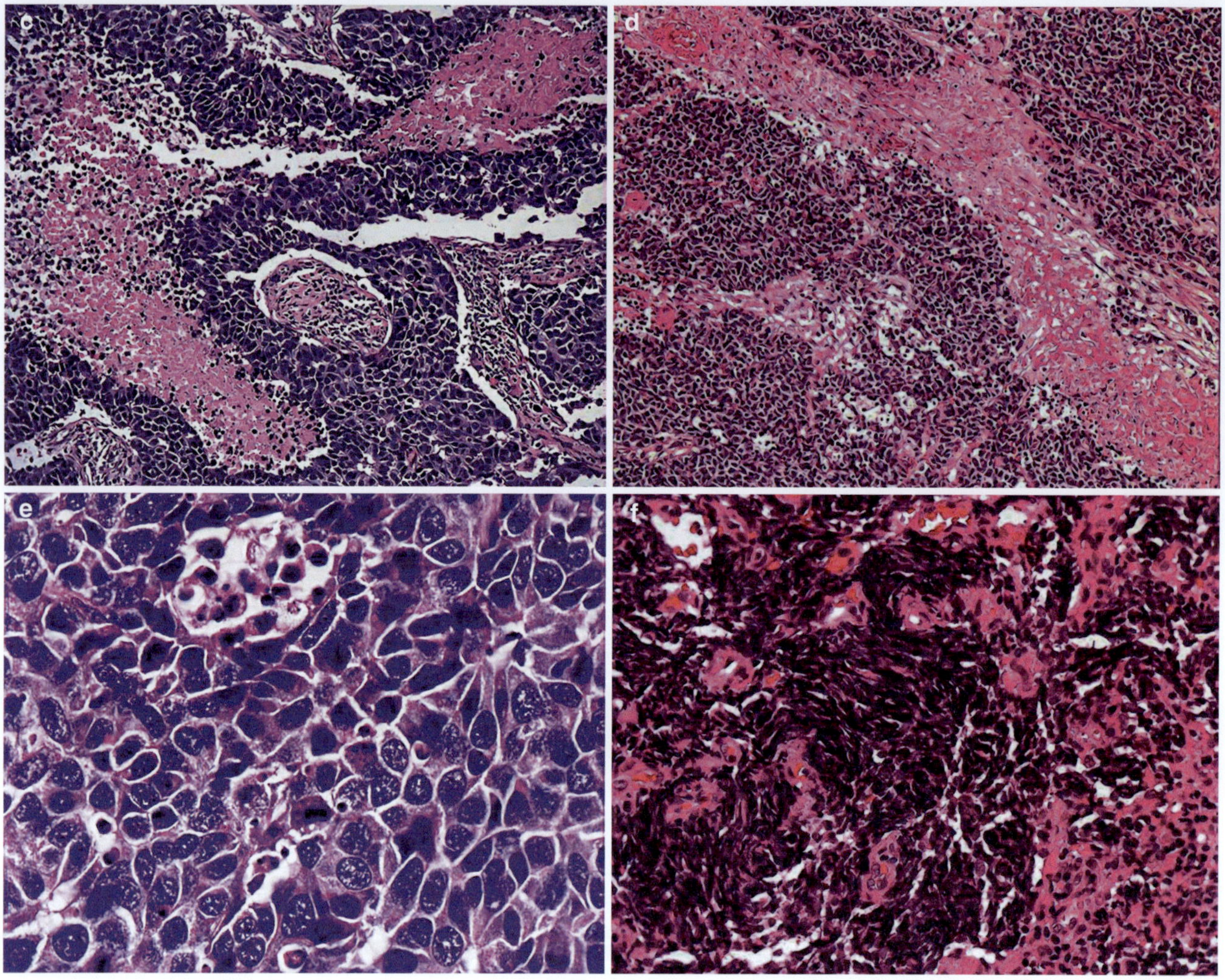

Sections show infiltration of pulmonary tissue by small, oval, rounded, and fusiform cells with scarce cytoplasm, large nuclei having irregular borders, fine granular chromatin, and inconspicuous nucleoli. The cells generally have nuclear molding and an increased number of mitoses. Necrosis is extensive.

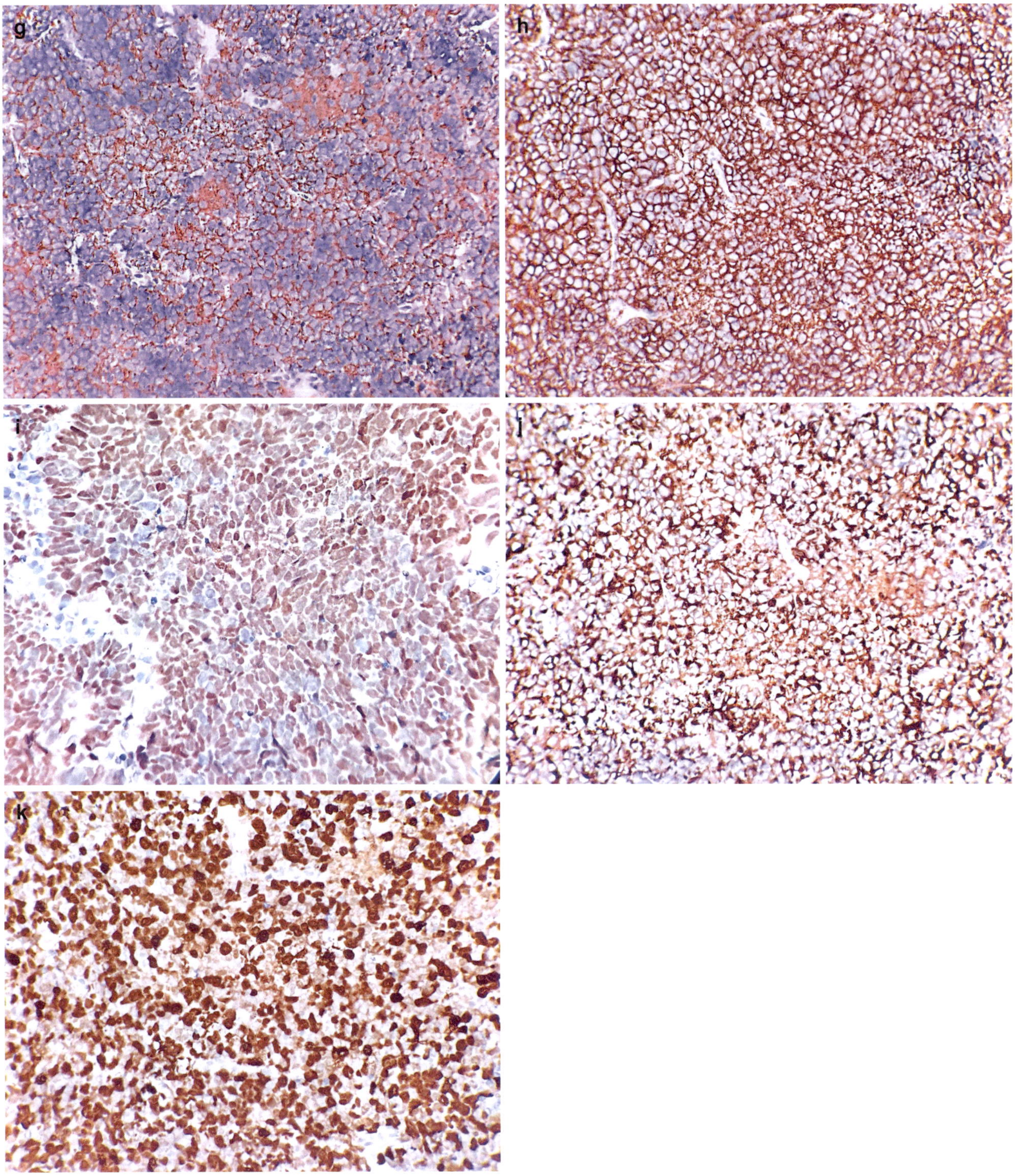

Ancillary Tools

The current WHO classification of lung cancer states that a diagnosis of SCLC can be reliably made on routine histological and cytological grounds, but immunohistochemistry (IHC) may be required, particularly in cases in which histologic features are equivocal and in cases in which the pathologist wants to increase confidence in diagnosis.

IHC [4]:

Synaptophysin (**g**),

CD56 (**h**)

TTF1 (**i**) (negative in 15–20%)

CK7 (**j**) (punctate, not strong/diffuse)

Ki67 (**k**) will show a high proliferation index useful for differentiating between low and high-grade neuroendocrine carcinomas

Chromogranin A, INSM1 (90–100% specificity, low sensitivity)

p16, SOX2, CD117, PAX5, p53, calretinin (48%), CK8

Molecular/cytogenetics description [5]:

Deletion of 3p → loss of MLH1, VHL

p53 mutations due to deletion at 17p (90%)

RB1 loss of function at 13q14 (80–100%)

PTEN mutation (15–20%)

Wild-type c-KIT upregulation (80–90%)

MYC (MYC, MYCL1, or MYCN) amplification (20%)

Telomerase activation (90%)

Rare EGFR mutations and ALK rearrangements

Bronchogenic Carcinoma (Central Type)

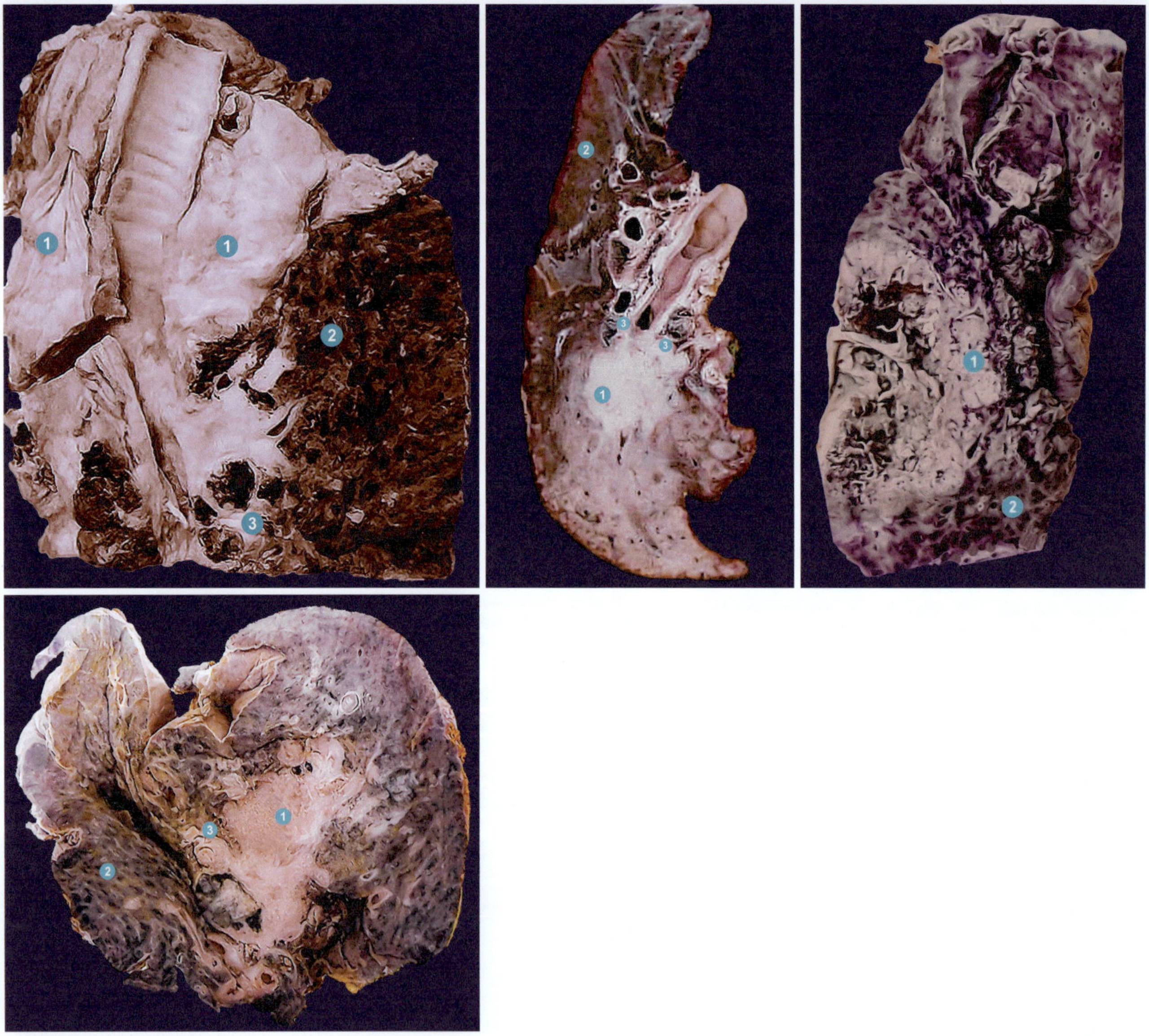

Lung bisected longitudinally is mounted.

1. The main bronchus is infiltrated and destroyed by irregular, white, necrotic tumor tissue, which also spreads along the bronchi and infiltrates the surrounding lung tissues and pleura.
2. The rest of the lung shows atelectasis.
3. The hilar lymph nodes are enlarged and infiltrated by tumor tissue.

Bronchogenic Carcinoma (Central Type) (a, b)

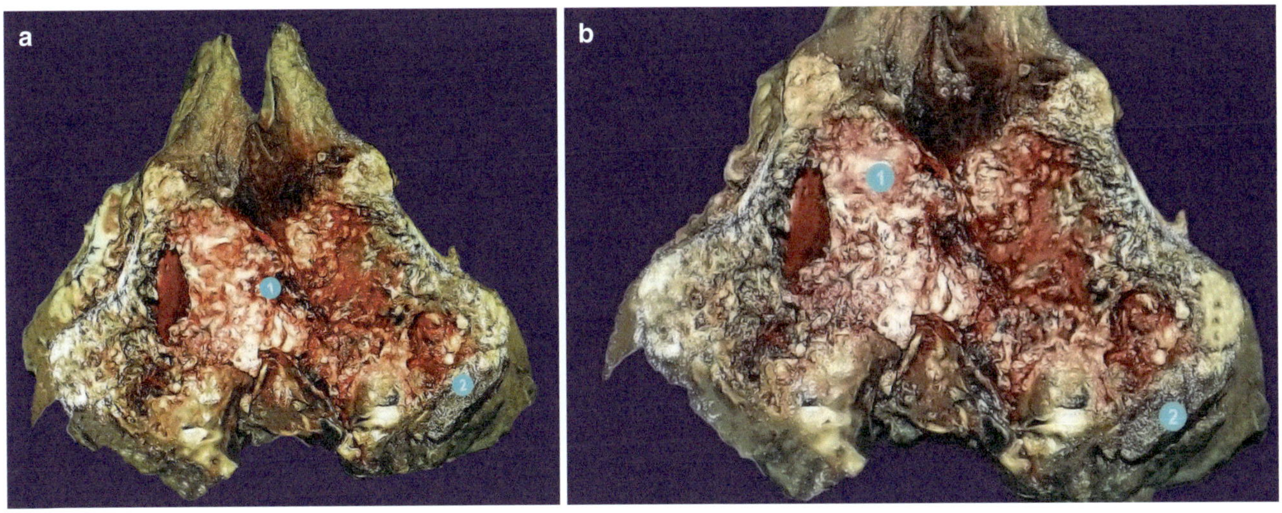

Lung bisected longitudinally is mounted.

1. The main bronchus is infiltrated and destroyed by an irregular, white, necrotic tumor tissue, which also infiltrates the surrounding lung tissues with extensive hemorrhage and necrosis.
2. The rest of the lung shows atelectasis.

Bronchogenic Carcinoma (Peripheral Type)

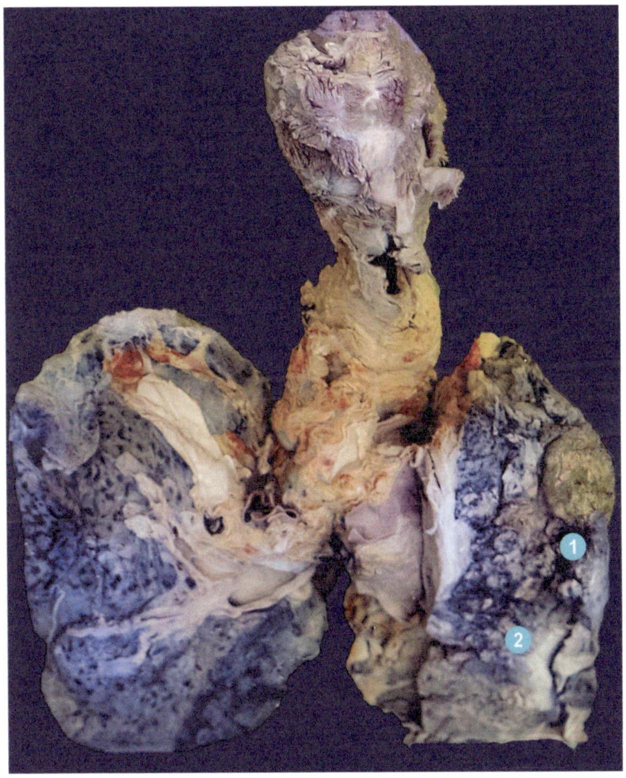

Both lungs and trachea are mounted.

1. A subpleural, peripheral, single, round, well-defined but nonencapsulated mass with a tan-white cut surface with a central area of scar or necrosis
2. The rest of the lung shows atelectasis.

Microscopic Picture of Bronchogenic Carcinoma (Adenocarcinoma) (a–p)

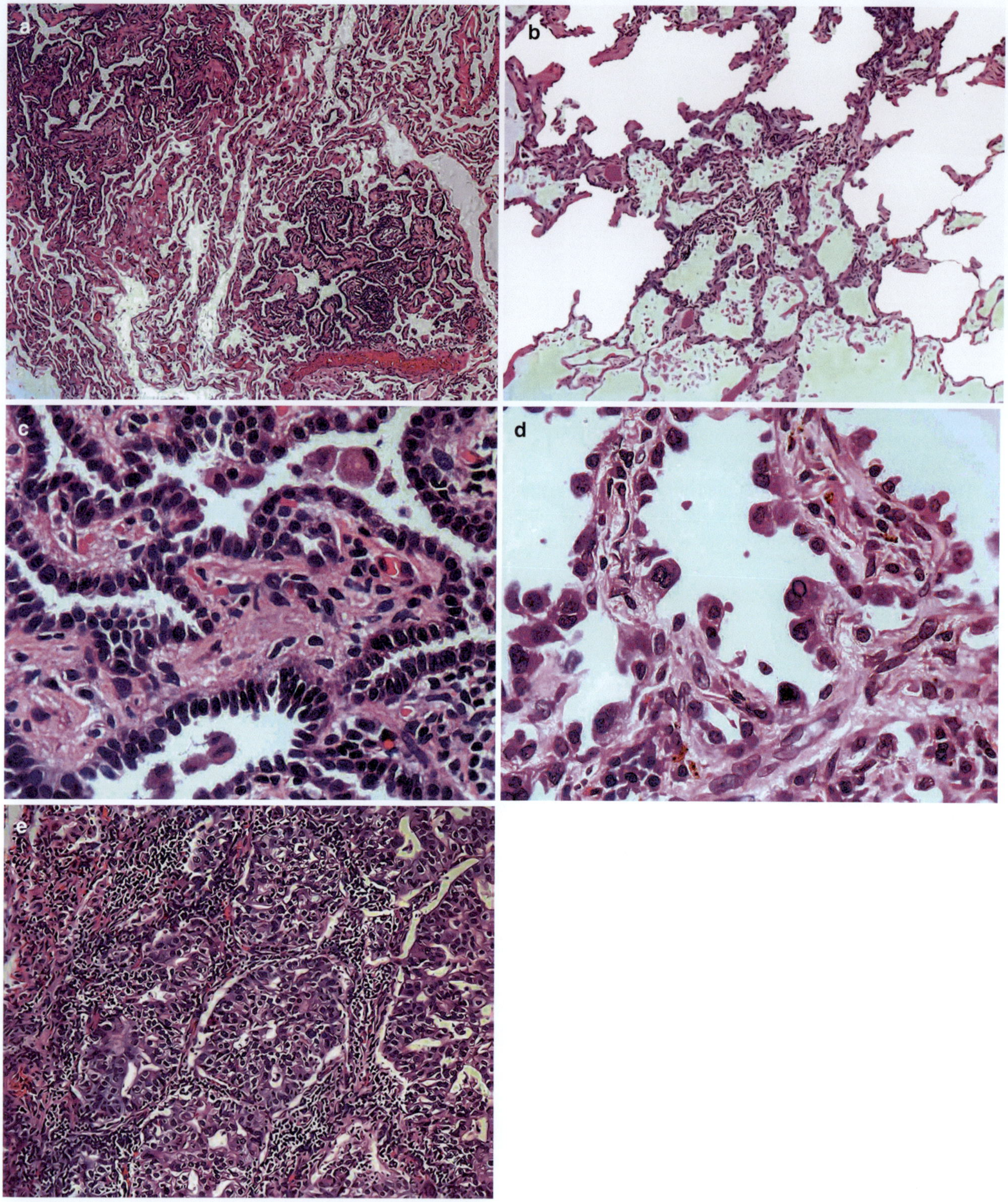

Sections are put to demonstrate the various types of pulmonary adenocarcinoma even with its preinvasive (adenocarcinoma in situ) state.

(a–d): **Adenocarcinoma in situ**: showing a non-mucinous type with lepidic growth pattern only: back-to-back neoplastic cells growing along pre-existing alveolar

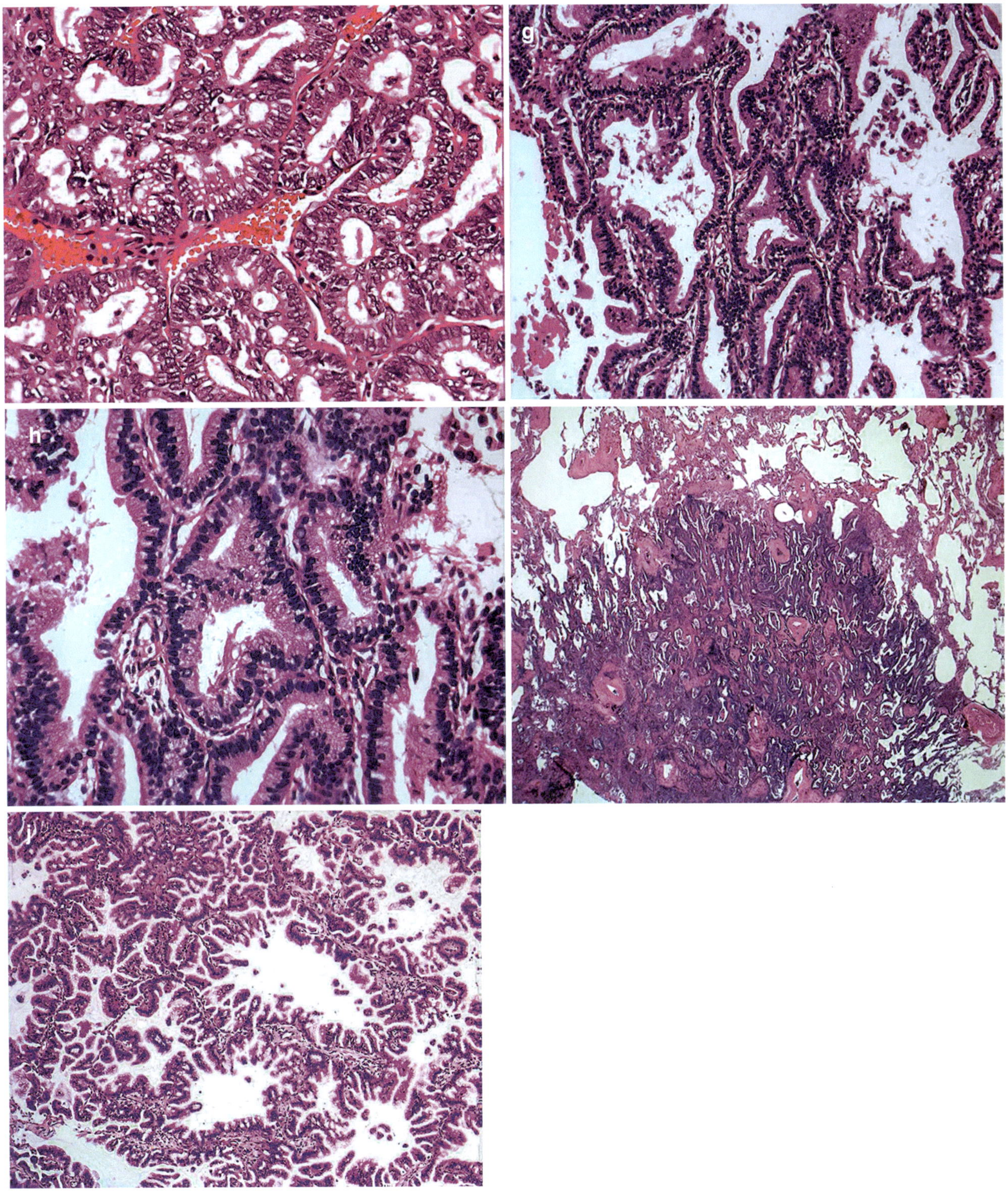

structures only. No stromal, vascular, or pleural invasion; and no necrosis. The tumor cells show moderate atypia in the form of nuclear membrane irregularity, intranuclear pseudoinclusions, nuclear grooves, hyperchromasia, anisocytosis, small nucleoli, increased nuclear to cytoplasmic ratio, and hobnailing.

(e–o) Invasive Adenocarcinoma.

- e: **Acinar Pattern**: gland-forming; round/oval glands, or irregularly shaped malignant glands with central lumina and a hint of cribriform architecture invading the fibrous stroma with complex glandular formation.

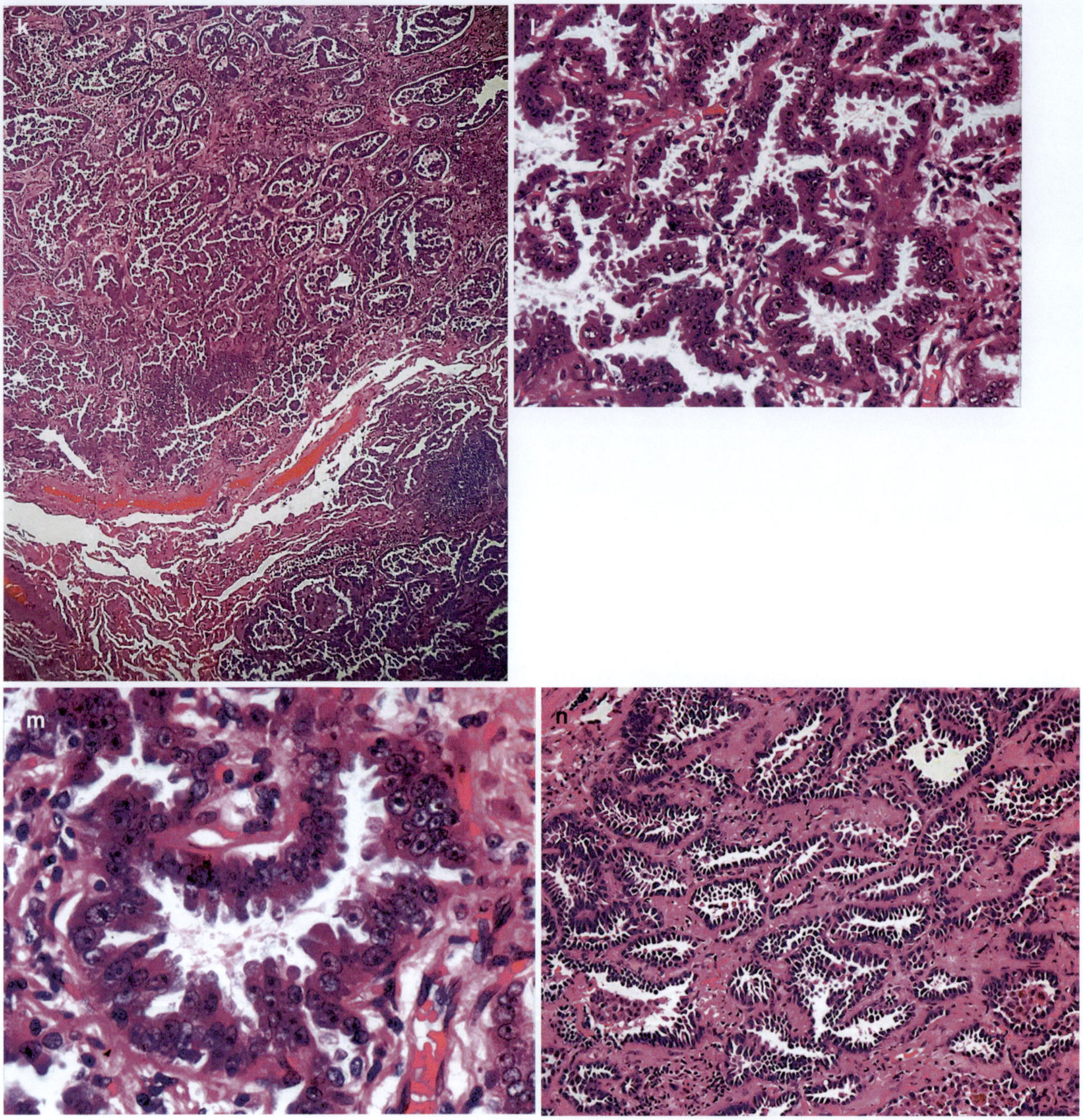

- f–h: **Mucinous pattern**: in which the tumor cells are columnar and abundant intracytoplasmic apical and intra-alveolar mucin.
- i, j: **Papillary Pattern**: malignant cuboidal/columnar cells replace alveolar lining; contains fibrovascular cores.
- k–m: **Micropapillary Pattern**: ill-defined projection/tufting that lacks fibrovascular cores. The filigree micropapillary growth pattern has recently been defined as "tumor cells growing in delicate lace-like narrow stacks of cells without fibrovascular cores." The **filigree pattern** differs from the classical micropapillary pattern by the absence of floret tufts.

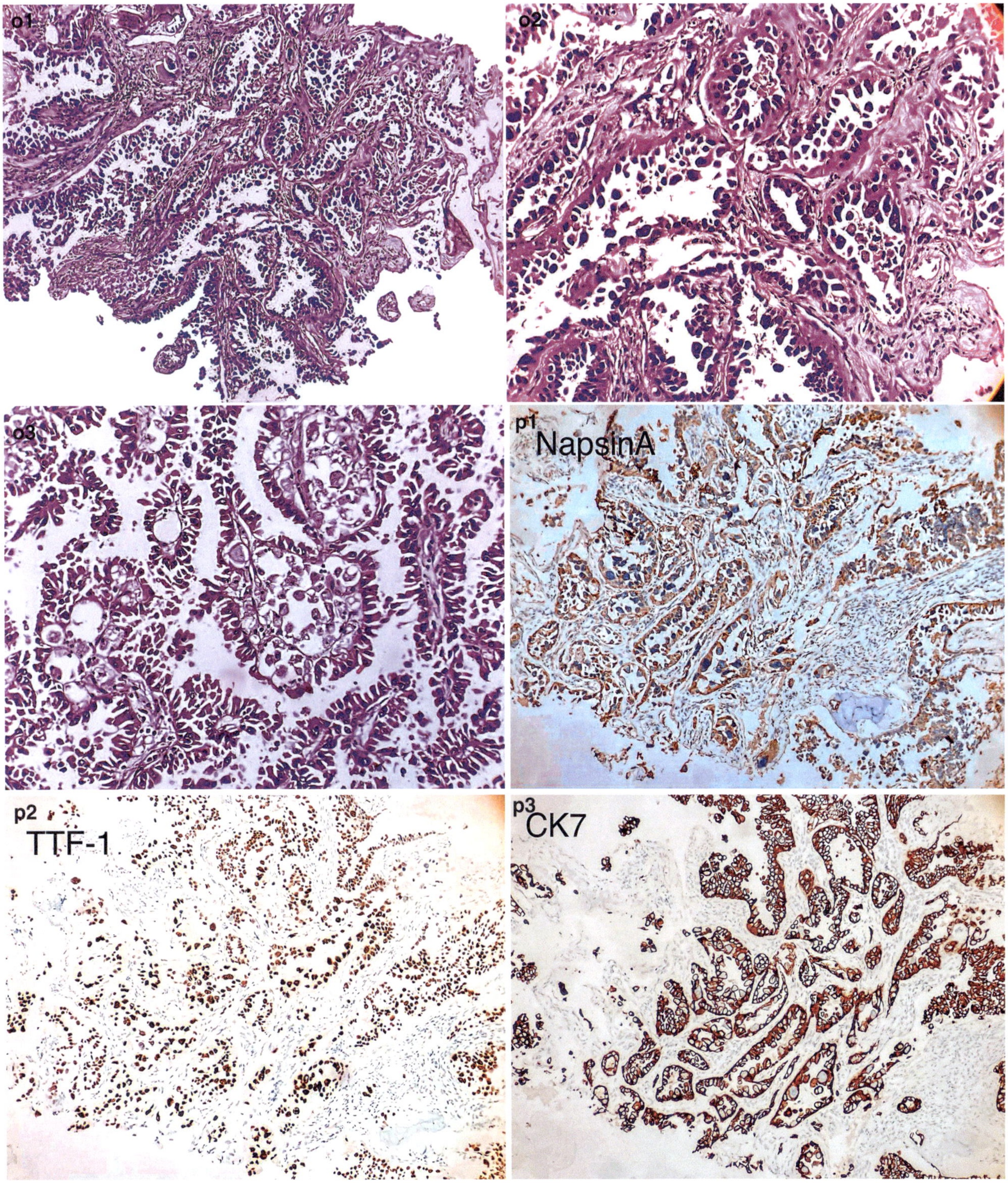

- n and o(1–3): **Lepidic pattern**: in which there is proliferation of cells similar to type II pneumocytes along the surface of alveolar septa and alveolar walls.

Ancillary Tools [6]

IHC includes:

Napsin A (**p1**)

TTF1 (**p2**)

CK7 (**p3**)

AE1/AE3

Beta catenin, TTF1 clone 8G7G3/1 is more specific but less sensitive compared with SPT24 and SP141.

Molecular/cytogenetics description:

EGFR mutation: 10–15% overall, 49% in Asia, rare in mucinous subtype

KRAS mutation: 20–25% overall, 76% of mucinous subtype

ALK rearrangement: 4%

ROS1 gene fusions: 1–2%

BRAF mutation: 1.5–3.5%, V600E most common

NTRK mutation: 2–3%

RET fusion: 0.4–2%

HER2 amplification: 13–22.8%

MET amplification: 2–4%

SMARCA4 loss of function: 5%

Superior Pulmonary Sulcus (Pancoast) Tumor (a, b)

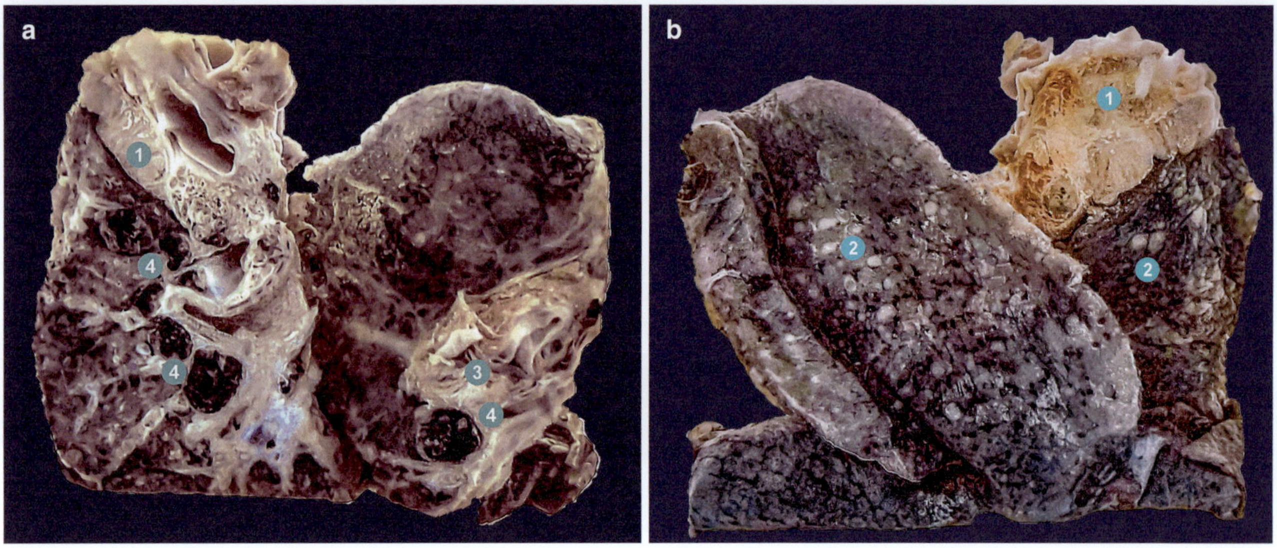

Both lungs are mounted.

1. The upper lobe of the left lung is replaced by a large malignant tumor mass infiltrating and destroying the lung tissue, bronchi, and pleura.
2. Nodules of a malignant tumor are seen under the pleura, infiltrating the rest of the lung and the right lung.
3. The pleura is thickened and covered with fibrin (pleurisy).
4. Hilar lymph nodes are enlarged and have a white cut section as they are infiltrated by the tumor.

Pearls

Overall, the majority of Pancoast tumors are non-small cell lung carcinomas. The possibility of a small cell carcinoma at this site is very rare (only up to 5%). Close to 50% of the cases are adenocarcinomas, and the rest are squamous cell carcinomas (historically squamous cell carcinoma was predominant, but increasing cases of adenocarcinomas are now seen) [7].

Diffuse Malignant Mesothelioma of Pleura (a–c)

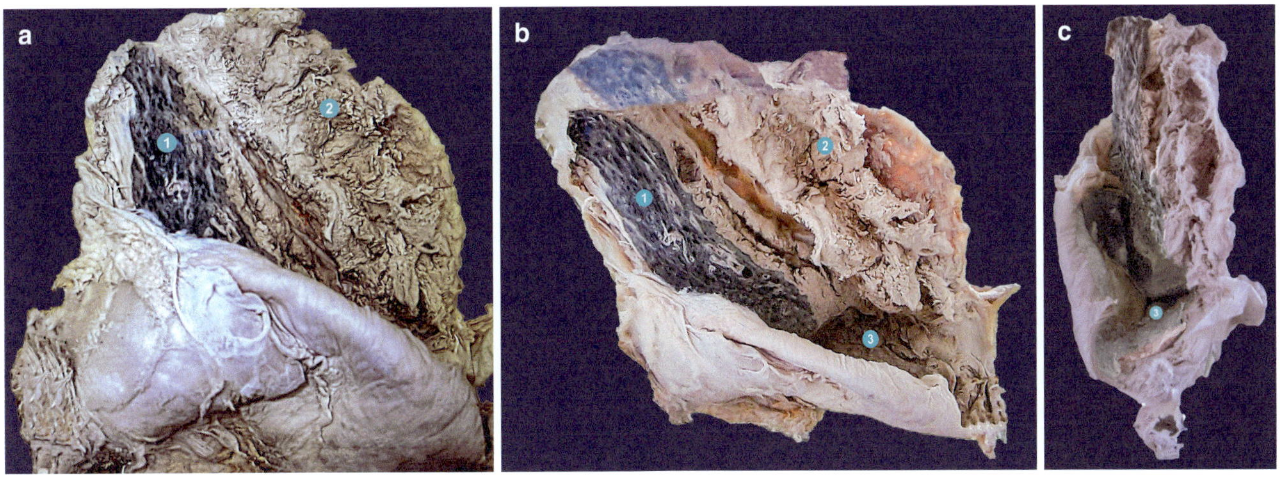

The left lung is mounted.

1. The lung has collapsed.
2. There is diffuse, white, irregular, solid, friable malignant tissue covering both visceral and parietal pleura.
3. The pleural sac appears enlarged and filled with a malignant tumor, which can also be seen in fissures between lung lobes.

Microscopic Picture of Malignant Mesothelioma of Pleura

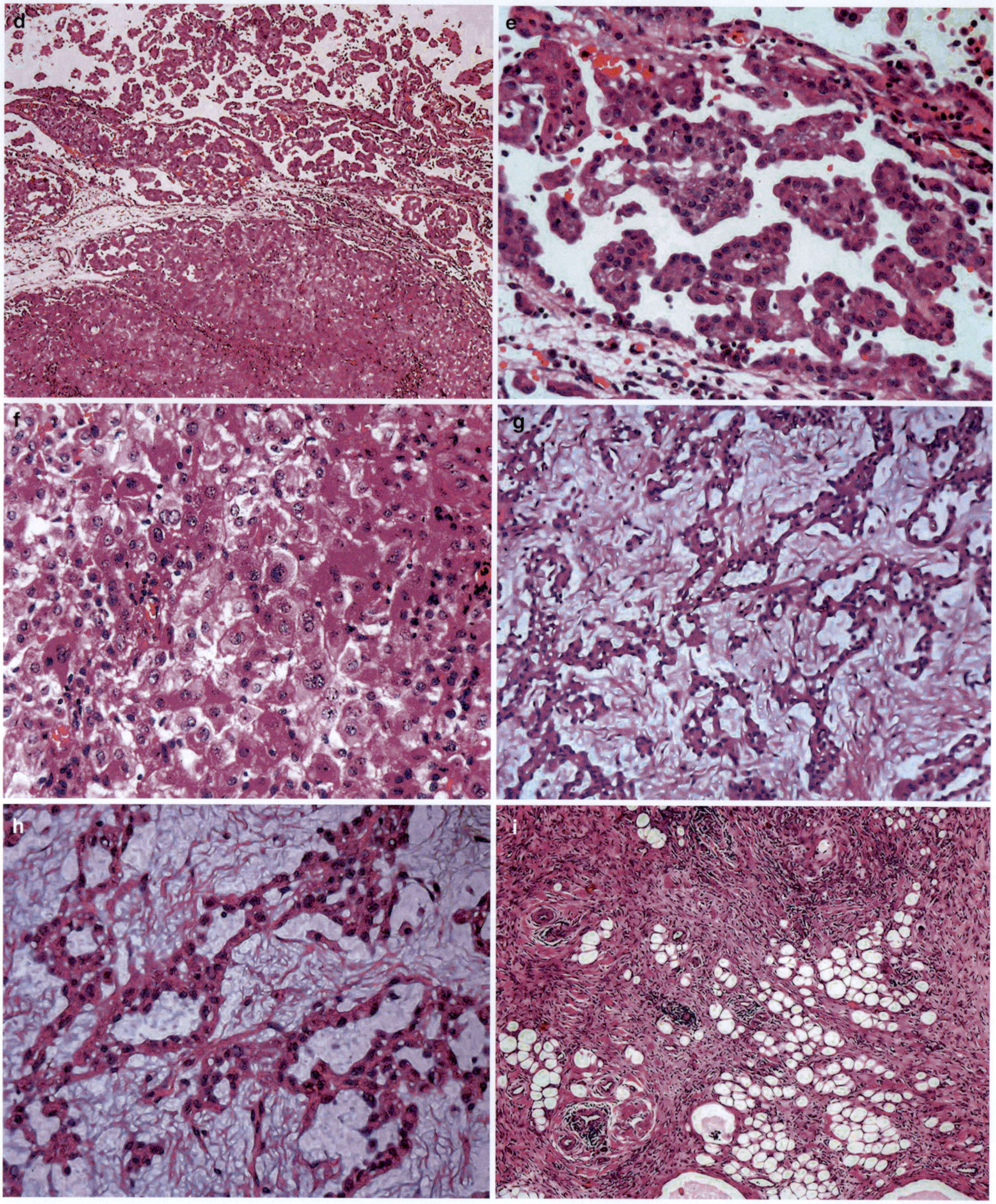

- (d–f) **Micropapillary epithelioid mesothelioma**: sections show cohesive masses of malignant mesothelial cells thrown into micropapillae and invading the stroma as sheets of round to oval malignant mesothelial cells. Tumor cells are polygonal, oval, or cuboidal with distinct cell borders, abundant cytoplasm, and round to oval nuclei. Mitoses are infrequent.
- (g, h) **Acinar pattern**: in which malignant epithelioid cells may be arranged in the form of acini with irregular lumina embedded in a myxoid stroma.

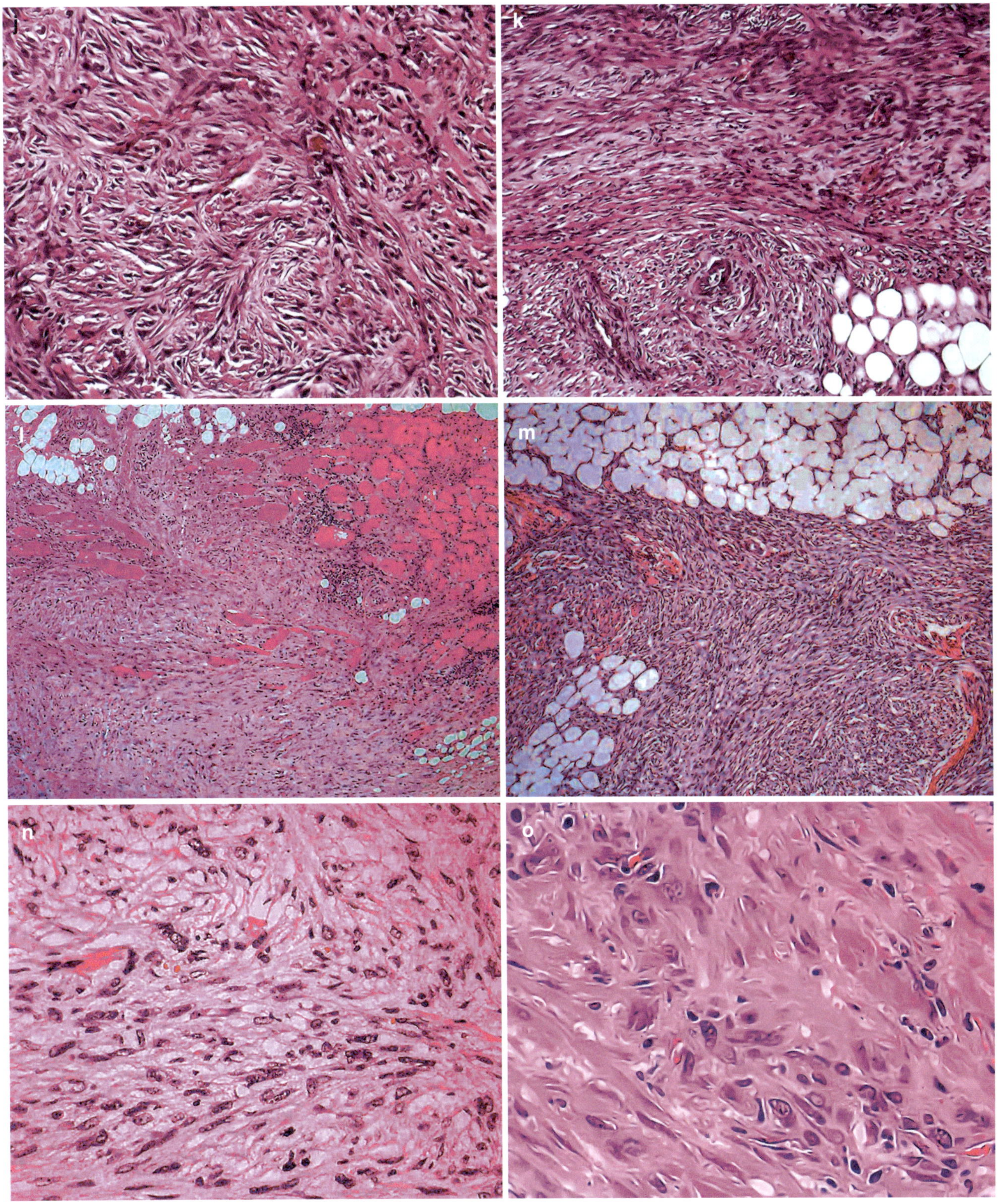

- (i–l) **Desmoplastic mesothelioma**: showing characteristic dense collagenized tissue separated by atypical cells arranged in a storiform or haphazard pattern with focal infiltration of the muscle and fatty tissues.
- (m–o) **Sarcomatoid mesothelioma:** shows infiltrative malignant spindle cells arranged in fascicles or having a haphazard distribution.

Pearls

22021 WHO Classification of Tumors of the Pleura and Pericardium: Essential and Desirable Diagnostic Criteria [8].

Mesothelioma		
• Localized pleural mesotheliomas	• Presentation as a solitary localized mass by imaging, surgical findings, and histology • Examination of a surgical resection specimen revealing a lack of invasion beyond the circumscribed borders of the tumor • Histologic features of diffuse mesothelioma • Immunohistochemical evidence of mesothelial origin	• Multidisciplinary discussion to confirm the diagnosis
• Diffuse pleural mesotheliomas	• Diffuse pleural thickening by a malignant neoplasm with epithelioid, sarcomatoid, or biphasic histology • Invasion of adjacent structures (i.e., adipose tissue, skeletal muscle, and/or lung parenchyma), tumor necrosis, or formation of unequivocal malignant tumor nodules • Desmoplastic mesothelioma is characterized by dense collagenized tissue separated by malignant mesothelial cells arranged in a storiform or so-called patternless pattern, which must be present in ≥50% of the tumor in definitive resection specimens • Biphasic mesothelioma is mesothelioma revealing ≥10% each of epithelioid and sarcomatoid patterns in definitive resection specimens or any percentage of each component in smaller biopsy and cytology specimens • Immunohistochemistry confirming mesothelial origin	• Loss of BAP1 and/or MTAP by immunohistochemistry and/or *CDKN2A* loss by FISH • Or mutations in *BAP1* or *CDKN2A* demonstrated by next-generation sequencing

Ancillary Tools

Markers that aid in the distinction between reactive and malignant mesothelial proliferation [9, 10].

Markers	Sensitivity	Specificity
Loss of expression of nuclear BAP1		100
All mesothelioma	27–67	
Epithelioid mesothelioma	56–81	
Sarcomatoid mesothelioma	0–63	
Loss of expression of cytoplasmic MTAP		100
Epithelioid mesothelioma	37	
Sarcomatoid mesothelioma	80	
Homozygous deletion of CDKN2A (p16) by FISH		100
All mesothelioma	58–62	
Epithelioid mesothelioma	48–78	
Sarcomatoid mesothelioma	67	
Loss of BAP expression or homozygous deletion of CDKN2A		100
All mesothelioma	58–92	
Epithelioid mesothelioma	92	
Sarcomatoid mesothelioma	67–100	
Loss of expression of BAP1 or MTAP		100
All mesothelioma	76–90	
Sarcomatoid mesothelioma	90	

Commonly used immunohistochemical stains for the diagnosis of malignant pleural mesothelioma [11].

Immunohistochemical stain	Frequency of expression in malignant mesothelioma, %	Relevant other neoplasms that might express that marker at least in a subset of cases
Keratin AE1/AE3	84–100	Carcinomas
CAM 5.2	98–99	Carcinomas
WT1 (nuclear)	64–82	Carcinomas of the gynecologic tract (e.g., serous carcinomas), Wilms tumor
Calretinin (nuclear and cytoplasmic)	55–90	Granulosa cell tumor, squamous cell carcinoma
CK5, CK5/6[a]	28–93	Squamous cell carcinoma, NUT carcinoma, breast carcinoma, urothelial carcinoma
Podoplanin (D2–40)	43–80	Squamous cell carcinoma, follicular dendritic cell tumor, angiosarcoma, seminoma, serous carcinoma

3.7 Metastatic Lung Disease

Pulmonary Metastases (a, b)

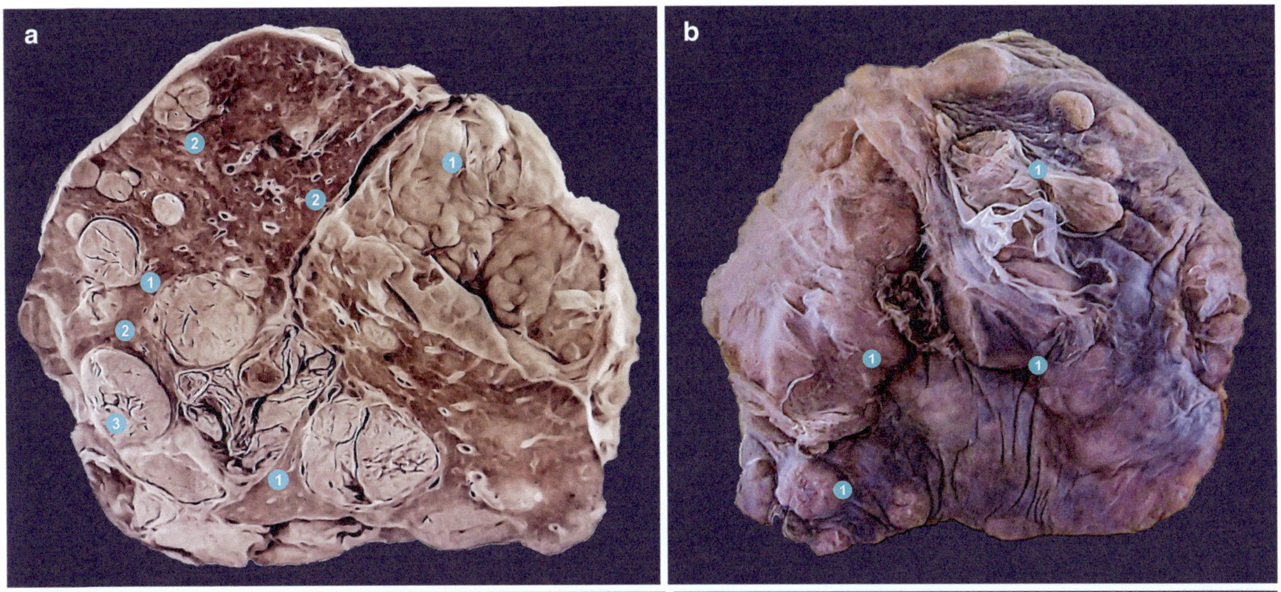

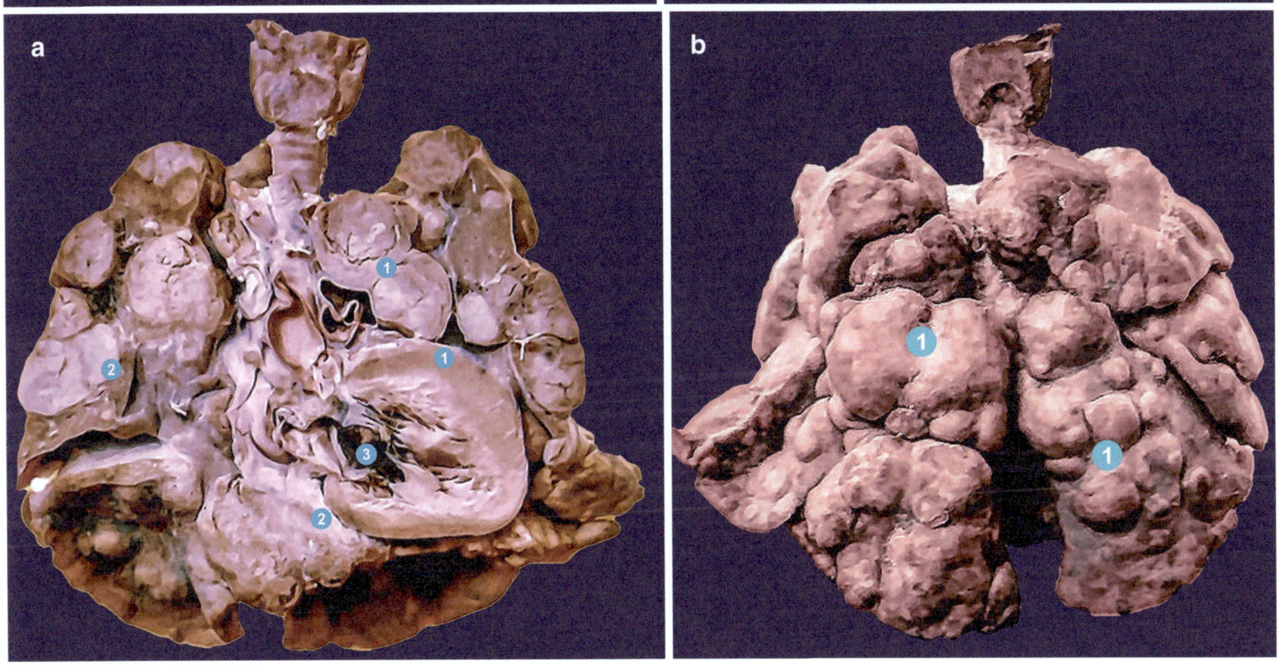

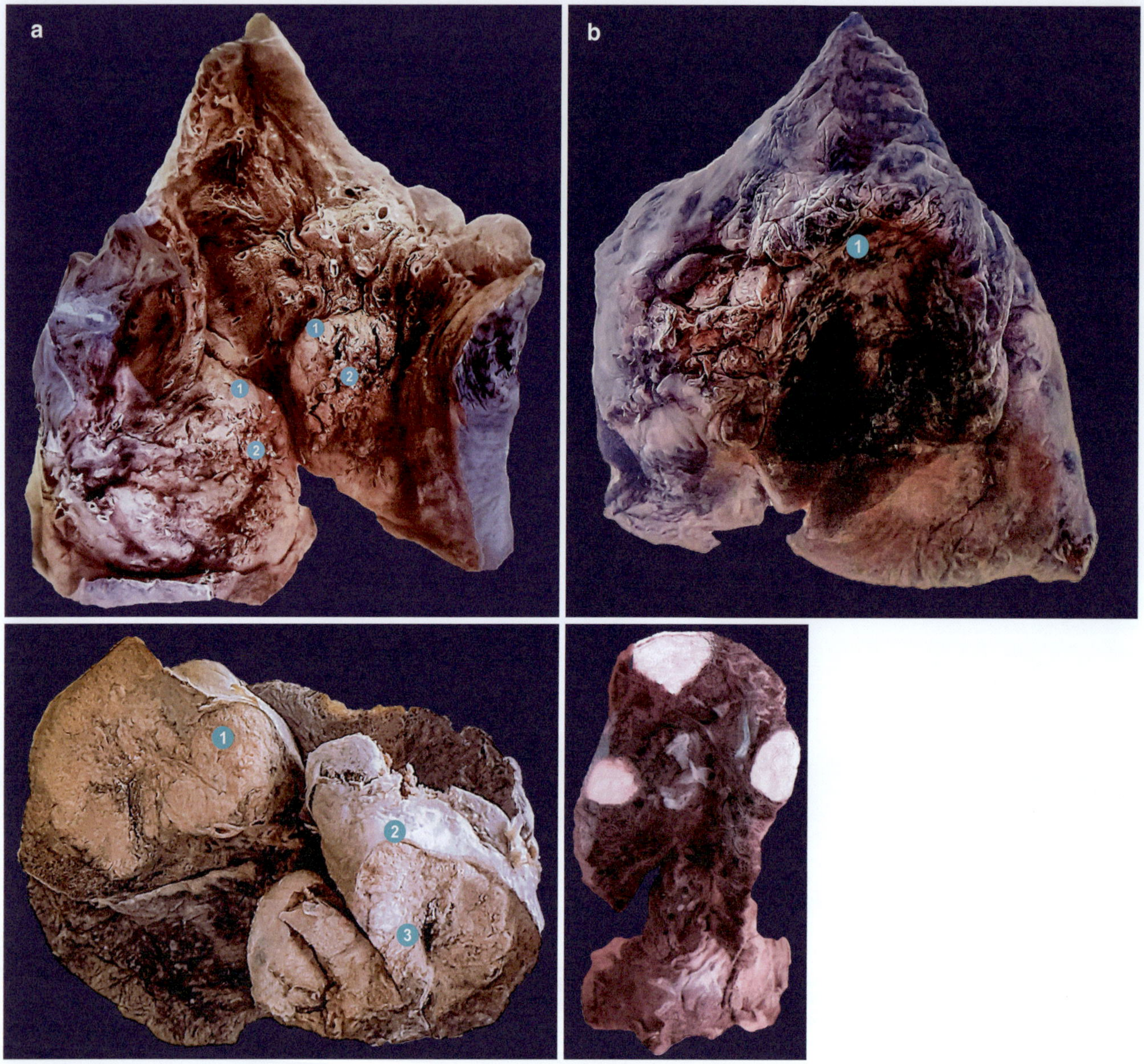

The lung is mounted.

1. It shows multiple, round, tan-gray nodules variable in size. The nodules appear demarcated from the surrounding lung tissue and projecting under the pleura.
2. Lung tissue compressed around the nodules, forming a false capsule.
3. Some nodules show central necrosis.

References

1. Lyoda A., et al. (2021). A novel finding related to bulla and bleb formation in patients with primary spontaneous pneumothorax. BMC Pulm Med. 21(1):20. doi: https://doi.org/10.1186/s12890-021-01402-z. PMCID: PMC7797130.
2. Brower K.S., Del Vecchio M.T., Aronoff S.C. (2014).The etiologies of non-CF bronchiectasis in childhood: a systematic review of 989 subjects. BMC Pediatr. 10:14:4. doi: https://doi.org/10.1186/s12887-014-0299-y. PMCID: PMC4275950.

3. Gagno G. et al. (2022). Pulmonary Embolism Presenting with Pulmonary Infarction: Update and Practical Review of Literature Data. J Clin Med. 11(16):4916. doi: https://doi.org/10.3390/jcm11164916. PMID: 36013155; PMCID: PMC9409643.
4. Thunnissen E., et al. (2017): The Use of Immunohistochemistry Improves the Diagnosis of Small Cell Lung Cancer and Its Differential Diagnosis. An International Reproducibility Study in a Demanding Set of Cases. Journal of Thoracic Oncology. 12, (2): 334-346. https://doi.org/10.1016/j.jtho.2016.12.004.
5. Nong J. et al. (2018). Circulating tumor DNA analysis depicts subclonal architecture and genomic evolution of small cell lung cancer. Nat Commun. 9(1):3114. doi: https://doi.org/10.1038/s41467-018-05327.w.
6. Alidousty C. et al. (2019). Advance of theragnosis biomarkers in lung cancer: from clinical to molecular pathology and biology. J Thorac Dis.11(Suppl 1):S3-S8. doi: https://doi.org/10.21037/jtd.2018.12.03.
7. Villgran V.D. et al. (2024). Pancoast syndrome. In: StatPearls [Internet]. Treasure Island (FL): StatPearls Publishing; 2024. Available from: https://www.ncbi.nlm.nih.gov/books/NBK482155/
8. Sauter J.L., et al. (2022). The 2021 WHO Classification of Tumors of the Pleura: Advances Since the 2015 Classification. Journal of Thoracic Oncology.17,(5):608—622. https://doi.org/10.1016/j.jtho.2021.12.014.
9. Cigognetti M., et al. (2015). BAP1 (BRCA1-associated protein 1) is a highly specific marker for differentiating mesothelioma from reactive mesothelial proliferations. Mod Pathol. 28(8):1043-57. doi: https://doi.org/10.1038/modpathol.2015.65. PMID: 26022455.
10. Kinoshita Y., et al. (2018). A combination of MTAP and BAP1 immunohistochemistry is effective for distinguishing sarcomatoid mesothelioma from fibrous pleuritis. Lung Cancer. 125:198-204. doi: https://doi.org/10.1016/j.lungcan.2018.09.019. PMID: 30429020.
11. Stang N.L. et al. (2020). Differential Diagnosis of Epithelioid Malignant Mesothelioma with Lung and Breast Pleural Metastasis: A Systematic Review Compared With a Standardized Panel of Antibodies-A New Proposal That May Influence Pathologic Practice. Arch Pathol Lab Med: 144(4):446-456. doi: https://doi.org/10.5858/arpa.2018-0457-OA. PMID: 31389715.

4 Diseases of the Gastrointestinal Tract

4.1 Introduction

The human gastrointestinal (GI) tract, a complex, interconnected system that plays a vital role in digestion, absorption, and metabolism, is susceptible to a myriad of disorders that manifest in various pathological changes. This chapter, "Diseases of the Gastrointestinal Tract," offers an in-depth exploration of the broad spectrum of diseases that affect the GI tract, their gross and microscopic pathological features, and how these appearances can guide our understanding of disease mechanisms.

The chapter's structure will mirror the anatomical arrangement of the GI tract, starting from the esophagus, followed by the stomach, small intestine, large intestine, and finally the rectum and anus. For each disease, we will describe its typical gross and microscopic pathologic features.

This chapter will provide you with a comprehensive overview of the fascinating field of gastrointestinal gross and microscopic pathology. It aims to not only enrich your knowledge base but also hone your skills in the accurate interpretation of gross and microscopic pathological findings within the context of GI diseases. As we navigate the dynamic landscape of gastrointestinal pathology, you will find that understanding the "gross" can indeed lead to an appreciation of the "subtle."

The chapter will be organized according to the following order:

1. Esophageal Lesions
   (a) Congenital esophageal atresia with trachea-esophageal fistula
   (b) Esophageal varices
2. Gastric Lesions
   (a) Inflammatory lesions
      - Atrophic gastritis
      - Hypertrophic gastritis
      - Gastric ulcer
   (b) Neoplastic lesions
      - Peritoneal Inclusion Cysts (Benign Multicystic Peritoneal Mesothelioma)
      - Gastric carcinoma
3. Small Intestine Lesions
   (a) Congenital lesions
      - Meckel's diverticulum
   (b) Inflammatory lesions
      - Tuberculosis
      - Typhoid ulcer
   (c) Mechanical lesions
      - Strangulated hernia
      - Intussusception
   (d) Neoplastic lesions
      - Neuroendocrine tumor (NET)
      - Duodenal carcinoma
      - Periampullary carcinoma
4. Appendiceal Lesions
   (a) Inflammatory lesions
      - Acute suppurative appendicitis
      - Mucocele of appendix
5. Colorectal Lesions
   (a) Inflammatory lesions
      - Anal Fistula
      - Miliary tuberculosis
      - Pseudomembranous colitis
      - Bilharziasis
      - Chronic ulcerative colitis
   (b) Neoplastic lesions
      - Benign tumors: Lipoma, Adenomatous polyps, Rectal NET, Colonic GIST
      - Malignant tumors: Carcinoma

G. Dawood, *Color Atlas of Human Gross and Microscopic Pathology*, https://doi.org/10.1007/978-3-031-76007-5_4

4.2 Esophageal Lesions

Congenital Esophageal Atresia with Trachea-Esophageal Fistula (EA/TEF)

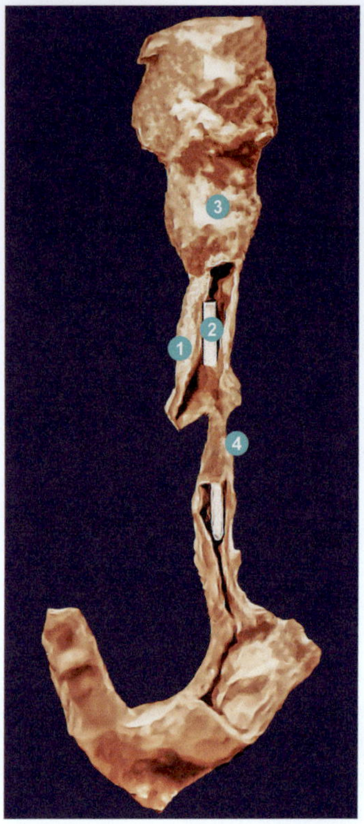

1. Esophageal Atresia: The esophagus exhibits a blind-ending pouch, where a portion of the esophagus is absent. The site of atresia is located proximal to the stomach.
2. Trachea-Esophageal Fistula (white rod): A fistulous connection between the trachea and the esophagus is present. This abnormal communication allows air to pass from the trachea into the esophagus, which can cause respiratory distress and gastric distension.
3. Distended Upper Esophageal Segment: The segment of the esophagus that is proximal to the atresia site is dilated and usually filled with accumulated secretions, mucus, and saliva. This dilation occurs because swallowed fluids cannot pass through the atretic portion of the esophagus.
4. Lower Esophageal Segment: The segment of the esophagus that is distal to the atresia site is dilated to some extent.

Pearls

Congenital esophageal atresia with trachea-esophageal fistula may result from combined genetic and environmental factors. It may be associated with other congenital anomalies, such as cardiac defects, vertebral abnormalities, gastrointestinal malformations, and other anomalies of the respiratory or urinary systems. These associated anomalies may also be evident during the gross examination [1].

Esophageal Varices (a, b)

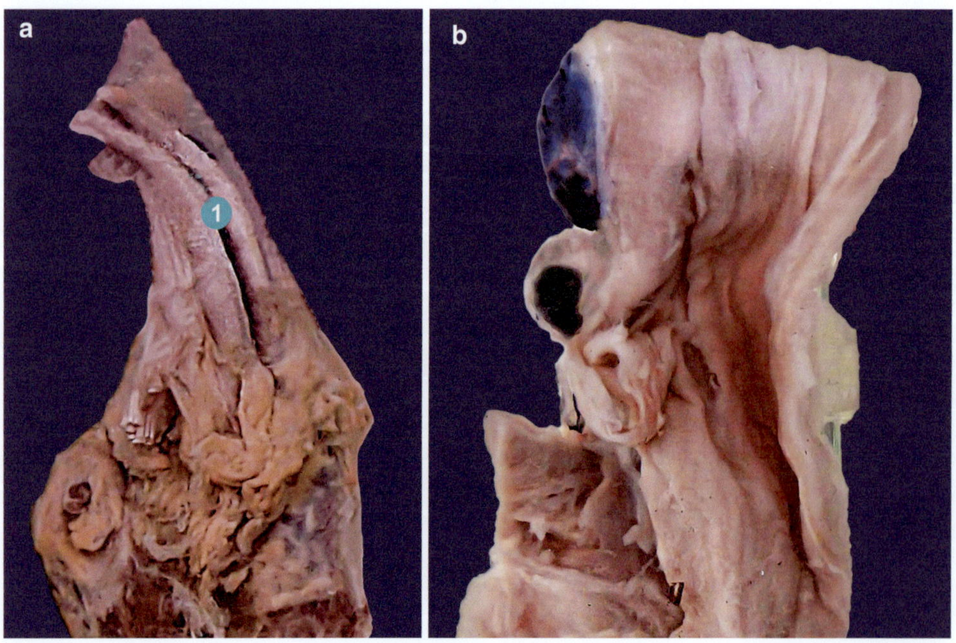

The esophagus has been opened longitudinally.

1. Numerous tortuous, submucosal dilated veins are seen.

Microscopic Picture of Esophageal Varices (c–f)

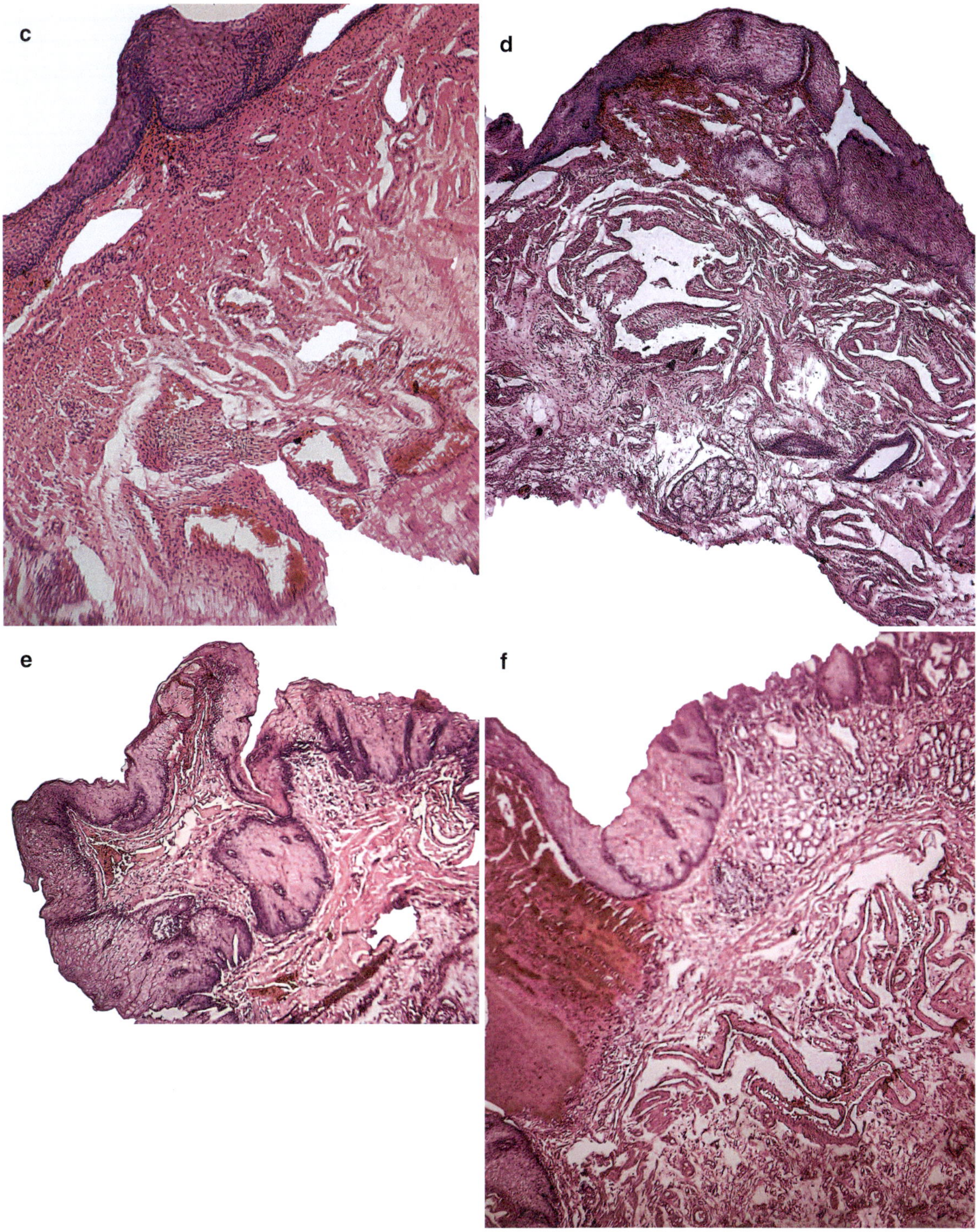

Sections show gastroesophageal junction. Multiple dilated, tortuous, and thin-walled fragile veins with irregular lumens are seen within the submucosa of the esophagus and stomach. A subepithelial extensive interstitial hemorrhage is observed.

4.3 Gastric Lesions

4.3.1 Inflammatory Lesions

Atrophic Gastritis

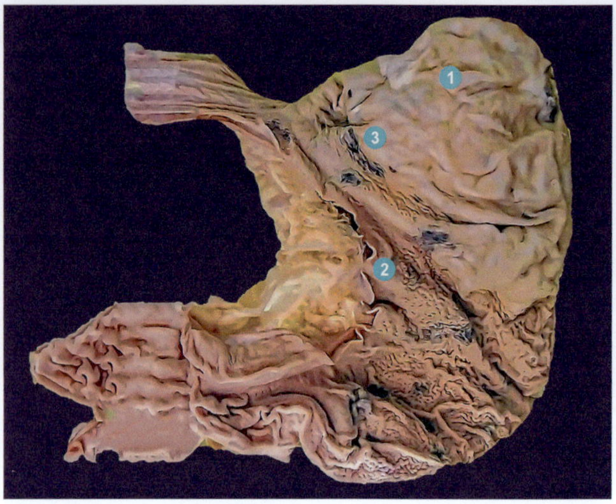

An opened stomach is mounted.

1. The upper two-thirds of the stomach show thin and atrophic gastric mucosa with loss of the normal rugal folds. The surface of the stomach appears smooth and flattened.
2. The walls of the stomach appear thinner than normal.
3. A small gastric ulcer

N.B. The specimen was obtained from a 40-year-old female with achylia gastrica, pernicious anemia, and subacute combined degeneration of the spinal cord.

Pearls

Besides the above-mentioned lesions, atrophic gastritis is a risk factor for the development of other conditions such as gastric ulcers, gastric polyps, and gastric cancer. These complications may be observed during gross examination if present [2].

Hypertrophic Gastritis (Menetrier's Disease)

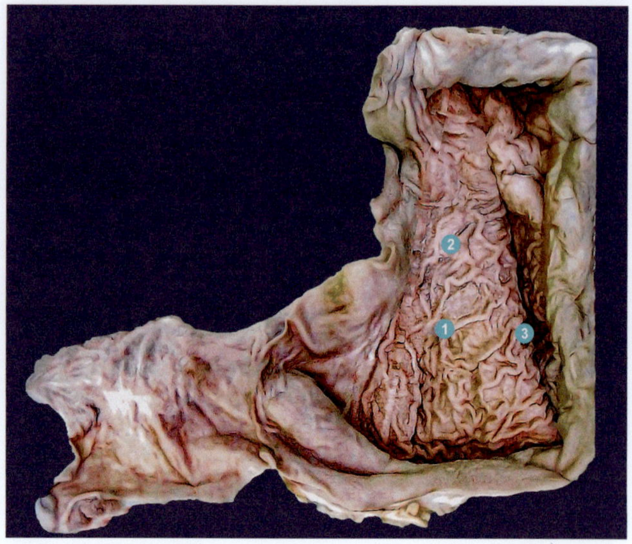

An opened stomach is mounted.

1. The gastric mucosa appears diffusely thickened, resulting in a "cobblestone" or "rugae-like" appearance. This thickening is most prominent in the body and fundus of the stomach.
2. Giant Rugae: The gastric rugae may be dramatically enlarged, giving a "honeycomb" or "brain-like" appearance. "These giant rugae can extend across the entire stomach."
3. The gastric mucosa appears reddened or congested due to increased blood flow.

Pearls

Hypertrophic gastritis is a rare form of chronic gastritis. It is associated with excessive growth factor production and is believed to have an autoimmune or allergic component [3].

Microscopic Picture of Hypertrophic Gastritis (Menetrier's Disease) (a, b)

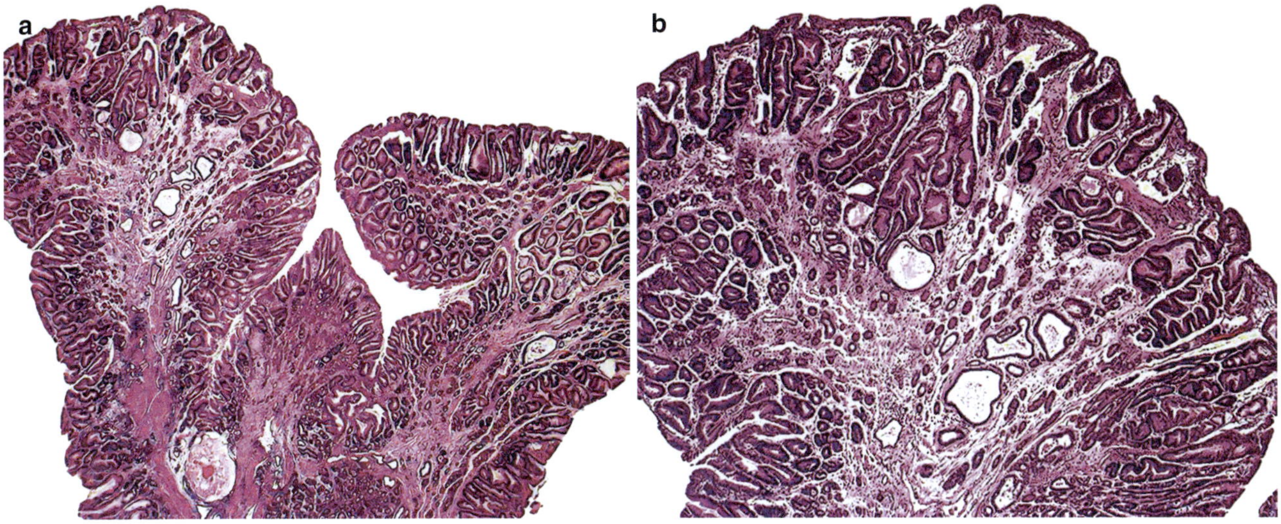

Sections show enlarged gastric folds, foveolar hyperplasia (elongation of the surface epithelium), thickening of the mucosa, and glandular hyperplasia. Submucosa shows fibrosis and infiltration with lymphocytes and plasma cells.

Chronic Peptic Ulcers

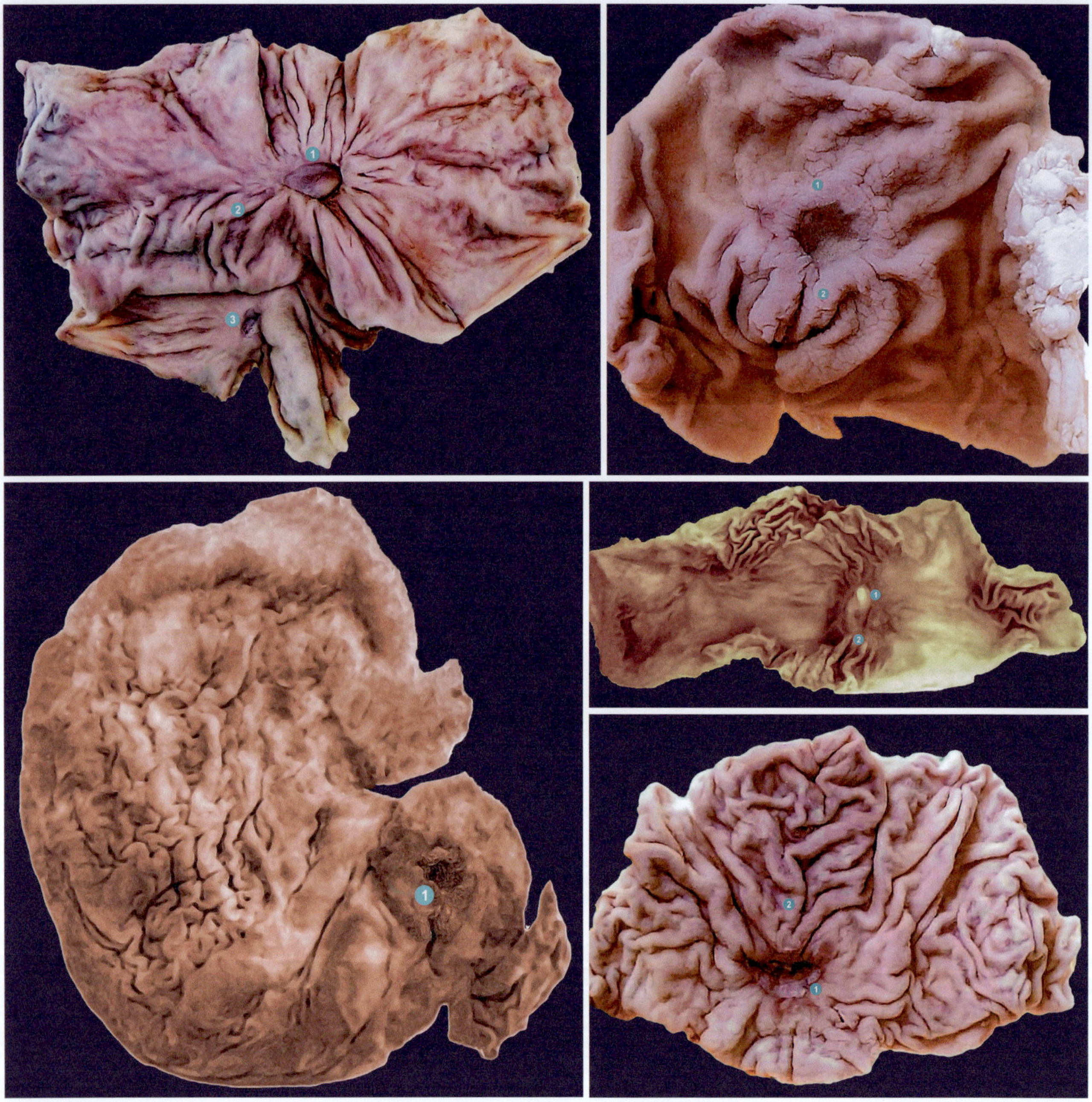

An opened stomach is mounted.

1. It shows a sharply demarcated, oval, 2 × 1 cm. ulcer with straight, sharp edges, and its base is composed of smooth but irregularly heaped-up granulation and scar tissue.
2. The mucosa around the ulcer is corrugated because of fibrosis at the base.
3. There is another smaller, more superficial ulcer at the lower part of the stomach, and its base is formed by the muscle layer.

Microscopic Picture of Chronic Peptic Ulcers (a–d)

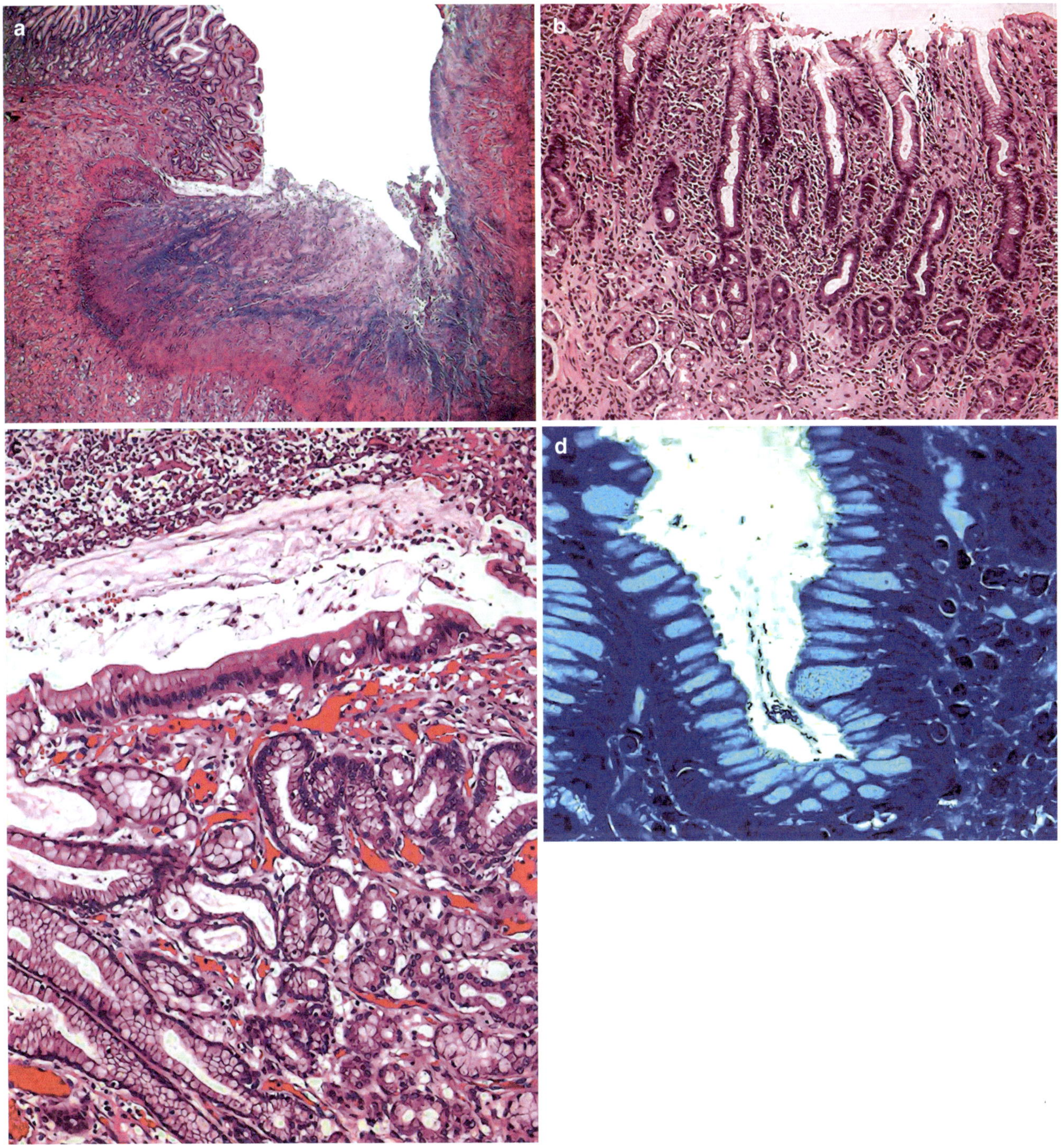

Sections show overhanging proximal gastric mucosa with the presence of chronic gastritis. The epithelium is ulcerated with the presence of surface neutrophils, bacteria, and necrotic debris. Fibrinoid necrosis is seen at the base and margins with the presence of granulation tissue infiltrated with chronic inflammatory cells. The ulcer is associated with *H. pylori* (stained with Giemsa stain) (d).

Perforated Peptic Ulcer (a, b)

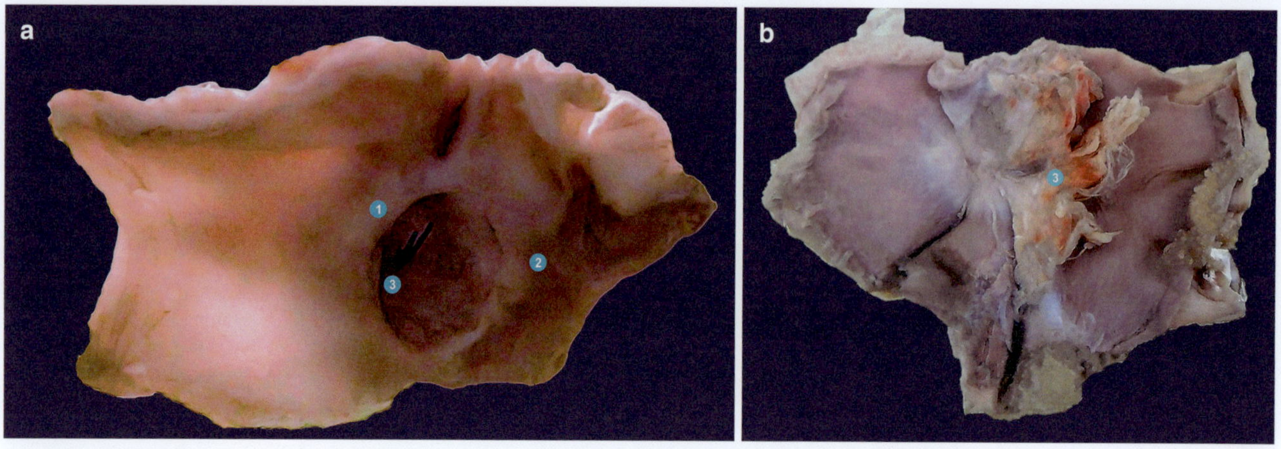

Part of the stomach is mounted.

1. An ulcer with a sharply demarcated, oval edge, 2 × 1 cm. with straight sharp edges, and its base is composed of smooth but irregularly heaped-up granulation and scar tissue.
2. The mucosa around the ulcer is corrugated because of fibrosis at the base.
3. In this specimen, while a small area of granulation tissue remains at the border of the ulcer, perforation has occurred (straw). The serosa overlying the ulcer is fibrous.

4.3.2 Neoplastic Lesions

Peritoneal Inclusion Cysts (Benign Multicystic Peritoneal Mesothelioma)

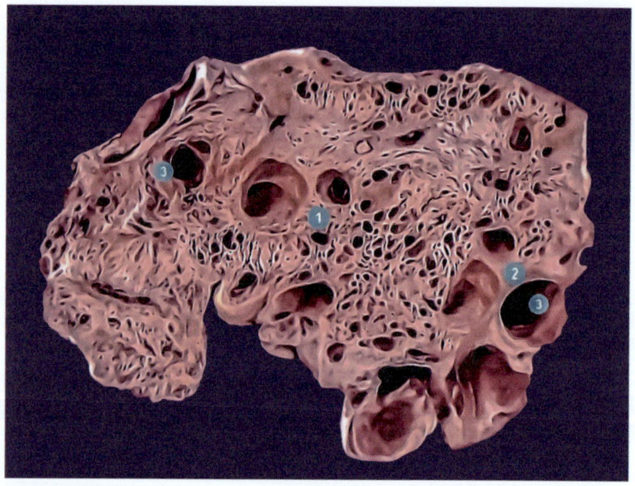

A piece of the peritoneum is mounted.

1. Multiple, separate (multiloculated) cysts are distributed throughout the peritoneum, forming a confluent mass. These cysts vary significantly in size, ranging from a few millimeters to several centimeters.
2. The walls of the cysts are thin and opaque.
3. Some locules contain hemorrhagic fluid.

Microscopic Picture of Peritoneal Inclusion Cysts (Benign Multicystic Peritoneal Mesothelioma) (a–c)

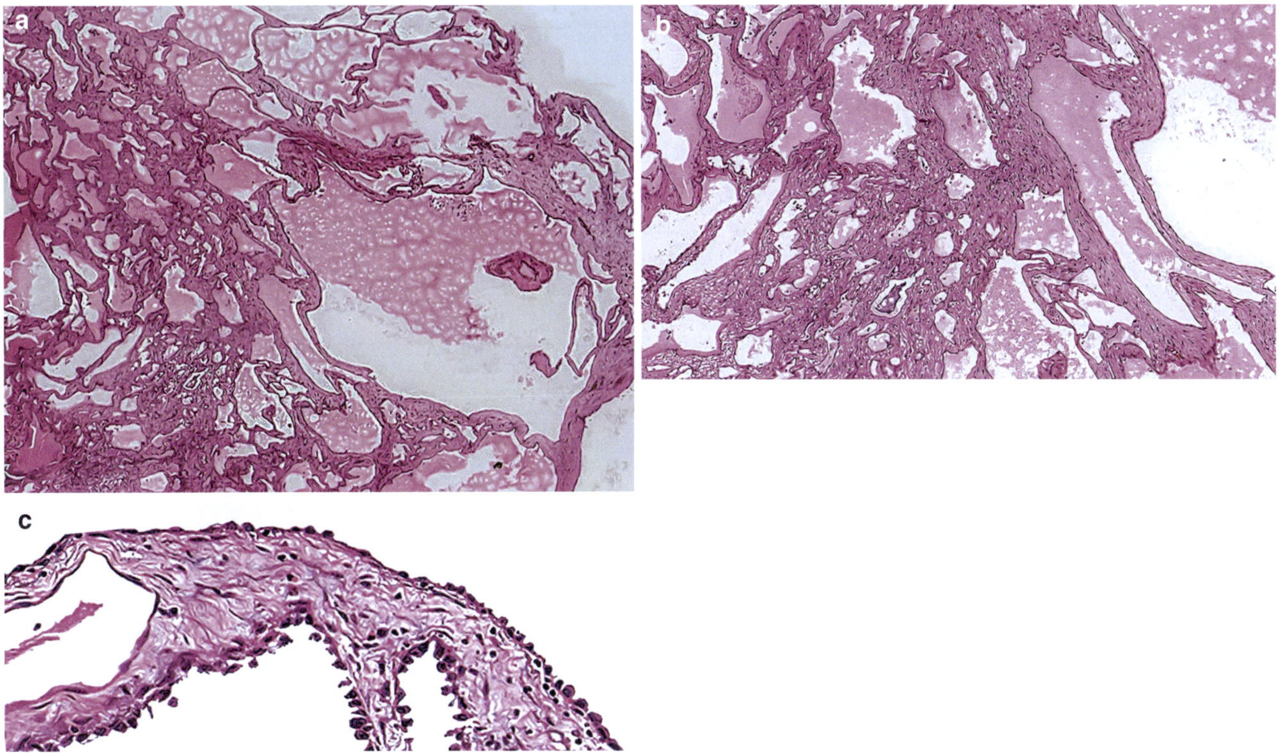

Sections show multiple and variably-sized cystic structures lined by a single layer of cuboidal-flat mesothelial cells and embedded among loose fibrous stroma. The cysts are filled with clear or slightly cloudy eosinophilic fluid.

Ancillary Tools

IHC include [4]:

- Cytokeratin
- Calretinin
- CK5/6
- WT1
- D2-40
- BAP1 (normal/retained)
- MTAP (normal/retained)

Pearls

The nature of peritoneal inclusion cysts (benign multicystic peritoneal mesothelioma), whether neoplastic or reactive, is unclear.

- **Factors favoring neoplastic pathogenesis** [5]
  - The progressive nature of untreated cases
  - Rare transformation to malignant mesothelioma
  - Inconstant association with prior surgery or inflammatory process
  - Occasional co-occurrence with adenomatoid tumor or well-differentiated papillary mesothelioma
- **Factors favoring reactive pathogenesis** [6]
  - Frequent association with prior surgery, pelvic inflammatory disease, endometriosis, or peritoneal dialysis

Ulcerative Carcinoma of the Stomach

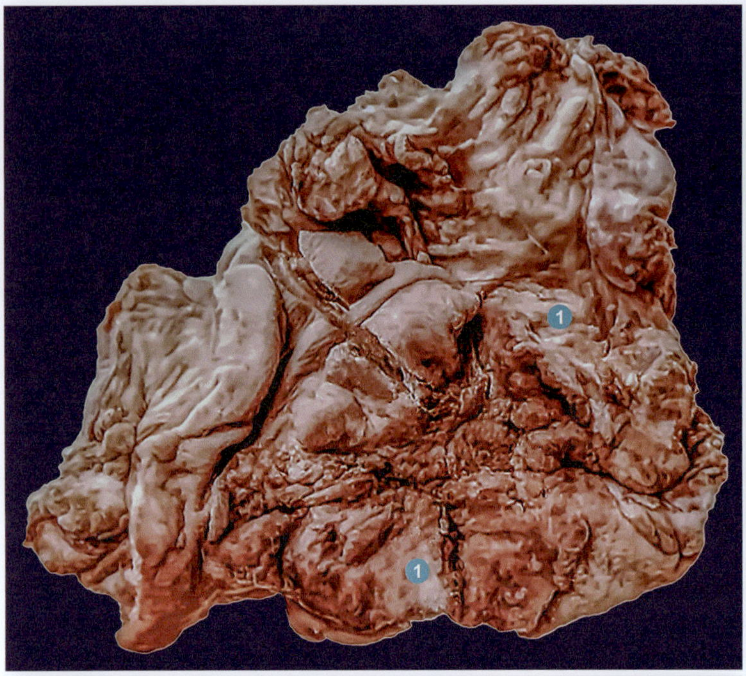

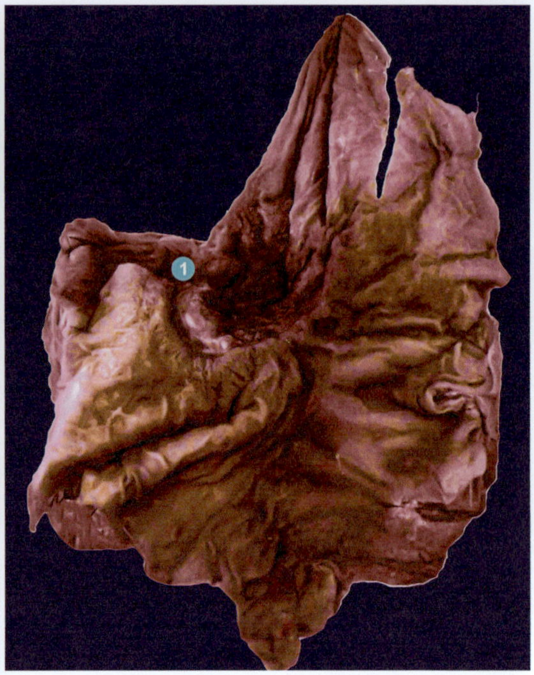

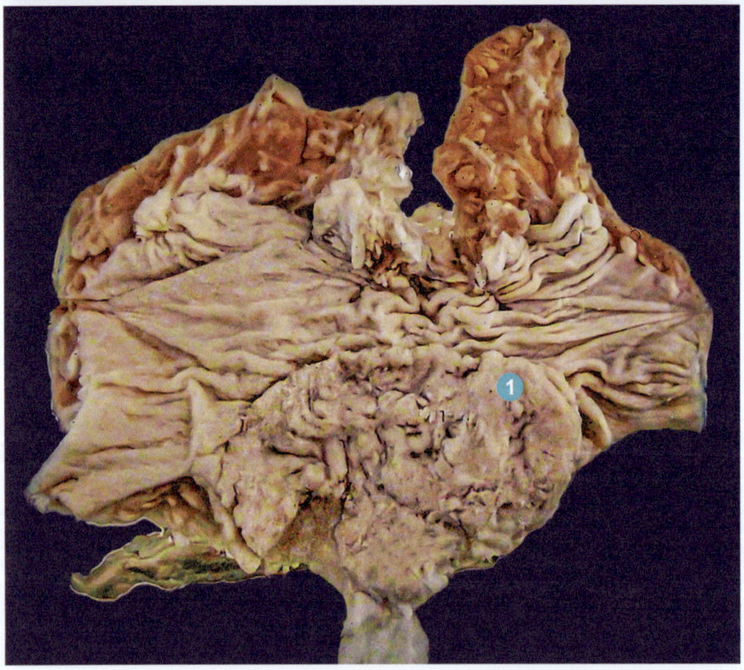

An opened stomach is mounted.

1. A malignant ulcer is seen near the lesser curvature. The ulcer is oval with a raised everted edge, round margin, and necrotic floor.

Polypoid Carcinoma of the Stomach (a, b)

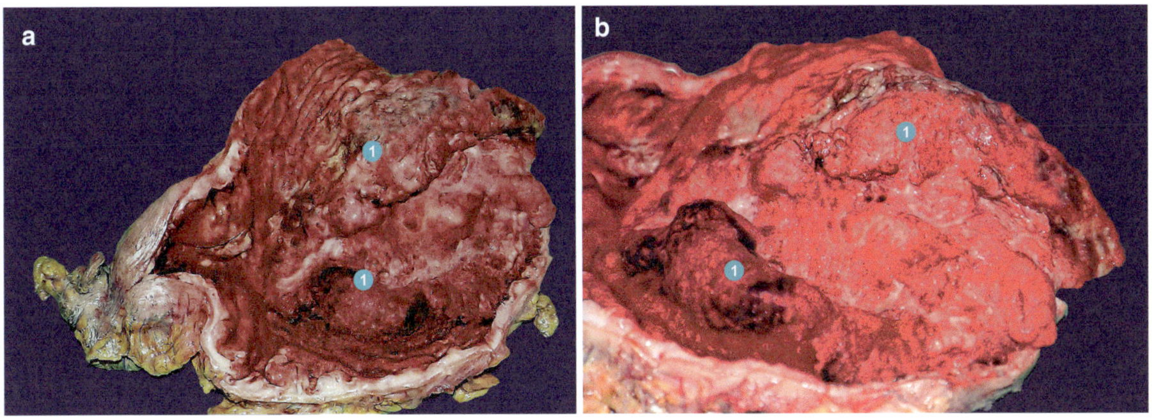

An opened stomach is mounted.

1. A large polypoid ulcerated and hemorrhagic mass with areas of necrosis projecting into the lumen.

Microscopic Picture of Polypoid Carcinoma of the Stomach (c–i)

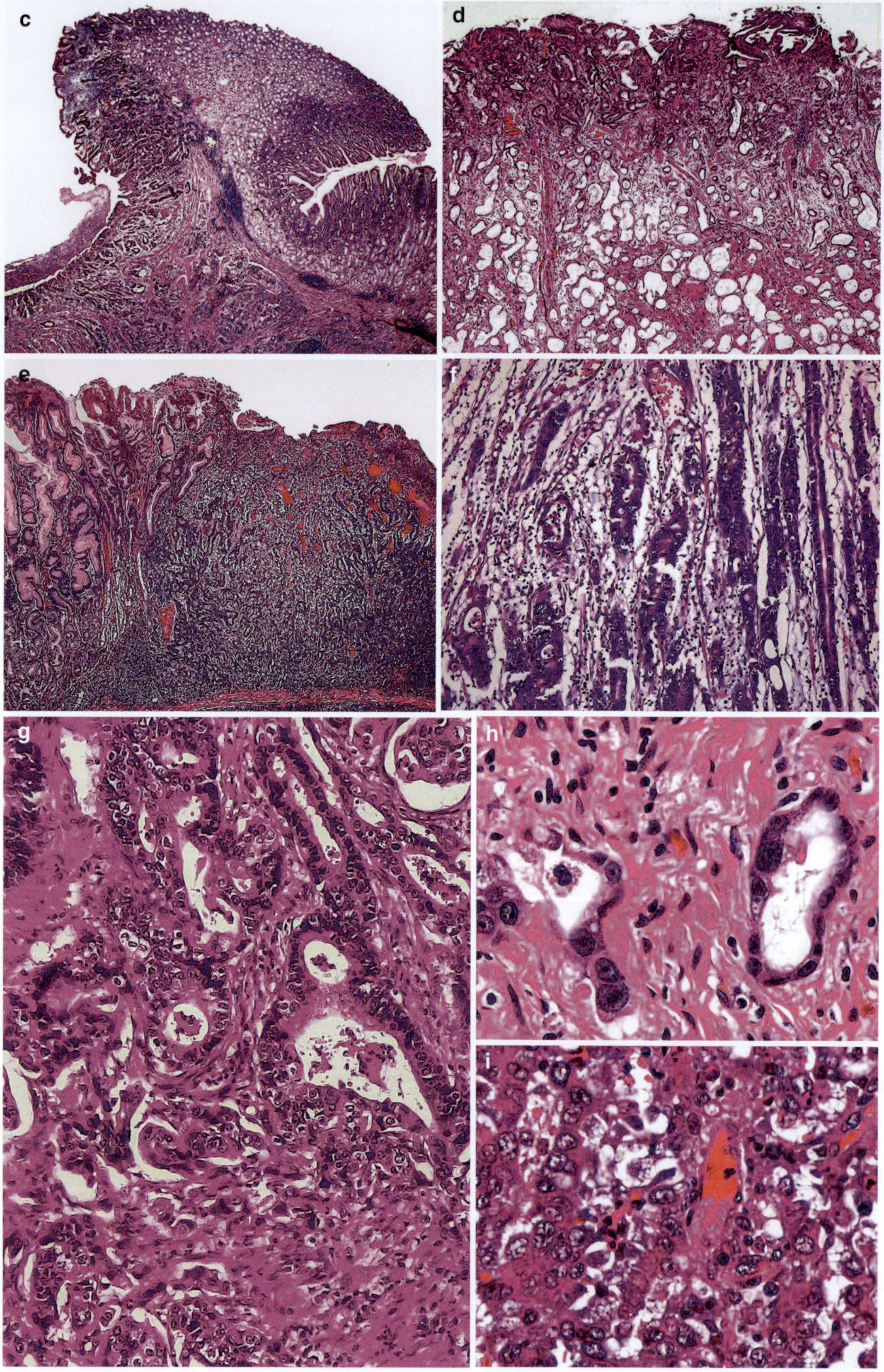

Sections show irregularly distended, fused, or branching malignant gastric glands variable in sizes and shapes and embedded in fibrous stroma infiltrated with chronic inflammatory cells. Tumor cells infiltrate upward, causing ulceration of the gastric mucosa, and downward to infiltrate the muscle layer. The tumor cells are pleomorphic with an increased nuclear/cytoplasmic ratio and prominent nucleoli.

Ancillary Tools

IHC [7]:

IHC is not usually required to make the diagnosis.

IHC is used to confirm the HER2 status and the PDL1 status (with HER2 in situ hybridization if required), although HER2 expression is heterogenous in 40% of gastric cancers and multiple biopsies are recommended to obtain a meaningful result.

Molecular/cytogenetics description [8]:

Next-generation sequencing for microsatellite instability (MSI), high tumor mutational burden (TMB), or NTRK gene fusions can be performed to guide targeted therapeutic agents.

Infiltrating Carcinoma of Pylorus

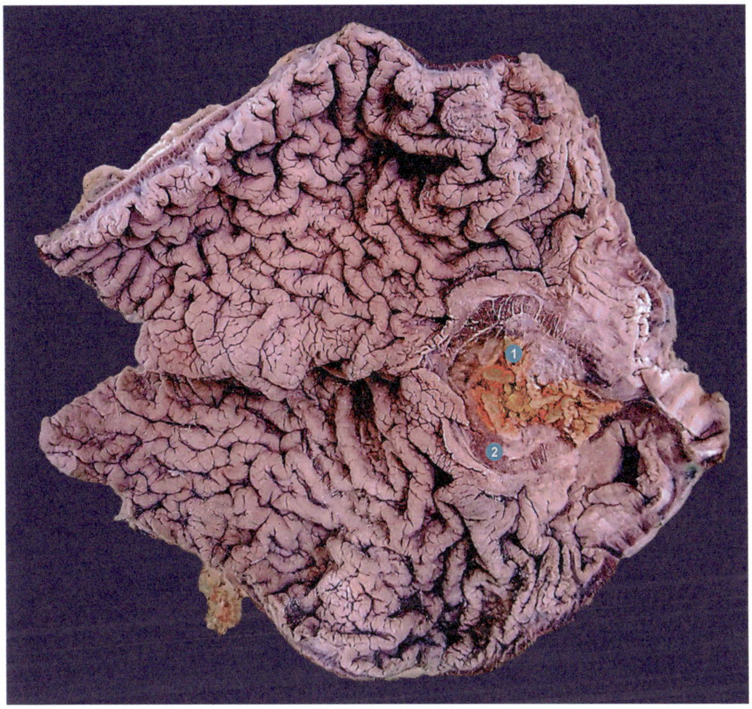

An opened stomach is mounted.

1. The pyloric part is diffusely infiltrated by tumor tissue, producing thickening of the wall and narrowing of the pyloric canal.
2. The tumor infiltrates the muscle layer.

Localized Infiltrating Carcinoma

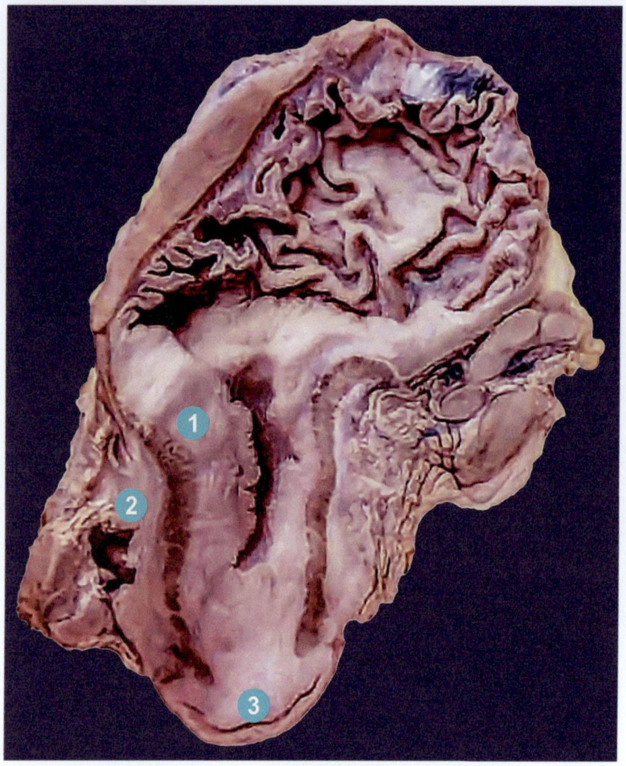

The distal half of the stomach is mounted.

1. An extensive thickening of the wall by a pale tumor mass diffusely infiltrates the layers of the gastric wall.
2. The tumor insinuates between the muscularis propria into the serosa.
3. The tumor obstructs the gastric outlet.

Linitis Plastica

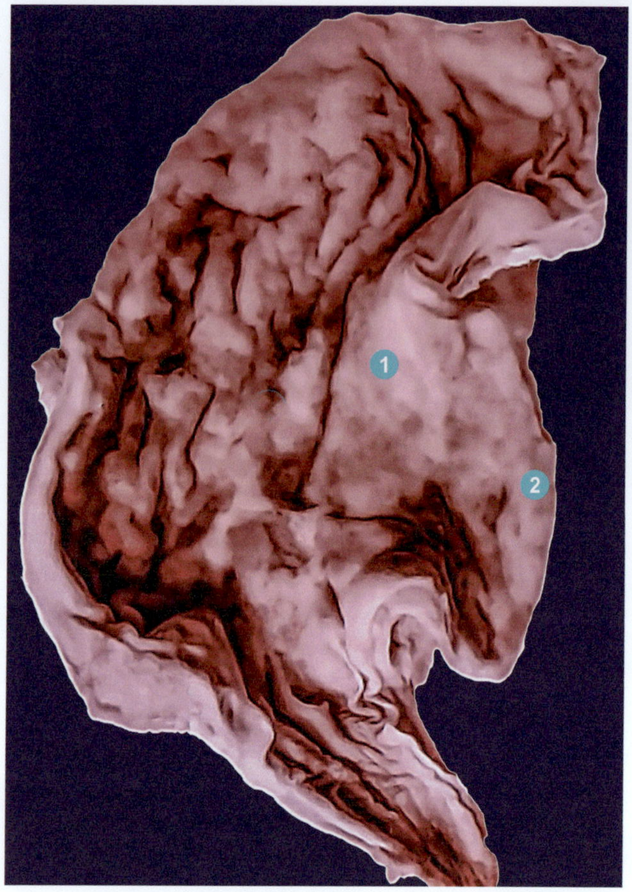

An opened stomach is mounted.

1. The stomach at lesser curvature shows an extensive thickening of the wall by a pale tumor mass diffusely infiltrating the layers of the gastric wall.
2. The tumor insinuates between the muscularis propria into the serosa.

Microscopic Picture of Linitis Plastica (a–c)

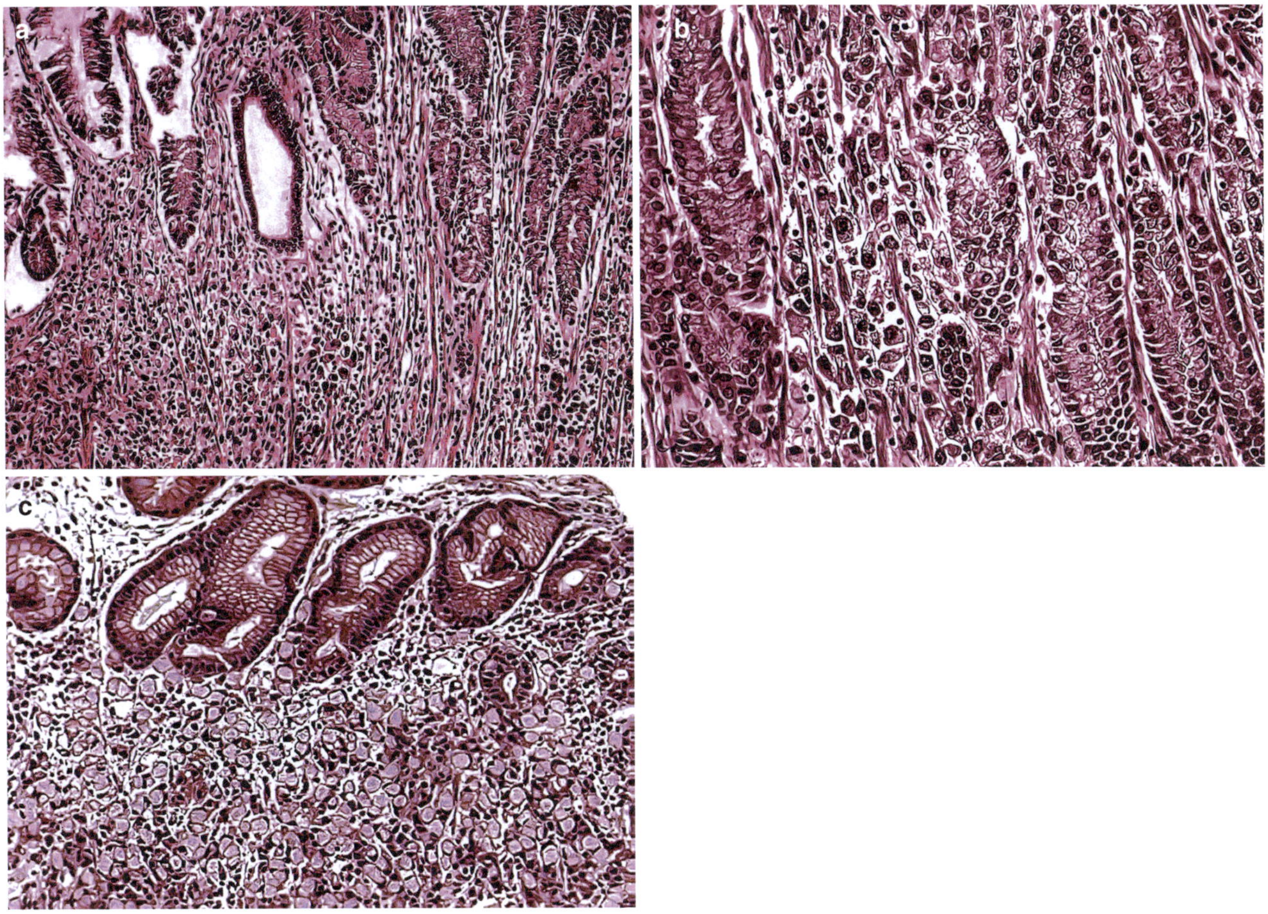

Sections show diffuse infiltration of the submucosa by poorly differentiated malignant tumor cells with abundant cytoplasmic mucin, giving them a signet ring appearance.

Ancillary Tools [7]

IHC:

Cytokeratin AE1/AE3, CEA, EMA, keratin, villin.

Molecular/cytogenetics description:

Mutations in the CDH1 gene leading to reduced E-cadherin expression

Activated ErbB2/ErbB3 complex in signet ring cell carcinoma binds PI3K, leading to phosphorylation of tyrosine residues and activation of downstream pathways, including p38 MAP kinase.

Activation of p38 MAP kinase leads to loss of cell-to-cell contact by disruption of adherent junctions. MUC4 has been reported to increase activation of the ErbB2/ErbB3 complex. MUC4 belongs to the family of mucins that are normally expressed in gastric mucosae (MUC1, MUC5AC, MUC6) or expressed de novo in gastric cancer (MUC2, MUC4).

4.4 Small Intestine Lesions

4.4.1 Congenital Lesions

Meckel's Diverticulum

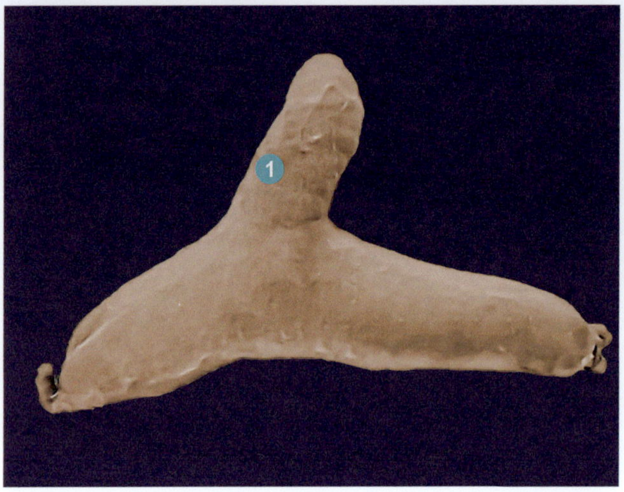

A piece of ileum is mounted.

1. A blinded end diverticulum arising from antimesenteric border of ileum.

Microscopic Picture of Meckel's Diverticulum containing Gastric Mucosa (a)

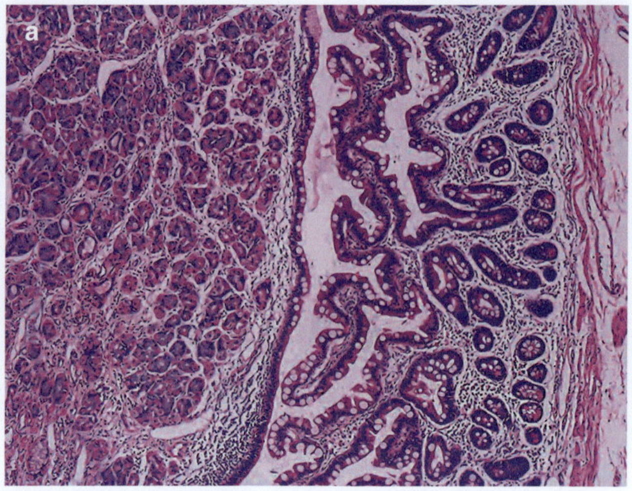

The section shows the wall of the diverticulum lined with small intestine mucosa (on the right-hand side). The other part shows benign-looking gastric mucosa.

Pearls

Meckel's diverticulum is a remnant of the omphalomesenteric duct, which connects the developing embryo to the yolk sac during early fetal development. Normally, this duct disappears by the seventh week of gestation, but in some individuals, it fails to close completely, leading to the formation of Meckel's diverticulum. In most cases, Meckel's diverticulum does not cause any symptoms and goes unnoticed throughout a person's life. However, in some cases, it can lead to complications and cause abdominal pain, gastrointestinal bleeding, or other symptoms [9].

4.4.2 Inflammatory Lesions

Tuberculous Lymphadenitis of the Ileocecal Region (a, b)

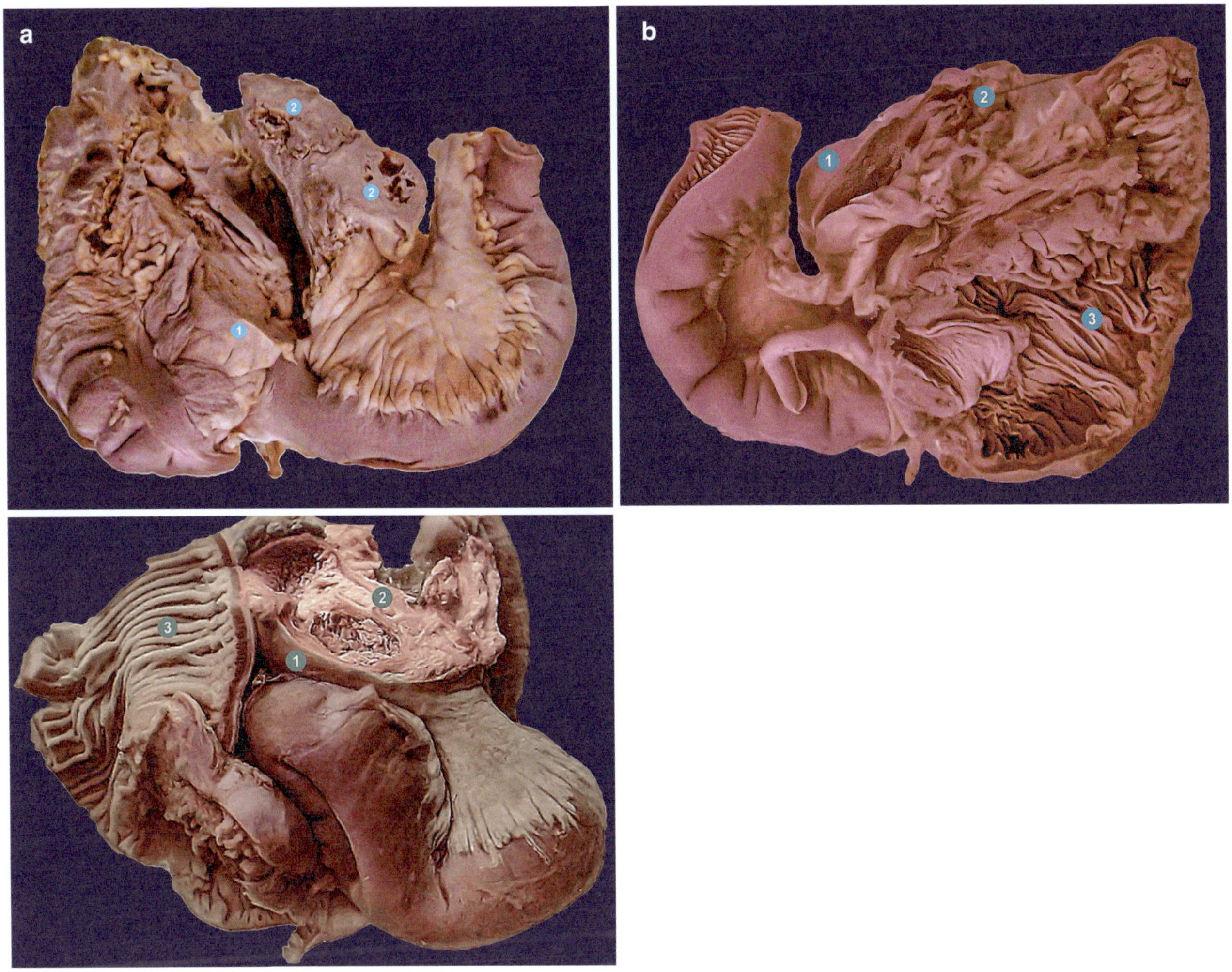

The specimen is formed of the terminal part of the ileum, cecum, and appendix.

1. A mass of matted lymph nodes is seen at the ileocecal junction.
2. The cut section is yellow with caseation and focal tiny cavitation resulting from fallen caseous material.
3. No apparent lesions are seen in the mucosa.

The patient presented with a mass in the right iliac fossa, which was removed for fear of neoplasia.

Tuberculous Ulcers of the Small Intestine

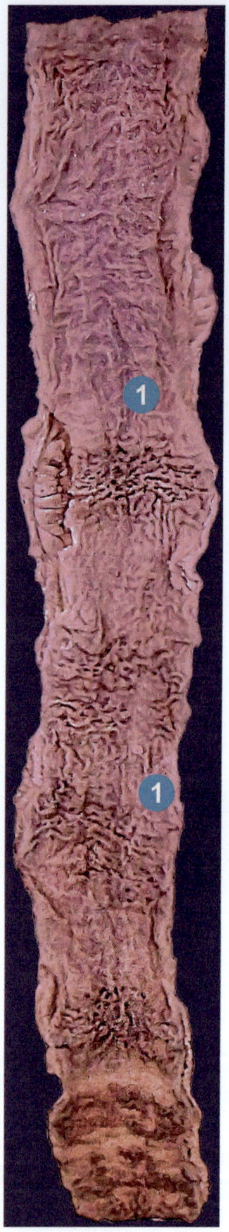

A loop of the small intestine is mounted.

1. It shows multiple transverse mucosal ulcers lying perpendicular to the long axis of the bowel wall (girdle ulcers).

The ulceration has occurred at the sites of necrosis and fibrosis of lymphatics.

Microscopic Picture of Tuberculous Ulcers of Small Intestine (a)

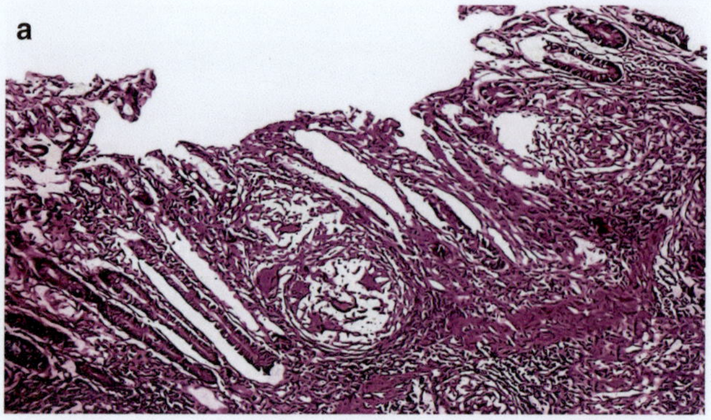

The section shows multiple epithelioid granulomas in the submucosa with focal ulceration of epithelium. Granulomas are formed of epithelioid cells, multinucleated Langhans giant cells, and lymphocytes with focal caseation necrosis and fibrosis of the surrounding stroma.

Typhoid Ulcers of the Small Intestine

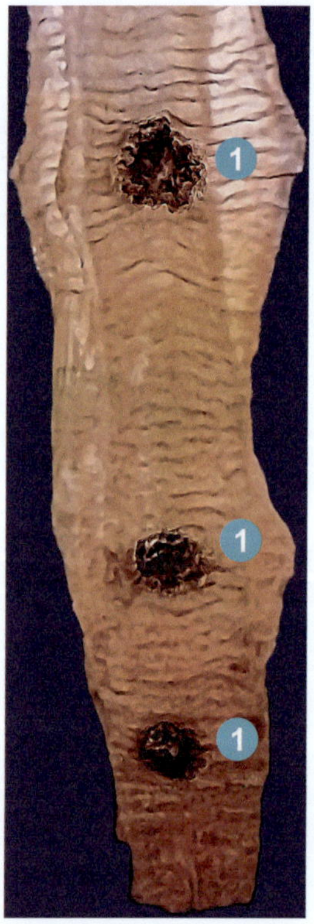

An opened segment of the small intestine is mounted.

1. Several ovoid mucosal ulcers lying parallel to the bowel wall are seen.

The ulceration has occurred at the site of necrosis of Peyer's patches.

4.4.3 Mechanical Lesions

Strangulated Hernia (a, b)

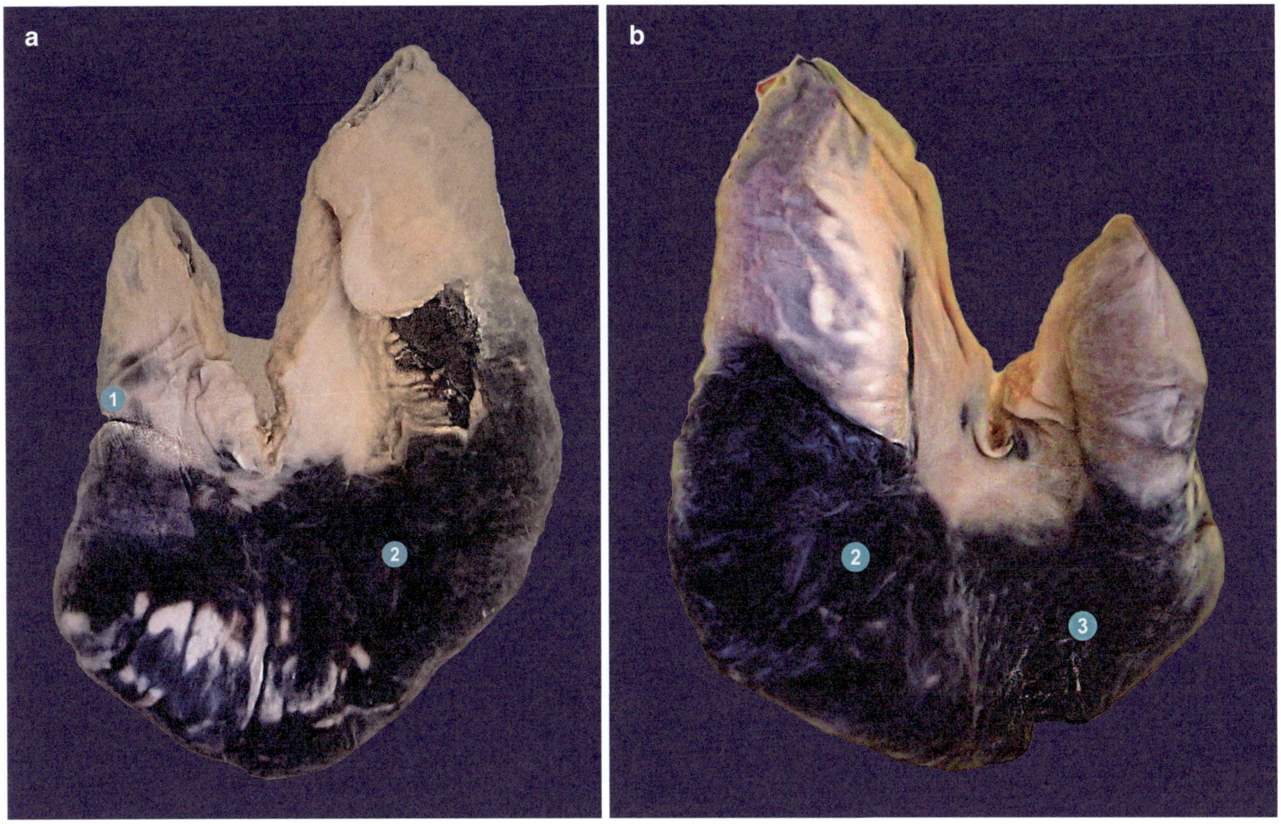

A loop of the small intestine with mesentery is mounted.

1. It shows constriction at its upper part, where it was compressed by the inguinal ring.
2. The loop is swollen, gangrenous, and black-red.
3. An area of perforation.

The patient presented with manifestations of acute intestinal obstruction (acute constipation, vomiting, and shock).

Ileoileal Intussusception (a, b)

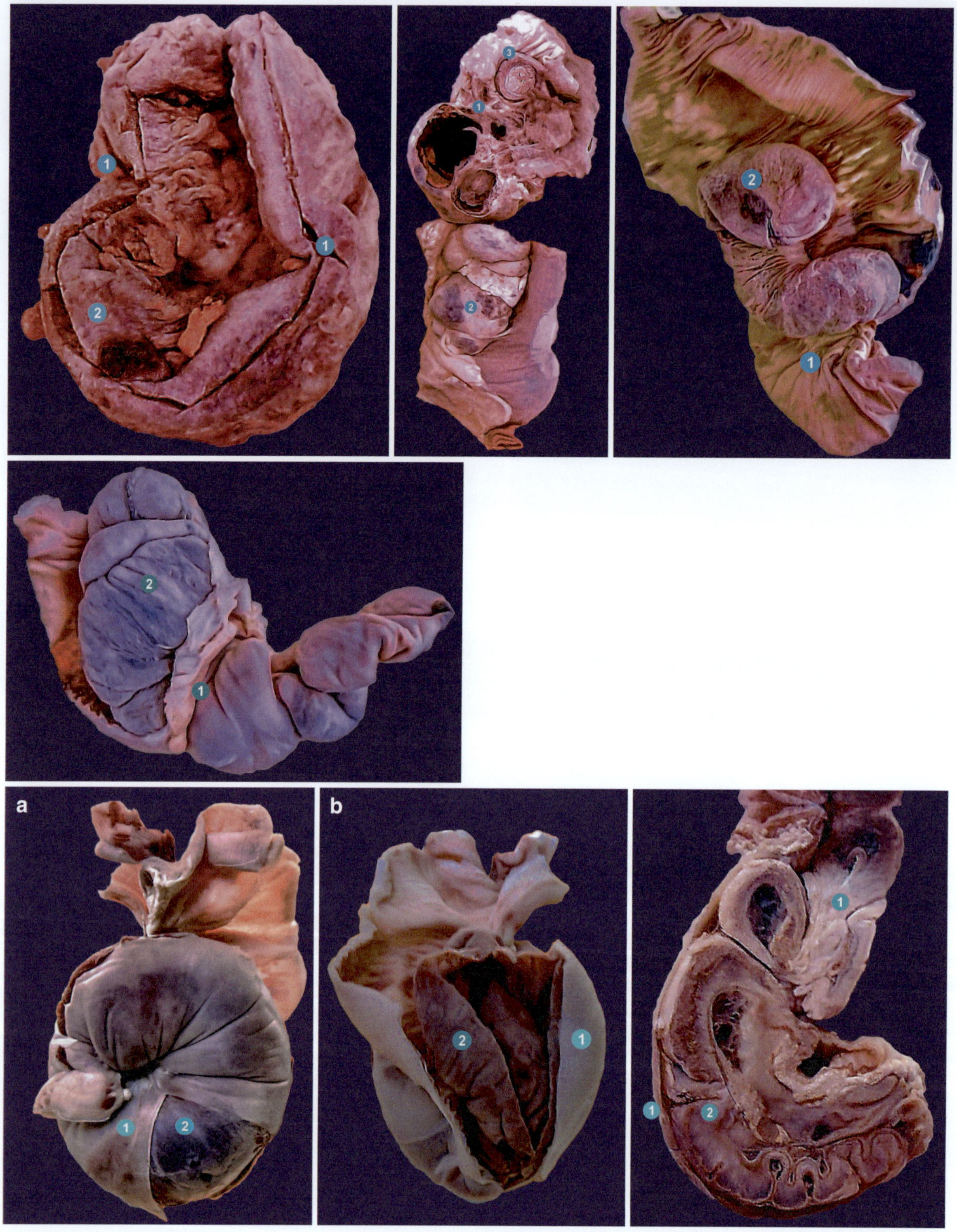

A loop of the small intestine is mounted.

1. Invagination of one part of the ileum telescoping into another part of the ileum. The invaginated outer part (intussuscepien) is partially removed to expose the inner part (intussusceptum).
2. Intussusceptum appears swollen, macerated, and black because of gangrene.
3. A round encapsulated benign tumor is displayed. It was the cause of irregular peristalsis, which results in the condition. It was proved microscopically to be a GIST.

Ileocecal Intussusception

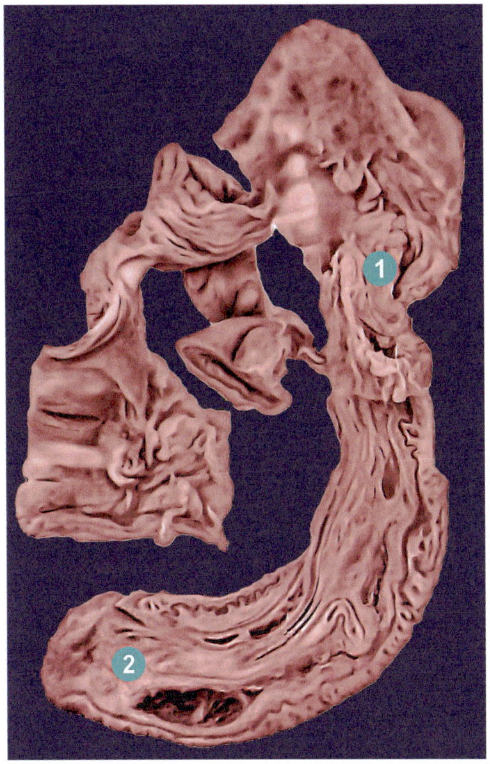

A loop of the small intestine is mounted.

1. There is an invagination of the ileum into the cecum. The invaginated outer part (intussuscepien) is partially removed to expose the inner part (intussusceptum).
2. The intussusceptum appears swollen and congested.

4.4.4 Neoplastic Lesions

Neuroendocrine Tumor (NET) of Small Intestine

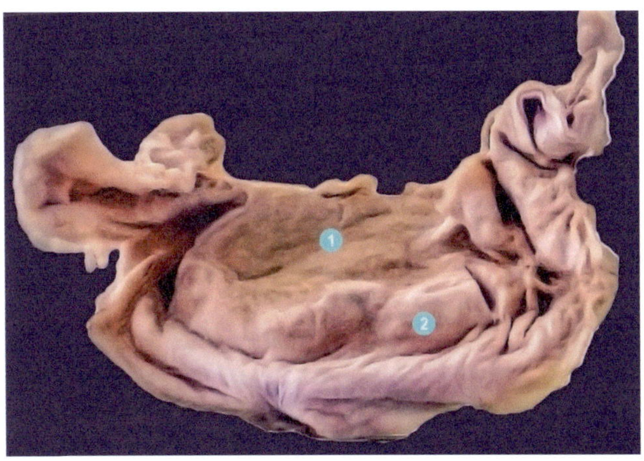

A loop of small intestine is mounted.

1. There is a submucosal, well-defined, encapsulated, ovoid, solid mass projecting in the lumen.
2. The tumor is covered by an intact mucosa.

Ileal Neuroendocrine Tumor (NET)

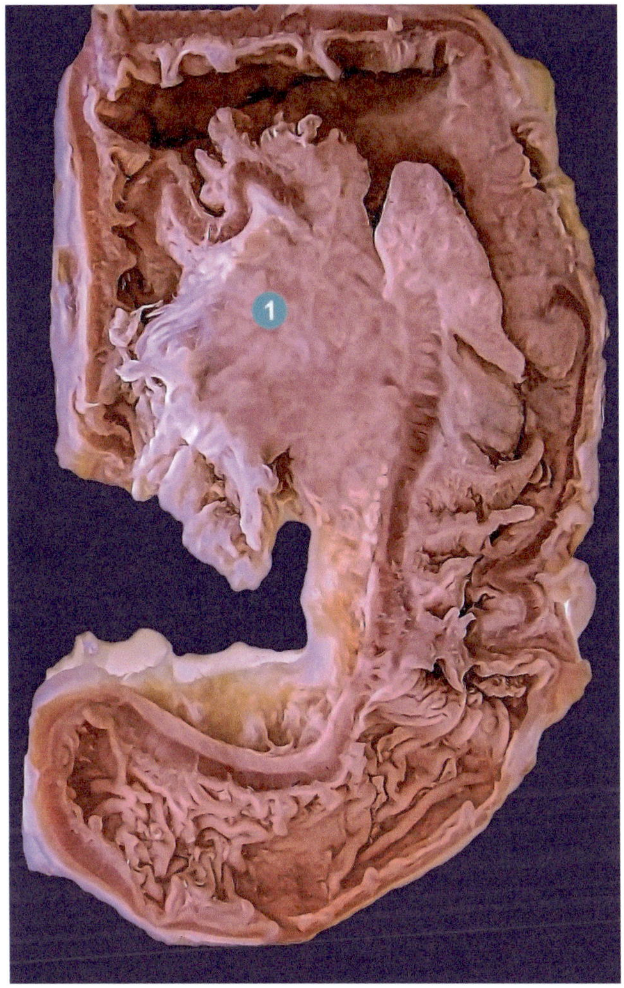

Part of the ileum, cecum, and appendix are sectioned longitudinally.

1. There is a homogenous, well-defined mass at the ileum protruding through the mucosa as a polypoid lesion with intact overlying mucosa causing mild obstruction of the lumen of the ileum.

Microscopic Picture of Neuroendocrine Tumor (NET) of Small Intestine (a–c)

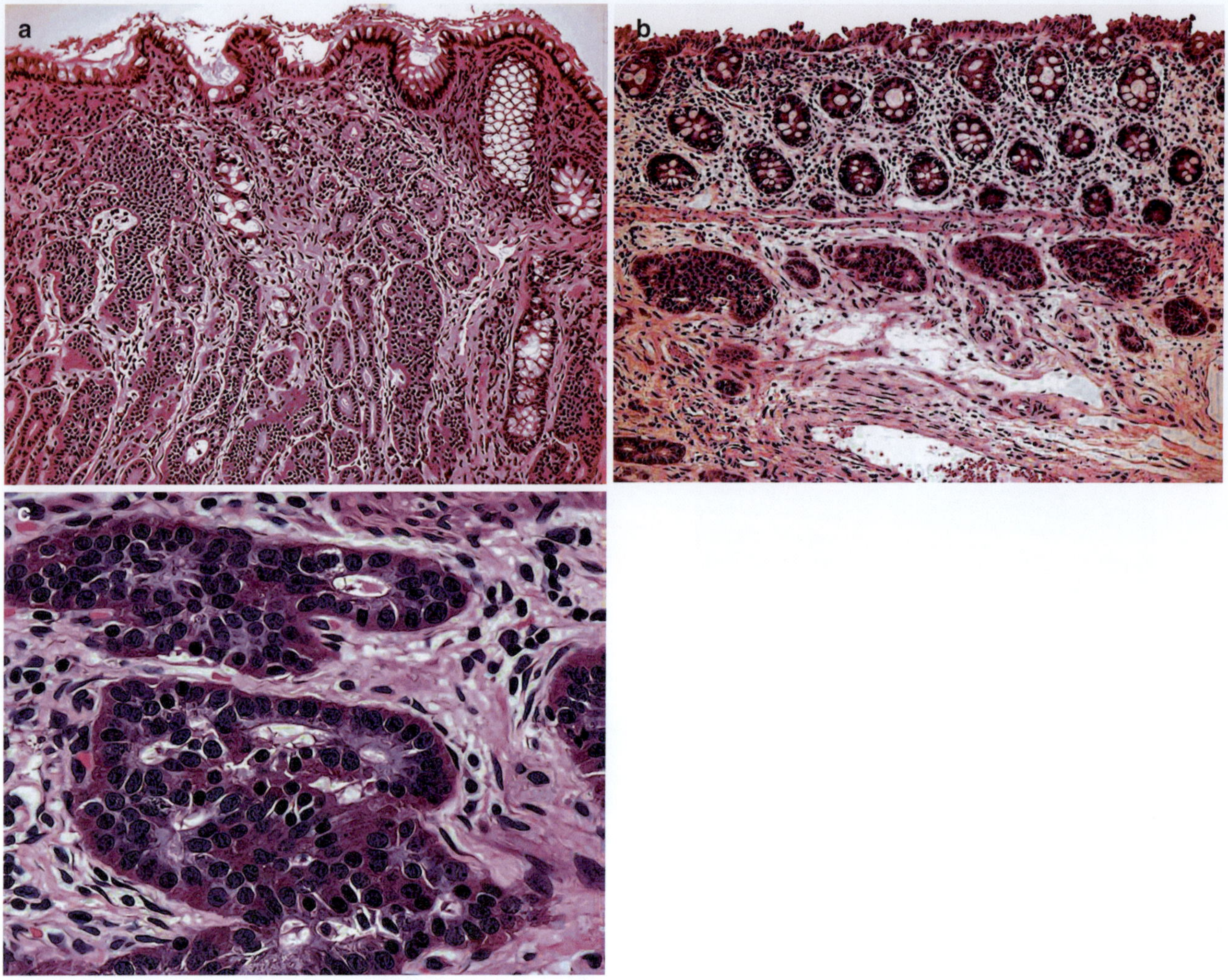

Sections show monotonous uniform tumor cells showing round to oval nuclei with salt and pepper chromatin present in the submucosa of the small intestine. The tumor cells are arranged in a trabecular and glandular pattern and separated by fibrovascular tissue.

Ancillary Tools

IHC [10]:

AE1/AE3, CAM5.2

Chromogranin A, synaptophysin

Somatostatin-expressing NETs are less likely to express chromogranin A

CDX2 and SSTR2A are positive in serotonin-producing EC cell NETs

Molecular/cytogenetics description [11]:

Small intestinal NETs have a complex genomic landscape:

- 60–90% of jejunoileal NETs show chromosome 18 deletion
- Chromosome 14 gain in advanced lesions and metastases
- CDKN1B mutations in ≤10% of ileal NETs
- Epigenetic changes are common

>50% of ileal NETs are CpG island methylator phenotype

Substantial epigenetic dysregulation found in 70–80% of tumors

- 3 molecular subgroups with potential prognostic impact
- Favorable prognosis: small intestinal NET with chromosome 18 loss (55%). Correlates with CpG island methylator phenotype negativity and CDKN1B mutation
- Intermediate prognosis: small intestinal NET with no whole arm copy number variation (19%). Correlates with CpG island methylator phenotype positivity
- Poor prognosis: small intestinal NET with multiple whole arm copy number variations (26%)

Infiltrating Carcinoma of the Duodenum

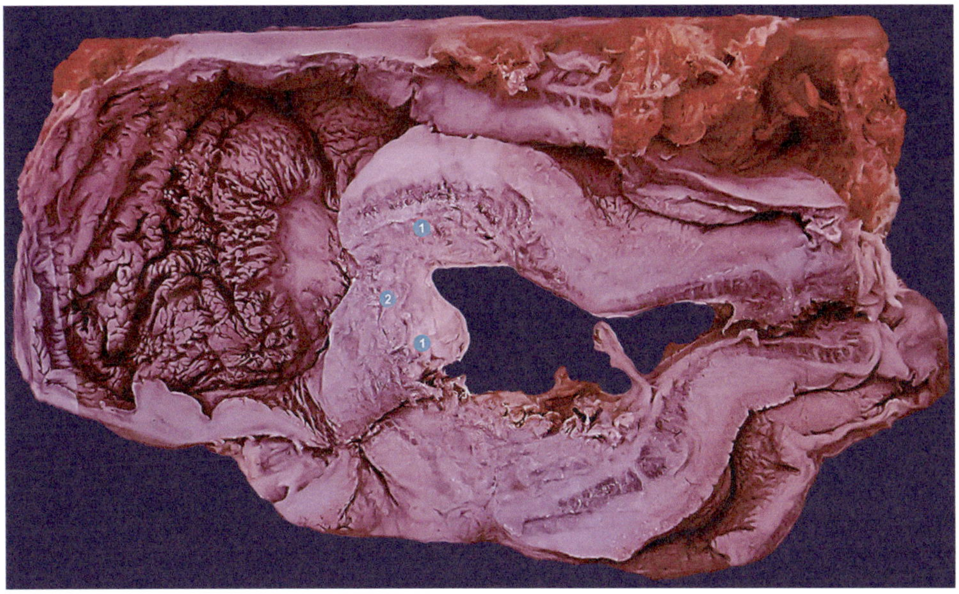

The third part of the duodenum was opened and mounted.

1. A large exophytic mass obstructs the lumen partially with dilatation of the duodenum above the obstruction.
2. The tumor infiltrates the muscle layer in areas.

Microscopic Picture of Moderately and Poorly Differentiated Adenocarcinoma of Duodenum (Intestinal Type) (a, b)

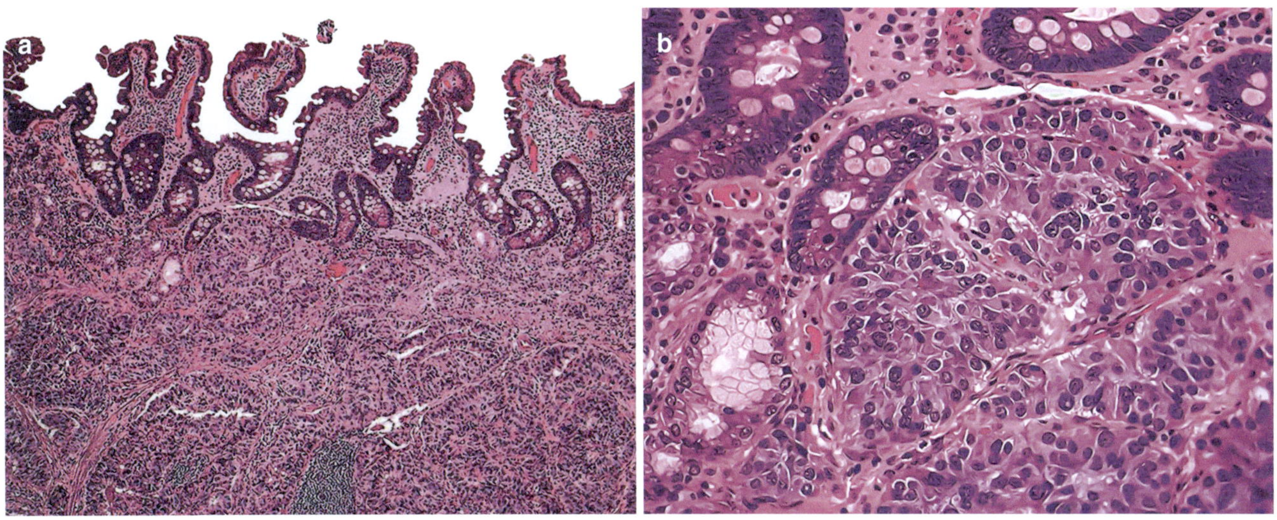

Sections show malignant columnar epithelial cells with elongated, pseudostratified nuclei forming poorly formed glands, complex glandular architecture, cellular and nuclear pleomorphism, and loss of epithelial polarity.

Ancillary Tools

IHC [12]:

CK7, CK20 (variable)

CDX2 in up to 70% of cases

SATB2 in up to 46% of cases, with patchy and weak staining in most cases and strong and diffuse staining in <10% of cases

MUC1 (EMA): positive in up to 53% of cases

MUC2: positive in up to 57% of cases

Villin: positive in up to 67% of cases (can be focal)

Small intestinal mucin antigen (SIMA): variably positive in up to 50% of cases

p53: strong, diffuse overexpression, or completely negative (mutated phenotype) in a subset of mutated tumors

MUC5AC: focally in up to 40% of cases

MUC6: focally in up to 30% of cases.

Molecular/cytogenetics description [13]:

Two well-defined molecular pathways are reported in small bowel adenocarcinomas, similar to colorectal adenocarcinoma tumorigenesis.

The first pathway includes APC, KRAS, and TP53. The prevalence of mutations in KRAS is similar between colorectal and small bowel adenocarcinomas, typically 30–60%. The prevalence of TP53 mutations is also comparable, 20–50%. Fewer than 20% of small bowel adenocarcinomas have mutations in APC, in contrast to 80% of colorectal carcinomas.

The second pathway includes inactivation of mismatch repair (MMR) genes, either by germline mutations (Lynch syndrome) or promoter hypermethylation (sporadic), which occurs in up to 38.5% of small bowel adenocarcinomas.

Several other genetic alterations have been reported in small bowel adenocarcinomas, including mutations in CTNNB1, SMAD4, IDH1, CDH1, KIT, FGFR2, FLT3, NPM1, PTEN, MET, AKT, RET, ERBB2 (HER2), NOTCH1, and ERBB4.

Pearls

Tumors arising in the non-ampullaryV (extra-ampullary) segment of the duodenum are considered true "duodenal cancers." These primary "duodenal" carcinomas are rare and constitute 35–50% of all small intestinal carcinomas. Their analysis is frequently combined with other small bowel, pancreatic, and distal bile duct cancers (periampullary cancers) that have caused marked confusion in the literature regarding their frequency and clinicopathologic characteristics [14].

Periampullary Carcinoma

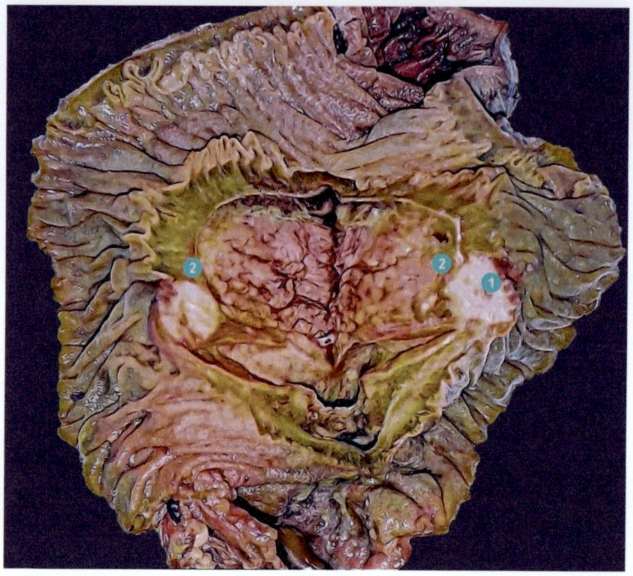

An opened piece of duodenum is mounted.

1. A small, exophytic mass arising from the duodenal aspect of the ampulla obscures the ampullary orifice.
2. The invasive component of the lesion extends beyond the ampulla to involve the adjacent duodenal wall.

Microscopic Picture of Pancreatobiliary Carcinoma (a–e)

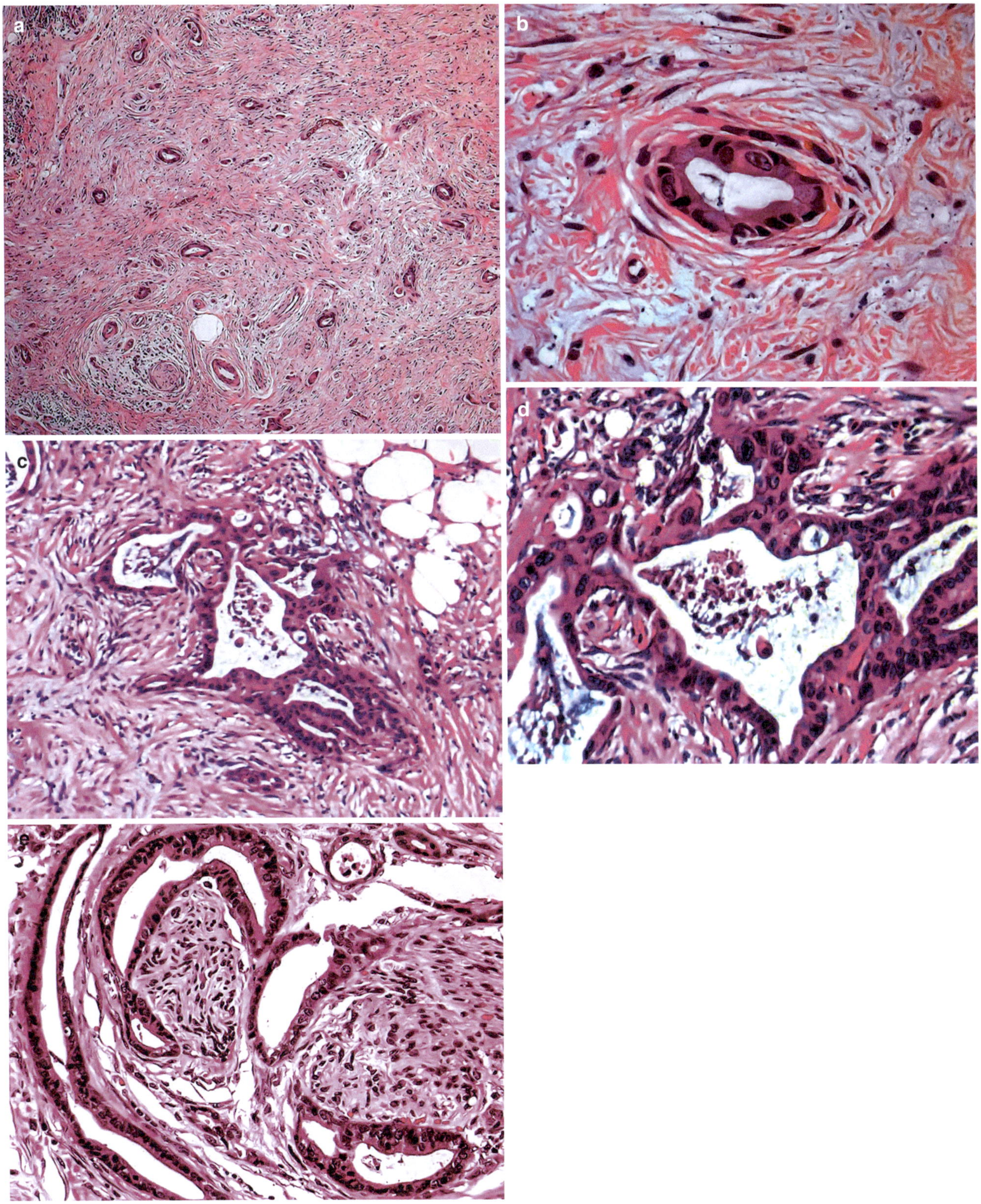

Sections show pleomorphic cuboidal cells forming small glands in a desmoplastic stroma with the presence of areas of perineural invasion.

Ancillary Tools

IHC:

Intestinal-type tumors are typically positive for CK20 (50%), CDX2 (> 25% of tumor staining, 89.5%), and S100P (63%) with variable CK7 (70–80%) Pancreatobiliary-type tumors are positive for MUC1 (100%), CK7 (91%) [15].

Molecular/cytogenetics description [16]:

KRAS mutations are present in 30–40%, may be associated with worse disease-free survival, and are more frequently found in pancreaticobiliary-type tumors.

TP53 is also a negative predictor of survival, regardless of phenotype.

Microsatellite instability is present in 10–15%, usually in intestinal-type tumors.

Other mutations detected include: APC, PIK3CA, SMAD4, BRAF, CDKN2A, FBXW7, TP53, APC, ELF3, and RAS mutations.

Targetable mutations have been identified in both intestinal and pancreatobiliary phenotype tumors.

General: ERBB, WNT, and PI3K

Intestinal phenotype: PI3/AKT

Pancreatobiliary phenotype: RAS/RAF and PI3/AKT

BRAF and KRAS are mutually exclusive.

4.5 Appendiceal Lesions

4.5.1 Inflammatory Lesions

Acute Suppurative Appendicitis

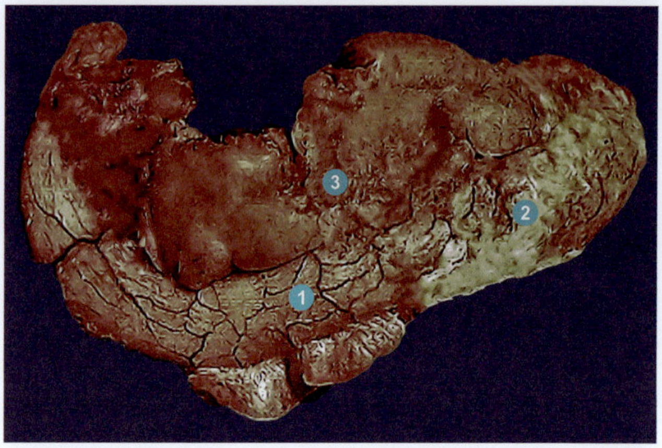

Appendix with mesoappendix is mounted.

1. The appendix is congested, edematous, and hyperemic with the presence of dilated congested vessels over the wall.
2. The wall shows an area of suppuration.
3. The mesoappendix is edematous and congested.

Microscopic Picture of Acute Suppurative Appendicitis (a, b)

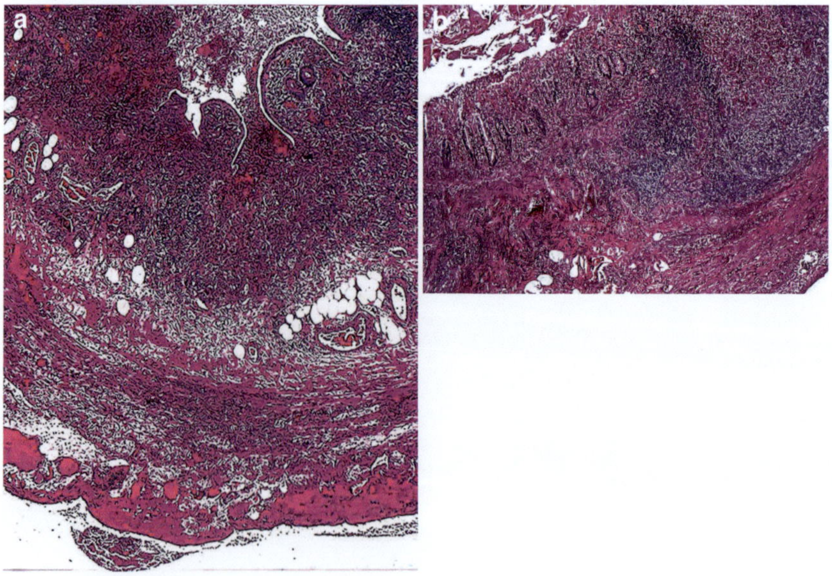

Sections show ulceration of the mucosa and diffuse infiltration of all appendiceal layers and peritoneum by acute inflammatory cells with the presence of dilated congested vessels and interstitial edema.

Simple Mucocele of Appendix

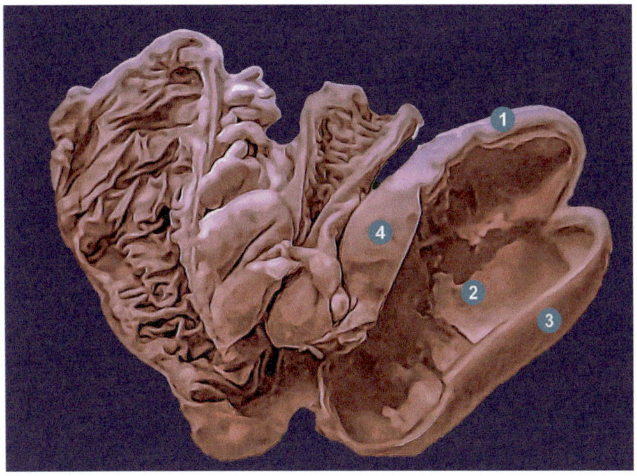

The appendix, opened longitudinally, is mounted.

1. The appendix appears significantly enlarged, distended, and cystically dilated.
2. The lumen of the appendix is filled with thick, gelatinous mucus. The mucus accumulation can lead to the distension of the appendix.
3. The wall of the appendix is translucent due to the accumulation of mucus.
4. The outer surface of the appendix is smooth and intact, without signs of inflammation or ulceration.

Microscopic Picture of Simple Mucocele of Appendix (a, b)

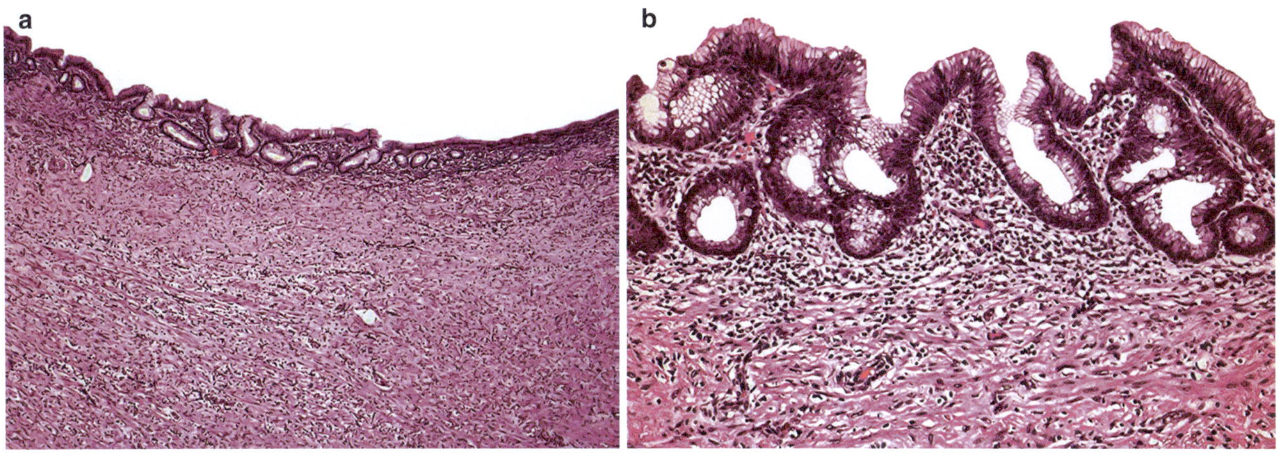

Sections show a dilated appendiceal lumen. The mucosa lining the appendix appears normal with focal atrophy. Submucosa shows interstitial edema and infiltration by sparse chronic inflammatory cells.

4.6 Colorectal Lesions

4.6.1 Inflammatory Lesions

Perianal Fistula (a, b)

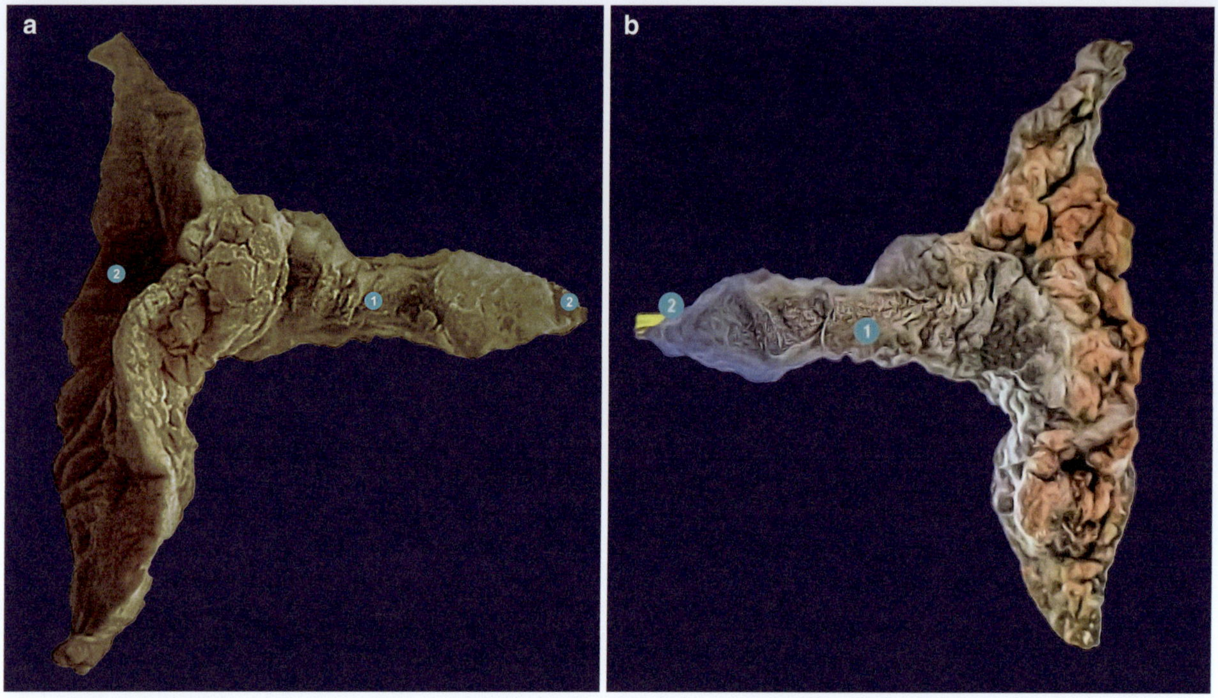

An excised fistula is mounted.

1. An irregularly shaped fibrous tissue excision with an inflamed sinus opening on one surface.
2. A probe followed from the fistula opening; cut surface shows the fistulous tract.

Microscopic Picture of Perianal Fistula (c, d)

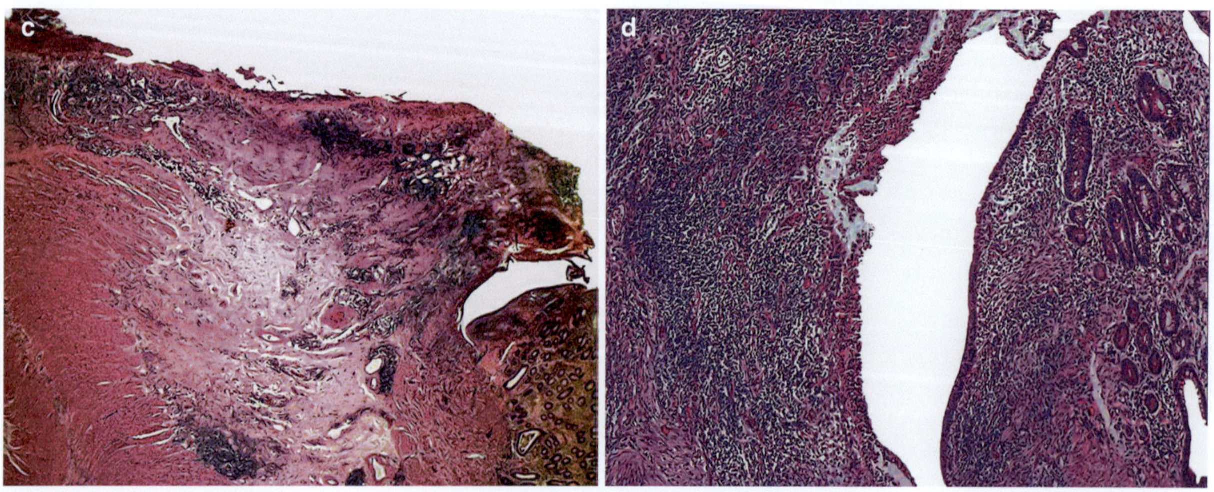

Sections show partially ulcerated colonic mucosa overlying granulation tissue infiltrated densely with acute and chronic inflammatory cells.

Miliary Tuberculosis of Large Intestine (a–g)

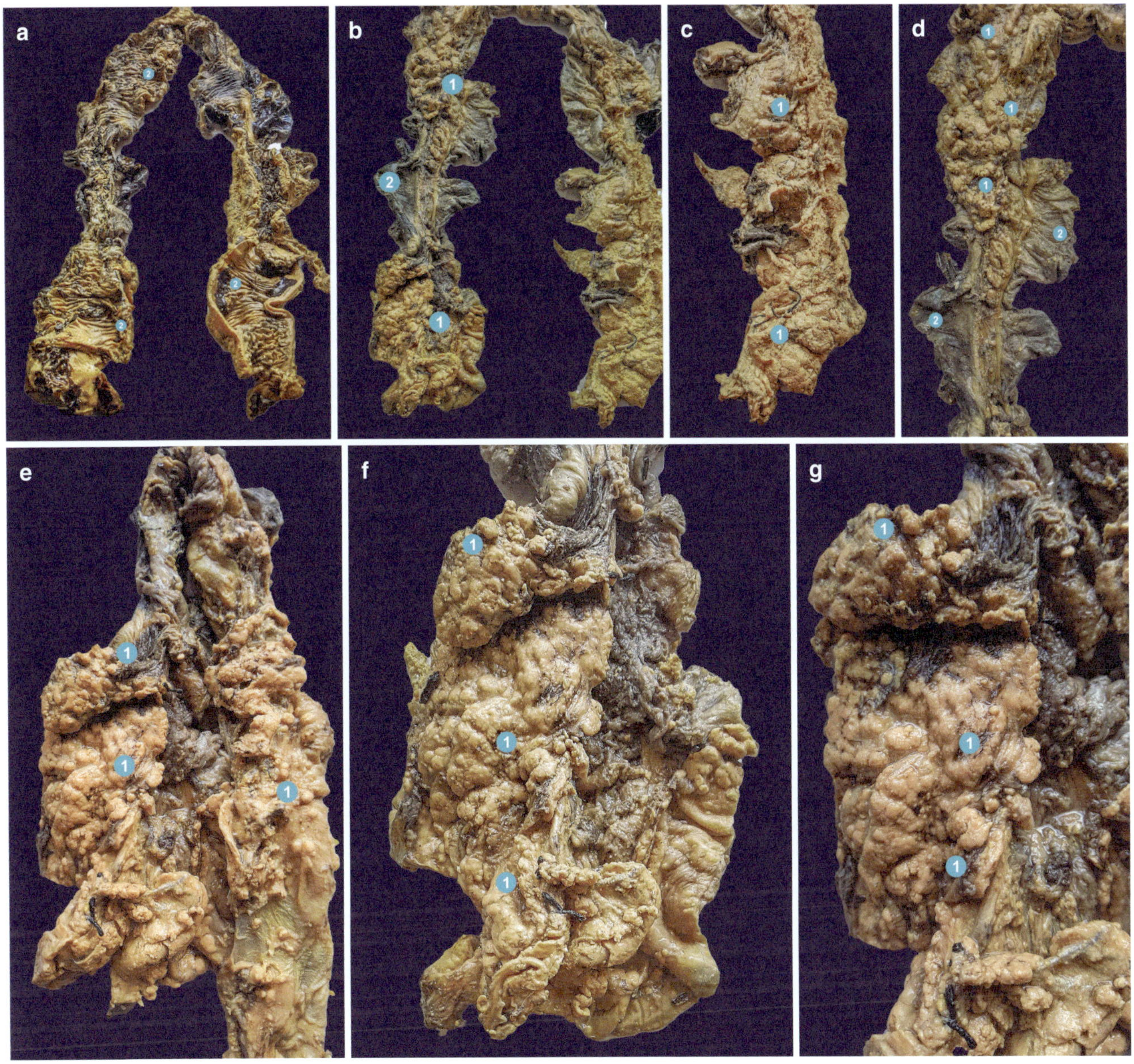

The whole length of the large intestine is mounted.

1. The serosa is extensively infiltrated by nodules of yellow and caseous foci variable in size.
2. The intestinal wall is atrophic and thin with irregular areas of necrosis and mucosal ulceration.

Pearls

Gastrointestinal tuberculosis (GTB) is defined as the involvement of any segment of the digestive tract, associated viscera, and peritoneum. In addition to the fact that its presentation is rare, representing around 1–3% of tuberculosis cases worldwide, the clinical presentation of GTB is nonspecific, so it can be confused with other infectious etiologies or inflammatory bowel disease (IBD) [17].

The presented case is a potential first to be reported with this extensive involvement of the whole large intestine by miliary tuberculosis. The presented case is the autopsy of a woman in her 50s with disseminated miliary tuberculosis, which also affected the entire large intestine. The patient presented with ileus. Despite surgery, the patient sadly passed away one week later.

Pseudomembranous Colitis (Bacillary Dysentery) (a, b)

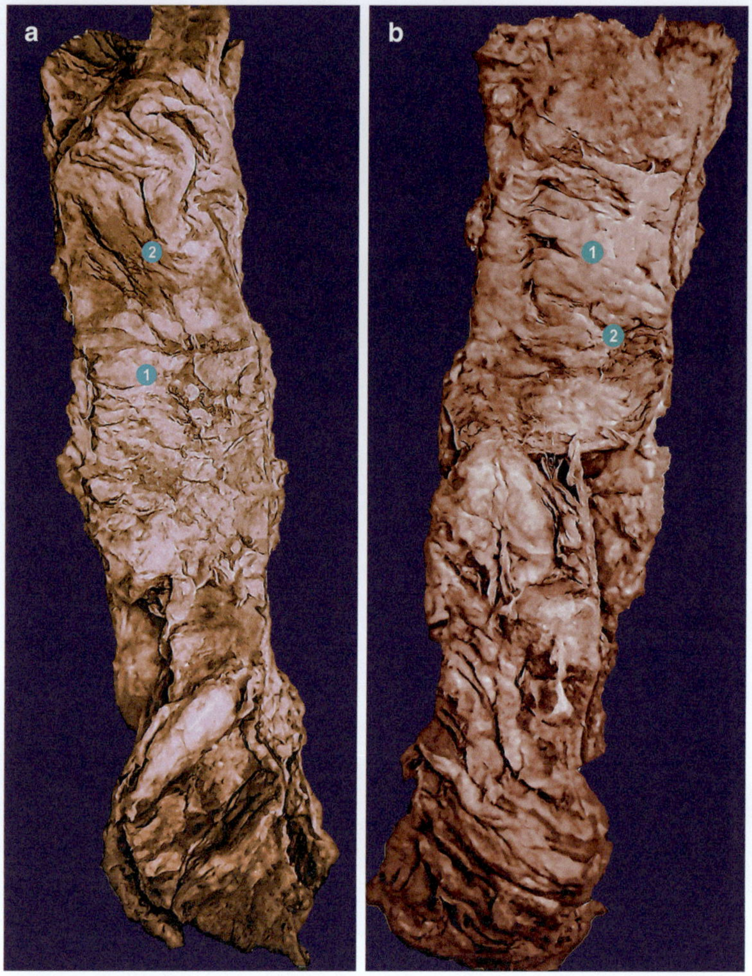

A loop of the large intestine is mounted.

1. The whole mucosa is congested and covered in parts by a dirty, gray-brown membrane.
2. Dark focal areas of ulceration are seen.

Microscopic Picture of Pseudomembranous Colitis (Bacillary Dysentery) (c–f)

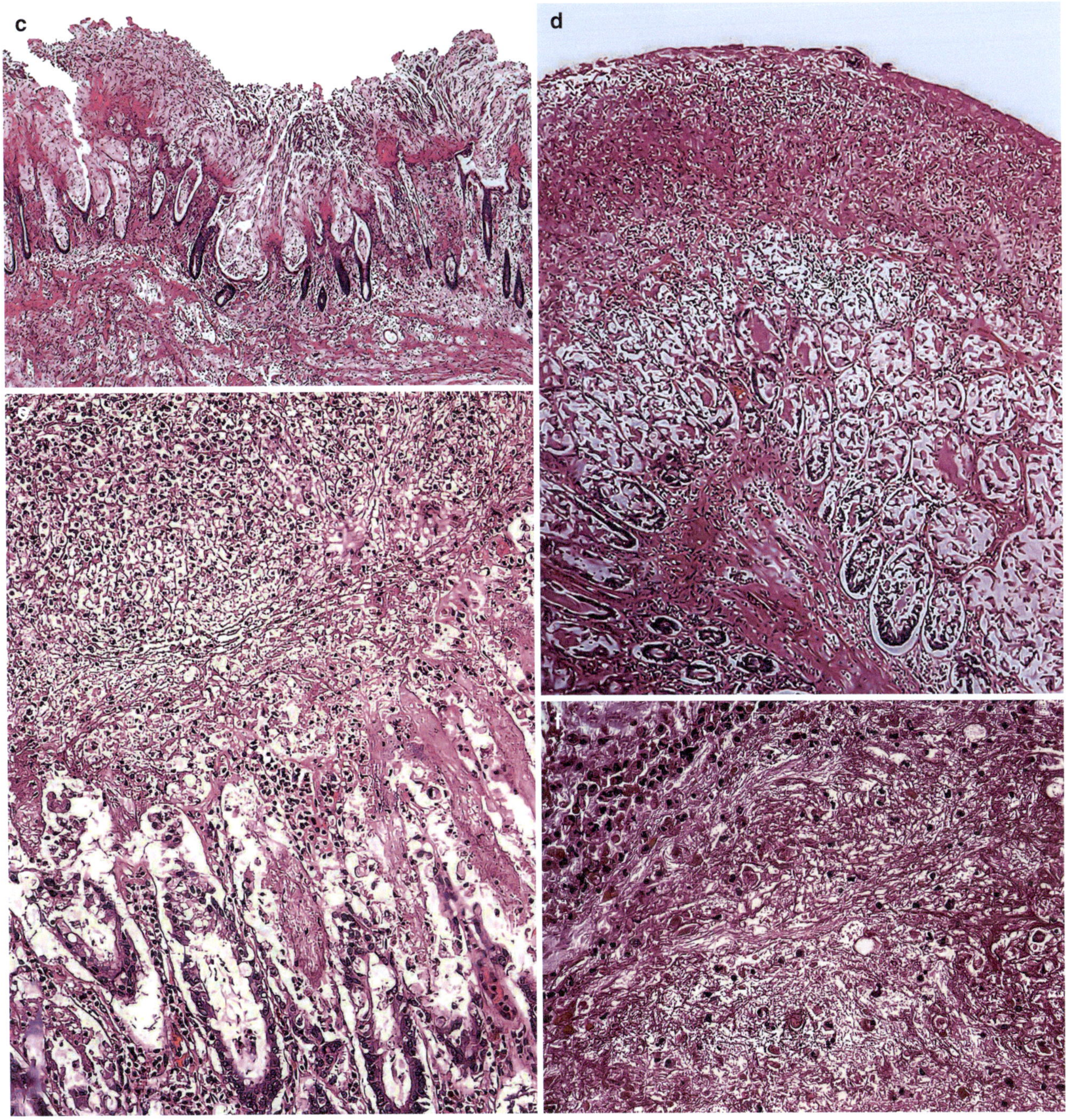

Sections show pseudomembrane on the surface of the ulcerated colonic mucosa, composed of fibrin, necrotic epithelial cells, inflammatory cells, and bacteria. There is necrosis of epithelial cells, erosion and ulceration of the mucosa, and infiltration of inflammatory cells rich in neutrophils into the lamina propria.

Amebic Colitis

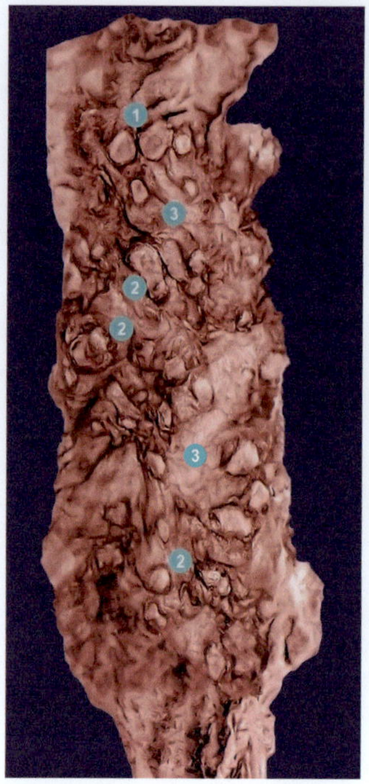

A loop of the large intestine is mounted.

1. Involvement of the entire loop by many necrotizing lesions and ulcers.
2. The lesions are discrete, sharply defined ulcers and erosions with smooth, irregularly shaped borders with white or yellow exudates. Ulcers may coalesce, resulting in larger lesions that may be necrotic in the center.
3. Normal intervening mucosa.

Bilharzial Polyposis of Large Intestine

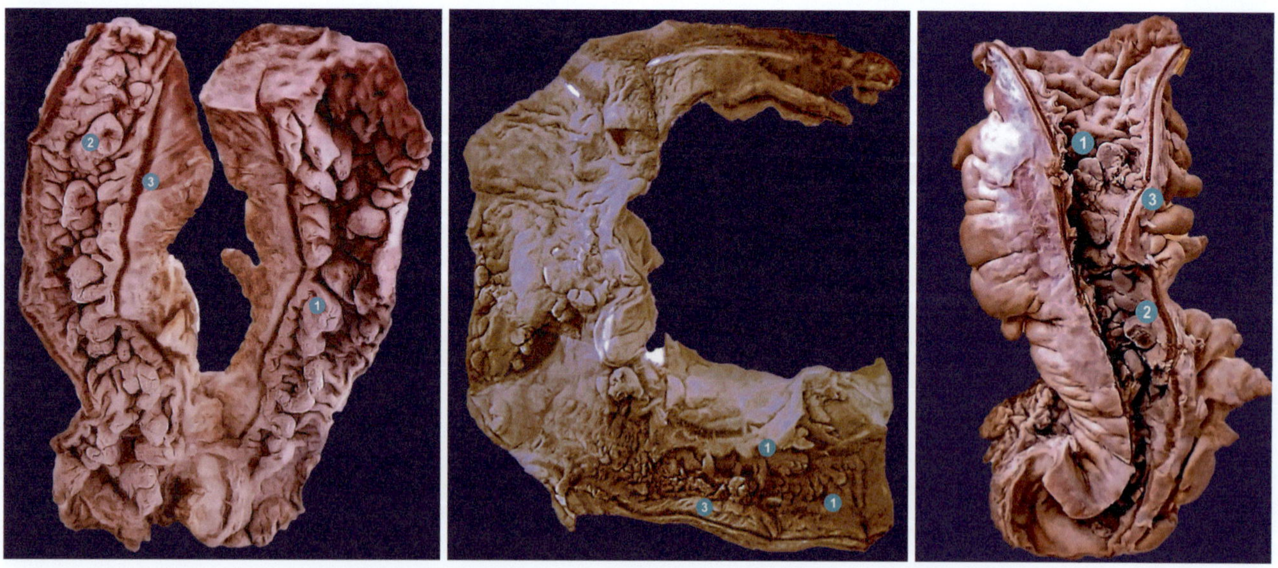

A strip of the rectosigmoid colon is mounted.

1. Numerous sessile and pedunculated polyps variable in size and shape nearly obstructing the lumen are observed.
2. Some polyps show superficial ulceration and hemorrhage.
3. The muscle coat is intact and not infiltrated.

Microscopic Picture of Bilharzial Polyposis of Large Intestine (a–d)

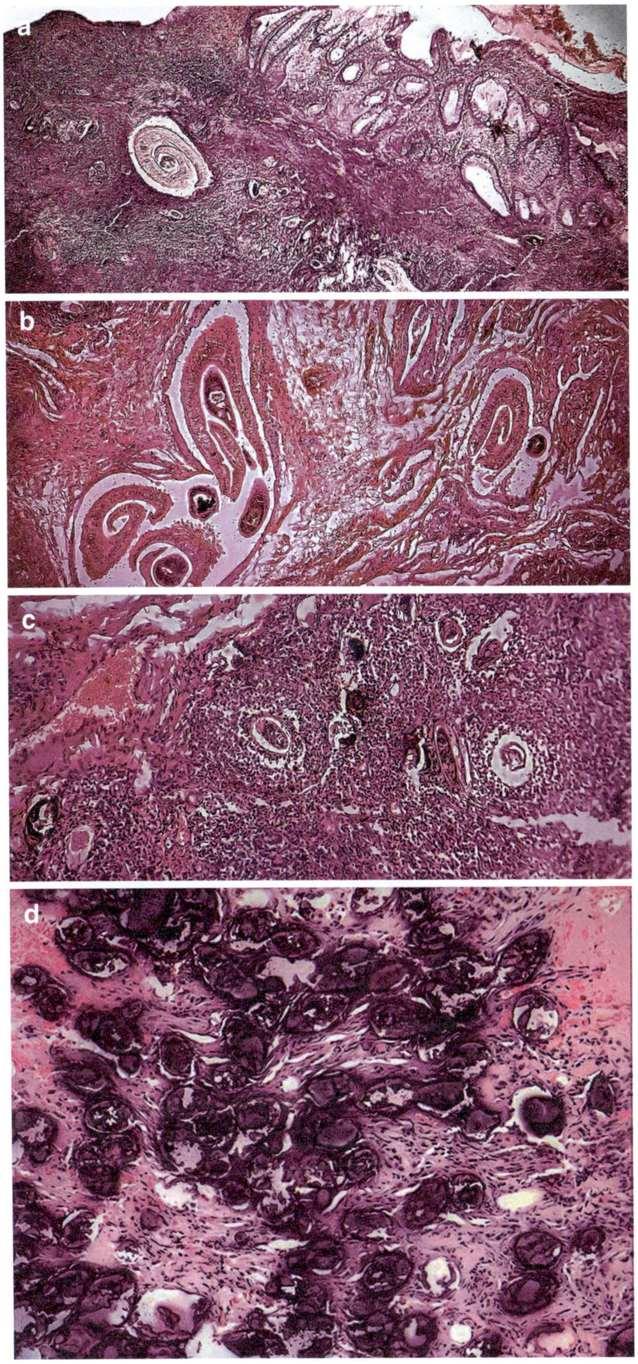

Sections show infiltration of lamina propria and submucosa by living, dead, and calcified bilharzial ova and worms embedded in a fibrous stroma and surrounded by chronic inflammatory cells, including foreign body giant cells.

Chronic Ulcerative Colitis

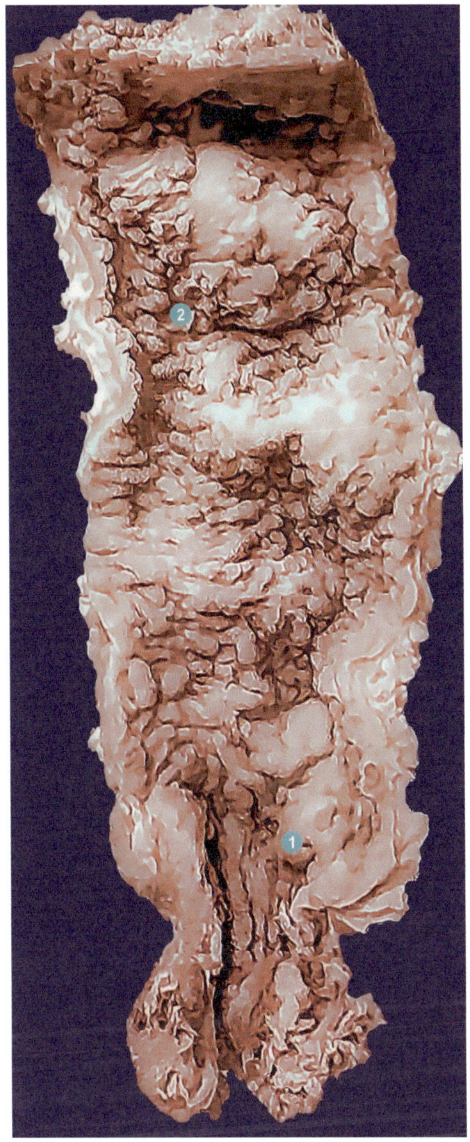

A segment of the rectosigmoid colon is mounted.

1. The distal portion of this rectum has a granular, almost velvety appearance with hemorrhage and shallow ulcers.
2. The segment of the large bowel shows mucosal congestion, and, besides, the mucosa is ‘thrown up’ into innumerable irregular polypoid protrusions. These are not true polyps but simply represent the effects of adjacent ulceration undermining the mucosa with granulation tissue formation. Even when the disease is in remission, these tags may persist as elevated areas between the healed atrophic foci of previously ulcerated mucosa.

Microscopic Picture of Chronic Ulcerative Colitis (a–d)

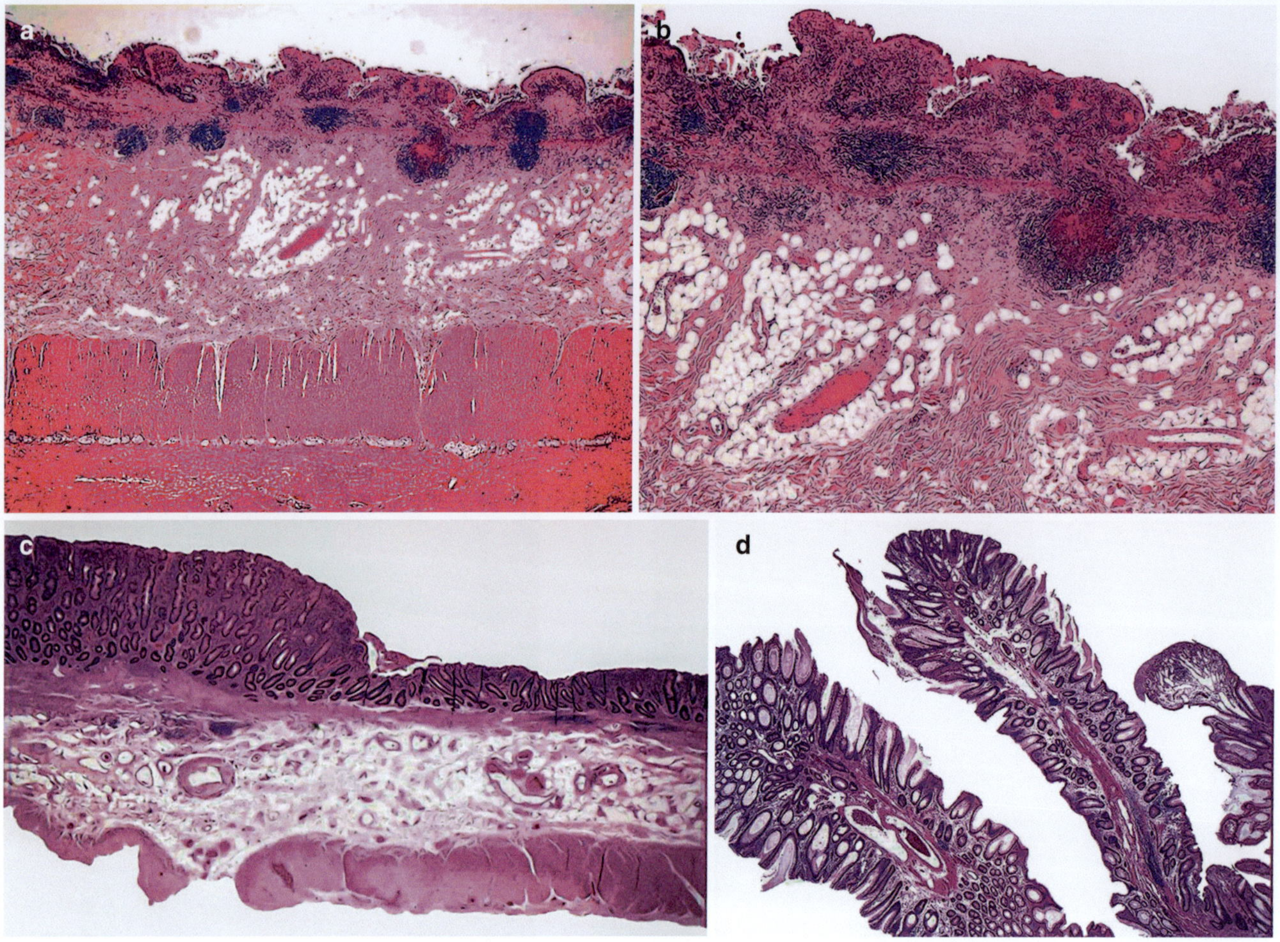

Sections show shallow mucosal ulcers with irregular borders. The remains of the mucosa between the ulcers are thrown into filiform polyps. The crypts are distorted with the presence of branching, shortening, and complete absence. There is infiltration of lamina propria and submucosa by chronic inflammatory cells with the presence of diffuse fibrosis.

4.6.2 Neoplastic Lesions

Lipoma of Colon (a, b)

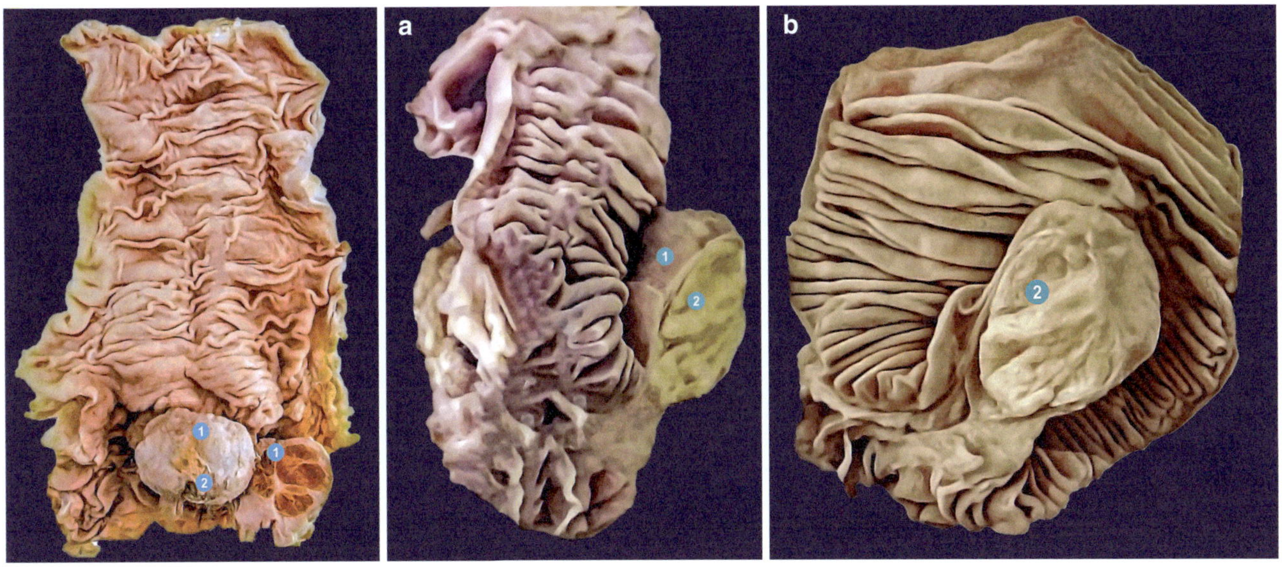

A strip of the colon is mounted.

1. It shows a sessile, well-defined, encapsulated globular polypoid mass with a lobulated yellow-cut section.
2. Surface ulceration is seen.

Microscopic Picture of Lipoma of Colon (c)

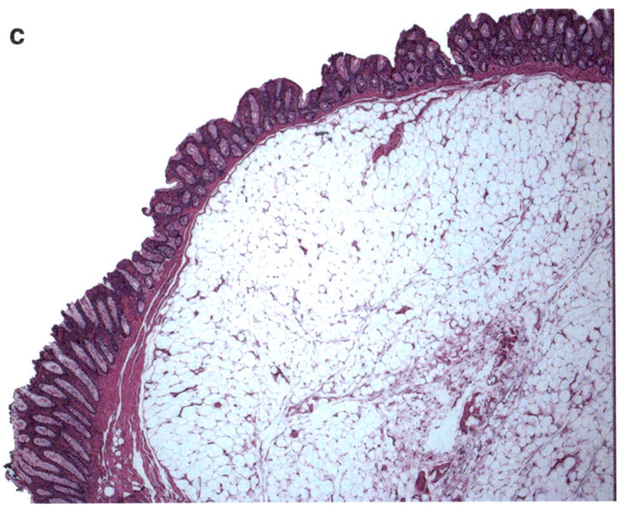

The section shows well-circumscribed lobules of mature fat cells, with signet-ring nuclei and clear cytoplasm, covered by colonic mucosa. The fat lobules are separated from each other by thin fibrovascular septa.

Colonic Polyps

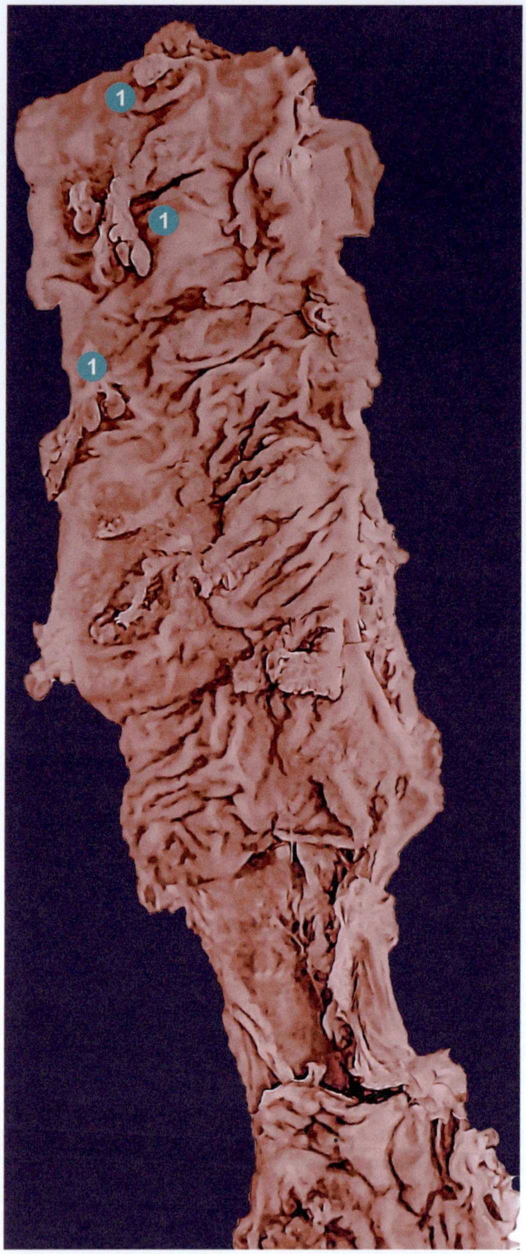

A strip of the large intestine is mounted.

1. Multiple, small, pedunculated polyps hanging from the mucosa are observed.

Microscopic Picture of Adenomatous Polyp (a–c)

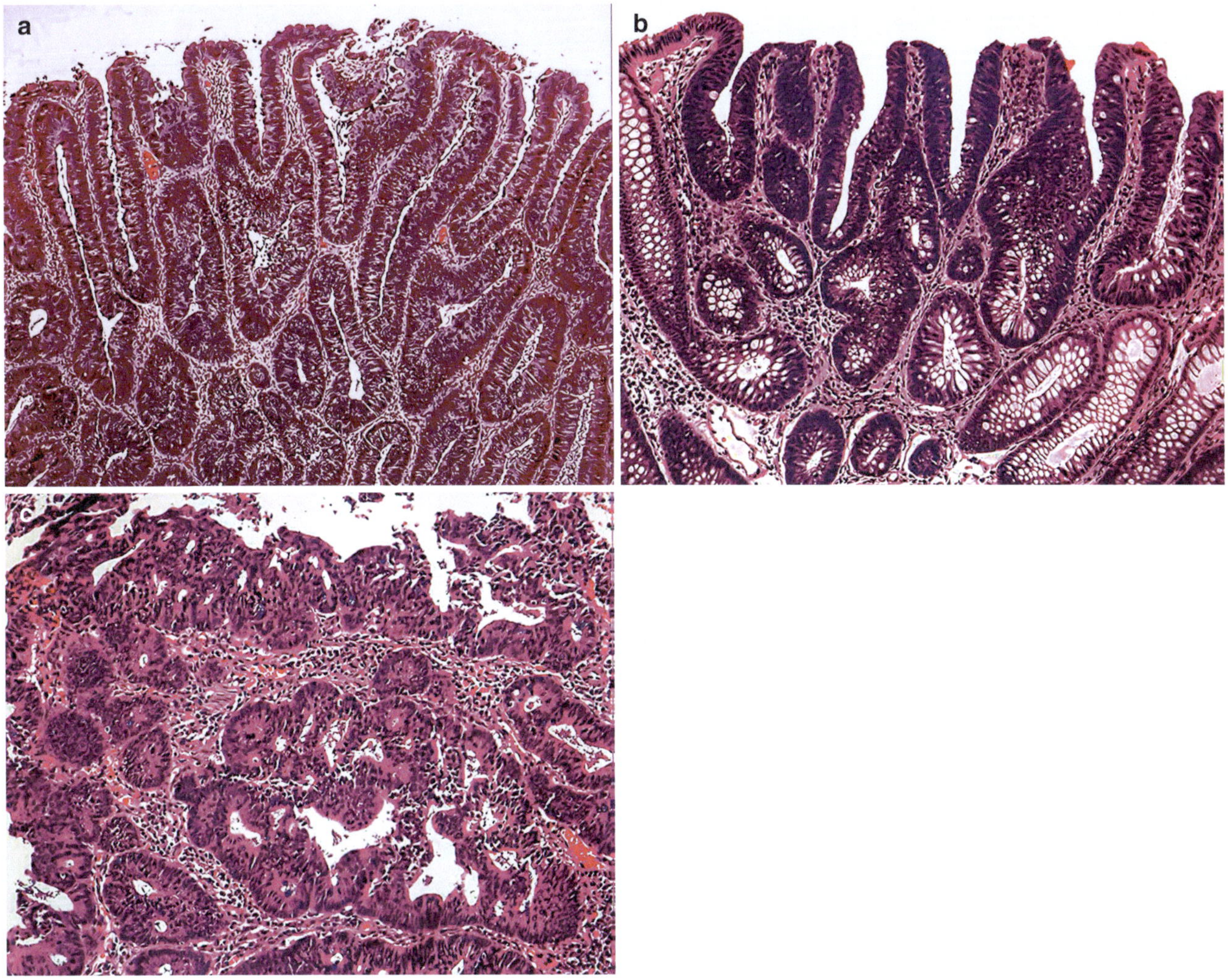

Sections show a polyp with a fibrovascular core. The polyp is composed of crowded glands (tubules) lined by hyperplastic epithelial cells with depleted cytoplasmic mucin and showing dysplasia in the form of increased size and number of nuclei and loss of normal cellular polarity.

Microscopic Picture of Hyperplastic Polyp (d, e)

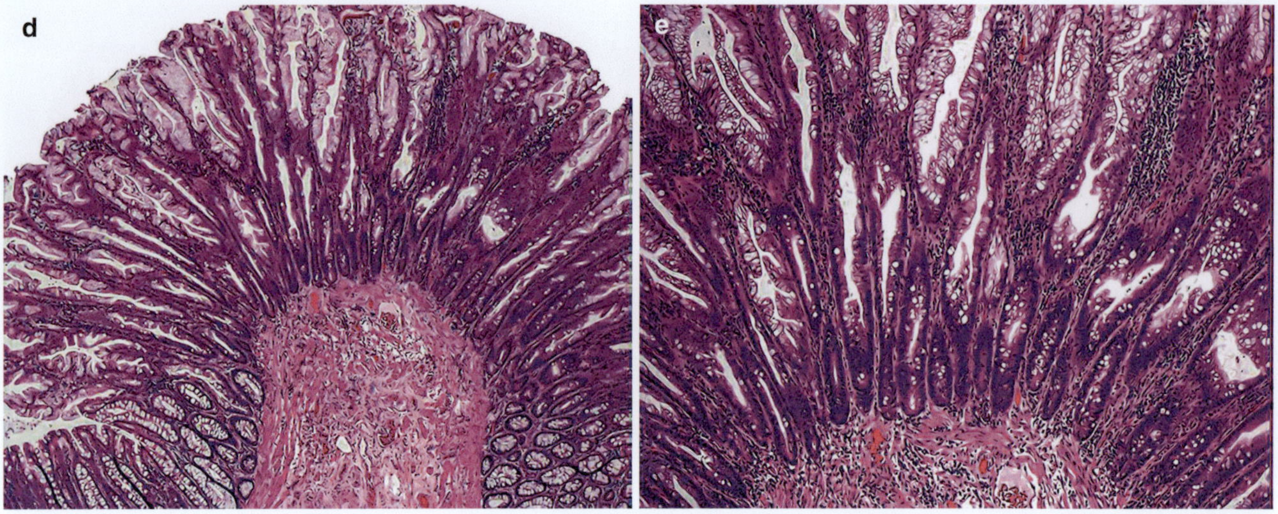

Sections show a sawtooth appearance, with serrations generally limited to the upper half of the crypts. Mild nuclear enlargement, stratification, and hyperchromasia are limited to the crypt bases. No dilated, branched, or horizontally spreading crypts. No evidence of conventional dysplasia.

Neuroendocrine Tumor (NET) of Rectum

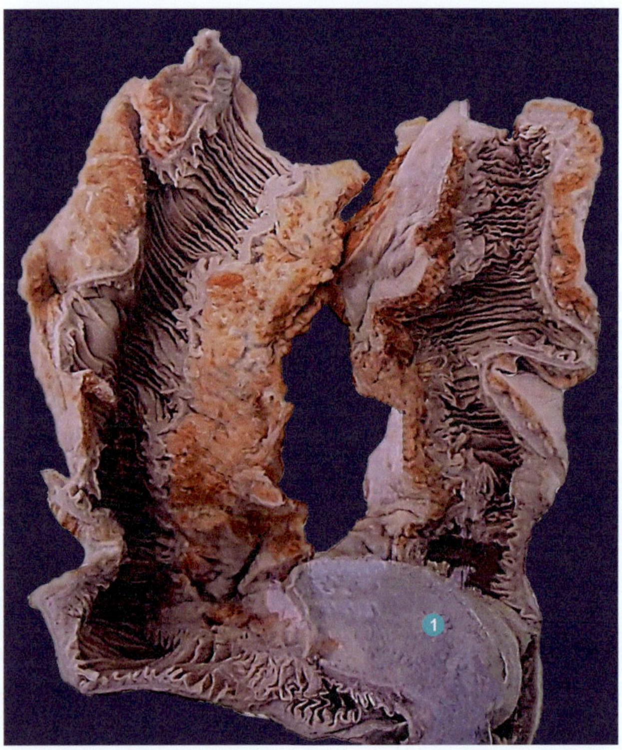

An opened segment of the sigmoid colon and rectum is mounted.

1. There is a submucosal, well-defined, encapsulated, polypoid, solid, and hemorrhagic mass in the rectum projecting in the lumen.

Microscopic Picture of Low-Grade Neuroendocrine Tumor (NET) of Rectum (a)

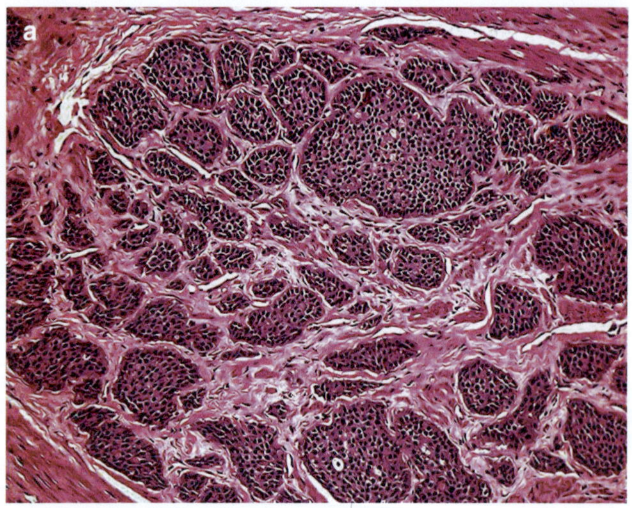

The section shows nests of monotonous small, oval-round tumor cells with round-oval nuclei and eosinophilic cytoplasm and minimal atypia. Tumor cells are embedded in a fibrovascular stroma.

Colonic Gastrointestinal Stromal Tumor (GIST) (a, b)

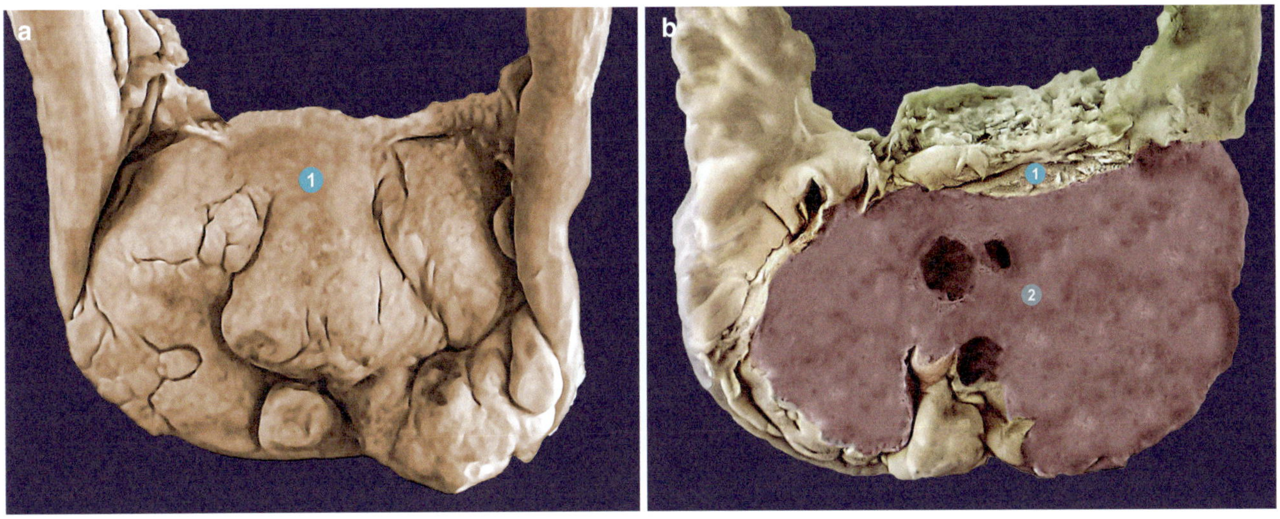

An opened segment of the colon and rectum is mounted.

1. There is a submucosal, well-defined, encapsulated, polypoid, solid, large, and bulky mass with an irregular multinodular surface projecting in the lumen.
2. The cut section has tannish brown parenchyma with hemorrhage, necrosis, and cystic softening.

Microscopic Picture of Gastrointestinal Stromal Tumor (GIST) (c–h)

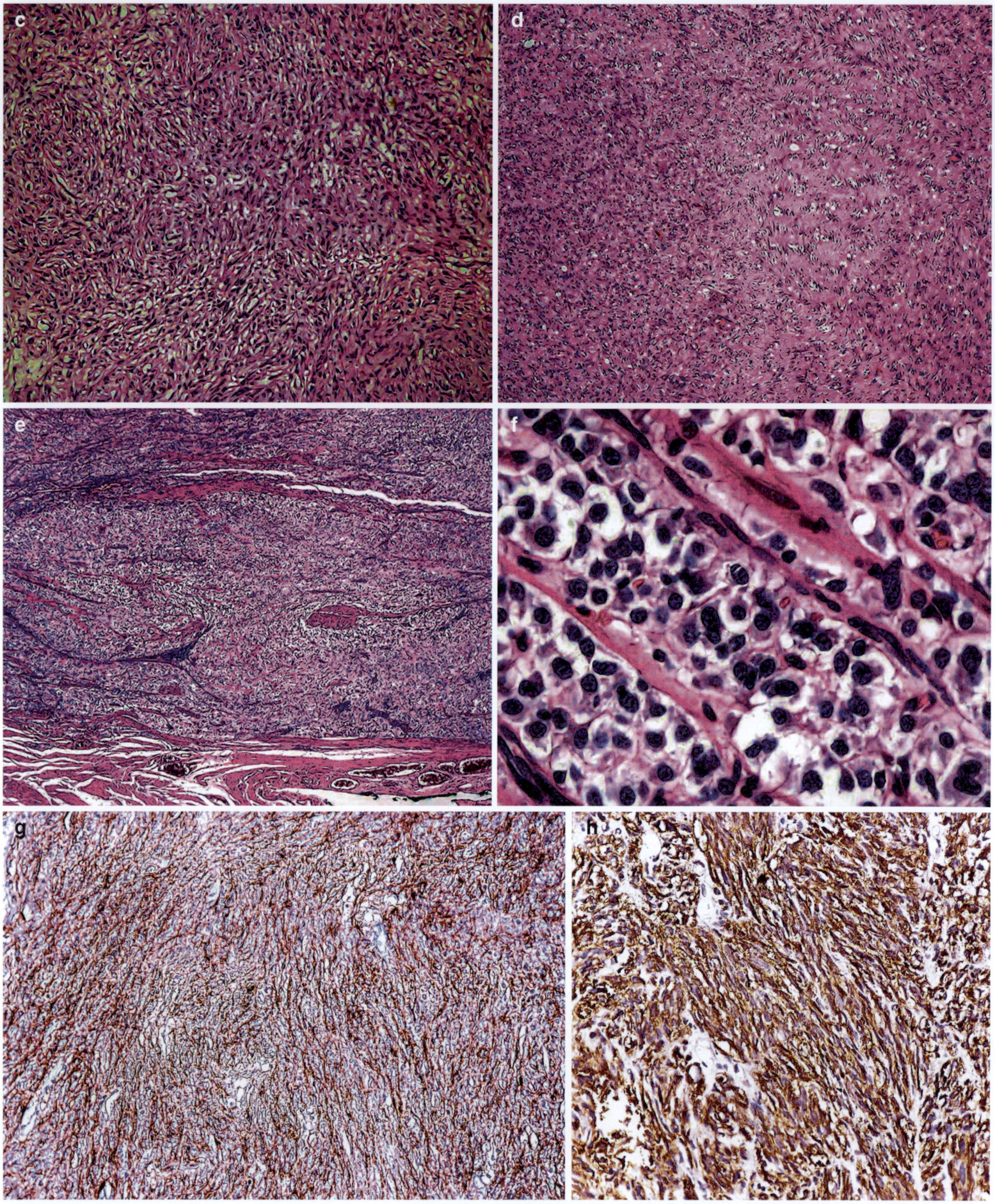

Sections show:

- (c, d) **Spindle cell type:** showing intersecting fascicles of plump spindled cells with eosinophilic cytoplasm within the variably hyalinized or edematous stroma.
- (e, f) **Epithelioid cell type:** showing round cells with clear to eosinophilic cytoplasm in sheets or nests; increased tendency for pleomorphism. The tumor cells stained positively with C-Kit (CD117) (g) and Dog-1 (h).

Pearls

Gastrointestinal stromal tumor (GIST), generally driven by oncogenic KIT or PDGFRA mutations, is the most common mesenchymal tumor of the gastrointestinal (GI) tract. GIST is most common in the stomach (60%) and small intestine (30%) but can occur anywhere in the GI tract and the intra-abdominal soft tissues. GIST can show spindle cell or epithelioid morphology, and mitotic count and tumor size are the most important prognostic parameters. GISTs in NF1 patients and children are distinctive clinicopathologic groups. Immunohistochemical testing for KIT and sometimes for DOG1/Ano 1 is essential in confirming the diagnosis [18].

Fungating Polypoid Carcinoma of Colon

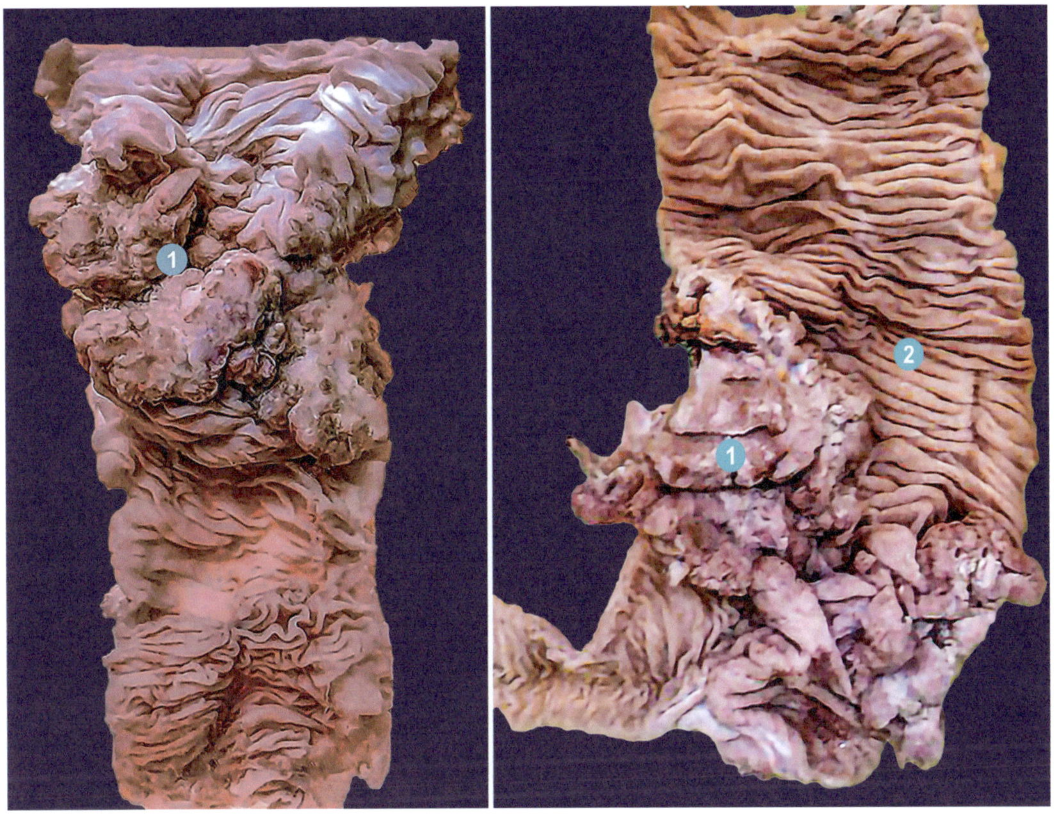

The specimen consists of a piece of the large intestine.

1. The mucosal surface shows an ulcerated polypoid infiltrative mass attached to the mucosa by a wide base. No lymph node metastases are evident.

Fungating Polypoid Carcinoma of Cecum

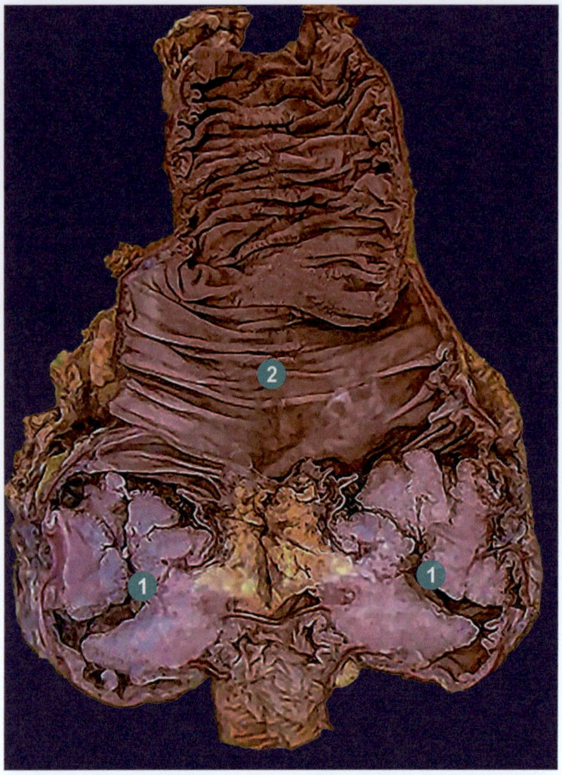

The specimen consists of a piece of the cecum and large intestine.

1. The mucosal surface shows an ulcerated polypoid infiltrative mass attached to the mucosa by a wide base.
2. The colon proximal to the obstruction is dilated.

Ulcerative Carcinoma of Colon

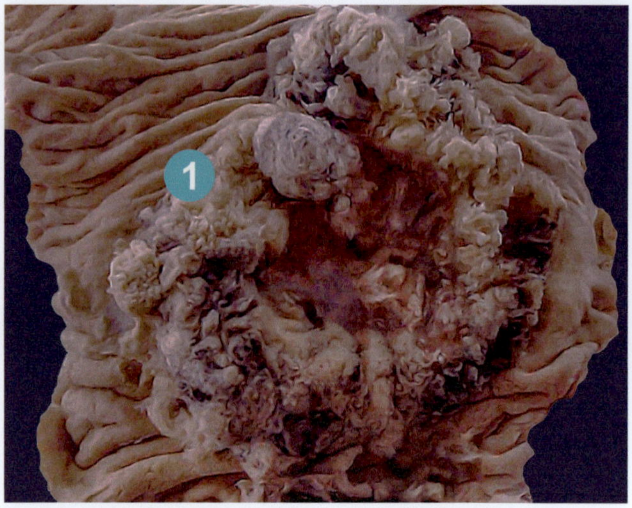

A strip of the large intestine is mounted.

1. A circular ulcer is seen. The ulcer has a raised and irregular everted edge, irregular margins, and a necrotic floor.

Ulcerated Annular Carcinoma of the Ano-Rectal Region

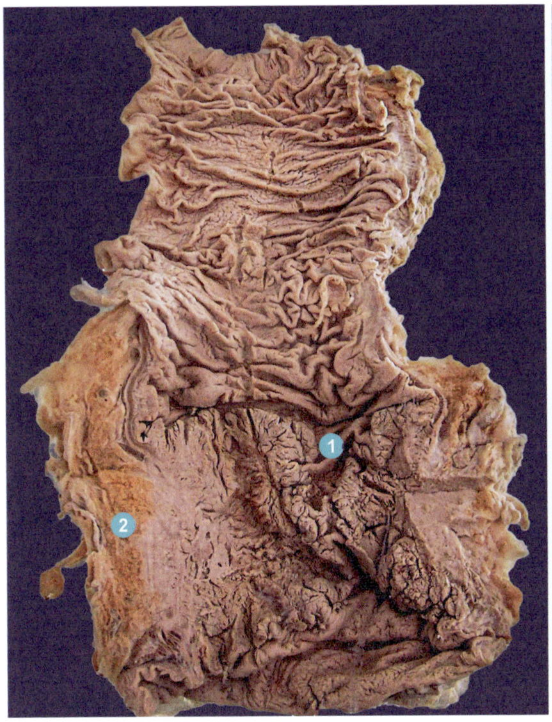

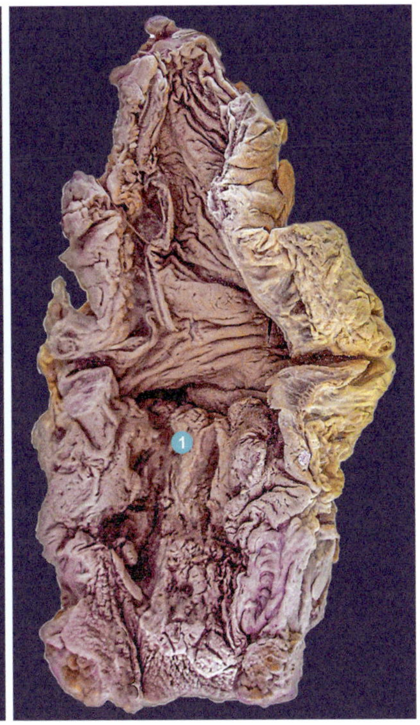

The specimen represents the rectum and anal canal.

1. A large longitudinal ulcer with a raised everted edge and a necrotic floor is seen near the anal orifice.
2. The tumor reaches the serosa and pericolic fat.

Ulcerative and Polypoid Fungating Carcinoma of Colon

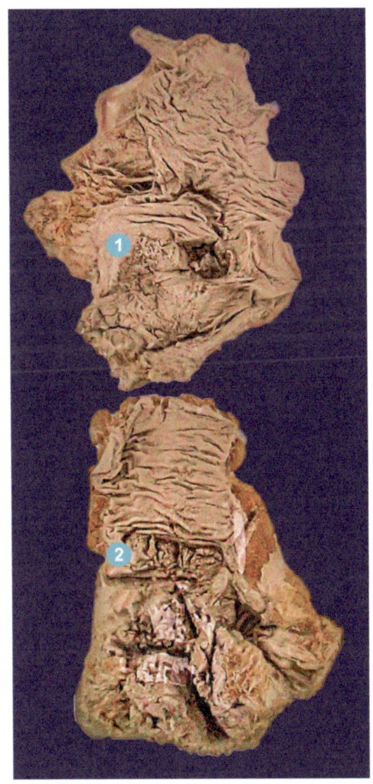

Two strips of the large intestine are mounted.

1. The upper one shows ulcerative carcinoma (case 51).
2. The lower strip shows polypoid-fungating carcinoma (case 50).

Microscopic Picture of Carcinoma of Colon (a–f)

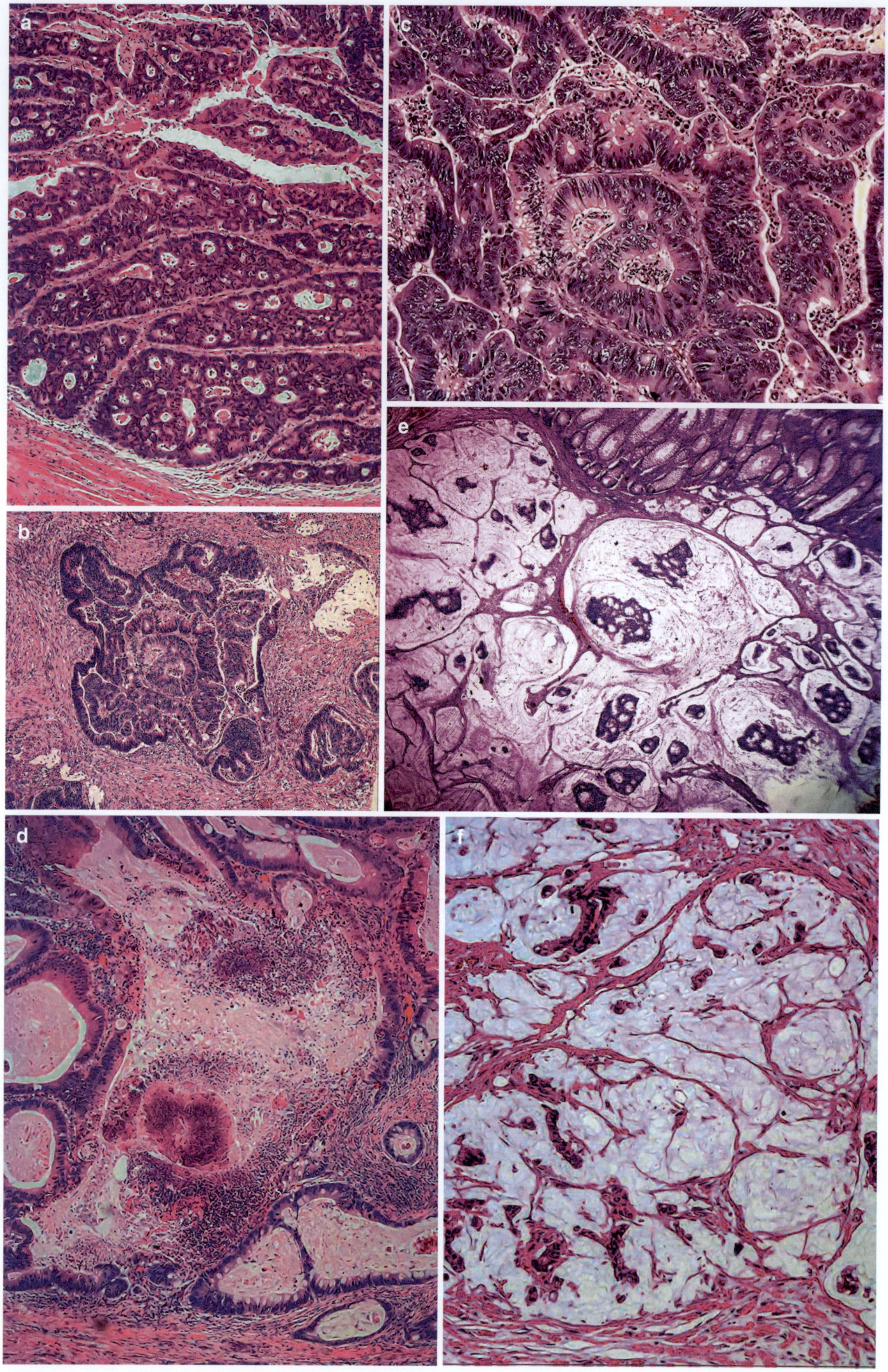

Sections show malignant acini infiltrating the mucosa, causing ulceration, submucosa, and musculosa. The malignant acini are lined with pleomorphic stratified epithelium with an increased number of mitoses and the presence of areas of necrosis.

Mucinous (colloid) carcinoma is presented (c–f) in which small tumor islands are embedded in pools of mucin with the presence of tumor necrosis. The tumor cells are embedded in a fibrous stroma infiltrated with chronic inflammatory cells with areas of mucoid secretion.

Ancillary Tools

IHC [19]:

CK20, CDX2, and AMACR

Sometimes estrogen receptor

CD10 in stromal cells

SATB2

Molecular/cytogenetics description [20]:

The most commonly mutated genes include APC, TP53, and KRAS

Tumors can be screened for microsatellite instability via immunohistochemistry for MLH1, MSH2, MSH6, and PMS2.

References

1. Gehlen J., et al. (2022). First genome-wide association study of esophageal atresia identifies three genetic risk loci at CTNNA3, FOXF1/FOXC2/FOXL1, and HNF1B. HGG Adv. 3(2): 100093. doi: https://doi.org/10.1016/j.xhgg.2022.100093. PMCID: PMC8844277.
2. Cheung D.Y. (2017). Atrophic Gastritis Increases the Risk of Gastric Cancer in Asymptomatic Population in Korea. Gut Liver. 11(5): 575–576. doi: https://doi.org/10.5009/gnl17356. PMCID: PMC5593317.
3. Almazar AE, et al. (2021). Survival Times of Patients with Menetrier's Disease and Risk of Gastric Cancer. Clin Gastroenterol Hepatol. 19(4):707-712. doi: https://doi.org/10.1016/j.cgh.2020.03.017. PMID: 32184187.
4. Amesse LS. et al. (2009). Peritoneal inclusion cysts in adolescent females: a clinicopathological characterization of four cases. J Pediatr. Adolesc. Gynecol. 22(1):41-8. doi:https://doi.org/10.1016/j.jpag.2008.02.003. PMID: 19232301.
5. Nizri E. et al. (2018). Multicystic mesothelioma: Operative and long-term outcomes with cytoreductive surgery and hyperthermic intraperitoneal chemotherapy. Eur J Surg Oncol. 44(7):1100-1104. doi: https://doi.org/10.1016/j.ejso.2018.03.004. PMID: 29703622.
6. Sawh RN, et al. (2003). Benign cystic mesothelioma of the peritoneum: a clinicopathologic study of 17 cases and immunohistochemical analysis of estrogen and progesterone receptor status. Hum Pathol. 34(4):369-74. doi: https://doi.org/10.1053/hupa.2003.31. PMID: 12733118.
7. Hu B. et al. (2012). Gastric cancer: Classification, histology, and application of molecular pathology. J Gastrointest. Oncol. 3(3):251-61. doi: https://doi.org/10.3978/j.issn.2078-6891.2012.021. PMID: 22943016. PMCID: PMC3418539.
8. Polom K. et al. (2018). Meta-analysis of microsatellite instability in relation to clinicopathological characteristics and overall survival in gastric cancer. Br J Surg. 105(3):159-167. doi: https://doi.org/10.1002/bjs.10663. PMID: 29091259.
9. Francis A., et al. (2016). Pediatric Meckel's Diverticulum: Report of 208 Cases and Review of Literature. Fetal Pediatr Pathol. 35(3):199-206.doi: https://doi.org/10.3109/15513815.2016.1161684. PMID: 27064958.
10. Albertelli M. et al. (2021). Pathology Reporting in Neuroendocrine Neoplasms of the Digestive System: Everything You Always Wanted to Know but Were Too Afraid to Ask. Front Endocrinol (Lausanne). 12:680305. doi: https://doi.org/10.3389/fendo.2021.680305. PMID: 33967966; PMCID: PMC8104083.
11. Karpathakis A. et al. (2016).Prognostic Impact of Novel Molecular Subtypes of Small Intestinal Neuroendocrine Tumor. Clin Cancer Res. 22(1):250-8. doi: https://doi.org/10.1158/1078-0432.CCR-15-0373. PMID: 26169971.
12. Wang H.L. et al. (2017).Practical Immunohistochemistry in Neoplastic Pathology of the Gastrointestinal Tract, Liver, Biliary Tract, and Pancreas. Arch Pathol. Lab. Med. 141(9):1155-1180. doi: https://doi.org/10.5858/arpa.2016-0489-RA. PMID: 28854347.
13. Arai M. et al. (1997). Mutations of the Ki-ras, p53, and APC genes in adenocarcinomas of the human small intestine. Int J Cancer. 70(4):390-5. doi: https://doi.org/10.1002/(sici)10970215(19970207)70:4<390::aid-ijc3>3.0.co;2-r. PMID: 9033644.
14. Xue, Y. et al. (2017). Non-ampullary–duodenal carcinomas: clinicopathologic analysis of 47 cases and comparison with ampullary and pancreatic adenocarcinomas. Mod Pathol 30, 255–266. https://doi.org/10.1038/modpathol.2016.174.
15. Ang D.C. et al. (2014). The utility of immunohistochemistry in subtyping adenocarcinoma of the ampulla of Vater. Am J Surg Pathol.38(10):1371-9. doi: https://doi.org/10.1097/PAS.0000000000000230. PMID: 24832159.
16. Mafficini A. et al. (2018). Ampulla of Vater Carcinoma: Sequencing Analysis Identifies TP53 Status as a Novel Independent Prognostic Factor and Potentially Actionable ERBB, PI3K, and WNT Pathways Gene Mutations. Ann Surg.267(1):149-156. doi: https://doi.org/10.1097/SLA.0000000000001999. PMID: 27611608.
17. Mantilla J.C. et al. (2023). Gastrointestinal tuberculosis: An autopsy-based study. Infectious Medicine. 2(2):122-127. https://doi.org/10.1016/j.imj.2023.04.007.
18. Miettinen M., Lasota J. (2011). Histopathology of gastrointestinal stromal tumor. J Surg Oncol. 104(8): 865–873. doi: https://doi.org/10.1002/jso.21945. PMCID: PMC7384443.
19. Fleming M. et al. (2012). Colorectal carcinoma: Pathologic aspects. J Gastrointest. Oncol. 3(3):153-73. doi: https://doi.org/10.3978/j.issn.2078-6891.2012.030. PMID: 22943008 PMCID: PMC3418538.
20. Gonzalez RS. Adenocarcinoma. PathologyOutlines.com website. https://www.pathologyoutlines.com/topic/colontumoradenocarcinoma.

5 Diseases of the Hepatobiliary System and Pancreas

The liver and gallbladder are integral components of the digestive system, playing pivotal roles in the metabolism of fats, proteins, and carbohydrates, detoxification, bile production, and storage, respectively. Disruptions in their structure or function can lead to a multitude of diseases, presenting in varied morphologies that we delve into in this chapter.

We will go through the range of pathological conditions that can afflict these organs. Emphasizing the gross and microscopic morphological changes that arise, we examine a host of hepatic conditions, from hepatic cirrhosis and fatty liver disease to various forms of hepatocellular carcinoma. Concurrently, we delve into gallbladder pathologies such as cholecystitis, cholesterol and pigment stones, and gallbladder cancer.

Throughout this chapter, illustrative images will enhance understanding of these disease processes, highlighting typical gross and microscopic appearances and discussing potential underlying mechanisms.

This chapter provides a comprehensive understanding of the pathology of the liver and gallbladder. Whether you are a medical student, a pathology resident, or an experienced practitioner, we trust this chapter will provide valuable insights and deepen your understanding of hepatobiliary pathology.

The hepatobiliary diseases discussed in this chapter will be arranged in this way:

1. Liver
   (a) Degenerative Lesions
   - Fatty Change of Liver
   - Hepatic Amyloidosis

   (b) Vascular Lesions
   - Chronic Venous Congestion

   (c) Inflammatory Lesions
   - Bacterial Infections
     - Tuberculosis
     - Syphilis (Hepar Lobatum)
   - Parasitic Infections
     - Amoebic Liver Abscess
     - Bilharzial Periportal Fibrosis
     - Hydatid Cyst

   (d) Cirrhosis
   - Micronodular Cirrhosis
   - Lennec Cirrhosis

   (e) Neoplastic Lesions
   - Primary Tumors
     - Hepatoblastoma
     - Pediatric Hepatocellular Carcinoma
     - Hepatocellular Carcinoma
   - Metastatic Tumors
2. Gallbladder
   (a) Inflammatory Lesions
   - Chronic Cholecystitis
   - Gallstone Disease

   (b) Neoplastic Lesions
   - Carcinoma of the Gallbladder
3. Pancreas
   (a) Neoplastic Lesions
   - Cancer Head of Pancreas

G. Dawood, *Color Atlas of Human Gross and Microscopic Pathology*, https://doi.org/10.1007/978-3-031-76007-5_5

5.1 Liver

5.1.1 Degenerative Lesions

Fatty Change of Liver

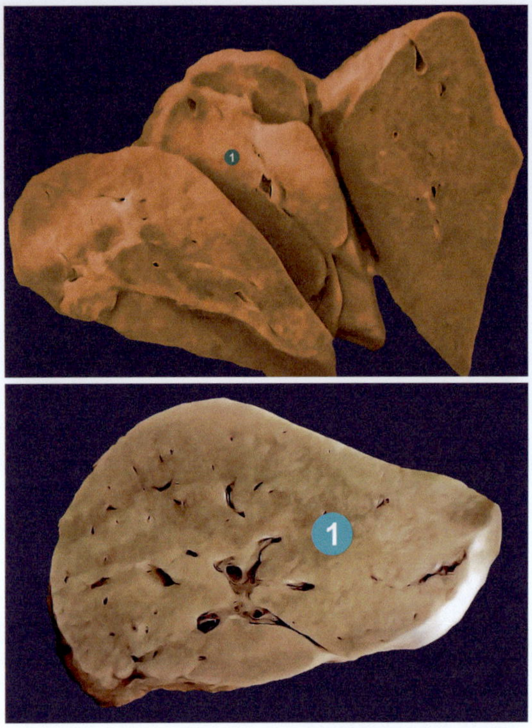

Slices of liver tissue are mounted.

1. They have a yellow, greasy, and smooth surface and rounded borders, indicating their soft consistency.

Microscopic Picture of Fatty Change of Liver (a, b)

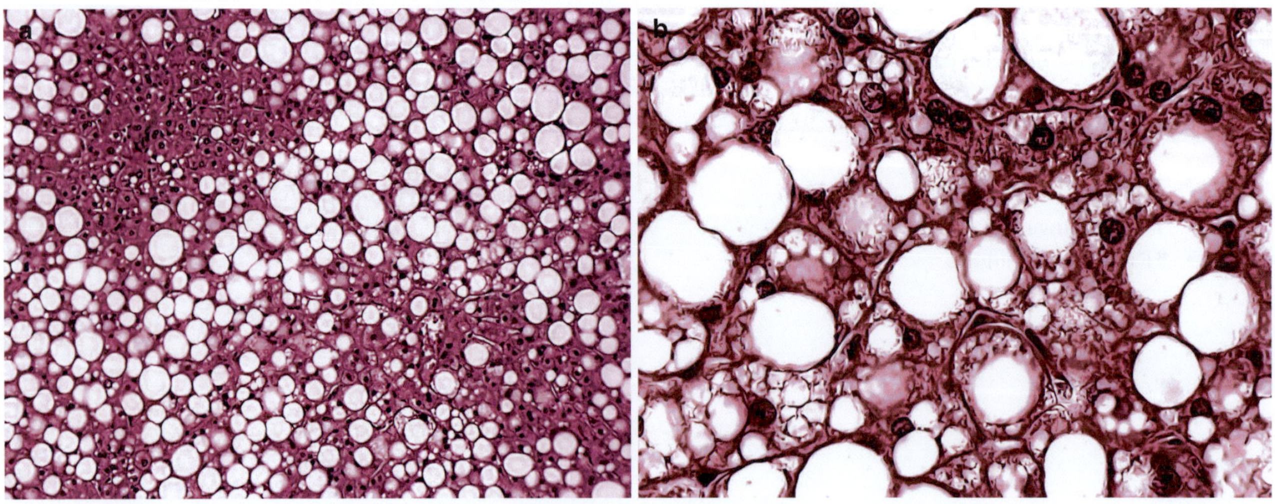

Sections show the normal-looking hepatic architecture. Some hepatocytes show an accumulation of small and large clear lipid droplets within hepatocytes (Micro- and Macrovesicular Steatosis). These lipid droplets displace the nuclei to the periphery of cells to cause hepatocyte enlargement and give them a signet-ring appearance.

Hepatic Amyloidosis

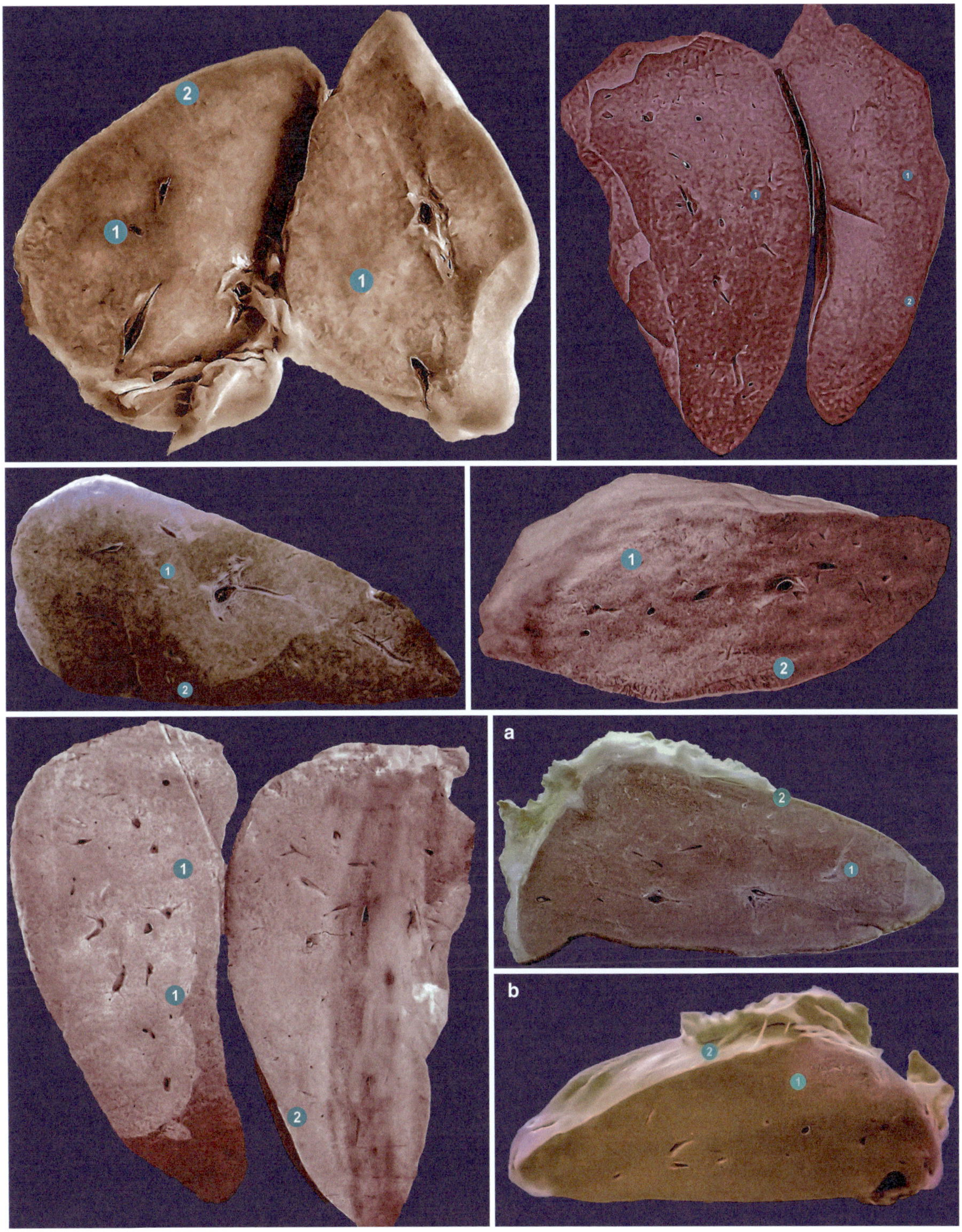

Slices of liver tissue are mounted.

1. Their large size indicates the large size of the liver from which they were taken. The surface is smooth with the presence of ill-defined pale-yellow areas among normal-colored liver.
2. The hepatic borders are sharp, indicating its firm consistency

Microscopic Picture of Hepatic Amyloidosis (c)

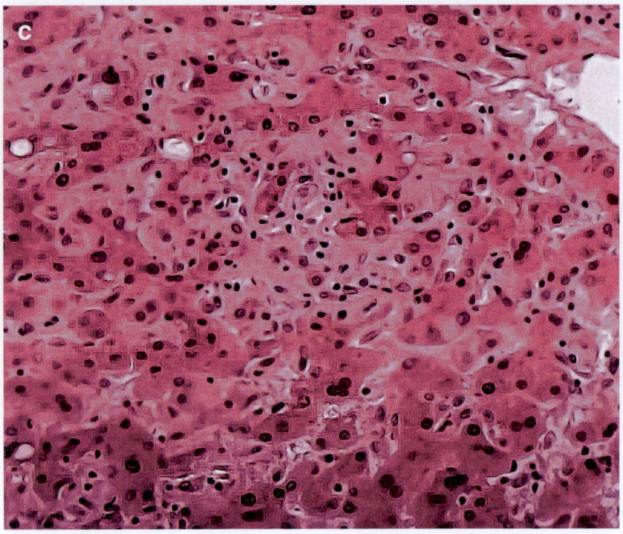

The section shows diffuse eosinophilic homogenous material throughout sinusoids with compressed and atrophic hepatocytes.

Ancillary Tools
Special Stains:

1. Congo red stain positive, showing apple-green birefringence on polarizing microscopy.
2. Metachromatic stains such as crystal violet and toluidine blue.
3. Fluorescent stains, e.g., thioflavin T or S.

IHC:

Anti-kappa and anti-lambda antibodies are useful in immunohistochemical classification and diagnosis of AL-type amyloidosis [1].

5.1.2 Vascular Lesions

Chronic Venous Congestion (Nutmeg Liver)

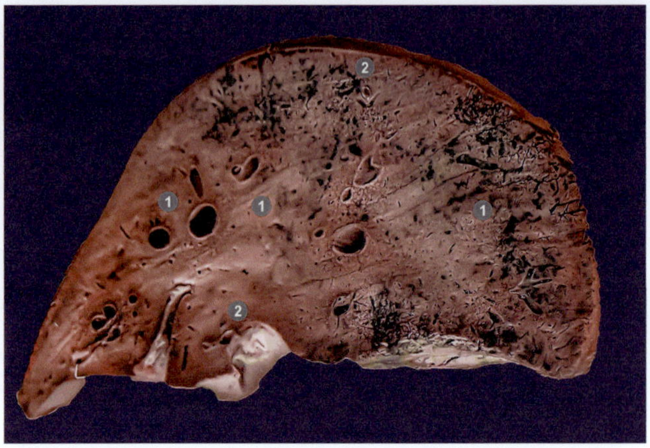

A slice of liver tissue with a smooth surface is mounted.

1. The large size indicates the large size of the liver from which it was taken. The surface is mottled by the presence of dark brown areas of congestion with periportal yellow areas of fatty change.
2. The borders are sharp, indicating firm consistency.

Microscopic Picture of Chronic Venous Congestion (a, b)

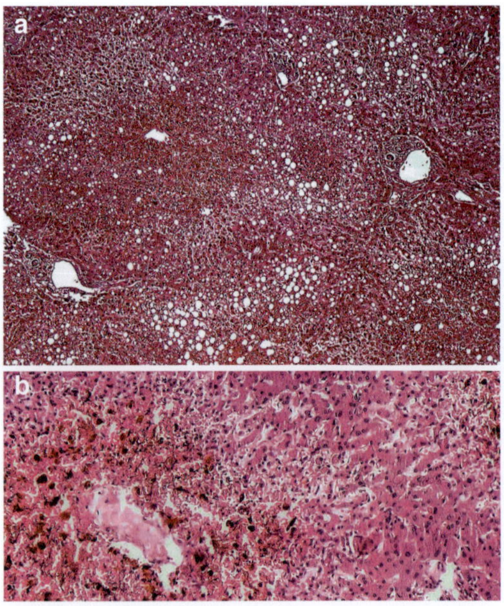

Sections show centrilobular hepatocyte necrosis and hemorrhage. Surviving hepatocytes undergo fatty change. The sinusoids are dilate and congested.

5.1.3 Inflammatory Lesions

5.1.3.1 Bacterial Infection

Miliary Tuberculosis of the Liver (a, b)

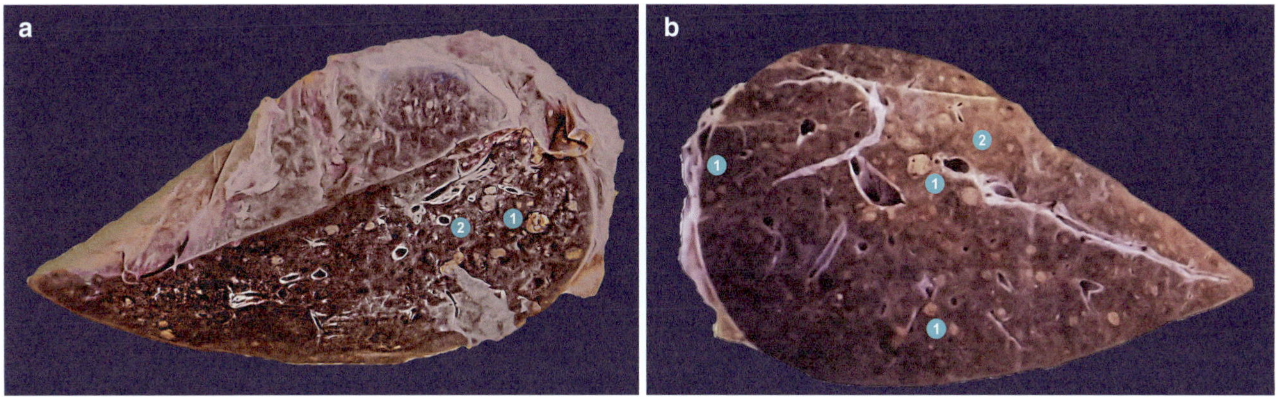

A slice of the liver is mounted.

1. The cut section shows multiple, small, yellow caseous foci.
2. The liver tissue in between shows the fatty change.

Multiple Tuberculomata of Liver (a, b)

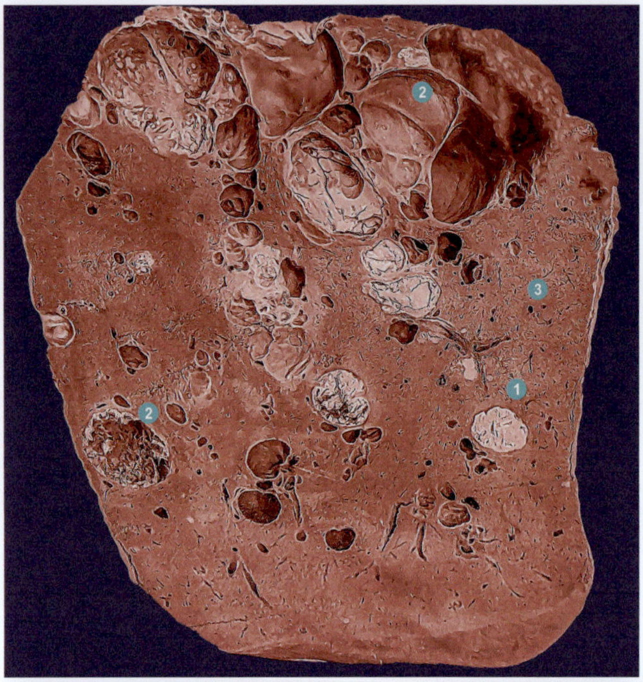

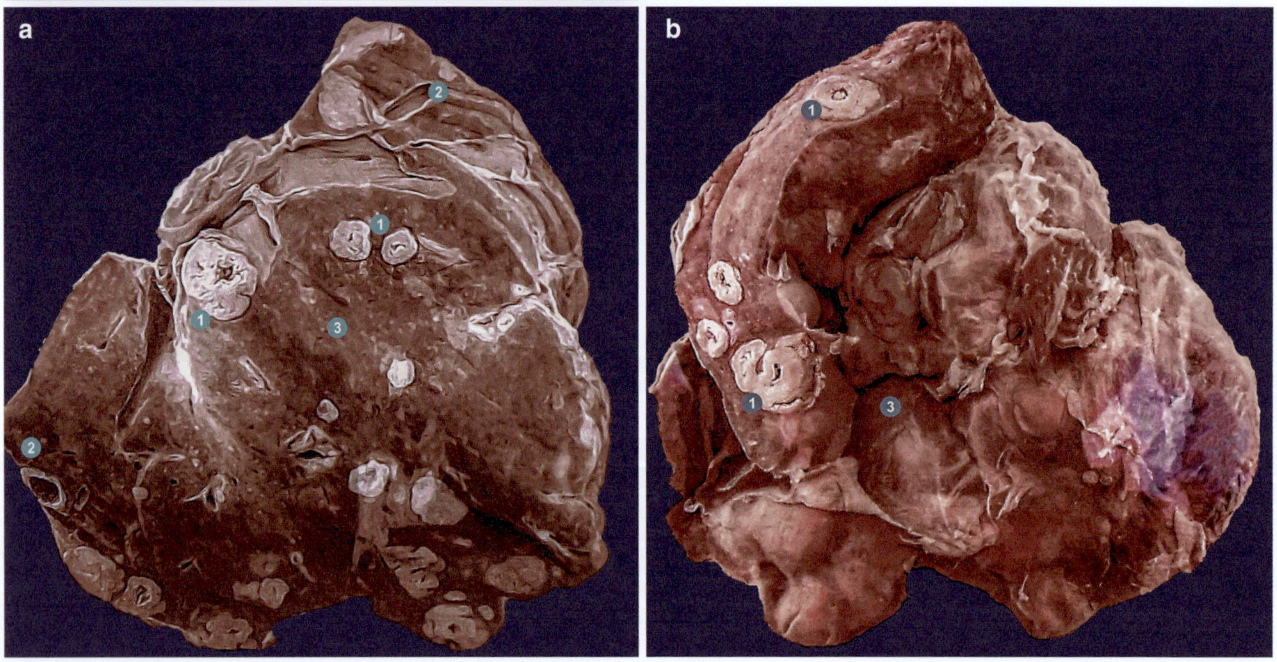

A slice of the liver is mounted.

1. Multiple yellow caseous foci, variable in size, fused in areas to form larger nodules are seen.
2. The caseous material fell from areas, leaving cavities lined with ragged walls while other cavities have smooth walls owing to fibrosis.
3. The intervening liver tissue is yellow owing to fatty change.

Microscopic Picture of Hepatic Tuberculosis (c, d)

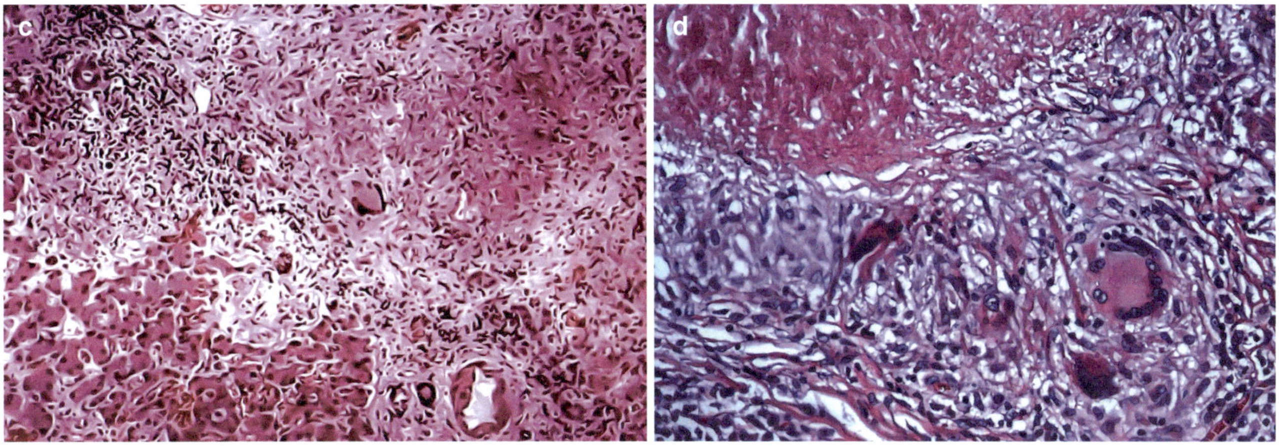

Sections show multiple tubercles with areas of caseation necrosis and fibrosis. Tubercles are formed of epithelioid cells, macrophages, Langhans multinucleated giant cells, and lymphocytes.

Hepar Lobatum (a, b)

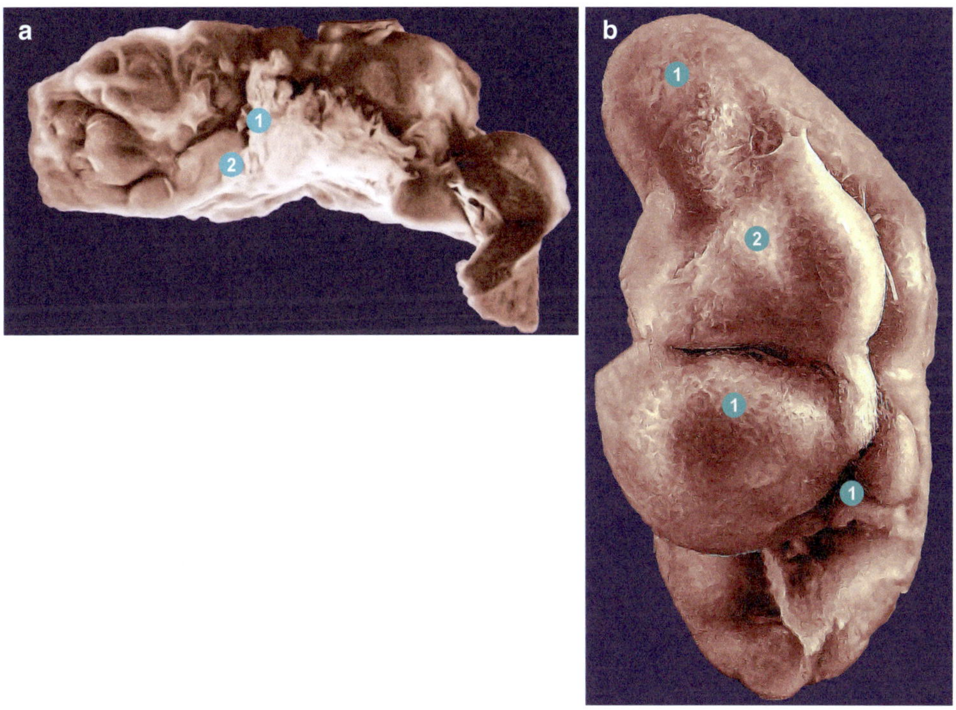

A liver is mounted.

1. It is shrunken, atrophic, and transformed into variably sized nodules (pseudolobules) separated from each other by dense fibrous tissues. Pseudolobulation of the liver is due to the in-drawing of the capsule by the fibrous scars.
2. The liver tissue is yellow-white due to fatty changes and fibrosis.

5.1.3.2 Parasitic Infection

Amoebic Liver Abscess (a, b)

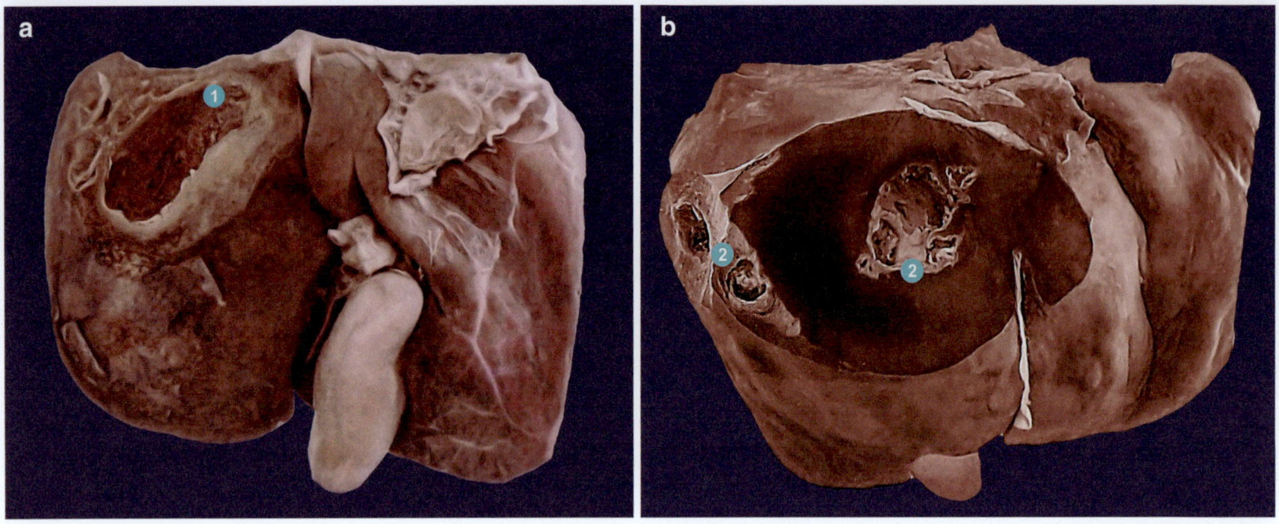

The liver of a child is displayed.

1. It shows a large cavity in the left lobe lined with an irregular necrotic yellow membrane.
2. The right lobe shows multiple smaller cavities. The cavities show characteristic roughened, necrotic inner lining of the abscesses.

Pearls

Note the absence of signs of acute inflammation around the lesions because the amebae produce substances to reduce the inflammatory response. Hemorrhage into an abscess may produce "anchovy sauce" pus. The abscesses may erode through the diaphragm to produce intrapulmonary lesions or pericardial tamponade.

Microscopic Picture of Amoebic Liver Abscess (c–f)

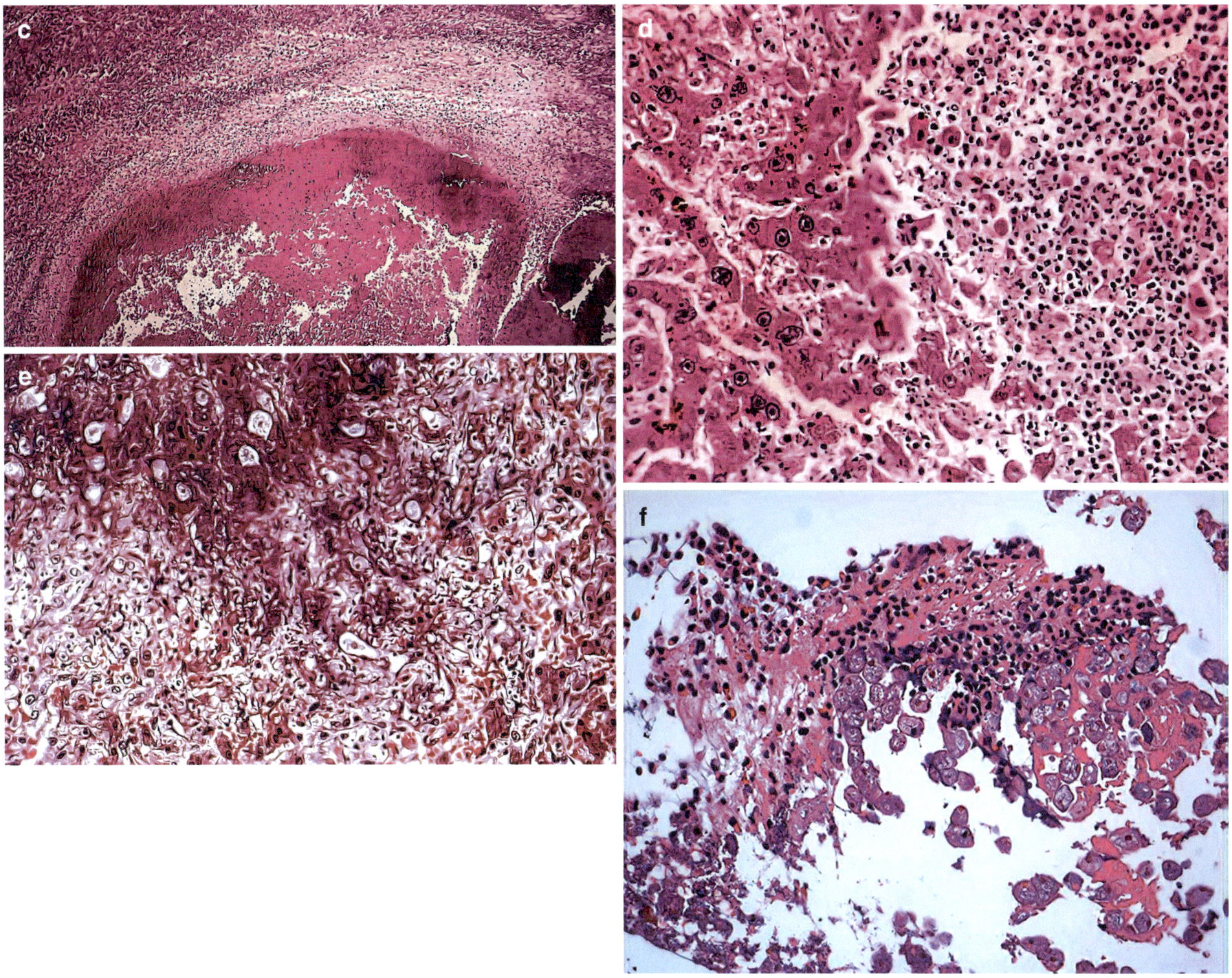

Sections show a central area of liquefactive necrosis infiltrated by inflammatory cells, including neutrophils, macrophages, and lymphocytes. Neutrophils are typically abundant in the early stages of infection. Trophozoites are seen in the necrotic area. Around the necrotic area, granulation tissue formation is seen characterized by fibroblasts, collagen deposition, and neovascularization.

Bilharzial Periportal Fibrosis

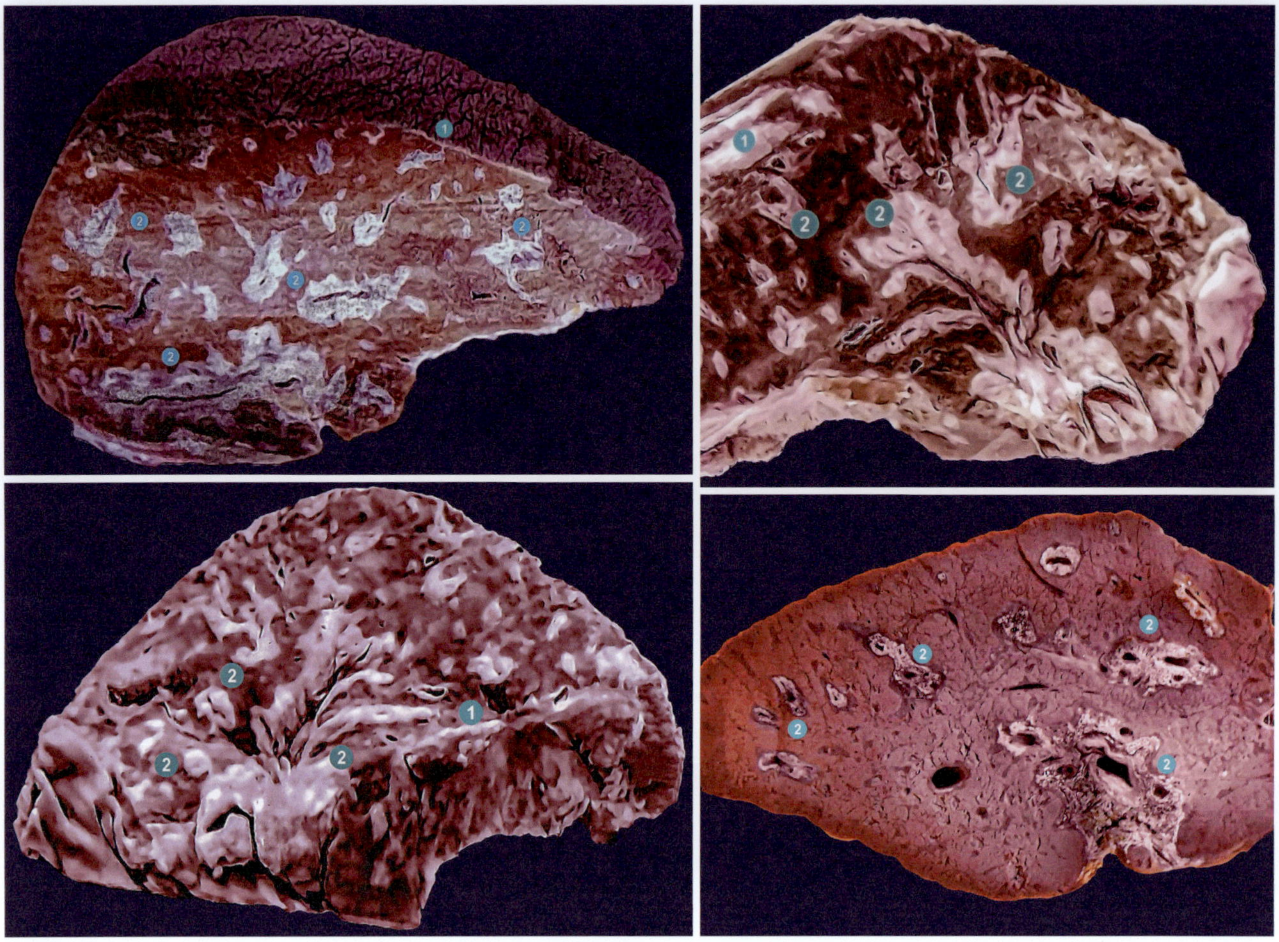

A slice of liver tissue is mounted.

1. It has a granular yellow surface and sharp borders.
2. Small and large portal tracts are thickened by gray-white fibrous tissue, which extends to affect the surrounding hepatic tissue.

Microscopic Picture of Bilharzial Periportal Fibrosis (a–g)

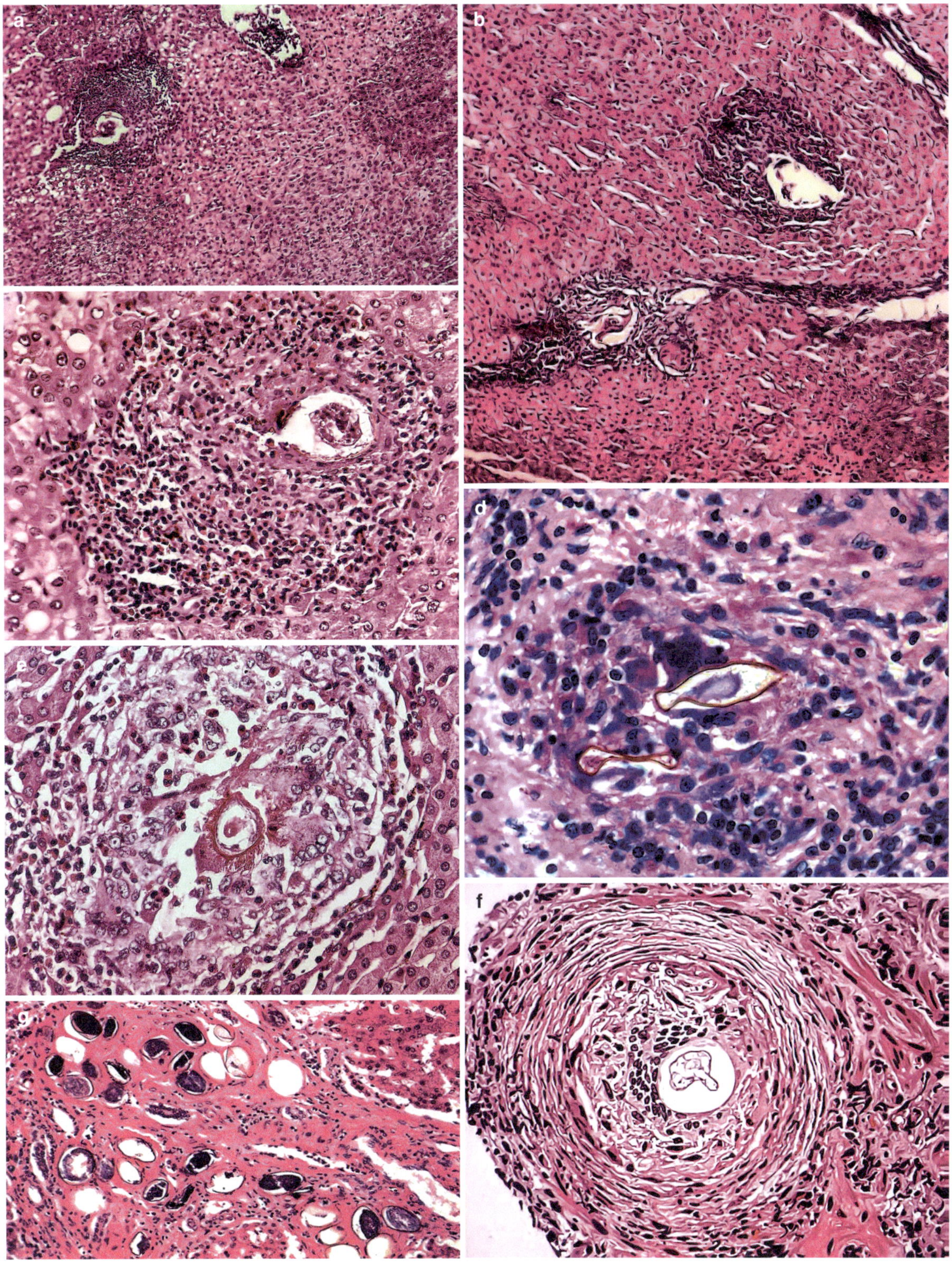

Sections show infiltration of portal tracts by chronic inflammatory cells around bilharzial ova with the presence of multinucleated giant cells around dead ova. With progression of the lesion, the infiltrate decreases with increased fibrous obliteration of portal tracts and calcification of bilharzial ova.

Hydatid Cysts of the Liver (a, b)

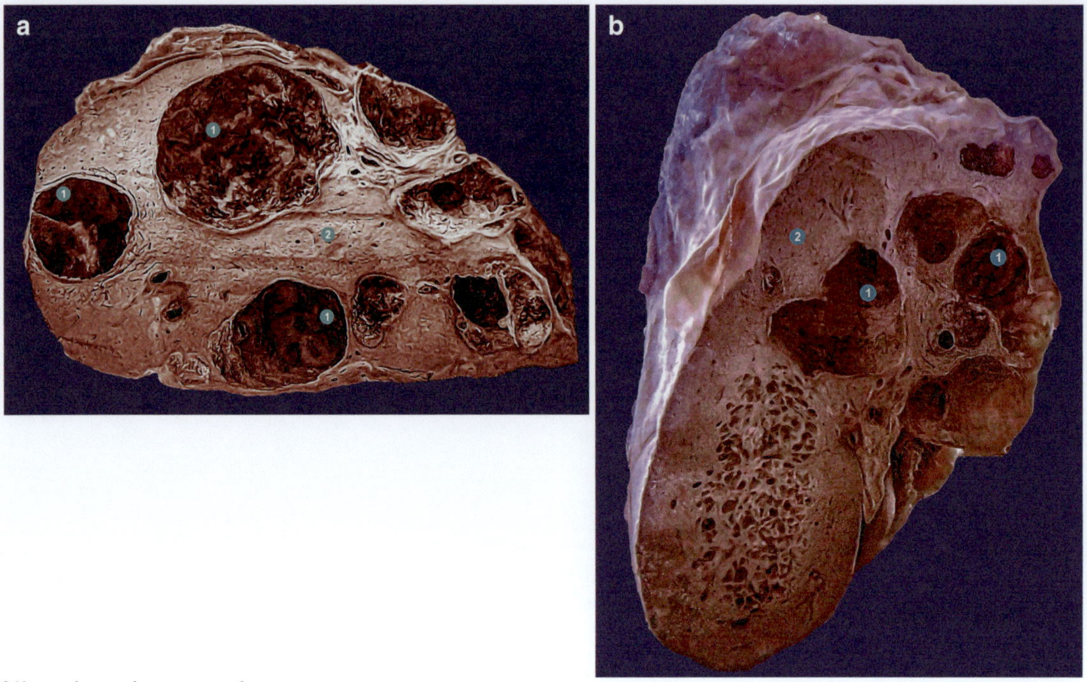

A slice of liver tissue is mounted.

1. Multiple cavities, variable in size, and lined with a smooth brown membrane are seen.
2. The intervening liver tissue shows a fatty change.

5.1.4 Cirrhosis

Micronodular Cirrhosis

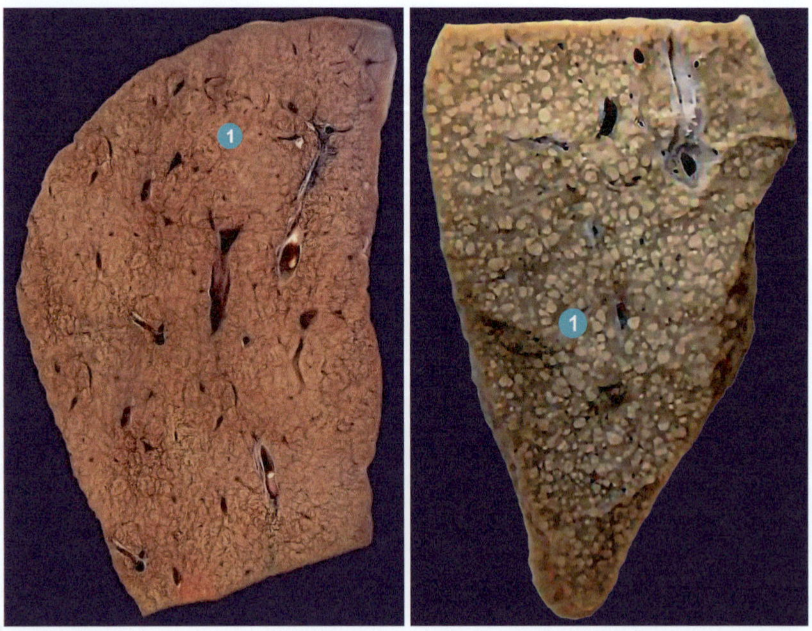

A slice of liver tissue is mounted.

1. The cut surface shows multiple small, pale yellow-brown nodules, which are rather uniform in appearance and <3 mm in diameter. The nodules are separated by thin fibrous bands.

Lennec Cirrhosis (a, b)

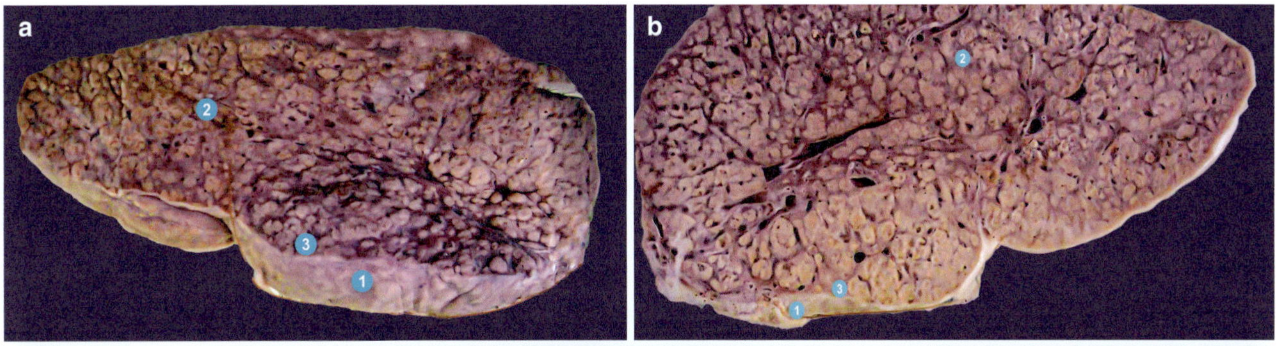

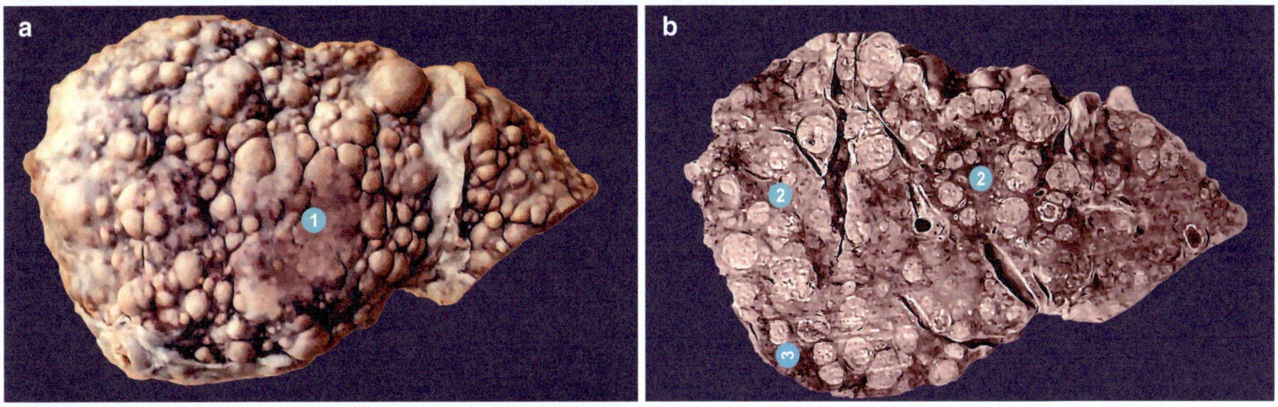

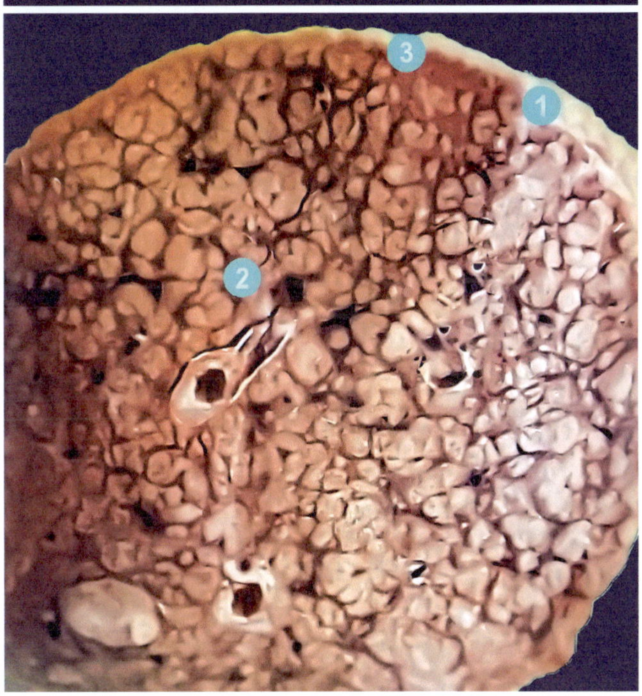

A slice of liver tissue is mounted.

1. The surface is nodular and yellow.
2. The cut section shows multiple pale-yellow nodules variable in size and shape separated from each other by bands of fibrous tissue.
3. The borders are sharp, indicating the firmness of tissue.

Microscopic Picture of Lennec Cirrhosis (a–e)

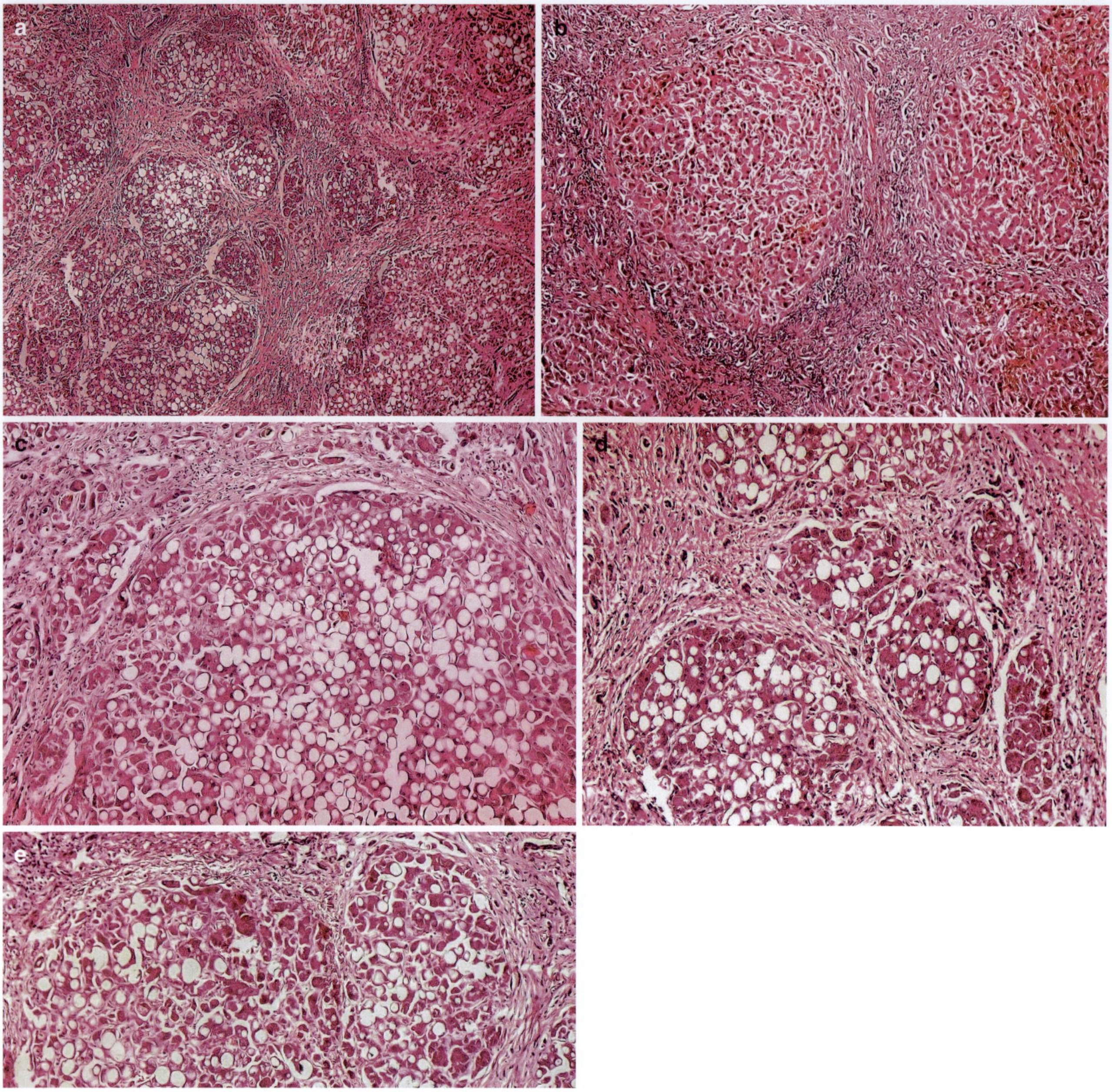

Sections show alteration of hepatic architecture by excessive fibrosis, turning hepatic lobules into regeneration nodules variable in size and shape. Fibrous septa are infiltrated by chronic lymphohistiocytic inflammatory infiltrate. Hepatocytes show ballooning degeneration, cytoplasmic vacuolization, and necrosis. The blood vessels within the liver are congested and dilated due to increased resistance to blood flow caused by fibrosis.

Pearls

The pathophysiology of cirrhosis involves:

1. A combination of processes:
   - Fibrosis: excessive production of collagen type I/III by hepatic stellate cells with or without portal fibroblasts through chronic inflammation (tumor necrosis factor [TNF] alpha, transforming growth factor [TGF] beta, IL1), cytokines from Kupffer cells, endothelial cells, bile duct cells, hepatocytes, and disruption of extracellular matrix and toxins

- Regeneration of hepatocytes through the proliferation of progenitor cells of the ductular reaction
- Parenchymal extinction due to vascular disruption [1]

2. Regression
   - Cirrhosis is potentially reversible after successful treatment of chronic liver disease, e.g., viral hepatitis.
   - Cessation of chronic damage allows hepatocyte recovery and modulates the microenvironment.
   - Shifting balance from inflammation to resolution results in phenotypic adjustments of immune cells.
   - Myofibroblasts are deactivated by senescence, apoptosis, and inactivation.
   - Matrix degradation also occurs [2]

5.1.5 Neoplastic Lesions

5.1.5.1 Primary Tumors

Hepatoblastoma

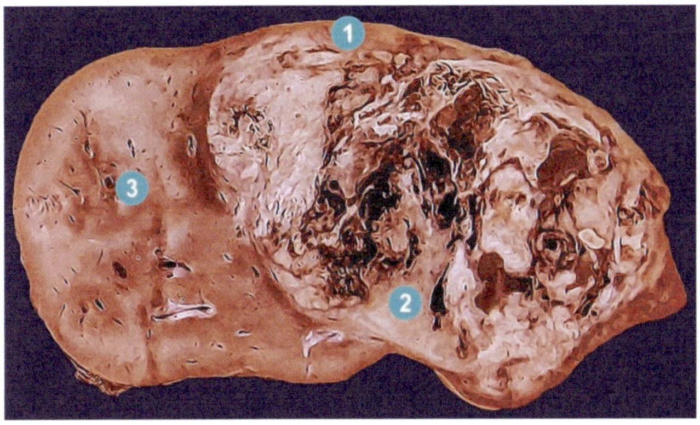

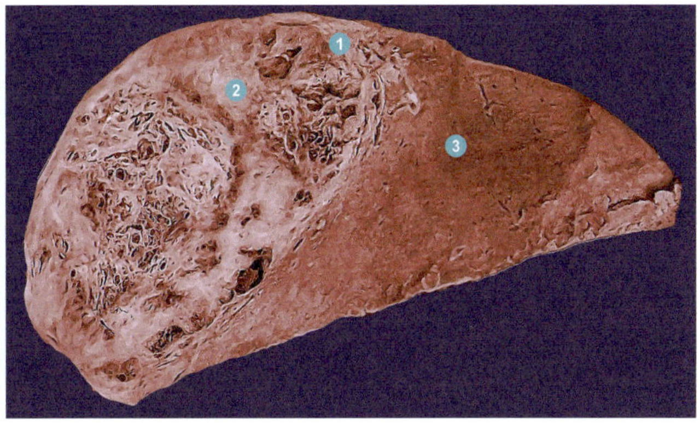

The liver of a child is mounted.

1. A large tumor mass occupies a significant portion of the right lobe of the liver.
2. The tumor is lobulated and well-circumscribed with a tan-yellow appearance with extensive areas of necrosis and hemorrhage.
3. The rest of the liver appears unremarkable.

Microscopic Picture of Mixed Epithelial and Mesenchymal Hepatoblastoma (a–e)

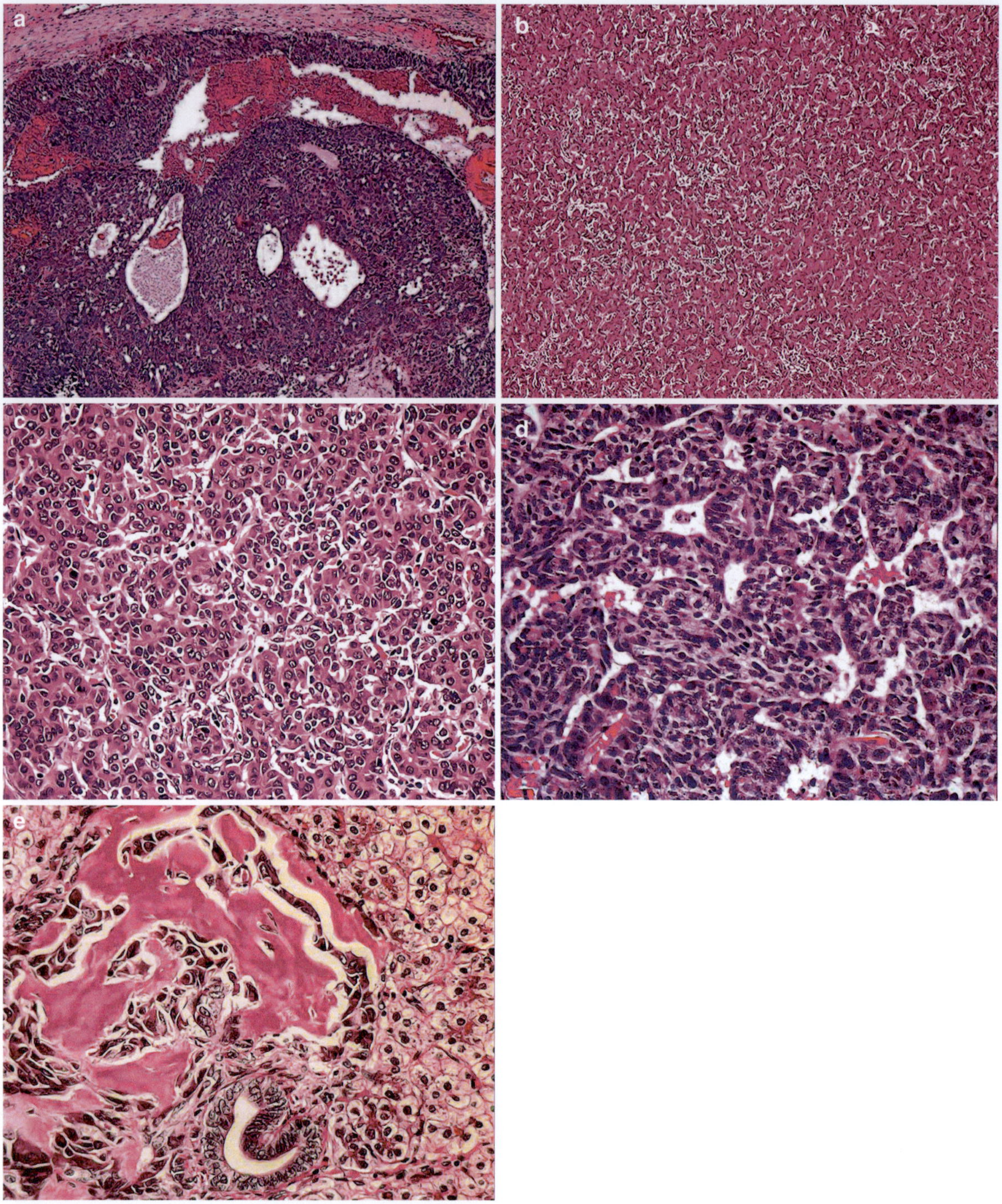

Sections show irregular clusters or sheets of cells reminiscent of embryonal and fetal liver tissue. These tumor cells form solid masses, interconnected structures resembling liver trabeculae, and gland-like arrangements mimicking bile ducts. The tumor cells exhibit variations in size and shape. They possess large, hyperchromatic nuclei, resulting in a high nucleus-to-cytoplasm ratio. Some tumor cells display differentiation towards liver cells, characterized by clear or eosinophilic cytoplasm, or towards bile duct epithelial cells. The tumor is embedded within a fibrous stroma. The mesenchymal component is seen in the form of osteoid production.

Ancillary Tools

IHC:

- Frequent beta-catenin and glutamine synthetase in the epithelial fetal (except the well-differentiated and low mitotic subtype) and mesenchymal patterns.
- AFP in the less differentiated epithelial components
- HepPar1 in the fetal pattern
- Polyclonal CEA
- Glypican 3 in the fetal and embryonal pattern
- Pancytokeratins have variable expression
- CK7 and CK19 in the cholangioblastic pattern
- INI1/SMARCB1 usually retained [3]

Molecular/cytogenetics description:

- High-risk tumors have upregulation of NFE2L2 activity, high LIN28B, HMGA2, SALL4, and AFP expression, and high coordinated expression of oncofetal proteins and stem cell markers
- Low-risk tumors have LIN28B and let-7 expression and high HNF1A activity [4].

Pearls

Hepatoblastomas are characterized by a complex pattern of chromosomal abnormalities, including gains or losses of genetic material on chromosomes 1q, 2q, 4q, 8, 11q, 17q, and 20. Genetic studies have identified several changes that contribute to the development of hepatoblastomas, affecting cell division, growth, cell death, signaling pathways, and differentiation. Among the alterations in key signaling pathways, the Wnt/β-catenin pathway is the most prominent. Mutations in the β-catenin gene are the most common genetic alteration in sporadic hepatoblastomas, occurring in at least 50% of cases and affecting both epithelial and mixed types of tumors [5].

Pediatric Hepatocellular Carcinoma (Fibrolamellar Type)

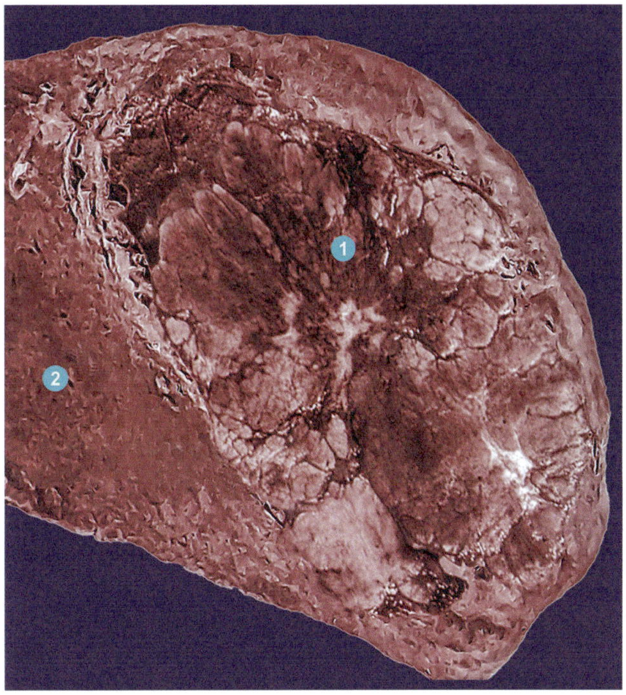

Part of the liver of a child is mounted.

1. A single, large, oval, well-circumscribed, and tan tumor mass with stellate scar and areas of hemorrhage and necrosis.
2. The rest of the liver appears unremarkable.

Microscopic Picture of Fibrolamellar Hepatocellular Carcinoma (a–c)

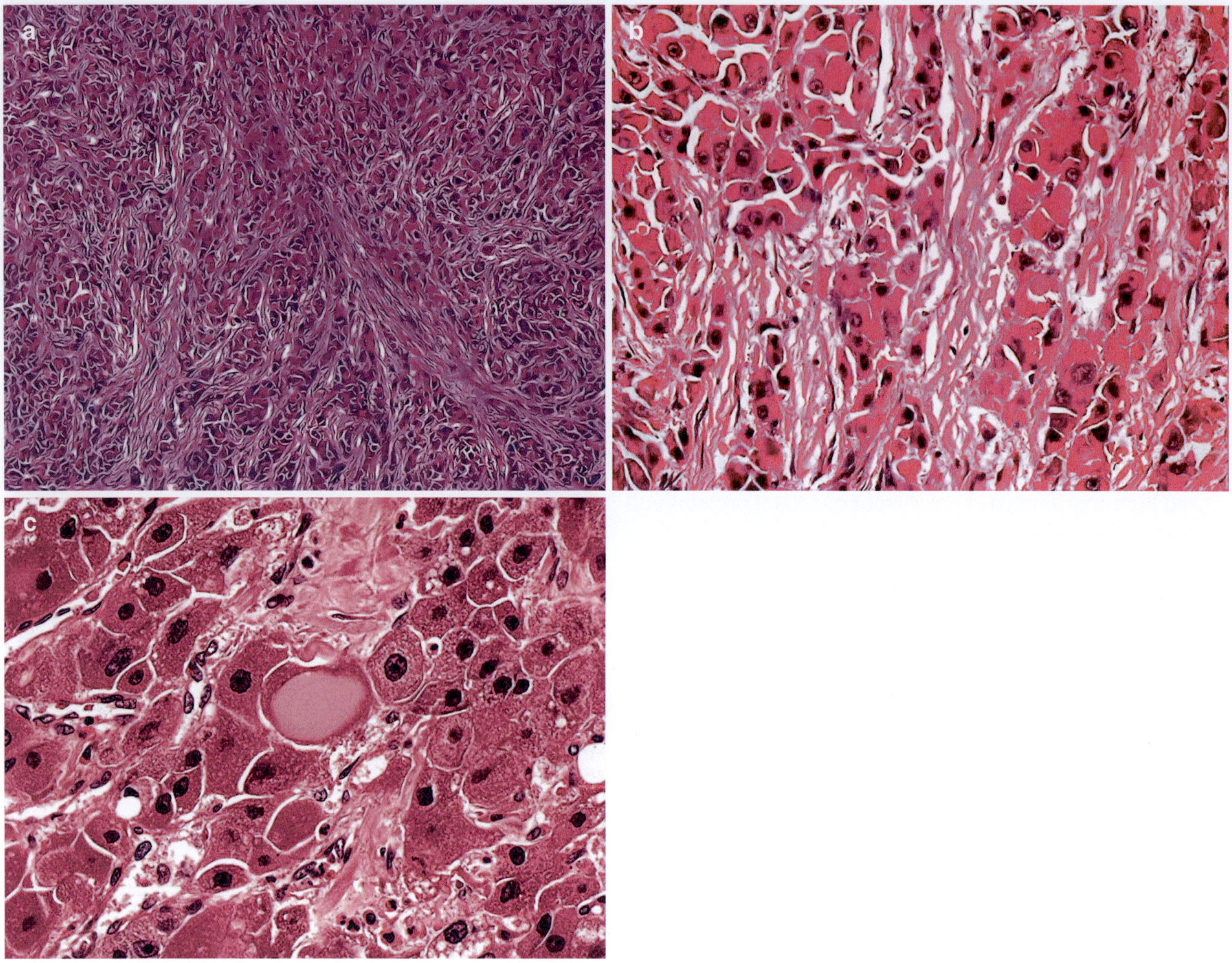

Sections show strands of large, polygonal cells with distinct borders. These cells have a granular, pink cytoplasm packed with mitochondria, often containing pale or pink bodies. Their nuclei have open chromatin and prominent large nucleoli. The surrounding tissue is dense with collagen fibers arranged in layers.

Ancillary Tools

IHC [6]:

HepPar1 and CK7

CD68

CK19

Fibrinogen (pale bodies), alpha-1 antitrypsin, polyclonal CEA, and CAM 5.2 (CK8/18)

Molecular/cytogenetics description [7]:

- Less than 95% of cases are characterized by the DNAJB1-PRKACA fusion gene; diagnostic tests exist.
- Rare cases are characterized by biallelic PRKAR1A loss (mostly in patients with the Carney complex) instead of the above fusion gene.
- Transcriptome has been published and revealed multiple insights.
- Overall fewer chromosomal abnormalities than in classic hepatocellular carcinoma.

Pearls

Pediatric hepatocellular carcinoma (HCC) is the second most common malignant liver tumor in children after hepatoblastoma. It differs from the adult HCC in the etiological predisposition, biological behavior, and lower frequency of cirrhosis. According to the SEER database, the most common histological subtype of pediatric HCC is non-fibrolamellar HCC, constituting 73% of cases, followed by fibrolamellar HCC in 25% and clear cell carcinoma in 2% of cases [8].

Hepatocellular Carcinoma, Nodular Pattern

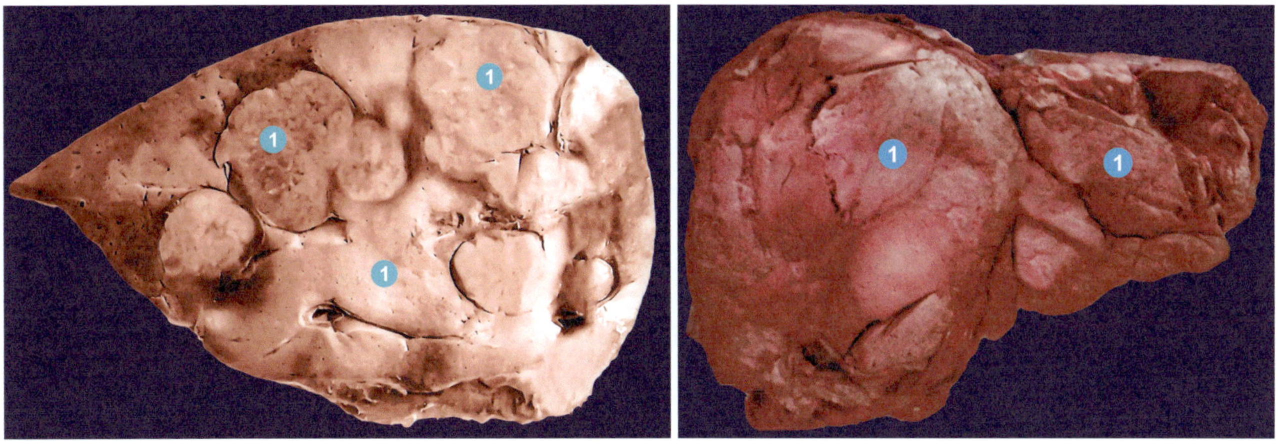

Part of the liver is mounted.

1. It is infiltrated by multiple masses well delineated from normal liver tissue with varying shades of yellow-tan to brown, paler than normal tissue.

Hepatocellular Carcinoma, Diffuse Pattern

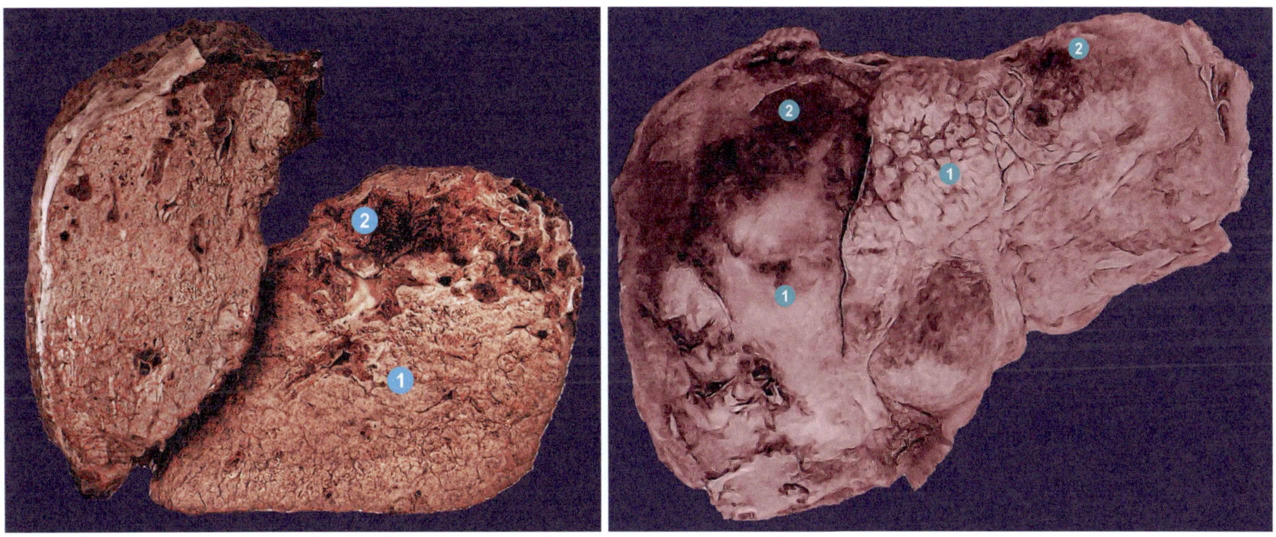

Part of the liver is mounted.

1. The tumor is composed of hundreds of small, light brown nodules that are grossly hard to differentiate from cirrhotic nodules.
2. Areas of hemorrhage and necrosis are seen.

Microscopic Picture of Hepatocellular Carcinoma (a–i)

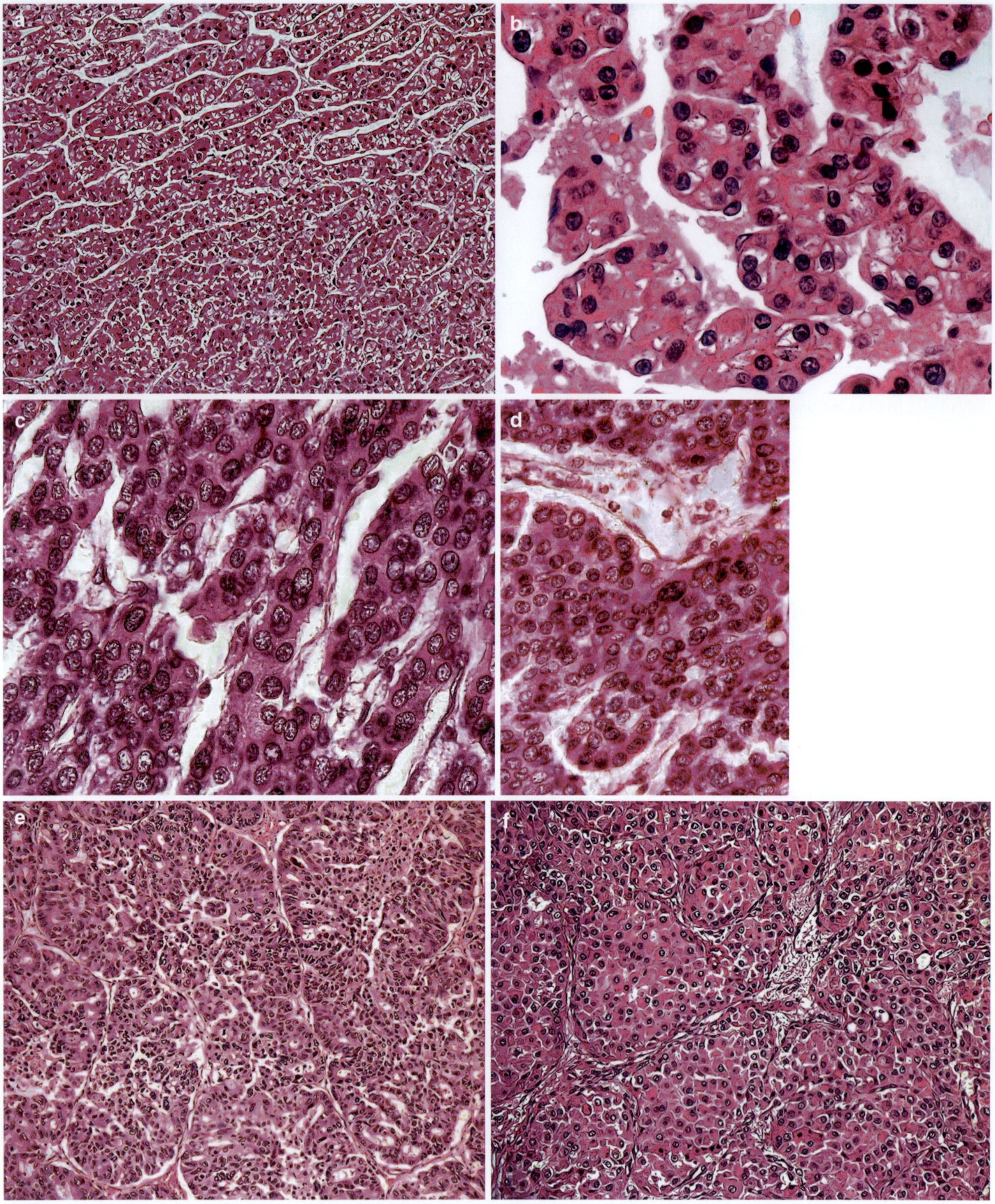

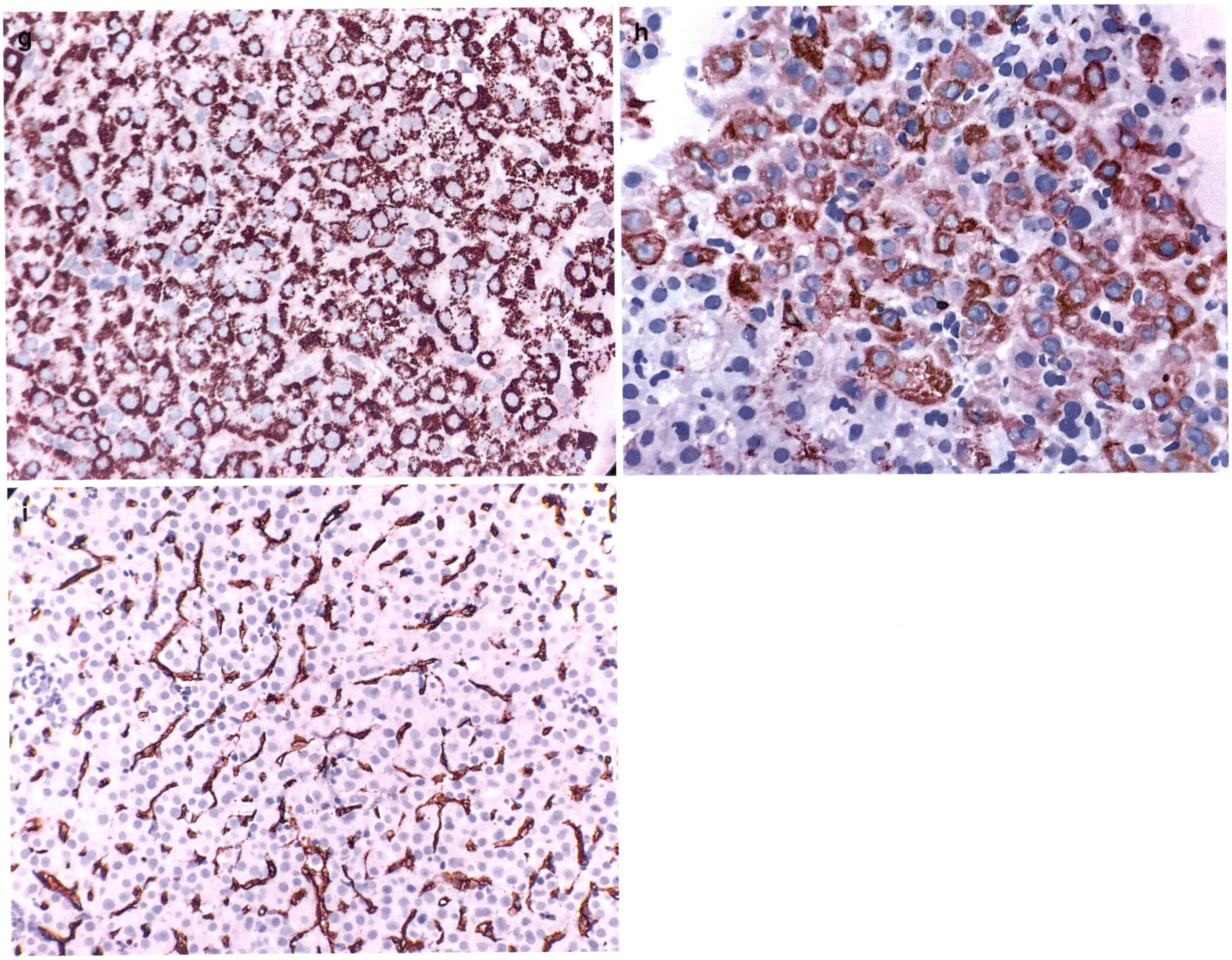

Sections show malignant hepatocytes arranged in trabecular, pseudoglandular, and solid patterns. The trabecular pattern is characterized by the arrangement of tumor cells in cords or trabeculae separated by sinusoidal spaces. The tumor cells show marked cellular atypia and invade adjacent liver tissue and blood vessels. The tumor cells are surrounded by fibrous stroma infiltrated by chronic inflammatory cells.

Hepatocellular Carcinoma with Peliotic Change

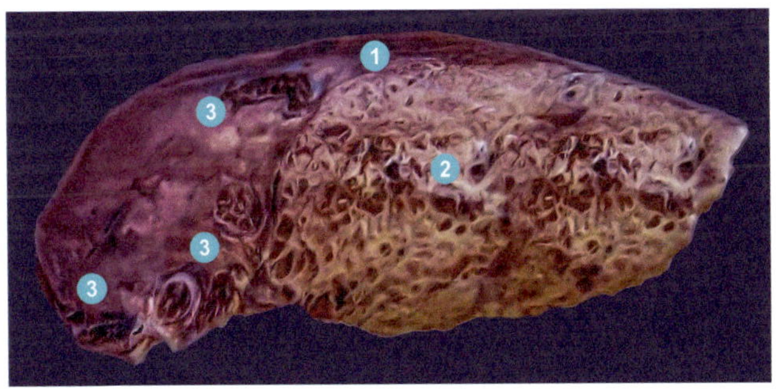

Part of the liver is mounted

1. An incompletely encapsulated large tumor occupying most of the resected hepatic tissue.
2. The tumor mass is solid at its periphery, but the rest of the mass shows peliotic change in the form of well-defined multiple cavities, giving the tumor a spongy appearance.
3. Intrahepatic metastases with a similar appearance are seen in the liver tissue near the periphery of the main tumor.

Microscopic Picture of Hepatocellular Carcinoma with Peliotic Change (a)

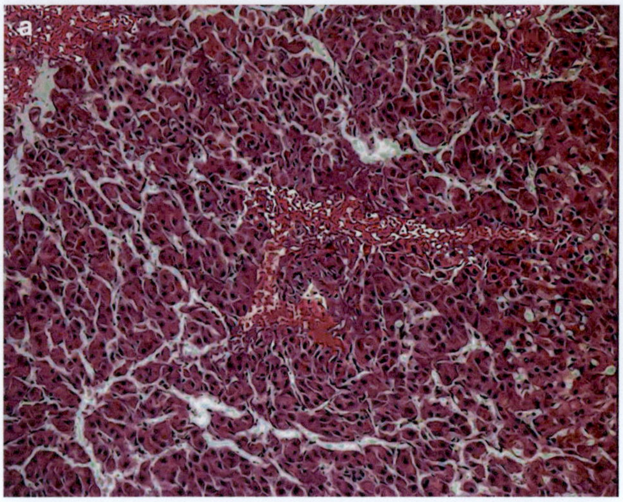

Sections show a well-differentiated HCC. In the main portion of the lesion dilated, sinusoid-like structures without an endothelial lining filled with red blood cells, suggestive of peliotic change, are observed, corresponding to the area of the tumor with a spongy appearance on macroscopic examination.

Pearls

Peliotic changes are frequently observed in HCCs. It is suggested that peliotic changes are different from hemorrhage. Degeneration and/or necrosis of tumor tissue cause hemorrhage in HCC. On the other hand, tumor tissues around peliotic changes are not degenerative or necrotic, and blood is localized within the spaces. The mechanism of peliotic change in HCC was explained by endothelial damage due to sinusoidal dilatation following increased intratumoral pressure [9].

Ancillary Tools

IHC [10]:

- HepPar1 (**g**): cytoplasmic and granular; overall highly sensitive, but 50% of poorly differentiated hepatocellular carcinomas lose expression.
- Glypican 3 (**h**): cytoplasmic; high sensitivity in poorly differentiated and scirrhous hepatocellular carcinoma but low sensitivity in well-differentiated hepatocellular carcinoma (nonneoplastic liver is negative).
- CD34 (**i**) is one of the most useful immunohistochemical markers in the distinction between benign and malignant hepatocellular lesions. Normal sinusoidal lining cells do not stain for CD34, whereas the abnormal capillaries of HCCs are diffusely CD34 positive.
- Arginase1: cytoplasmic or nuclear; useful in confirming hepatocellular differentiation; highly sensitive and specific, thus more useful than HepPar1 for poorly differentiated hepatocellular carcinoma.
- AFP: cytoplasmic; highly specific but low sensitivity; frequently negative in well-differentiated hepatocellular carcinoma
- Polyclonal CEA, villin, and CD10 reveal canalicular pattern and limited sensitivity in poorly differentiated hepatocellular carcinoma.
- Albumin ISH: high sensitivity for primary liver carcinoma, although this can also be positive in other adenocarcinomas not of biliary origin.
- Pancytokeratins (MNF116 or OSCAR) and CAM5.2 (CK8/CK18) are positive.

Molecular/cytogenetics description [11]:

The diagnosis of hepatocellular carcinoma often does not require molecular or cytogenetic testing, but these ancillary studies can aid in diagnosing difficult cases and identifying a specific subtype of hepatocellular carcinoma:

- Scirrhous subtype: TSC1/TSC2 mutations
- Steatohepatitic subtype: frequent IL6/JAK/STAT activation
- Macrotrabecular massive subtype: TP53 mutation and FGF19 amplification

Intrahepatic Cholangiocarcinoma (ICCA) (a, b)

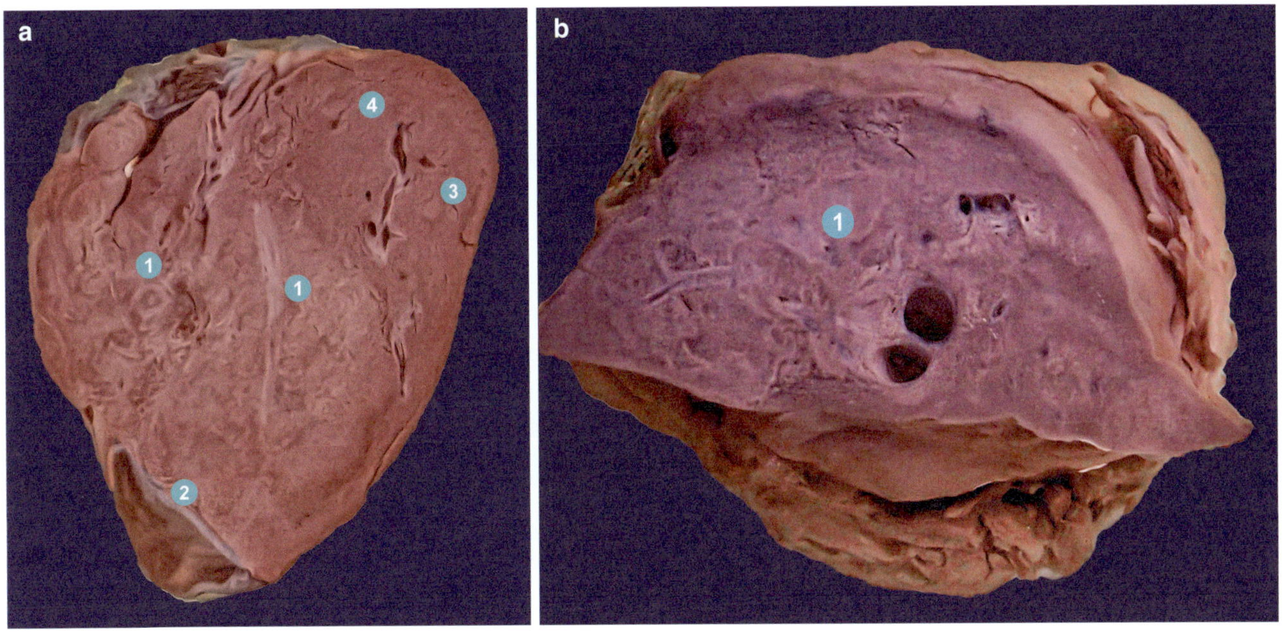

A part of the liver is mounted.

1. A large, firm, gray-white, and infiltrative tumor mass occupies most of the specimen.
2. The tumor is adherent to the gallbladder wall.
3. Satellite small gray-white tumor nodule is seen away from the tumor.
4. The rest of the liver tissue is unremarkable.

Microscopic Picture of Intrahepatic Cholangiocarcinoma (ICCA) (c–i)

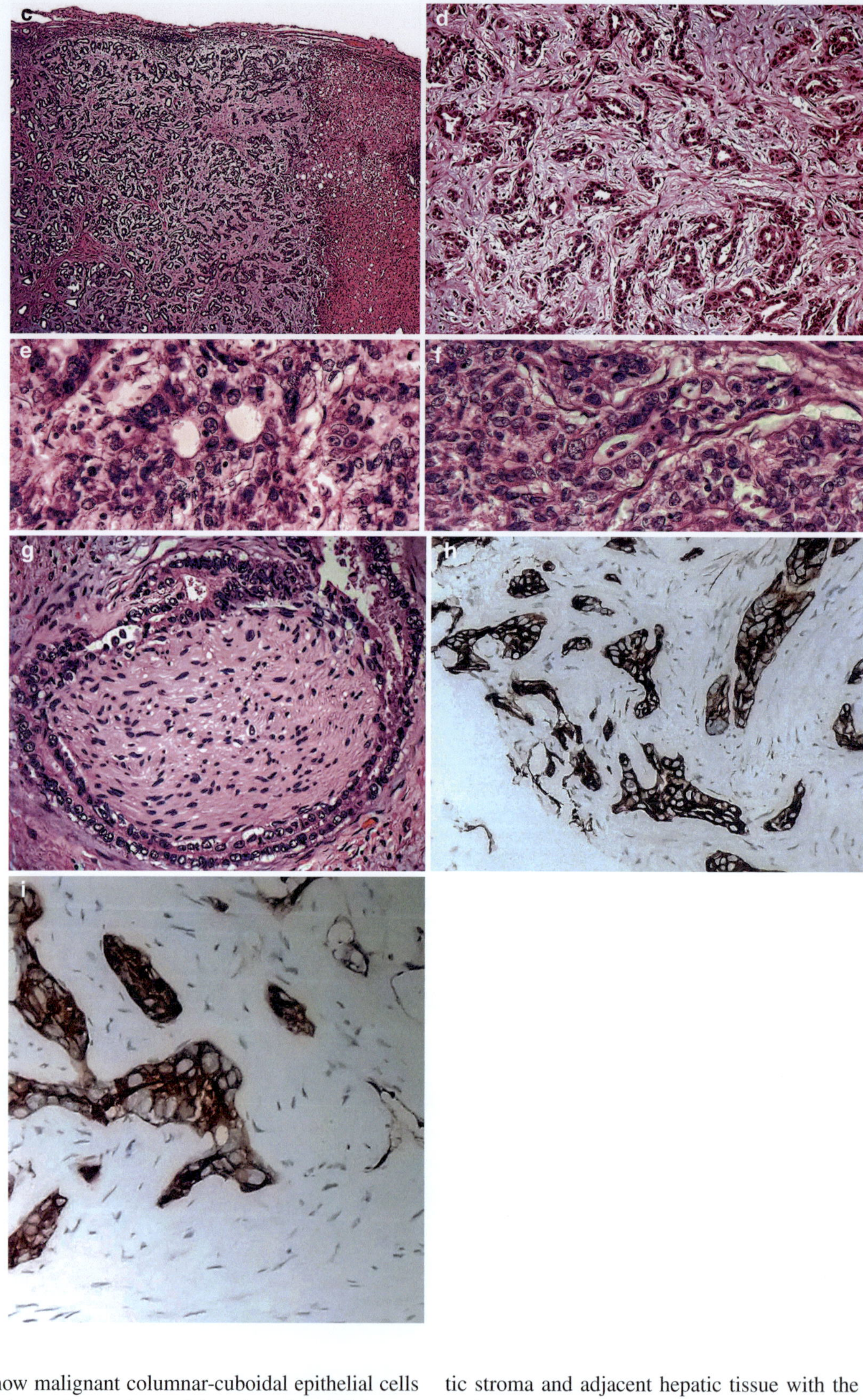

Sections show malignant columnar-cuboidal epithelial cells with large hyperchromatic nuclei and eosinophilic cytoplasm, forming small acini and cords infiltrating desmoplastic stroma and adjacent hepatic tissue with the presence of perineural invasion.

Ancillary Tools

IHC [12]:

CK7 (h)

CK19 (i)

CK17, CAM 5.2, MOC31, EMA, monoclonal CEA, polyclonal CEA (diffuse cytoplasmic pattern), claudin4, pVHL

Albumin RNA ISH (~80%) but does not differentiate iCCA from hepatocellular carcinoma

Glypican 3 and HepPar1 are occasionally positive in peripherally located iCCA

Molecular/cytogenetics description [13]:

Mutations in KRAS (22%), BRAF (7%), EGFR (2%), IDH1/IDH2 (14%), MET, activation of mTOR, overexpression of cyclin D1, overexpression of p21, inactivating mutations of DPC4/SMAD4 (13–15%) and TP53 (15%).

Chromosomal gains of 1q, 5p, 7p, 8q, 17q, and 20q and losses of 1p, 4q, 8p, 9p, 17p, and 18q

5.1.5.2 Metastatic Tumors

Multiple Metastases in Liver, Infiltrative Pattern

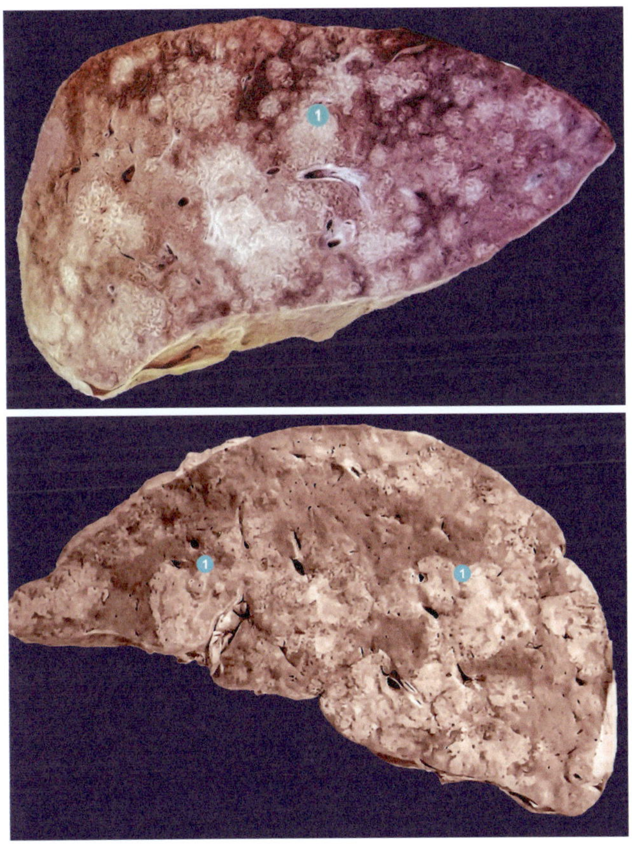

A slice of liver tissue is mounted.

1. The liver is diffusely infiltrated by multiple ill-defined nodular infiltrates demarcated from the surrounding liver tissue.

Microscopic Picture of Multiple Metastases in Liver (a)

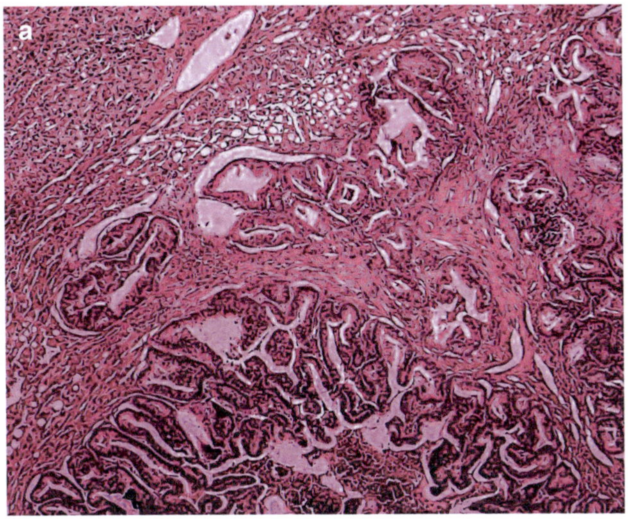

The section shows clusters of malignant acini embedded in a fibrous stroma and invading benign-looking hepatic tissue.

5.2 Gallbladder

5.2.1 Inflammatory Lesions

Chronic Acalcular Cholecystitis (a, b)

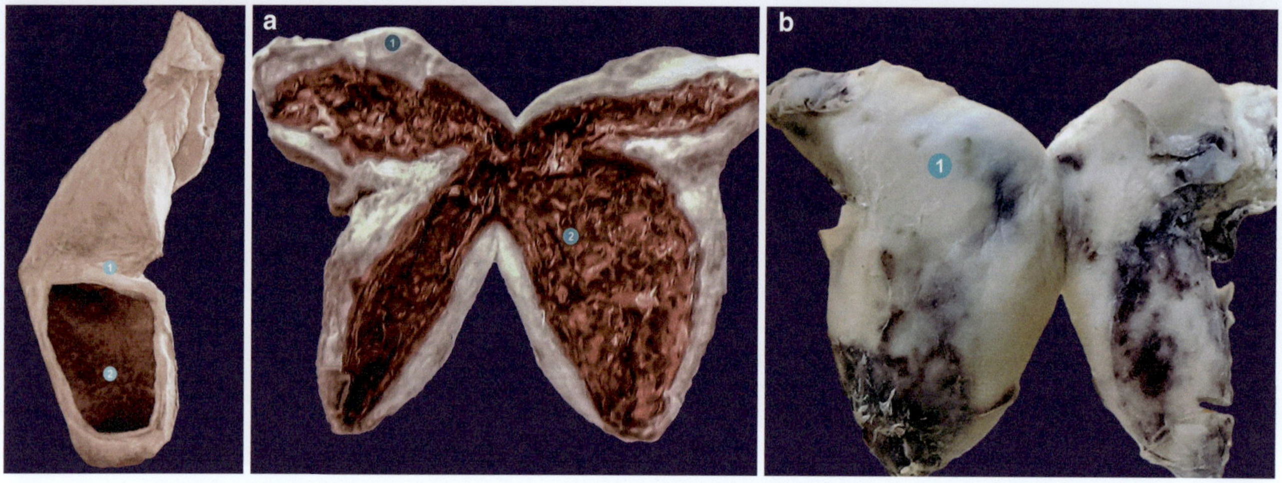

An opened gallbladder is mounted.

1. The wall is fibrous and thickened.
2. The mucosa is dark while the lumen shows brown biliary sludge.

Chronic Calcular Cholecystitis (a, b)

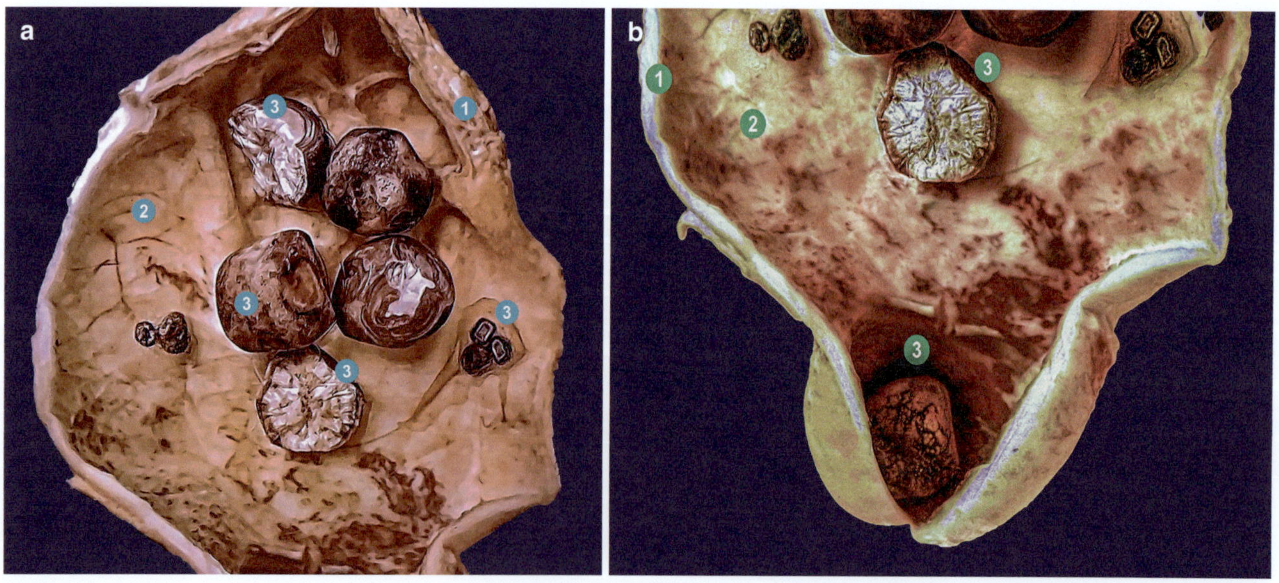

An opened gallbladder is mounted.

1. The wall is fibrous and thickened.
2. The lumen is dilated and shows multiple mixed gallstones.
3. The stones are variable in size and shape, with a brown faceted outer surface and radiating yellow-white cut section.

Microscopic Picture of Chronic Calcular Cholecystitis (c, d)

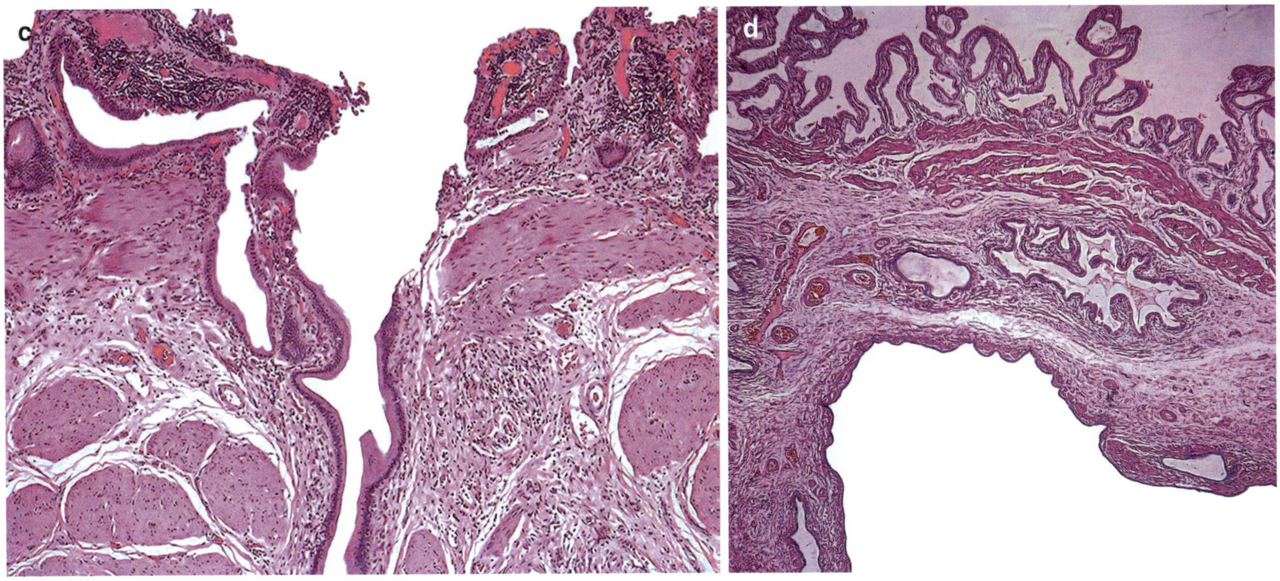

The section shows fibrosed subepithelial stroma infiltrated by chronic inflammatory cells. There is outpouching or invagination of the mucosal layer into the muscular layer of the gallbladder wall, forming the Rokitansky-Aschoff sinus.

Chronic Calcular Cholecystitis

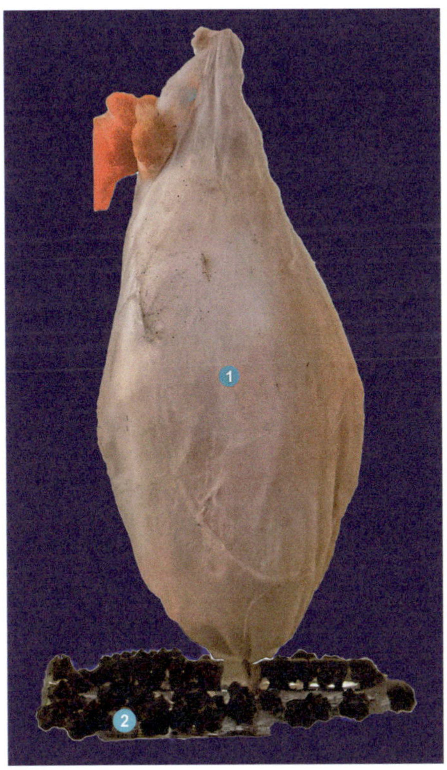

An opened gallbladder is mounted.

1. The wall is fibrous and thickened.
2. Multiple, small, hard, and black pigmented gallstones are seen.

Chronic Calcular Cholecystitis

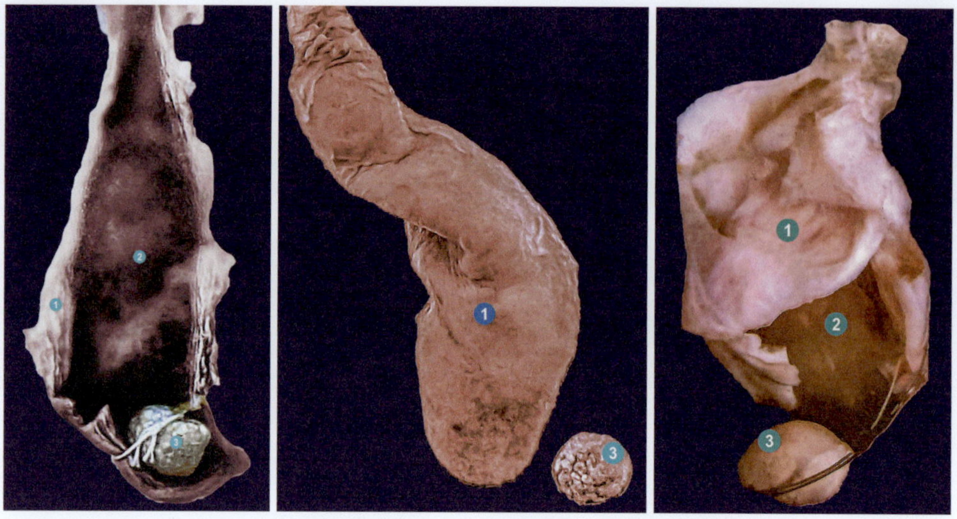

An opened gallbladder is mounted.

1. The wall is fibrous and thickened.
2. The lumen is dilated, lined with flat mucosa, and showing a single cholesterol stone.
3. The stone is single, large, yellow-white, with an irregular (a, b) or smooth (c) surface.

Cholesterol Stones

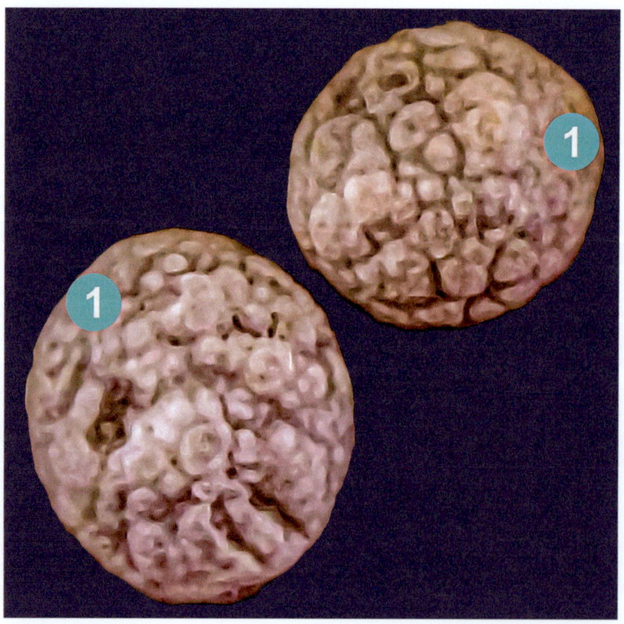

1. Two large, pale yellow, round stones with a mamillated surface.

Infected (Mixed) Stones

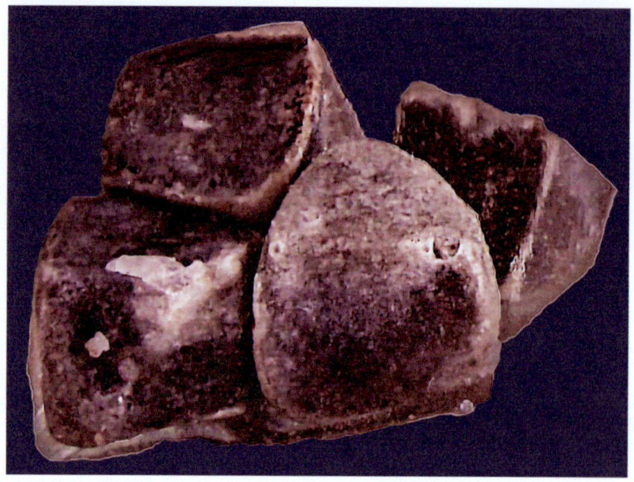

1. The stones are variable in size and shape, with a deep brown faceted outer surface

5.2.2 Neoplastic Lesions

Carcinoma of the Gallbladder with Chronic Cholecystitis

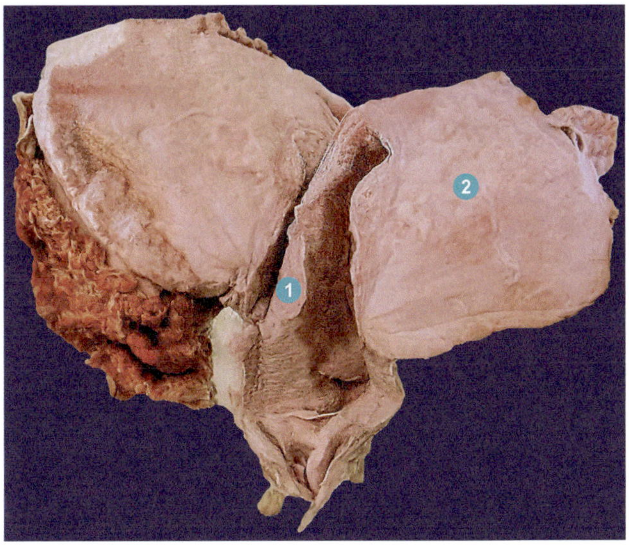

A dilated, opened gallbladder is mounted.

1. The wall is greatly thickened.
2. The fundus is occupied by a large, round, yellow-pink mass that infiltrates the gallbladder walls.

Papillary Carcinoma of the Gallbladder

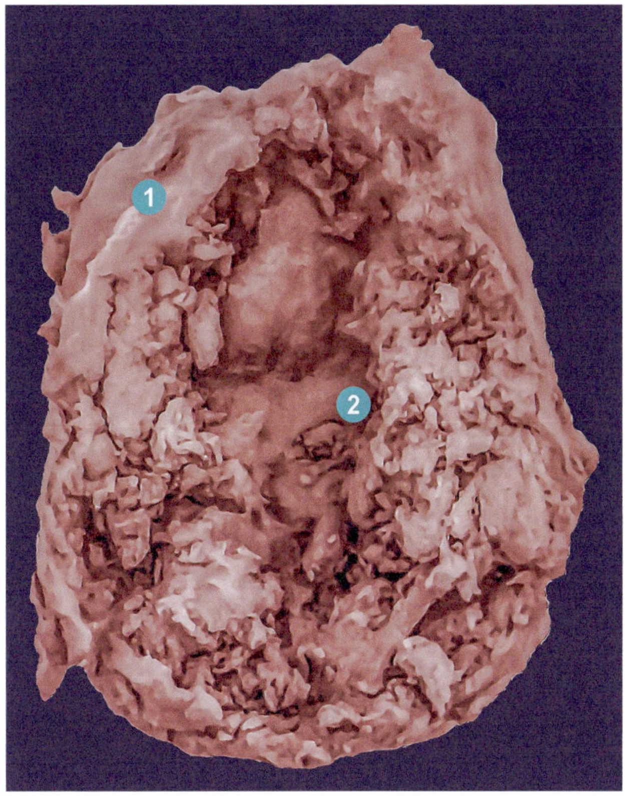

An opened gallbladder.

1. The wall is greatly thickened.
2. Multiple polypoid, friable masses covering the mucosa with areas of hemorrhage and necrosis.

Microscopic Picture of Biliary Type Papillary Adenocarcinoma of Gallbladder (a–e)

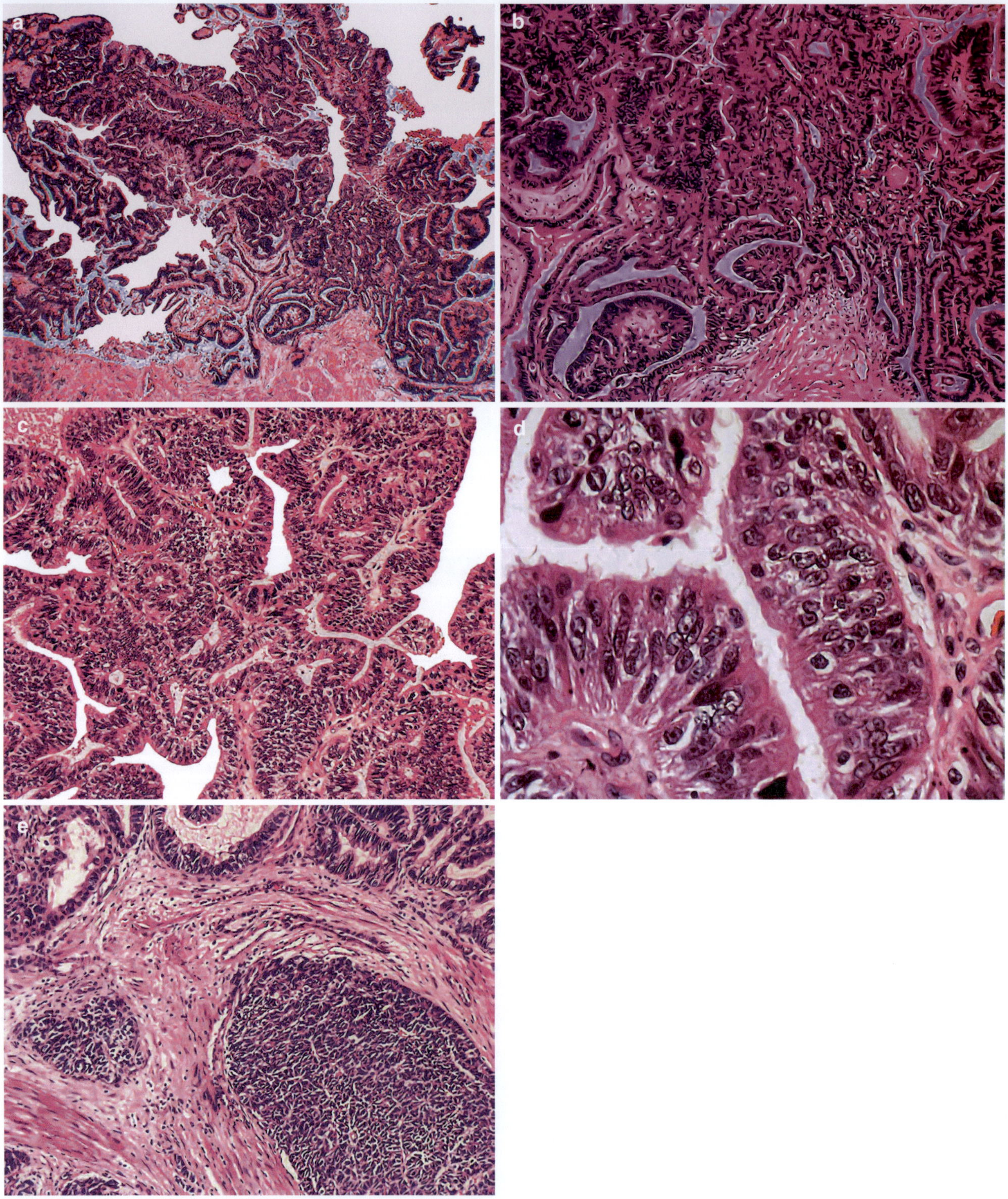

Sections show malignant cuboidal-columnar tumor cells forming papillae with fibrovascular cores. The tumor invades into the subepithelial stroma and muscularis propria. The tumor cells are surrounded by chronic inflammatory cells.

Ancillary Tools

IHC [14]:

CK7 (strong and diffuse), p53 (majority), CEA and CA19-9 (70–90%), IMP3 (80%), Maspin (60–100%), S100P and MUC1 (75%), HER2 (>60%), CK20, and CDX2 (focal)

Molecular/cytogenetics description [15]:

Common genetic alterations include TP53 (seen in >50% of cases), CDKN2A (20%), ARID1A (13%), PIK3CA (10%), and CTNNB1 (10%).

Amplifications of ERBB2 (HER2) have been reported in 16% of cases and microsatellite instability (MSI) in 10% of cancers, both of which have therapeutic implications. A higher KRAS mutation rate is noted in lesions related to pancreaticobiliary maljunction.

Pearls

Invasive papillary carcinomas have the most favorable prognosis than conventional nonpapillary gallbladder adenocarcinomas because they have an exophytic growth pattern, exhibit delayed invasion into the gallbladder wall, and are detected early due to obstructive symptoms [16]

Cancer Head of Pancreas

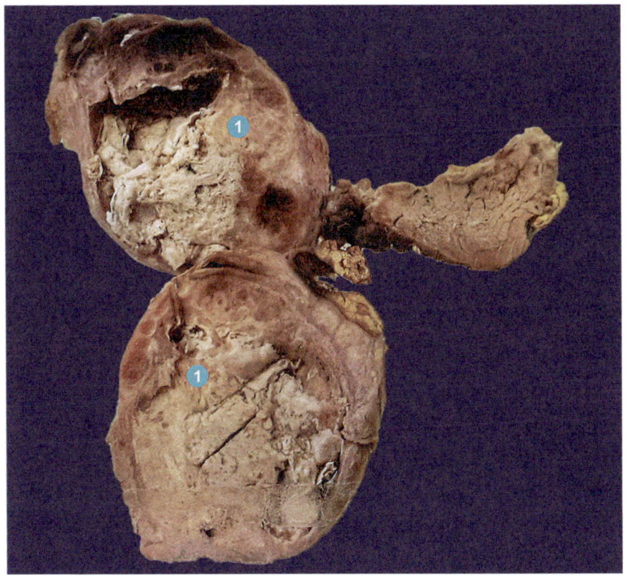

The pancreatectomy specimen is mounted

1. A large round, firm, well-defined, and yellow mass is present in the head of the pancreas with focal areas of hemorrhage and necrosis.

Microscopic Picture of Well-Differentiated Pancreatic Duct Adenocarcinoma (a–d)

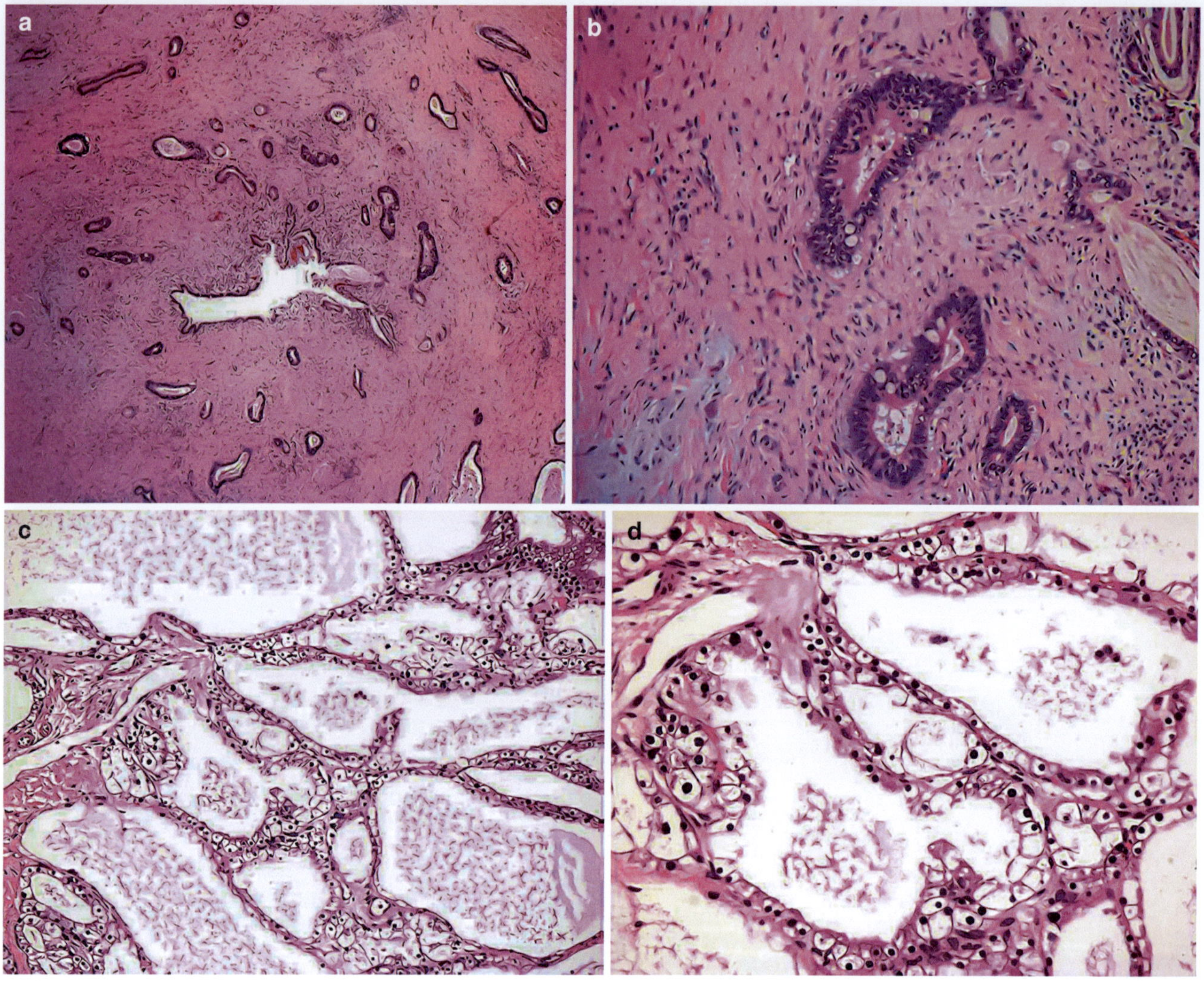

Sections show well-formed glands infiltrating singly in a haphazard fashion. The infiltrating glands are distributed in a disorganized fashion. The glandular structures show apical mucin granules, irregular in shape and distribution. Some glandular or ductal structures are lined with a single layer of polygonal clear cells with distinct cell borders and variable nuclear atypia. The stroma is desmoplastic and infiltrated with chronic inflammatory cells.

Ancillary Tools

IHC [17]:

Maspin, placental S100 (S100P), IMP3 (all positive in >90% PDACs).

p53 expressed in most cases.

CK7, CK8, CK18, CK19, MUC1, MUC3, MUC4, MUC5AC, CEA, B72.3, CA19-9, CA125 (48%)

Molecular/cytogenetics description [18]:

4 key driver gene mutations: KRAS: >95%, early event during carcinogenesis

CDKN2A (p16): 95%

TP53: 50–80%

SMAD4: 55%

50% overexpress HER2

Many core signaling pathways involved

~10% of pancreatic cancers have a familial basis

References

1. Sonthalia N. et al. (2016). Primary hepatic amyloidosis: A case report and review of literature World J Hepatol. 8(6):340-4. doi: https://doi.org/10.4254/wjh.v8.i6.340. PMID: 26962400.
2. Dezso K. et al. (2017). Human liver regeneration in advanced cirrhosis is organized by the portal tree. J Hepatol.66(4):778-786. doi: https://doi.org/10.1016/j.jhep.2016.11.014. PMID: 27913222.
3. Ranganathan S. et.al.(2020). Hepatoblastoma and Pediatric Hepatocellular Carcinoma: An Update. Pediatr. Dev. Pathol. 23(2):79-95. doi:https://doi.org/10.1177/1093526619875228. PMID: 31554479.
4. Nagae G, et al. (2021). Genetic and epigenetic basis of hepatoblastoma diversity. Nat Commun. 12: 5423. https://doi.org/10.1038/s41467-021-25430-9.
5. Tacke F., Trautwein C. (2015). Mechanisms of liver fibrosis resolution. J Hepatol. 63(4):1038-9. doi: https://doi.org/10.1016/j.jhep.2015.03.039. PMID: 26232376.
6. Ward S.C, et al. (2010). Fibrolamellar carcinoma of the liver exhibits immunohistochemical evidence of both hepatocyte and bile duct differentiation. Mod. Pathol. 23(9):1180-90. doi: https://doi.org/10.1038/modpathol.2010.105. PMID: 20495535.
7. Koehne de Gonzalez A.K. et al. (2015). Current concepts in the immunohistochemical evaluation of liver tumors World J Hepatol. 7(10):1403-11. doi:https://doi.org/10.4254/wjh.v7.i10.1403. PMID: 26052385.
8. Khanna R, Verma SK. (2018).Pediatric hepatocellular carcinoma. World J Gastroenterol. 24(35):3980-3999. doi: https://doi.org/10.3748/wjg.v24.i35.3980. PMID: 30254403; PMCID: PMC6148423.
9. Fujimoto M. et al. (2010). Clinicopathological study of hepatocellular carcinoma with peliotic change. Oncol Lett. 1(1):17-21. doi: https://doi.org/10.3892/ol_00000003. PMID: 22966249; PMCID: PMC3436385.
10. Calderaro J. et al. (2017).Histological subtypes of hepatocellular carcinoma are related to gene mutations and molecular tumor classification. J. Hepatol.67(4):727-738. doi: https://doi.org/10.1016/j.jhep.2017.05.014. PMID: 28532995.
11. Vyas M, Jain D. A. (2018). A practical diagnostic approach to hepatic masses. Indian J Pathol. Microbiol. 61(1):2-17. doi: https://doi.org/10.4103/IJPM.IJPM_578_17. PMID: 29567877.
12. Labib PL, Goodchild G, Pereira SP. (2019).Molecular Pathogenesis of Cholangiocarcinoma. BMC Cancer. 19(1):185. doi: https://doi.org/10.1186/s12885-019-5391-0. PMID: 30819129; PMCID: PMC6394015.
13. Wang HL. et al. (2017). Practical Immunohistochemistry in Neoplastic Pathology of the Gastrointestinal Tract, Liver, Biliary Tract, and Pancreas. Arch Pathol Lab Med.141(9):1155-1180. doi: https://doi.org/10.5858/arpa.2016-0489-RA. PMID: 28854347.
14. Goldin RD, Roa JC. (2009).Gallbladder cancer: a morphological and molecular update. Histopathology. 55(2):218-29. doi: https://doi.org/10.1111/j.1365-2559.2008.03192.x. PMID: 19490172.
15. Albores-Saavedra J. et al. (2005). Papillary carcinomas of the gallbladder: analysis of noninvasive and invasive types. Arch Pathol Lab Med.129(7):905-9. doi: https://doi.org/10.5858/2005-129-905-PCOTGA. PMID: 15974814.
16. Shi J. et al. (2013).Diagnostic utility of von Hippel-Lindau gene product, maspin, IMP3, and S100P in adenocarcinoma of the gallbladder. Hum Pathol. 44(4):503-11. doi: https://doi.org/10.1016/j.humpath.2012.06.010. PMID: 23079206.
17. Liu H. et al. (2012). Reevaluation and identification of the best immunohistochemical panel (pVHL, Maspin, S100P, IMP-3) for ductal adenocarcinoma of the pancreas. Arch Pathol Lab Med. 136(6):601-9. doi: https://doi.org/10.5858/arpa.2011-0326-OA. PMID: 22646265.
18. Cancer Genome Atlas Research Network. Integrated Genomic Characterization of Pancreatic Ductal Adenocarcinoma. (2017). Cancer Cell. 32(2):185-203.e13. doi: https://doi.org/10.1016/j.ccell.2017.07.007. PMID: 28810144; PMCID: PMC5964983.

6 Diseases of Kidney and Bladder

The urinary system is responsible for filtering waste from the body and maintaining a balance of salts, water, and electrolytes. It consists of the kidneys, ureters, bladder, and urethra.

This chapter will discuss the macroscopic and microscopic pathological changes that can occur in the urinary system. These changes can have significant implications for bodily function, often leading to symptoms or clinical conditions that require medical intervention.

We will examine each component of the urinary system in detail, focusing on various pathological conditions. This includes renal pathologies such as glomerulonephritis, pyelonephritis, and renal tumors; ureteral obstructions; and bladder abnormalities like bladder tumors.

The aim is to help readers develop an understanding of the key features of these diseases in the pathologic examination. By the end of this chapter, you should have a comprehensive understanding of the broad range of disorders that can affect the urinary system and how these manifest at a gross and microscopic pathological level. This knowledge will form a crucial foundation for diagnosing and treating these conditions and provide a springboard for a more in-depth study of the microscopic pathology of the urinary system.

The diseases of the urinary system discussed in this chapter will be arranged in this order:

1. **Kidney**
   (a) **Congenital Lesions**
   - APKD
   - Horseshoe Kidney
   - ARPK
   - Simple Renal Cyst

   (b) **Inflammatory Lesions**
   - GN
   - PN
   - Pyonephrosis
   - Pyemic Abscesses
   - Renal Tuberculosis
   - Urinary Bilharziasis

   (c) **Mechanical Lesions**
   - Hydronephrosis
   - Urolithiasis

   (d) **Fibrillar Lesions**
   - Renal Amyloidosis

   (e) **Vascular lesions**
   - Benign Nephrosclerosis
   - Malignant Nephrosclerosis

   (f) **Neoplastic Lesions**
   - Primary Tumors
     – Urothelial Papillomatosis
     – Nephroblastoma
     – Renal Cell Carcinoma
   - Renal Metastases
2. **Urinary Bladder**
   (a) **Neoplastic Lesions**
   - Carcinoma

G. Dawood, *Color Atlas of Human Gross and Microscopic Pathology*, https://doi.org/10.1007/978-3-031-76007-5_6

6.1 Kidney

6.1.1 Congenital Lesions

Adult Polycystic Kidney Disease (APKD) (a, b)

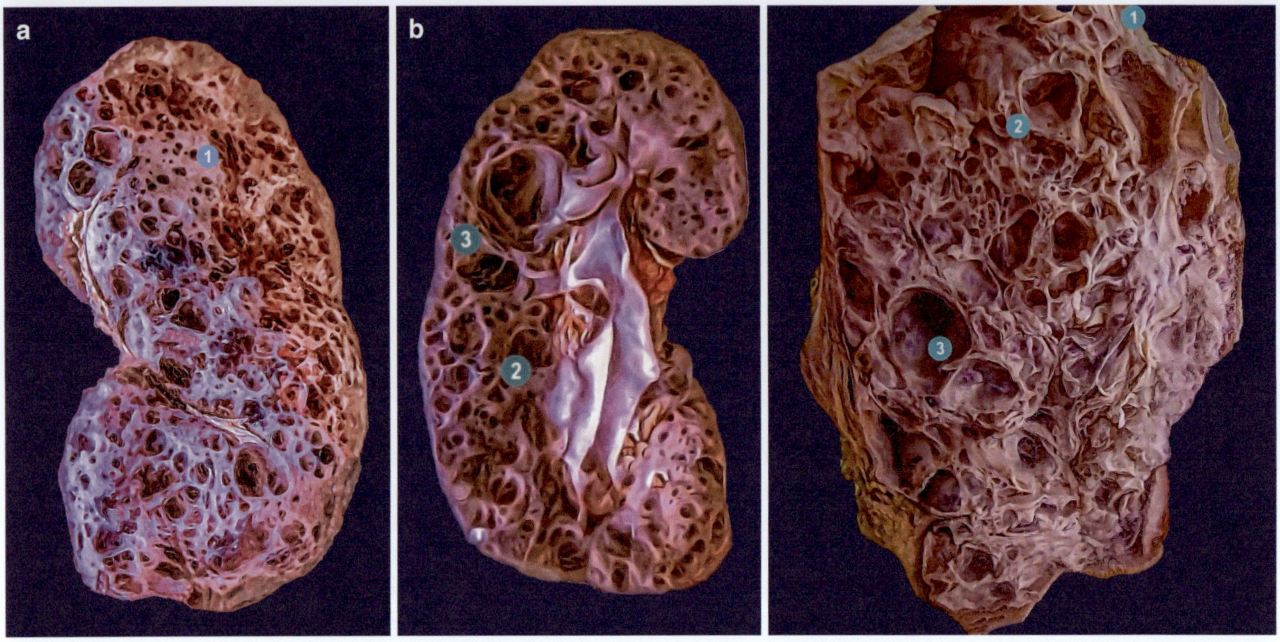

The kidney bisected longitudinally is mounted.

1. The kidney is enlarged.
2. Its normal tissue is replaced by multiple, communicating cysts variable in size and shape, with a smooth lining.
3. Some cysts contain clear or hemorrhagic fluid.

Adult Polycystic Kidney Disease (APKD) in Horseshoe Kidney (a–c)

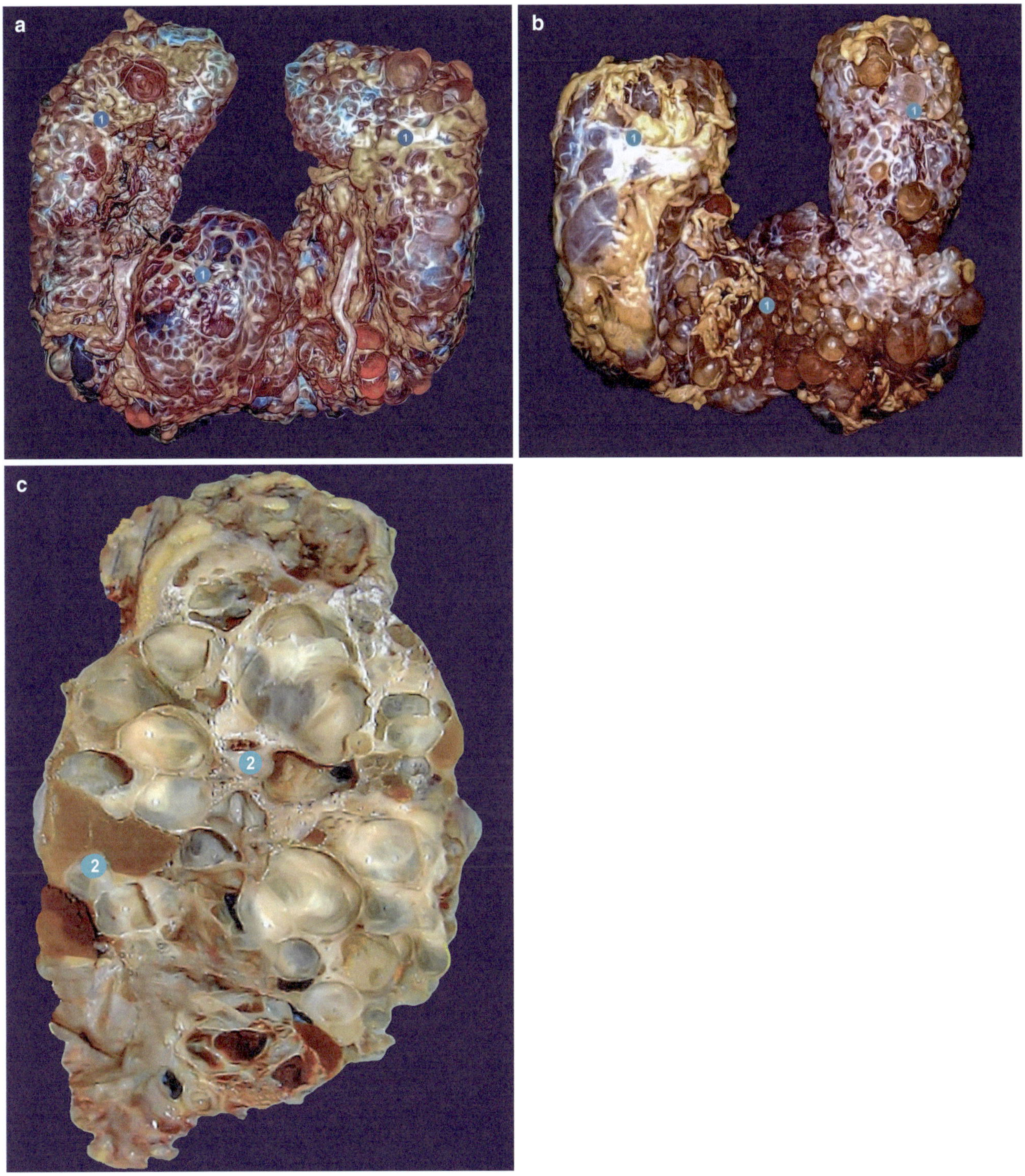

Two kidneys are mounted.

1. Kidneys are enlarged and fused at their lower poles by the isthmus.
2. The normal tissue is replaced by multiple, communicating cysts variable in size and shape, with a smooth lining, and contain clear or hemorrhagic fluid.

Pearls

About 20 patients with polycystic horseshoe kidneys have been reported in the literature. It is thought to represent two separate renal diseases. Horseshoe kidney is a renal fusion anomaly during embryogenesis; autosomal dominant polycystic kidney disease (ADPKD) is a hereditary disorder due to mutations in the genes responsible for the expression of the proteins polycystin 1 (ADPKD1) and polycystin 2 (ADPKD2). Horseshoe kidney occurs in 1 in 400–800 live births and ADPKD in 1 in 400–1000 live births. Polycystic horseshoe kidney occurs in 1 in 134,000 to 1 in 8,000,000 live births [2]. To date, no genetic association has been described between the ADPKD loci (PKD1 on chromosome 16 and PKD2 on chromosome 4) and horseshoe kidneys [1].

Autosomal Recessive Polycystic Kidney Disease (ARPKD)

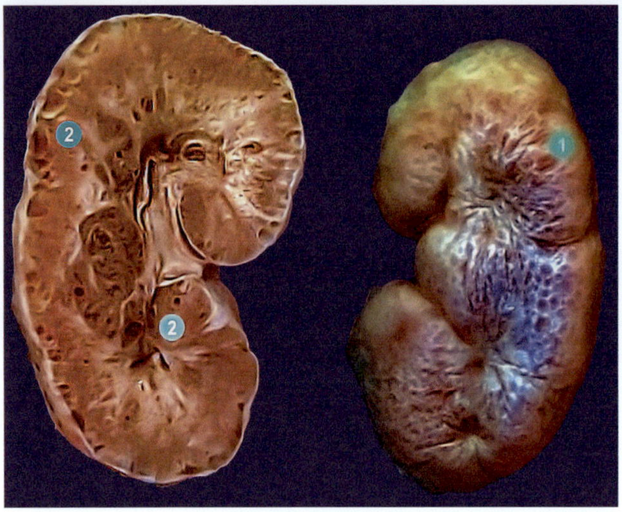

The kidney bisected longitudinally is mounted.

1. The kidney is enlarged with a smooth and spongy outer surface.
2. Cystic dilatations (microcysts) of the collecting tubules in the cortex and medulla. The cysts are fairly small but uniformly distributed throughout the parenchyma.

Simple Renal Cyst

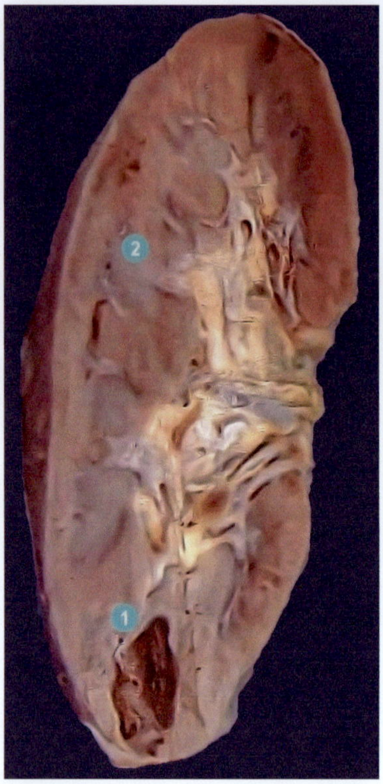

A kidney bisected longitudinally is mounted.

1. The lower pole shows a well-defined cyst with a smooth lining and red color.
2. The rest of the kidney looks normal.

6.1.2 Inflammatory Lesions

Acute Glomerulonephritis (AGN)

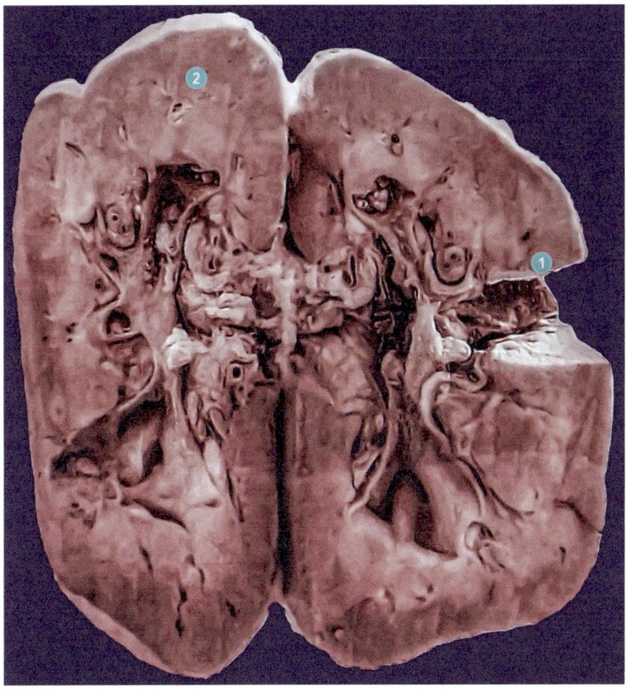

A kidney bisected longitudinally is mounted.

1. It is enlarged and firm (sharp cut section).
2. The cut section shows an expansion of the cortical area.

Chronic Pyelonephritis (a, b)

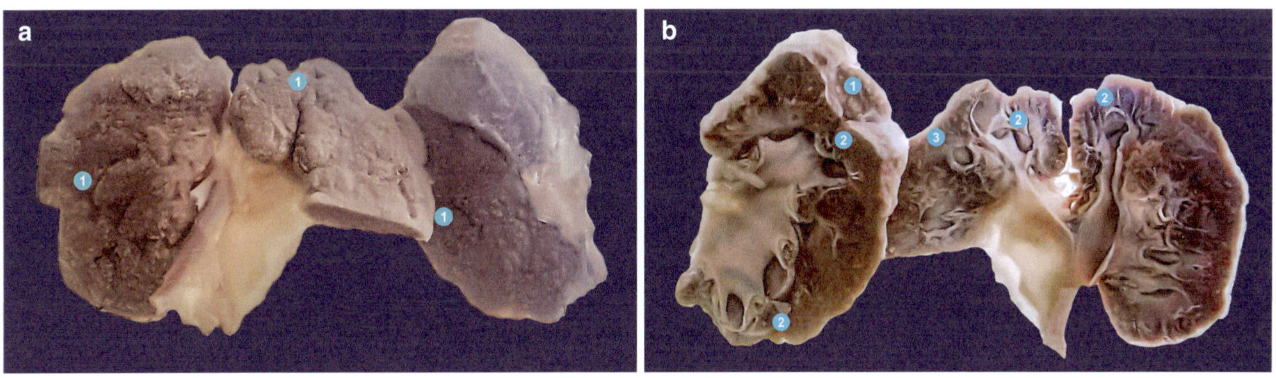

Two kidneys bisected longitudinally are mounted.

1. Their size is reduced and they have irregularly scarred surfaces.
2. Coarse discrete corticomedullary scars, especially at the upper and lower poles.
3. The cortex is thinned out.

Microscopic Picture of Chronic Pyelonephritis (c, d)

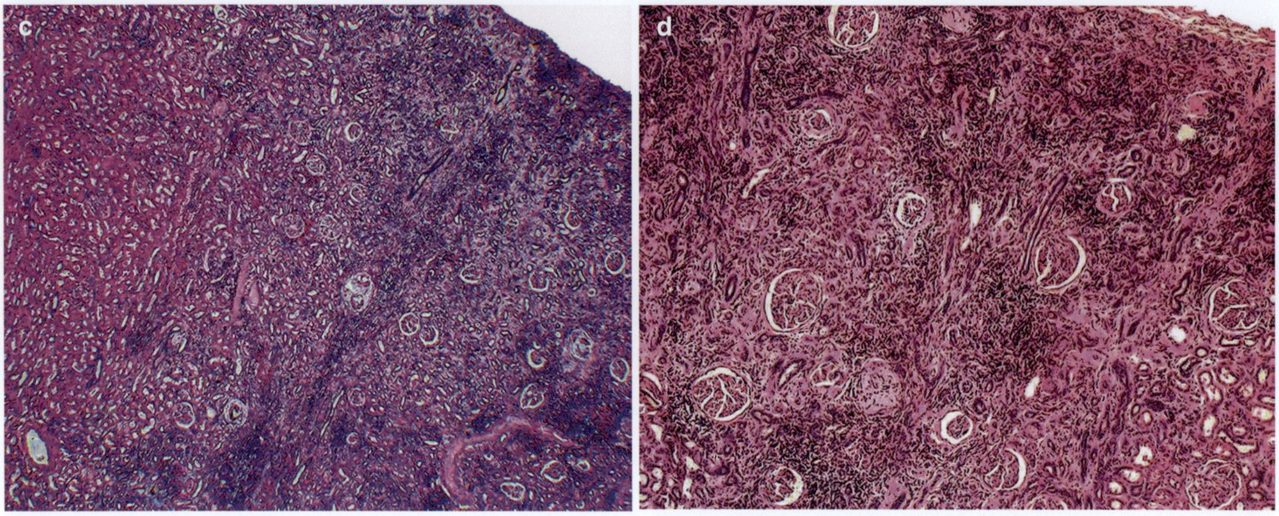

Sections show patchy scarring of the renal parenchyma, atrophy of tubules, and interstitial inflammation. Some glomeruli are atrophic with the presence of periglomerular and glomerular fibrosis. Interstitial tissue is infiltrated by lymphocytes, plasma cells, and macrophages.

Microscopic Picture of Xanthogranulomatous Pyelonephritis (e–g)

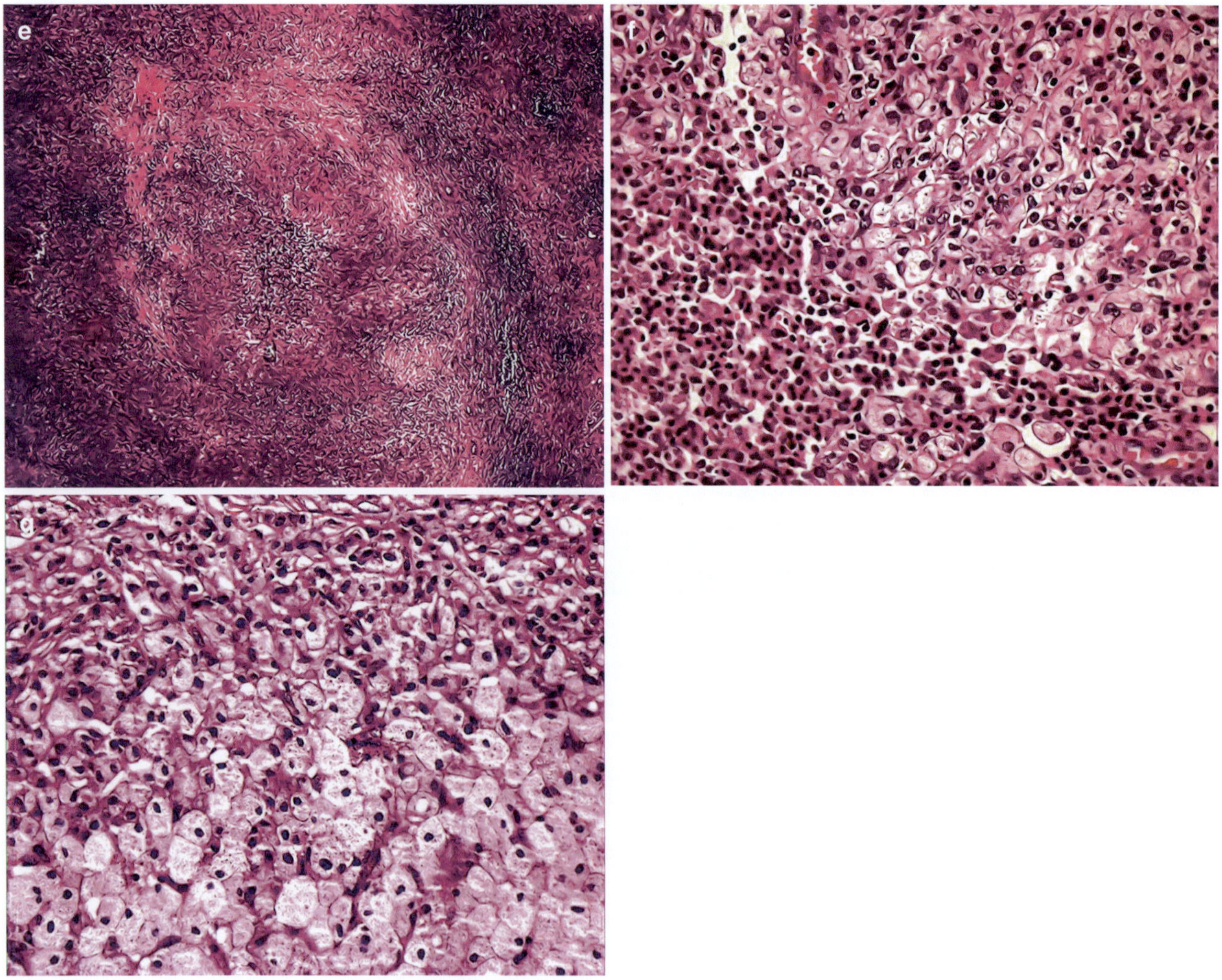

Sections show the zonal distribution of inflammation consisting of:

Inner zone: bacteria, inflammatory cells (neutrophils, lymphocytes, plasma cells), foreign body giant cells, foreign body granulomas,

Middle zone: (hallmark for the diagnosis): granulation tissues surrounded by lipid-laden foamy macrophages (xanthoma cells).

Outer zone: consists of giant cells, cholesterol clefts, and fibrous tissues with lymph follicles.

Pearls

Xanthogranulomatous pyelonephritis is a rare subtype of pyelonephritis, often occurring as a chronic consequence of nephrolithiasis or infections. Pathognomonic features are lipid-laden foamy CD68+ macrophages (xanthoma cells) that give the tissue a yellow-orange color on macroscopy. Rarely associated with renal cell carcinoma or urothelial carcinoma [2].

Pyonephrosis

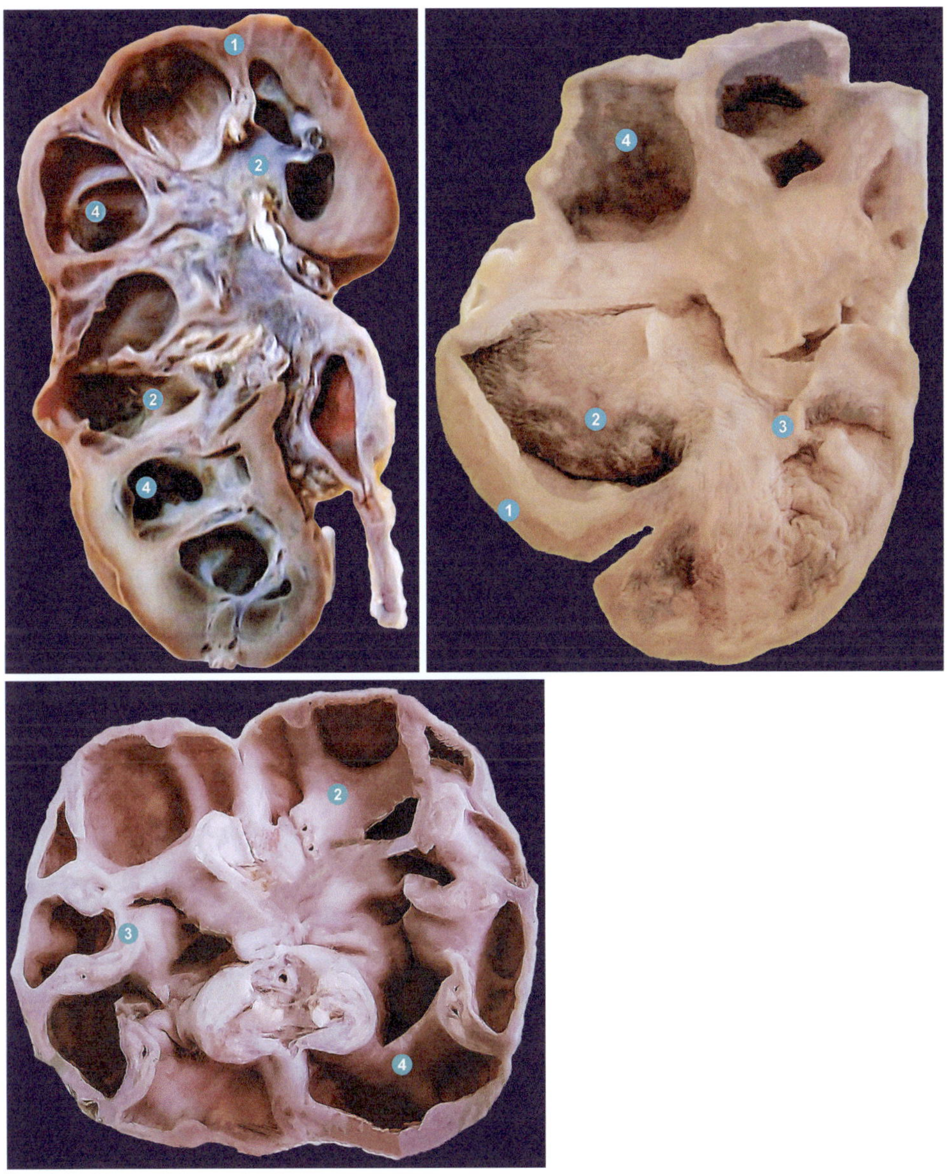

A kidney bisected longitudinally is mounted.

1. The entire kidney is pale and markedly enlarged with a flattened renal cortex.
2. Enormous dilation of the renal pelvis and calyces (was filled with pus).
3. Renal pyramids are grossly flattened.
4. The mucosa is dark red.

Pyonephrosis with Staghorn Calculus

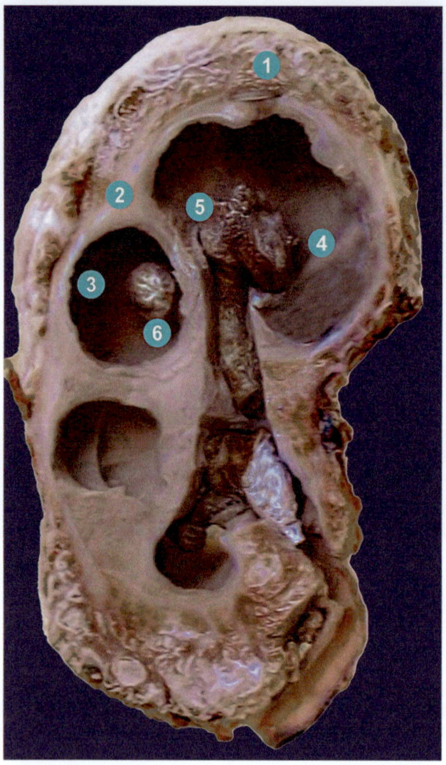

The kidney bisected longitudinally is mounted.

1. The kidney is markedly enlarged
2. The entire kidney is pale and atrophic with a flattened renal cortex.
3. The mucosa is dark red.
4. The pelvicalyceal system is dilated.
5. A stag horn stone with a yellow-brown surface is filling the dilated pelvicalyceal system.
6. Another round oxalate stone is present in a dilated calyx.

Pearls

Staghorn calculus is typically composed of struvite (a combination of magnesium, ammonium, and phosphate) and/or calcium carbonate apatite and inked to urinary tract infection by urease-producing pathogens [3].

Pyonephrosis with Oxalate Calculus

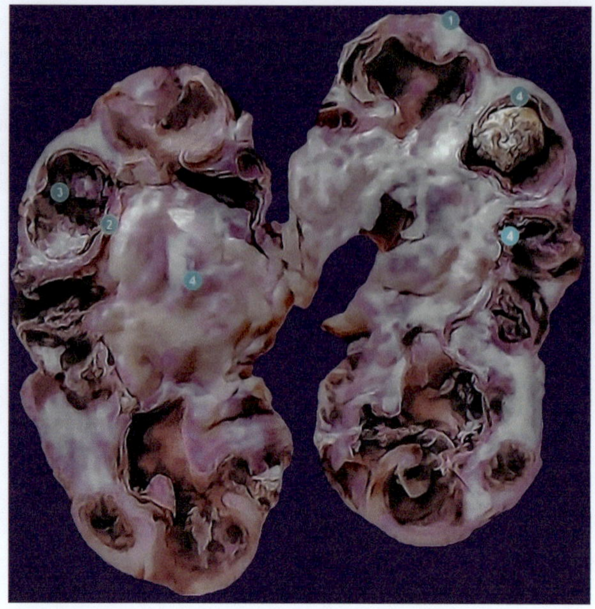

The kidney bisected longitudinally is mounted.

1. It is markedly enlarged.
2. The renal pyramids are grossly flattened, and the entire kidney is pale and atrophic with a flattened renal cortex.
3. The mucosa is dark red.
4. The pelvicalyceal system is dilated and filled with pus. An oxalate stone with a spikey, yellow-brown surface is present in the dilated calyces.

Renal Pyemic Abscesses

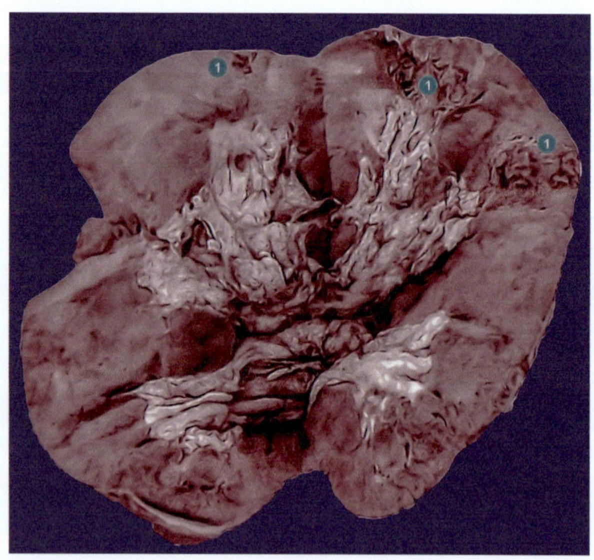

The kidney bisected longitudinally is mounted.

1. Multiple cortical lesions surrounded by a zone of congestion. The lesions are variable in size and shape.

Microscopic Picture of Renal Pyemic Abscesses (a)

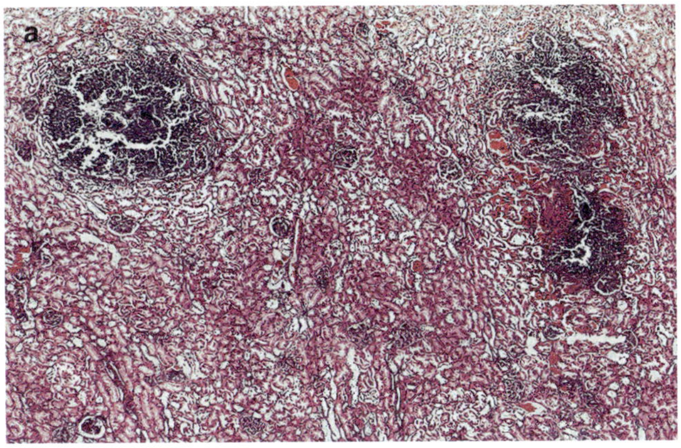

The section shows areas of necrosis that appear as basophilic debris surrounded by inflammatory cells such as neutrophils.

Renal Tuberculoma

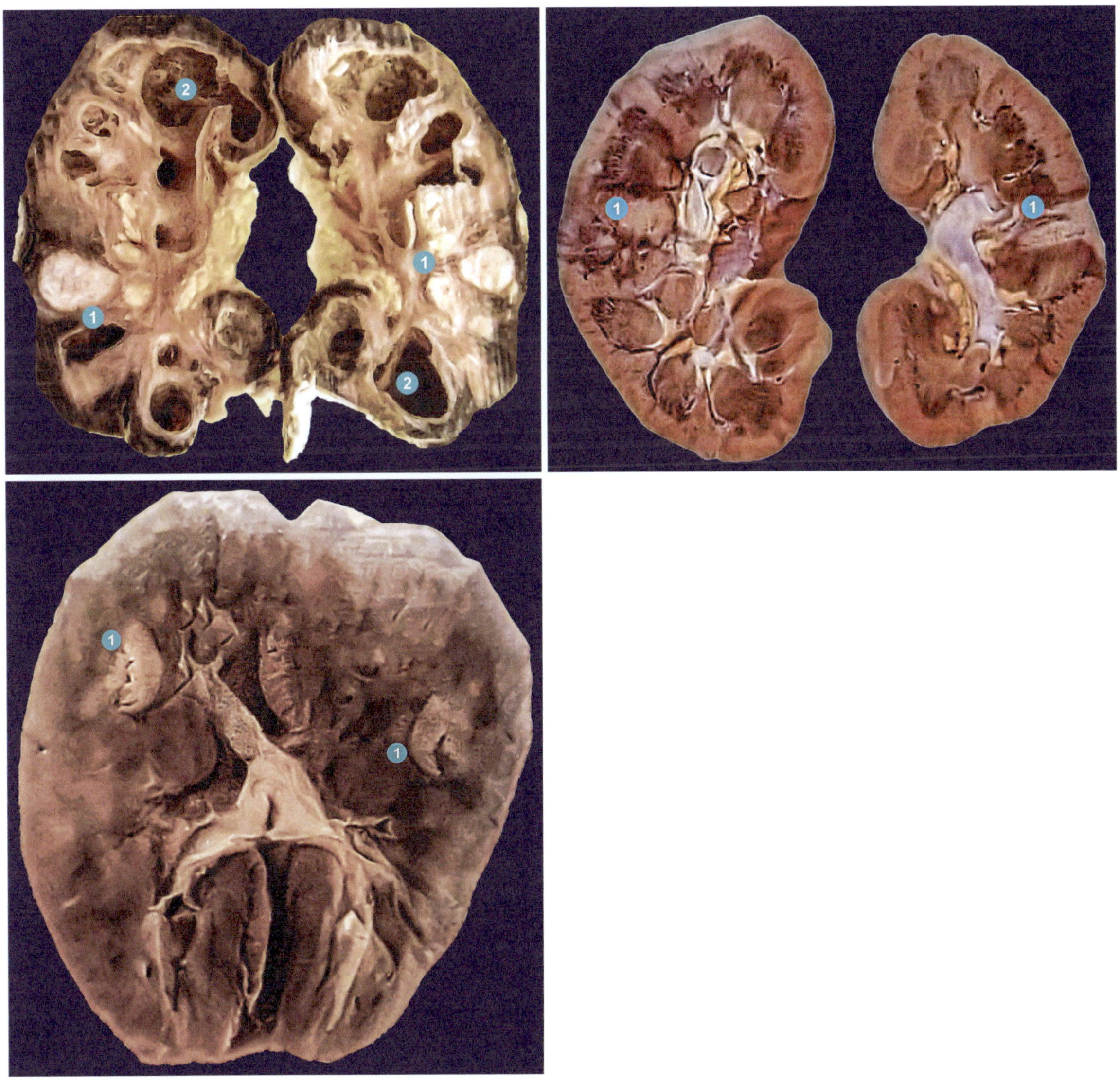

A normal-sized kidney is bisected longitudinally and mounted.

1. The cut section shows a yellow area of caseous necrosis at the tip of a pyramid near the corticomedullary junction.
2. The rest of the pelvicalyceal system is dilated with dark lining and remains of pus, indicating pyonephrosis.

Ulcerocaseous Tuberculosis of the Kidney (a, b)

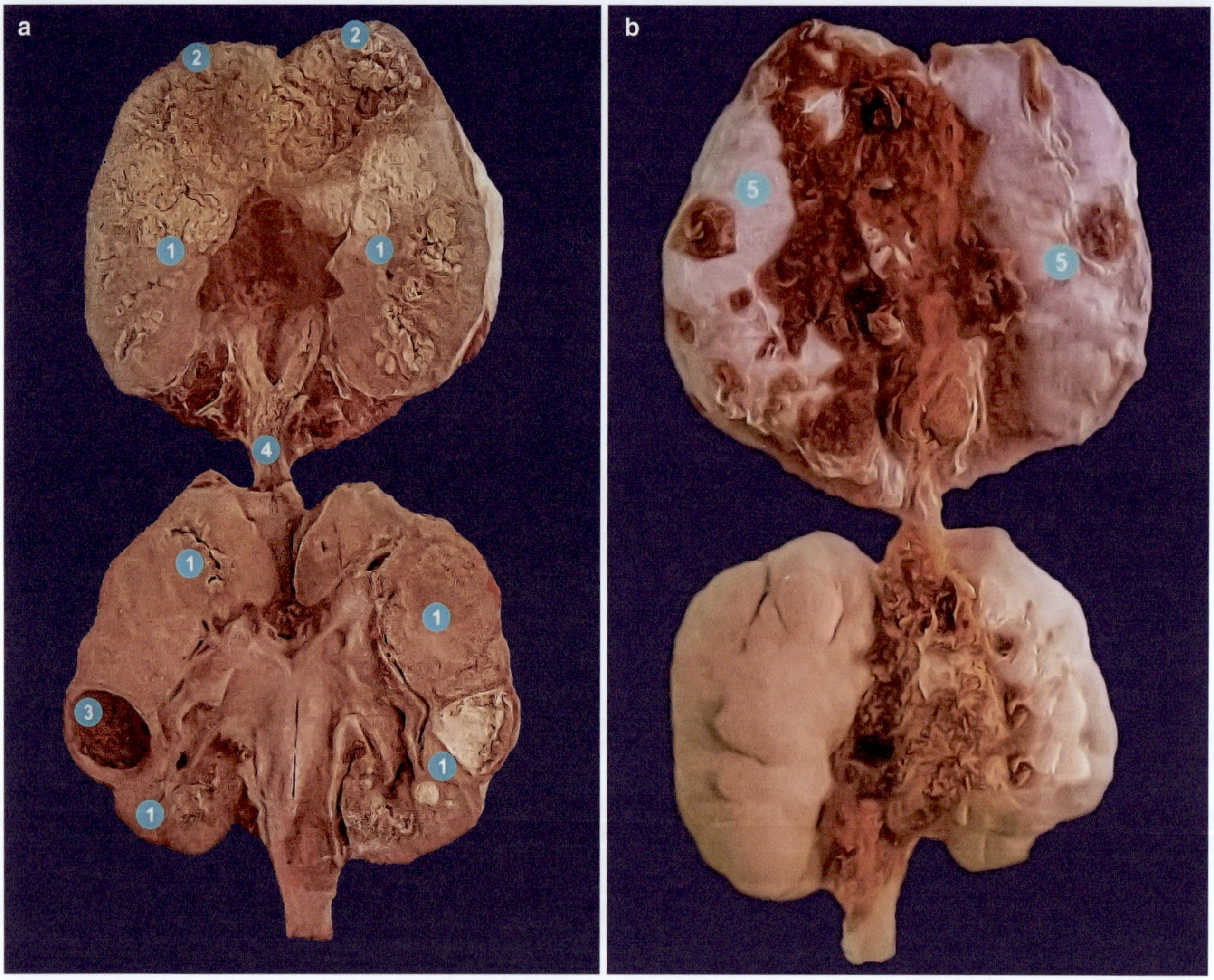

Two kidneys are bisected longitudinally and mounted.

1. Cut sections show multiple yellow foci of caseation necrosis.
2. Some caseous lesions ulcerated through the renal capsule.
3. Cavities: some of which have a smooth lining.
4. Ureters are thickened and dilated, and the upper specimen shows luminal caseation of the ureter.
5. The outer surface shows focal ulceration and a fibrosed capsule.

Microscopic Picture of Tuberculosis of Kidney (c)

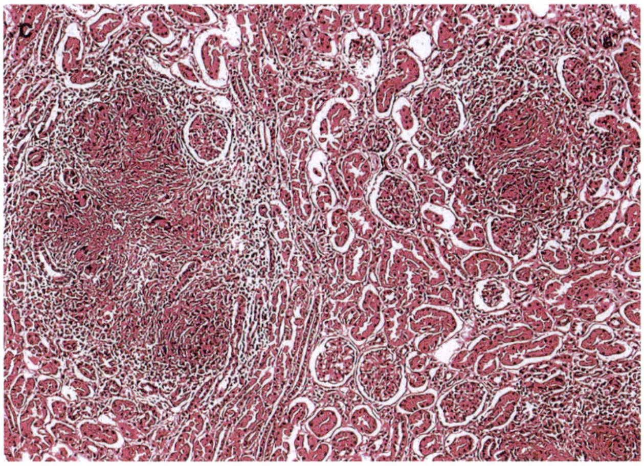

The section shows multiple tubercles, formed of epithelioid cells, Langhans giant cells, and lymphocytes with central areas of caseation necrosis, infiltrating renal interstitial tissue and destroying the renal parenchyma.

Bilharziasis of the Urinary Bladder and Ureters

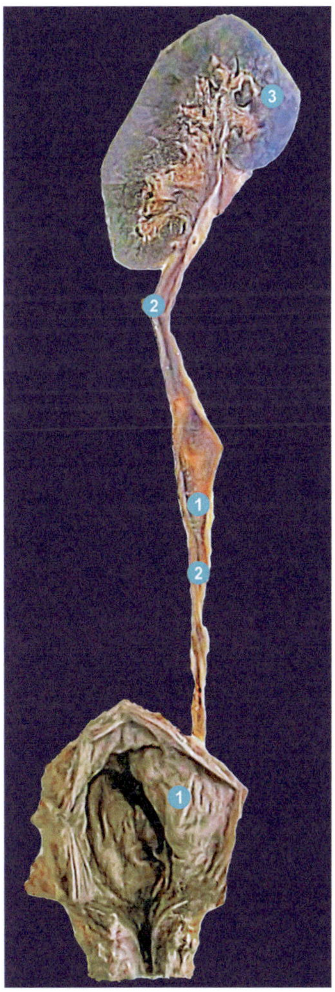

The left kidney, ureter, and urinary bladder are mounted.

1. The mucosa of the ureter and bladder is dirty brown.
2. The ureter has an irregular contour with areas of stricture and others of dilatation.
3. Renal papillae are round-concave with mild enlargement of the kidney

Bilharziasis of the Urinary Bladder and Ureters

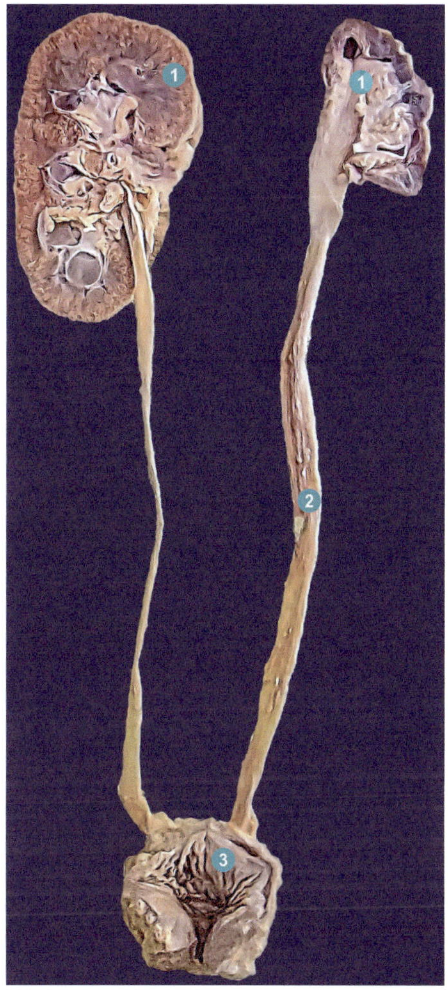

Sectioned kidneys, ureters, and an opened urinary bladder are mounted.

1. The left kidney shows manifestations of chronic pyelonephritis, while the right kidney shows compensatory hypertrophy.
2. Both ureters are dilated with the presence of small cysts along their course (ureteritis cystica) with stricture at the lower ends.
3. The bladder mucosa is dirty brown.

Microscopic Picture of Urinary Bladder Bilharziasis (a–g)

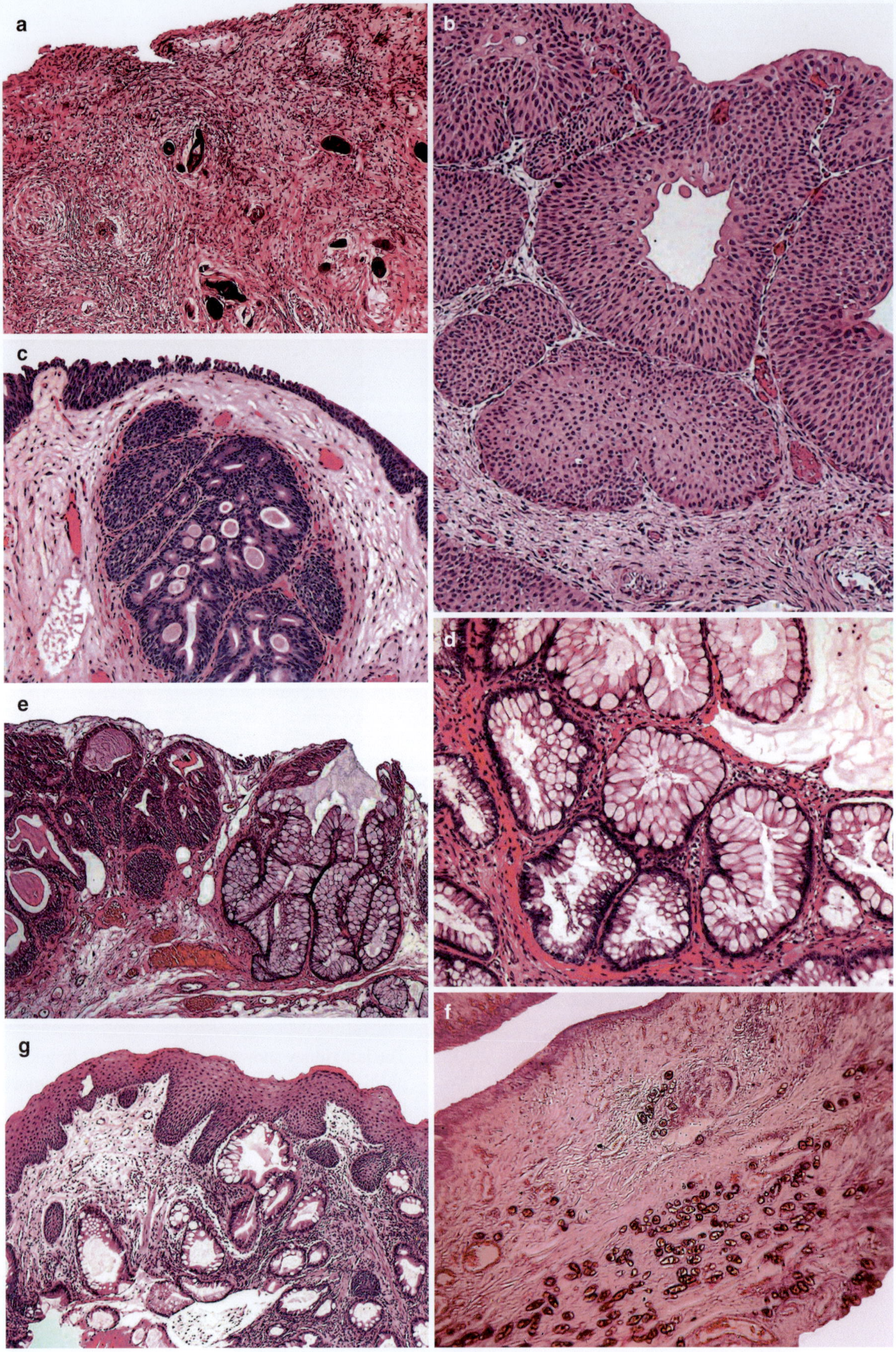

Sections show atrophic urothelium with a focal area of ulceration. The corium shows multiple calcified bilharzial ova, embedded in a hyalinized fibrous stroma infiltrated by chronic inflammatory cells. Additionally, due to chronic cystitis, the urothelial lining may show abnormal growth patterns, including:

(b) von Brunn nest hyperplasia: formation of rounded nests of urothelial cells pushing into deeper tissue layers.
(c) Cystitis cystica: presence of cyst-like structures filled with eosinophilic fluid.
(d) Cystitis glandularis: development of gland-like structures lined with epithelium (intestinal metaplasia is shown).
(e) A combination of the last two patterns can also occur.
(f) Urothelium may become greatly atrophic overlying a fibrous corium containing multiple calcified bilharzial ova.
(g) With continuation of chronic irritation, squamous metaplasia may occur, which may be associated with colonic metaplasia as observed in this example.

Bilharziasis of Urinary Bladder and Ureters, Pyonephrosis, and Pyoureter

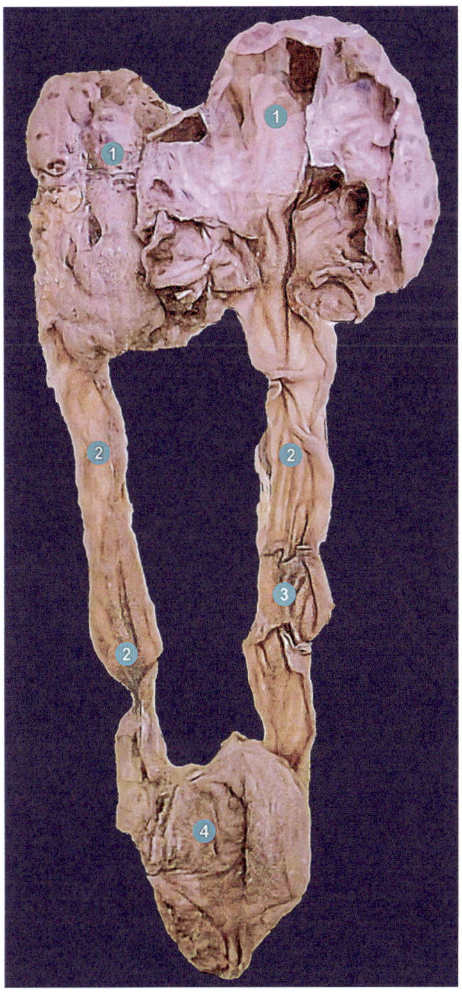

Sectioned kidneys, ureters, and an opened urinary bladder are mounted.

1. Both kidneys show manifestations of pyonephrosis.
2. Both ureters are dilated with the presence of small cysts along their course (ureteritis cystica) with stricture at the lower ends.
3. The left ureter shows 2 stenotic rings along its course.
4. The bladder mucosa is dirty yellow-brown.

6.1.3 Mechanical Lesions

6.1.3.1 Hydronephrosis

Hydronephrosis

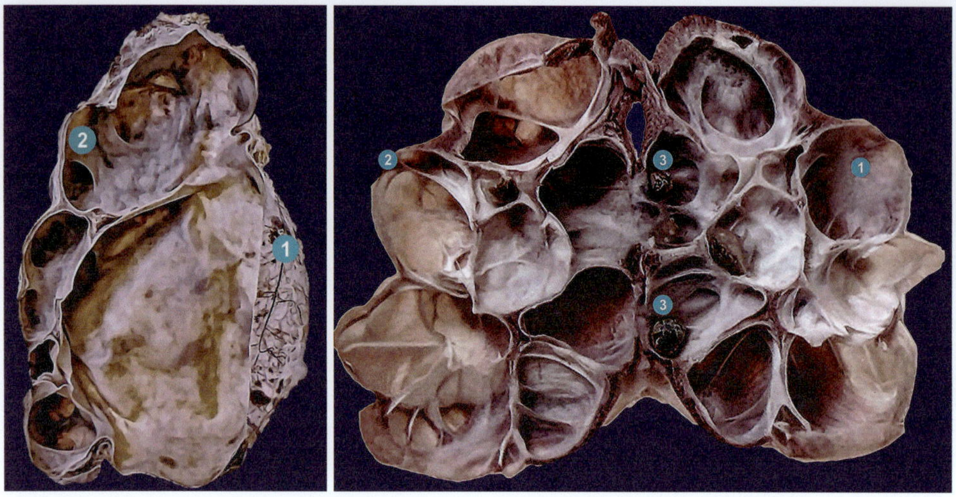

A kidney bisected longitudinally is mounted.

1. It is markedly enlarged and displays enormous dilation of the renal pelvis and calyces.
2. The renal cortex and pyramids are grossly flattened.
3. Two stones are observed I (6–22).

6.1.3.2 Urolithiasis

Oxalate and Urate Stones

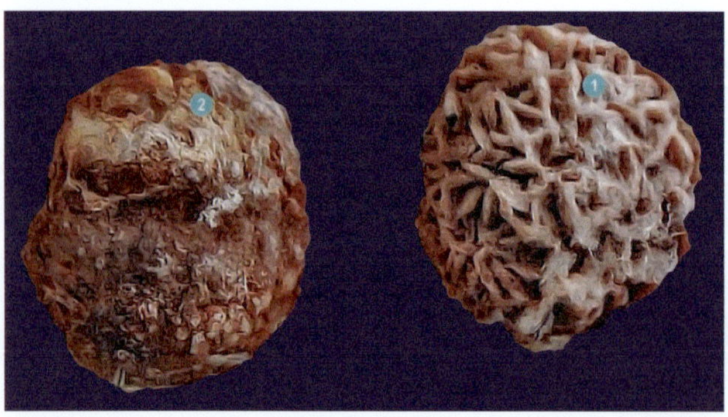

1. The right-sided oxalate stone is round with a spiny brown surface.
2. The left-sided stone is urate and is round with a yellow-brown irregular surface.

Oxalate Crystals (a)

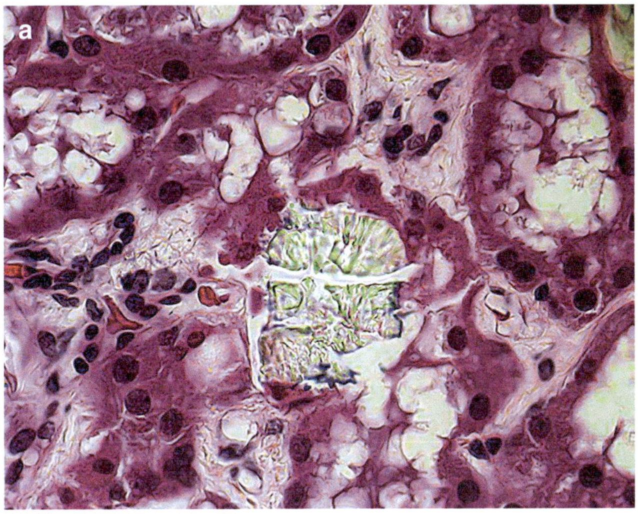

The section shows an intratubular accumulation of translucent polyhedral, rhomboid, and fan-like calcium oxalate crystals.

Urate Crystals (b)

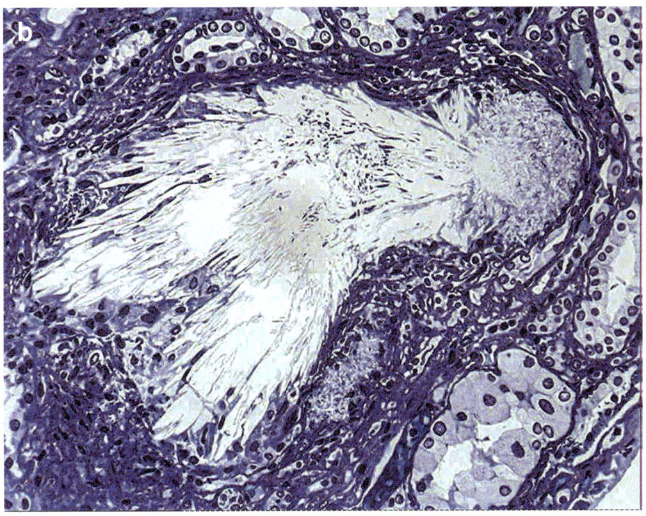

Interstitial accumulation of urate crystals, which appear as necrotic foci in which many fine needles (corresponding to crystals) are stained with methylene blue stain.

Oxalate Stones

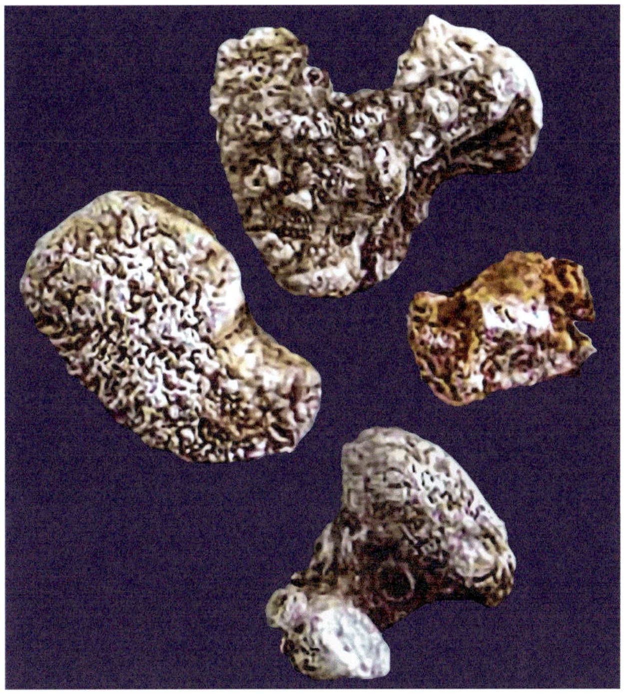

Several hard stones, some have a coralline appearance with a spiny brown surface.

6.1.4 Fibrillar Lesion

Renal Amyloidosis

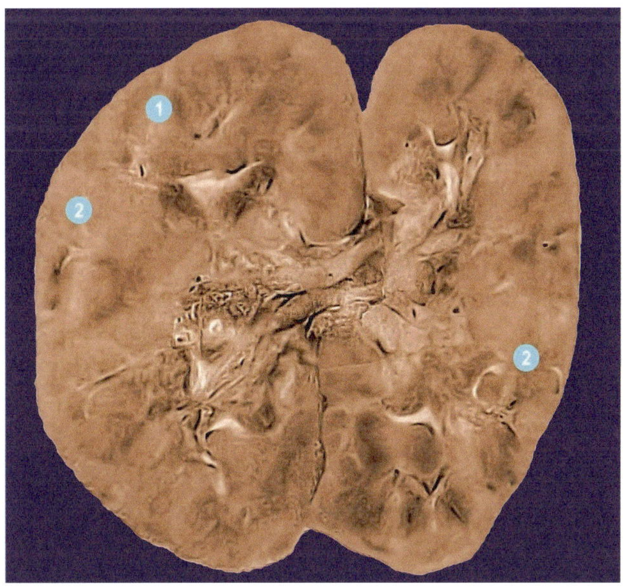

A bisected kidney is mounted.

1. The kidney is enlarged and has a pale waxy appearance.
2. On the cut surface, the cortico-medullary junction is indistinct.

Microscopic Picture of Renal Amyloidosis (a, b)

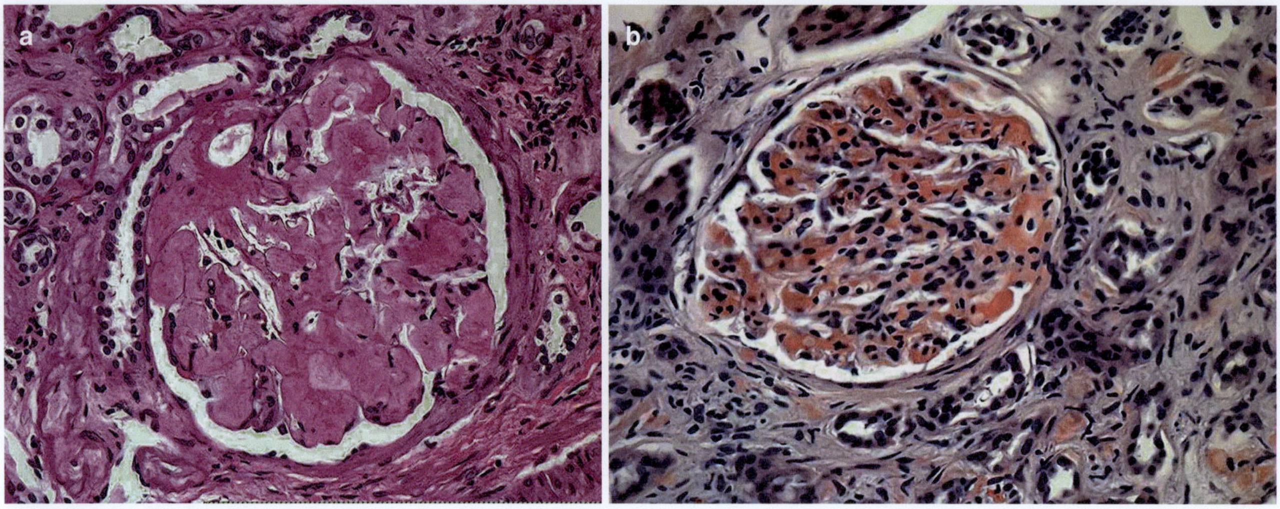

Sections show the expansion of mesangial regions with pale eosinophilic material (amyloid), which stained positively with Congo-red stain (b).

Pearls [4]

Amyloidosis is defined by the pathologic accumulation of extracellular proteins that adopt a beta-pleated configuration and share histochemical characteristics and fibrillary ultrastructure. Amyloidoses are a heterogeneous group of disorders with deposition of abnormally folded proteins in tissues. Amyloid deposits are formed from globular, soluble proteins that undergo misfolding and, subsequently, aggregate into insoluble fibrils, leading to progressive organ damage. By electron microscopy, amyloid fibrils appear rigid, are nonbranching, and typically measure 8–12 nm in diameter.

The three main biochemical forms are:

1. AL Protein: formed by light chains, mainly of lambda type, or by parts of them. This amyloid is associated with monoclonal proliferation of B cells or plasma cells; when proliferation of these cells is not identified, we call the disease "primary amyloidosis."
2. AA Protein: It is derived from a serum precursor denominated SAA (serum amyloid-associated), a protein synthesized in the liver and that circulates united to HDL lipoproteins. It is an acute phase reactant present in elevated levels in the serum of patients with chronic inflammatory conditions. Then, it is the amyloid deposited in amyloidosis secondary to chronic inflammations.
3. Beta-Amyloid: It is the amyloid found in cerebral lesions in Alzheimer's disease.

Other proteins that produce deposits of amyloid are:

Transthyretin (prealbumin): in some types of genetic disease and senile systemic amyloidosis; Beta2-microglobulin (a component of molecules of the major histocompatibility complex): amyloidosis associated with chronic hemodialysis.

Ancillary Tools

Cytogenetics [5]:

Mostly acquired with rare inherited forms

Hereditary forms: All show an autosomal dominant inheritance.

The transthyretin gene mutation is most common—Val30Met seen with renal involvement. Other gene mutations include fibrinogen alpha chain, apolipoprotein A1 and A2.

6.1.5 Vascular Lesions

Benign Nephrosclerosis (Arteriolosclerotic Kidney) (a, b)

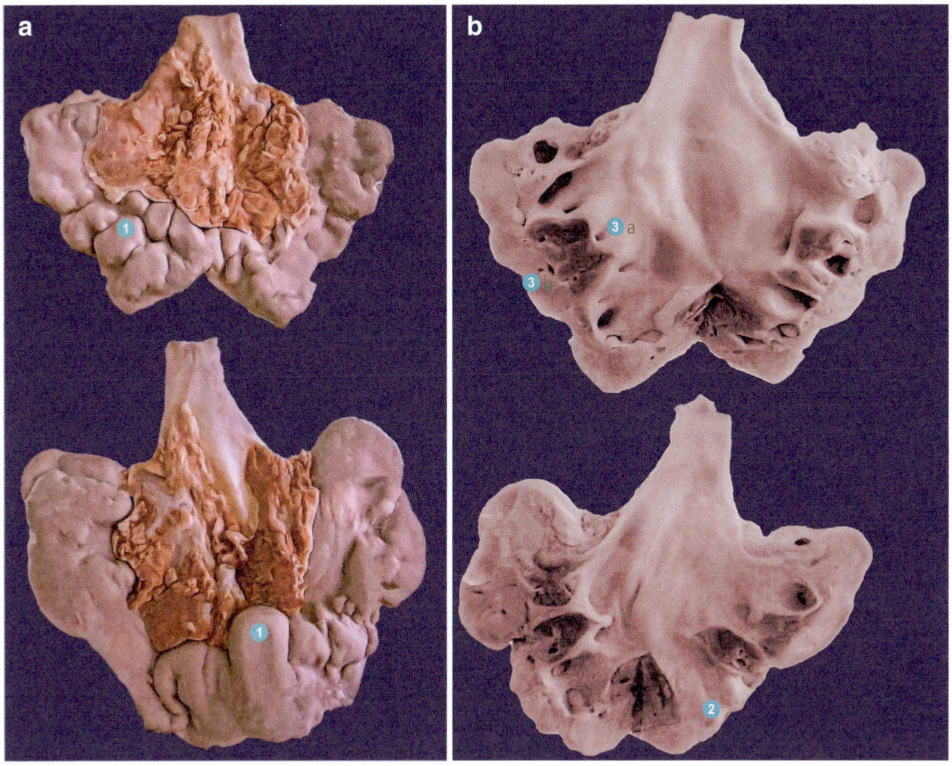

A kidney is bisected longitudinally and mounted.

1. The size is slightly reduced with a bossy surface.
2. The cut section shows an atrophic cortex.
3. Interlobar (a) and arcuate (b) arteries have thick walls, especially seen in the cut section.

Microscopic Picture of Arteriolonephrosclerosis (c–h)

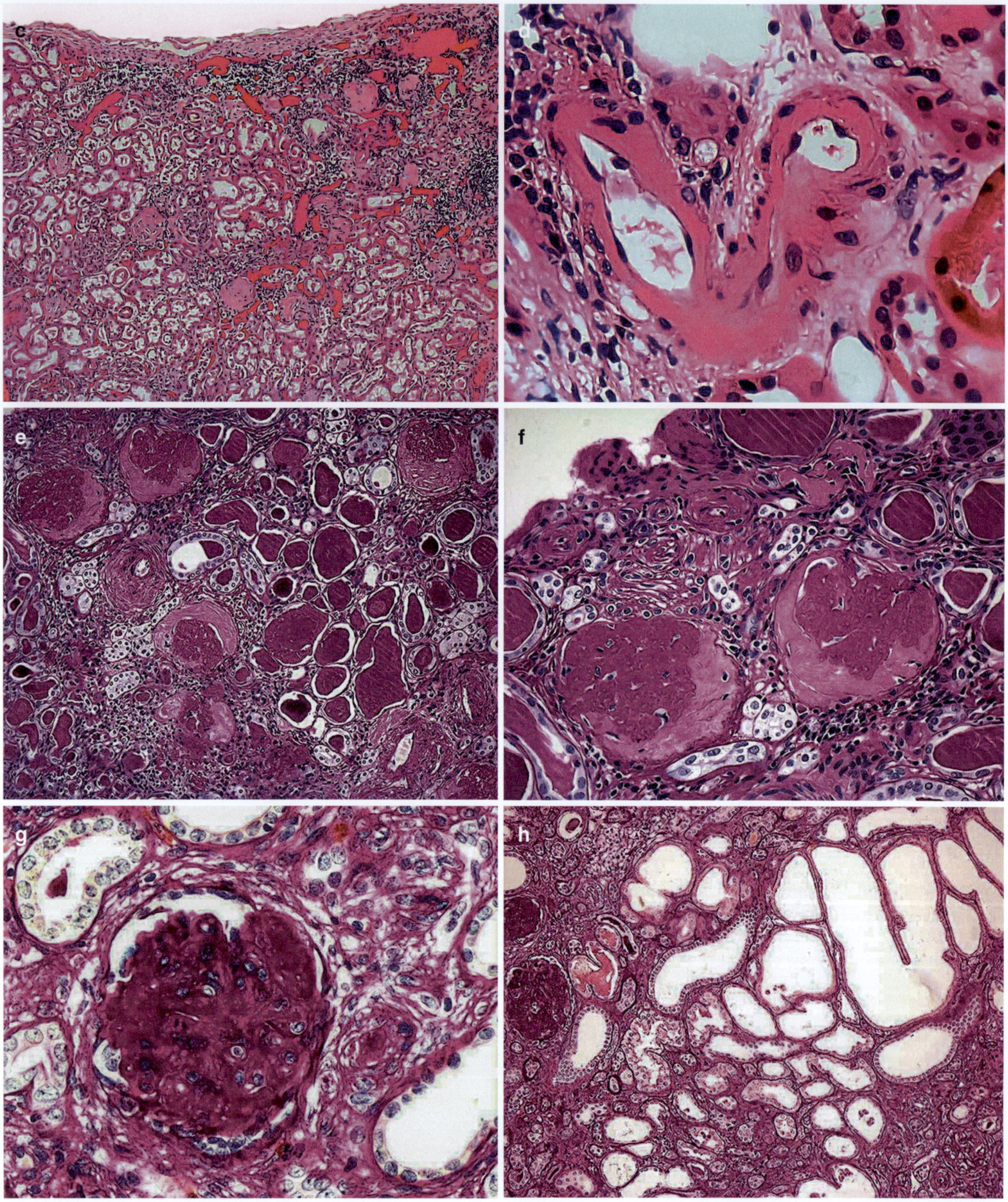

Sections show a partially and wholly collapsed glomerular tuft of capillaries with an accumulation of extracellular material in Bowman space. The arteriolar walls show hyaline arteriolosclerosis, predominantly involving the afferent arteriole, characterized by wall thickening due to the accumulation of homogeneous material that stains pink on H&E-stained slides. Arteries show medial thickening and subintimal fibrosis. This is accompanied by focal subcapsular scarring, proportional tubulointerstitial fibrosis, and microcystic tubular dilatation. PAS stain accentuates global glomerulosclerosis, fibrosis, scarring of the Bowman capsule, and hyaline arteriolosclerosis.

Malignant Hypertension and Accelerated Nephrosclerosis (Malignant Nephrosclerosis)

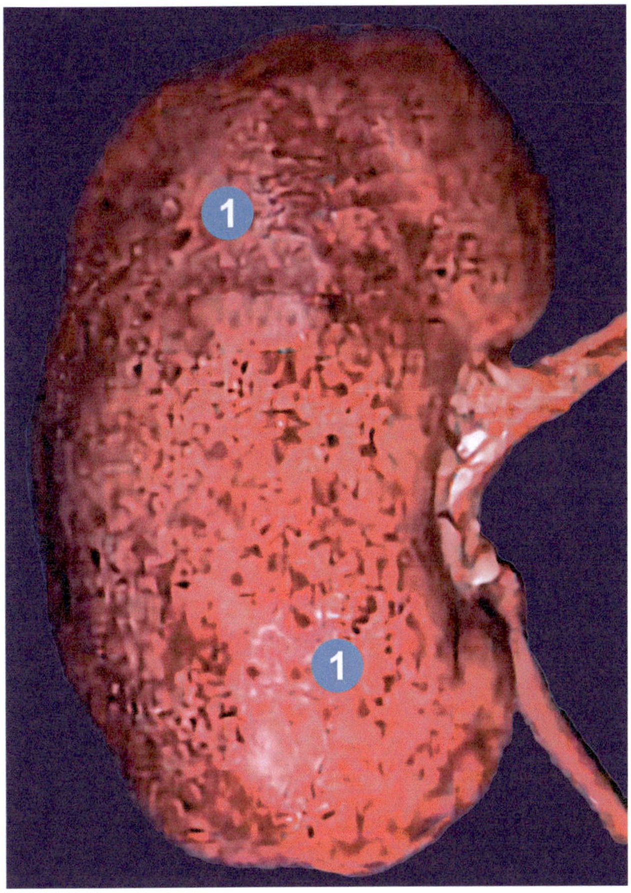

The whole kidney is mounted

1. The kidney shows capsular multiple focal petechial hemorrhages (flee-bitten kidney).

Microscopic Picture of Malignant Nephrosclerosis (a–c)

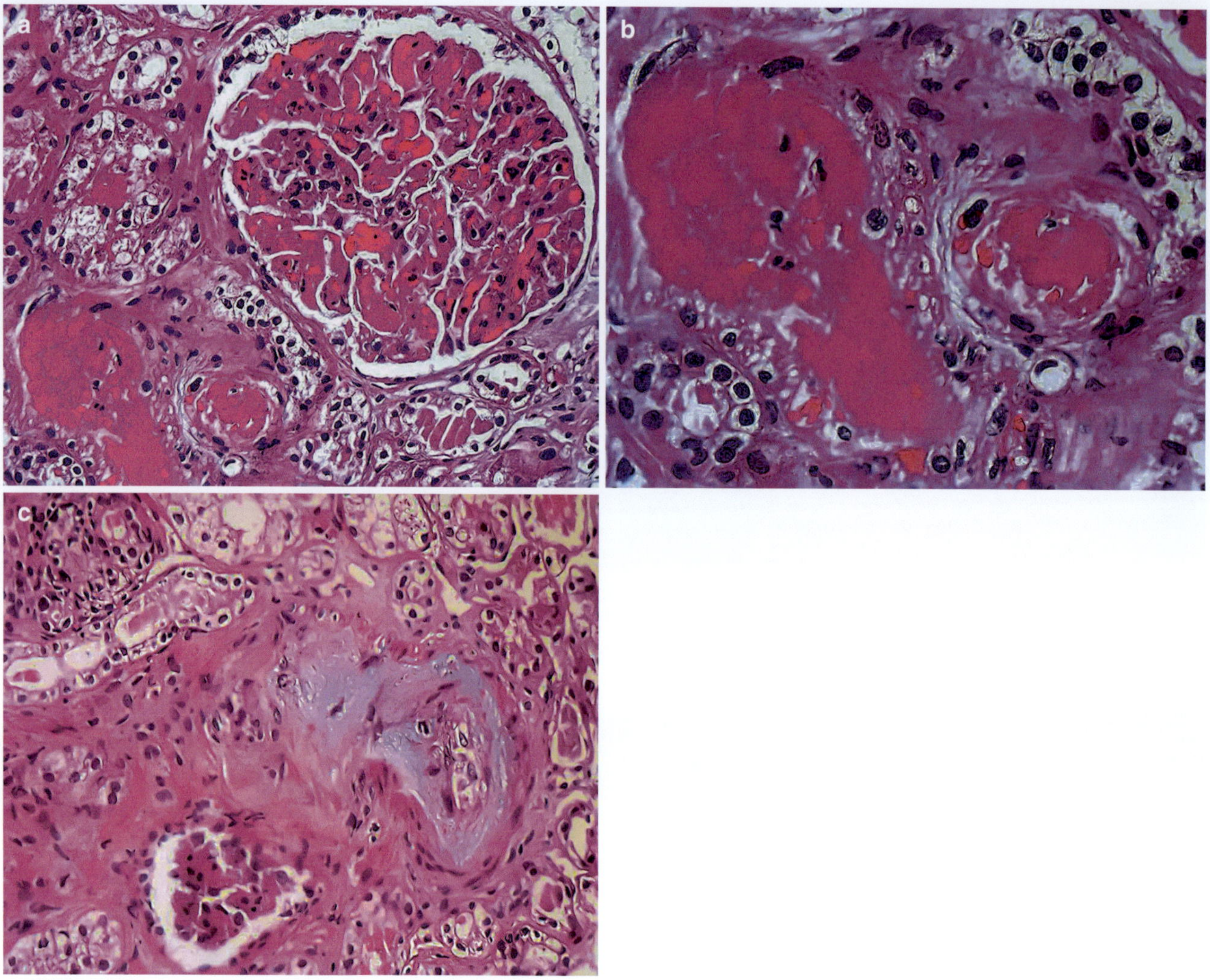

Sections show profound intimal thickening by myxoid connective tissue reducing lumen, vascular and glomerular thrombosis, necrosis, and glomerular congestion, and necrotizing arteriolitis: fibrinoid necrosis and thrombosis of afferent arteriole with media has deposits of deeply eosinophilic and fibrillar material containing fibrin and fibrinogen.

6.1.6 Neoplastic Lesions

Urothelial Papillomatosis of the Ureter and Renal Pelvis with Pyonephrosis

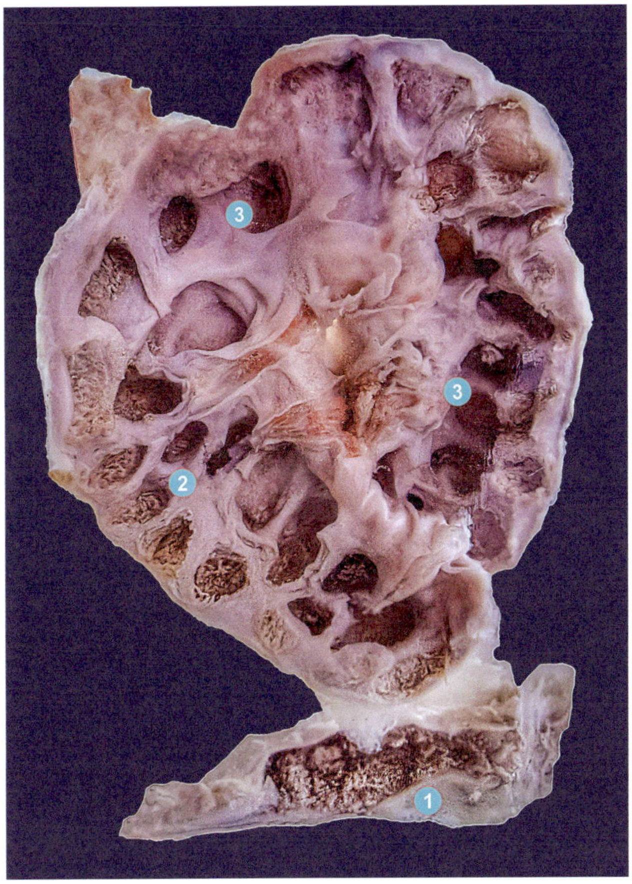

An opened kidney with the upper part of the ureter.

1. The ureter is dilated, thick-walled, and filled with multiple papillary excrescences with thin fronds.
2. The bisected kidney shows dilatation of the pelvicalyceal system with the presence of such thin papillae with the absence of the medulla and thinning of the cortex.
3. The mucosa is dark.

Microscopic Picture of Transitional Cell Papilloma (a–c)

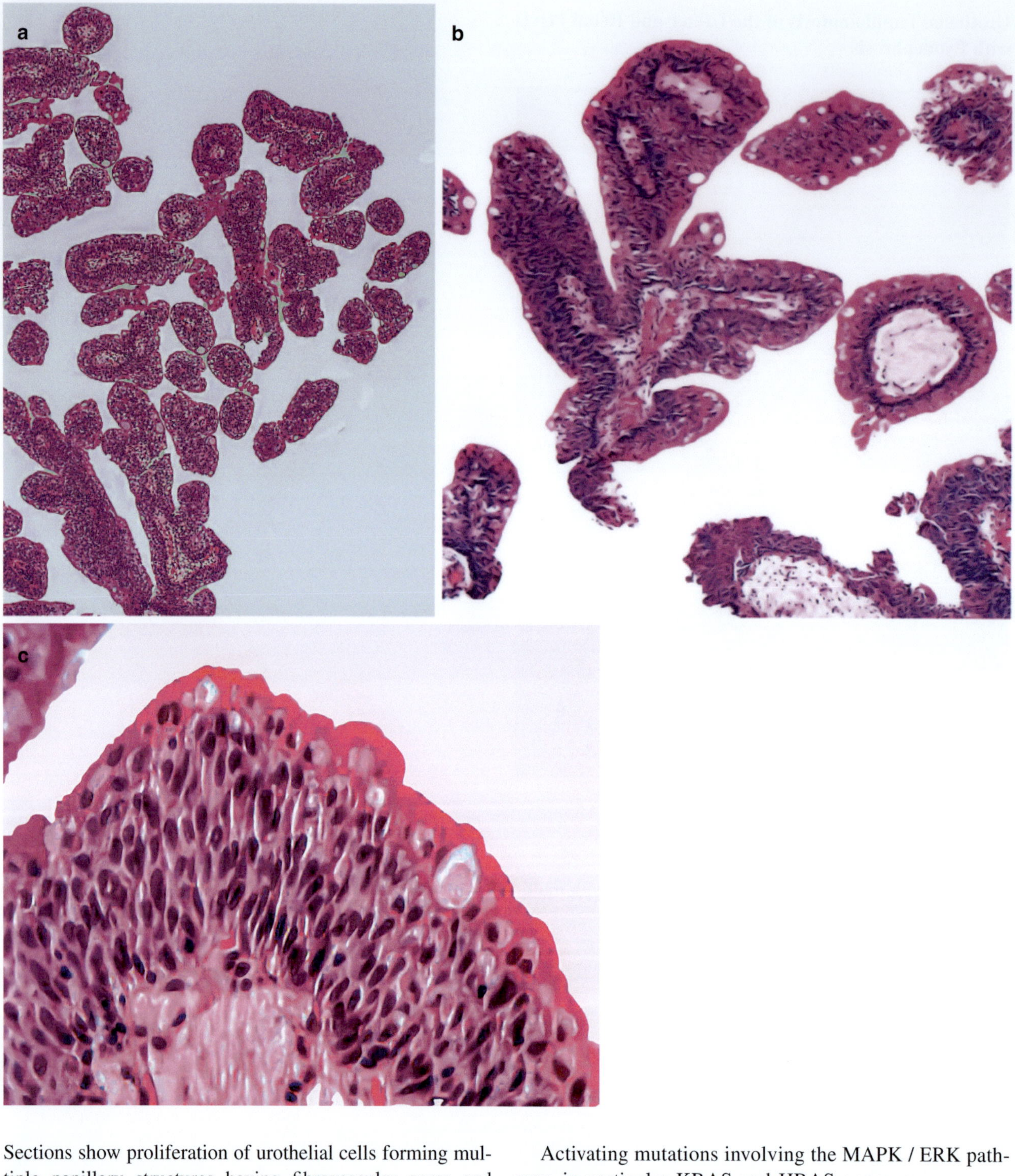

Sections show proliferation of urothelial cells forming multiple papillary structures having fibrovascular cores and loose stroma, without evidence of cellular atypia.

Ancillary Tools

IHC:

CK20 is positive in the umbrella cell layer.

Molecular/cytogenetics description [6]:

Targeted next-generation sequencing (NGS) and whole exome sequencing (WES) showed

Activating mutations involving the MAPK / ERK pathway, in particular KRAS and HRAS genes, are common alterations. KRAS mutations are more frequent than HRAS.

Mutations in chromatin modifiers (often associated with urothelial carcinoma) are rare.

Low tumor mutational burden

No APOBEC (apolipoprotein B mRNA editing catalytic polypeptide-like) mutational signature (identified in about 70% of muscle-invasive urothelial carcinomas).

Nephroblastoma (Wilm's Tumor, Embryoma) of Kidney

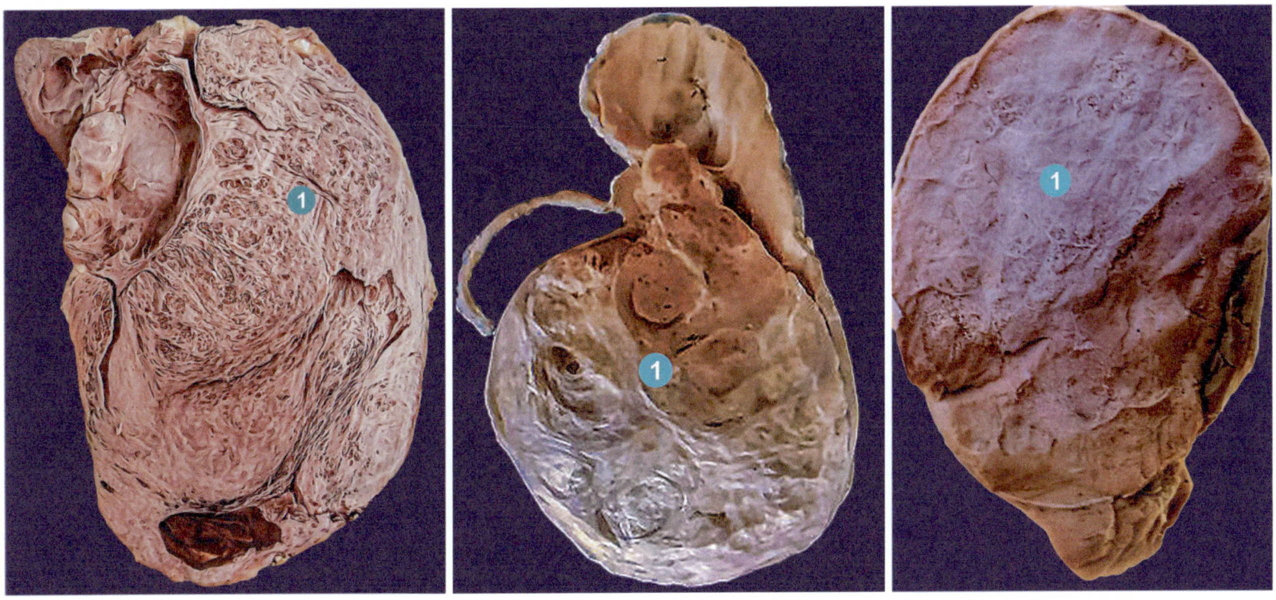

A kidney bisected longitudinally is mounted.

1. Kidney tissue is replaced with a solitary, large, sharply demarcated, lobulated, fleshy mass with a variegated pink-gray to gray-white color and areas of hemorrhage, necrosis, and cyst formation.

Microscopic Picture of Nephroblastoma of Kidney (a–e)

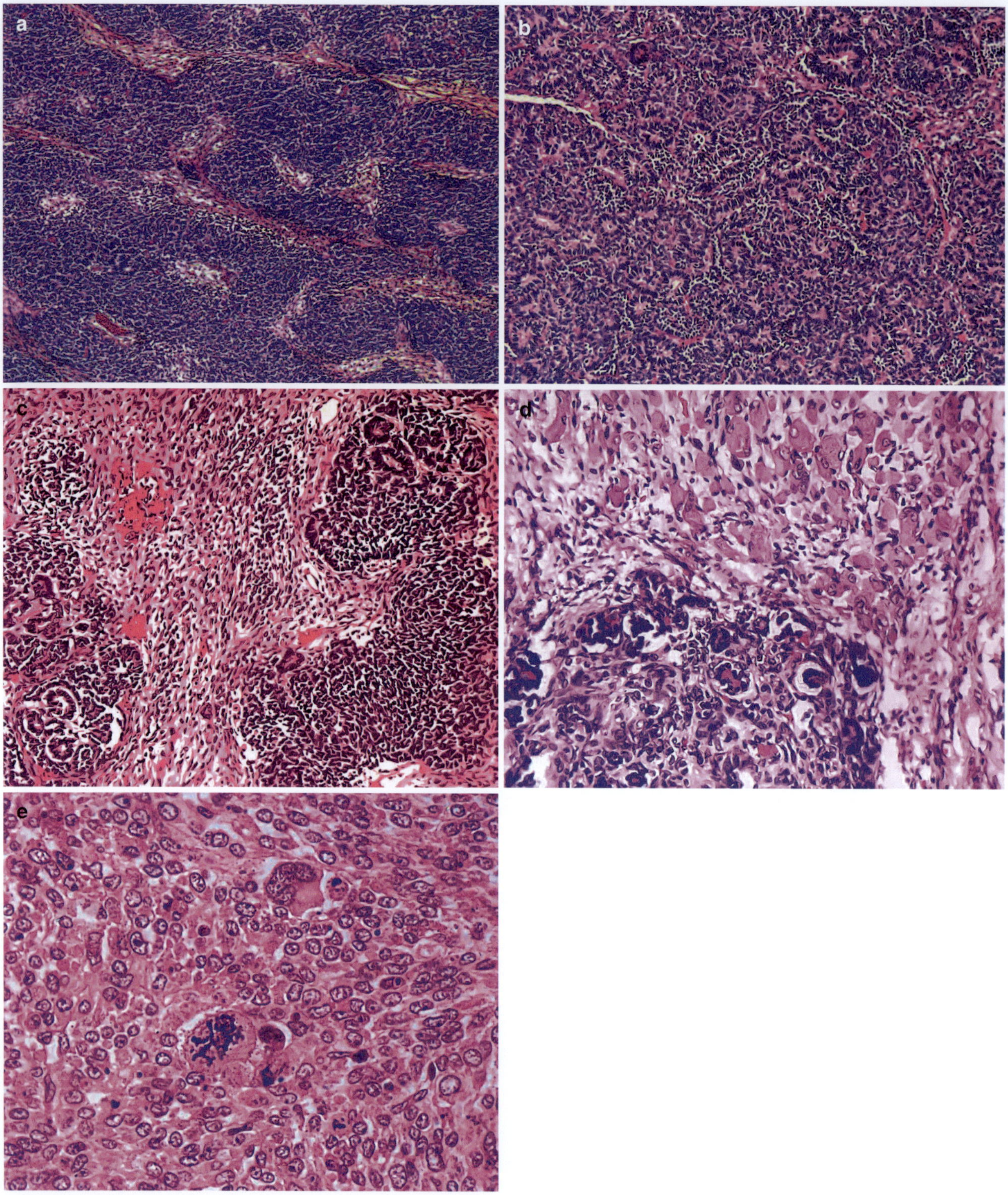

Sections show a triphasic tumor pattern formed of a blastemal component, epithelial component, and stromal component.

The blastemal component is the most primitive and undifferentiated part of the tumor. It consists of small, densely packed round or oval cells with hyperchromatic nuclei and scant cytoplasm arranged in a serpentine pattern (a).

The epithelial component consists of tubular structures lined by cuboidal or columnar epithelial cells (b). These structures may resemble embryonic renal tubules and are often surrounded by blastemal or stromal elements.

The stromal components are characterized by spindle-shaped cells resembling fibroblasts or heterologous elements, e.g., rhabdomyoblasts (c, d). In 5–10% of tumors, anaplasia is present (e). It is defined as the presence of enlarged, atypical, tripolar, or multipolar mitotic figures, marked nuclear enlargement, and hyperchromasia. All 3 features have to be present. May occur in any of the components. It may be focal or diffuse.

Ancillary Tools

IHC [7]:

WT1: The most sensitive and specific marker (positive in ~90% of cases). Only nuclear staining should be evaluated, seen with antibodies directed against the C terminal and N terminal. Cytoplasmic expression can be seen, especially using antibodies to the N terminal.

Blastema. Diffuse expression of WT1, PAX8, and vimentin

Variable CD56, CD57, cytokeratins, EMA, desmin

Epithelium

- Cytokeratin, EMA, CD56
- Variable PAX8, WT1
- Maybe focally cyclin D1 positive

Stroma

- Vimentin
- Variable BCL2, CD34
- WT1 is weak or absent
- Heterologous skeletal muscle component is reactive for desmin, myogenin, and MyoD1
- INI1 retained
- Glypican 3: expressed in the majority of Wilms tumors (blastema and epithelium)

Molecular/cytogenetics description [8]:

WT1 (11p13), prevalence 10–20%, early event, associated with stromal histology

CTNNB1 (3p22), prevalence ~15%, late event, not associated with nephrogenic rests

IGF2 (11p15), prevalence ~70%, early event, associated with perilobar nephrogenic rests and with epithelial and blastemal histology

TP53 (17p13), prevalence ~70%, associated with anaplasia and with reduced event-free and overall survival

MYCN (2p24), prevalence ~15%, associated with anaplasia and with reduced event-free and overall survival

1q gain, prevalence ~30–40%, associated with reduced event-free and overall survival.

Renal Cell Carcinoma (RCC)

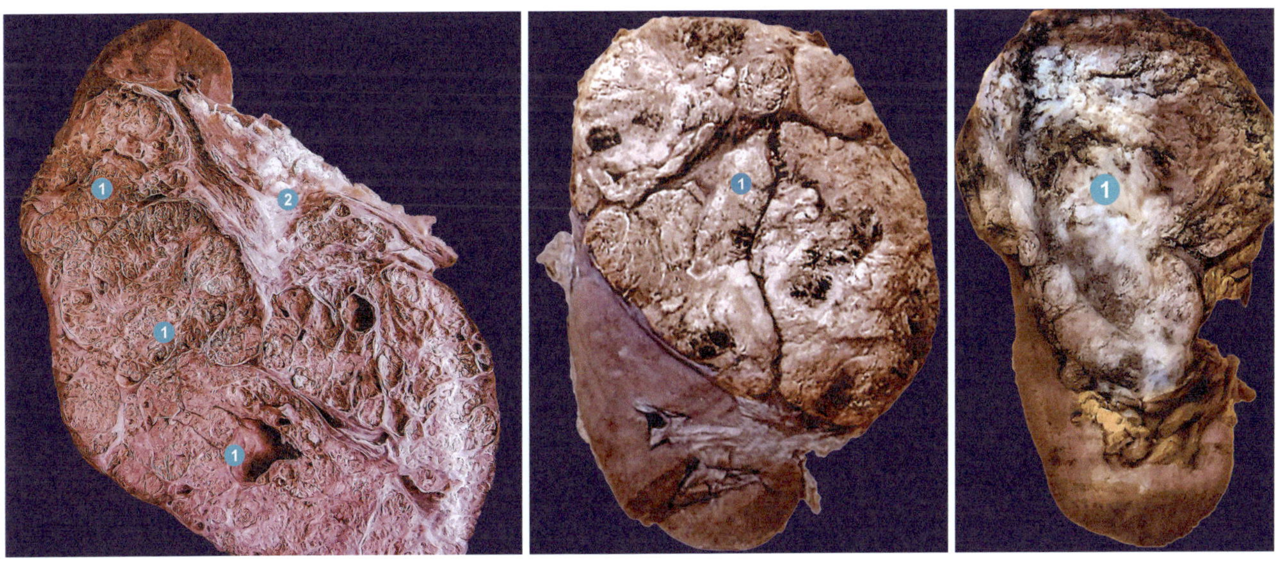

A kidney bisected longitudinally is mounted.

1. Renal tissue is replaced by a large, spherical tumor mass formed of yellow-grey tissue separated by bands of fibrous tissue with the presence of areas of hemorrhage, necrosis, and cyst formation.
2. Focal invasion of the renal capsule is observed.

Renal Cell Carcinoma

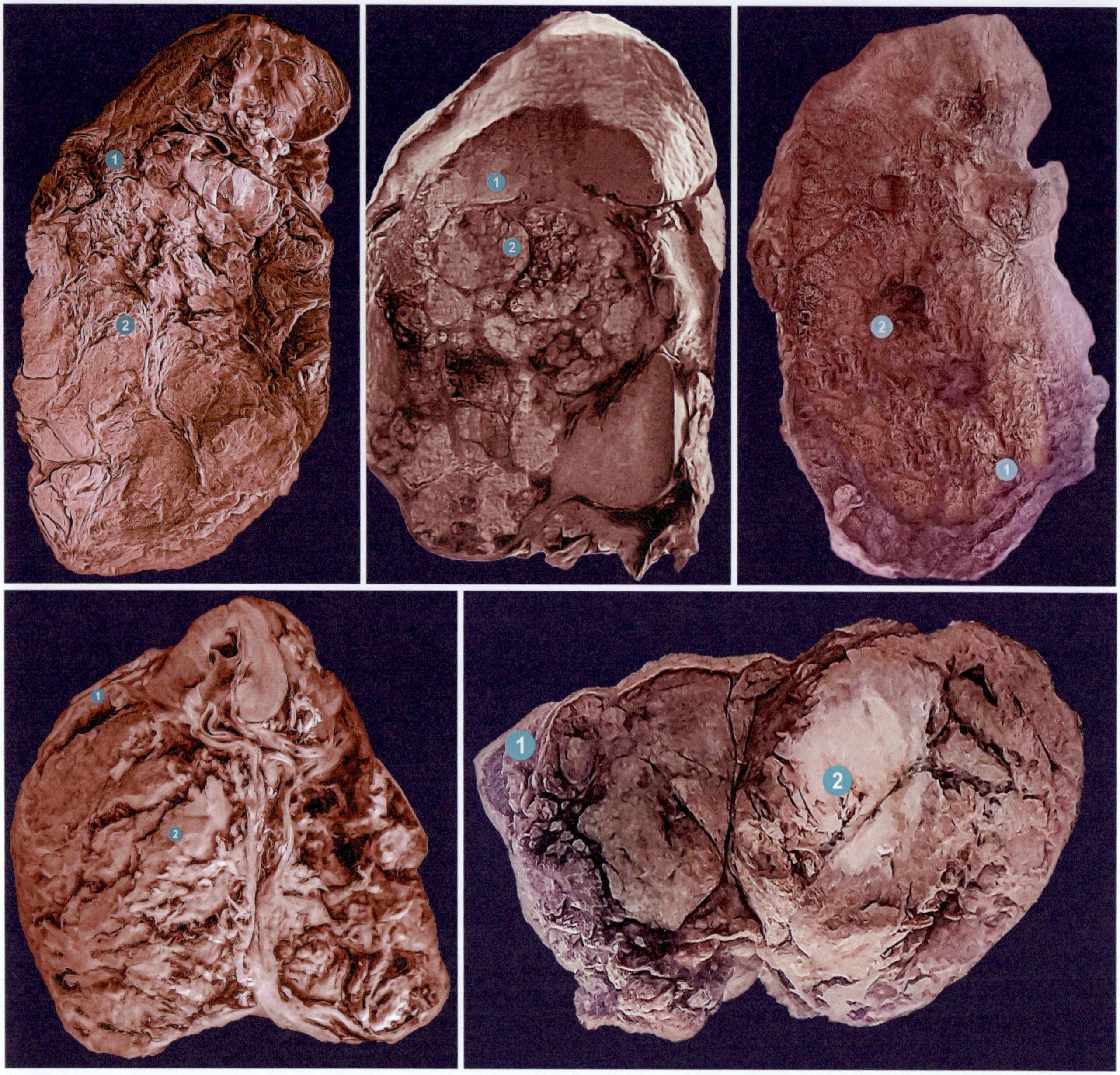

A kidney bisected longitudinally is mounted.

1. The cut section shows a large but still fairly circumscribed mass.
2. The cut surface has a variegated appearance with white, yellowish, brown, hemorrhagic red, and cystic areas.

Microscopic Picture of Renal Cell Carcinoma (RCC): Clear Cell Carcinoma (a, b)

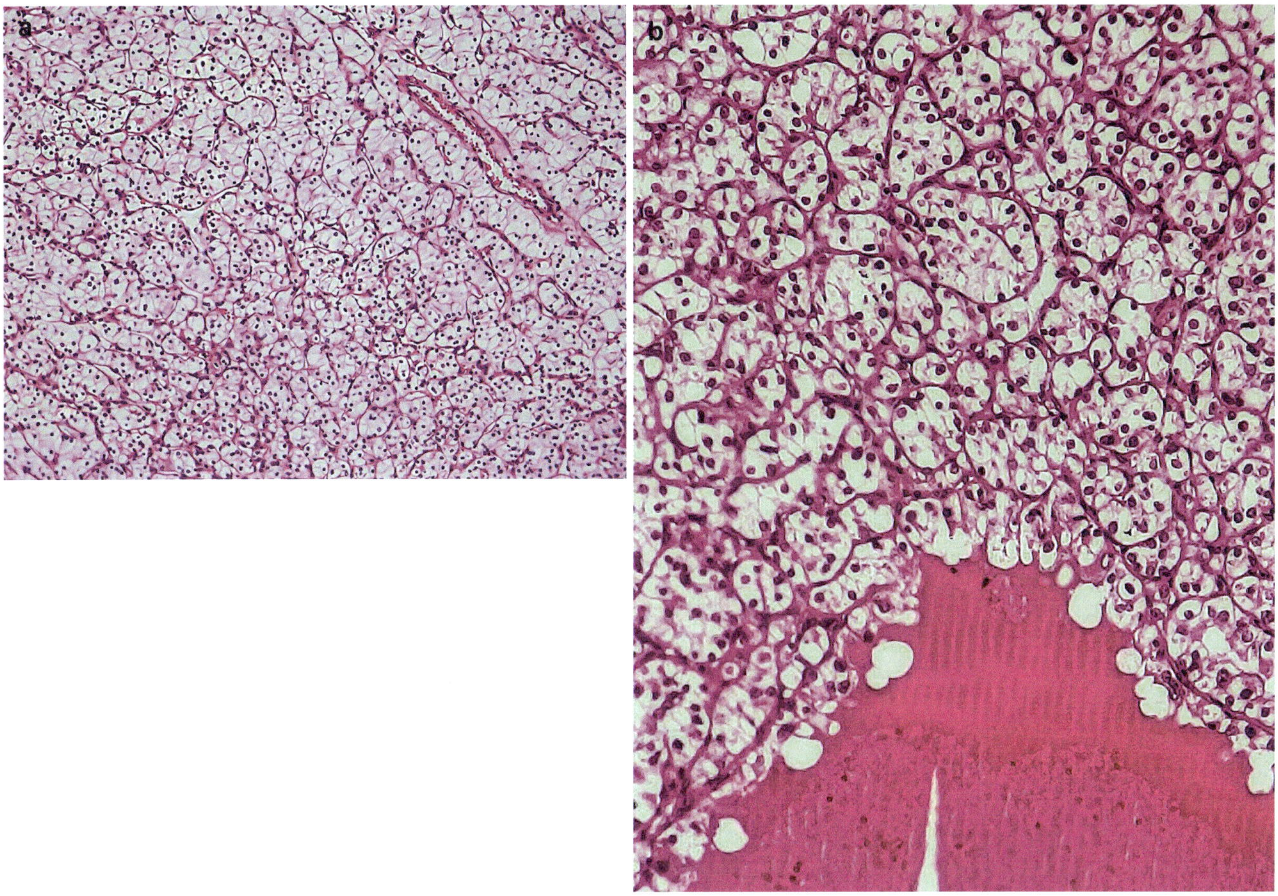

Sections show tumor cells arranged in solid nests and cords with a rich vascular network. Tumor cells are characterized by clear or pale cytoplasm due to the accumulation of glycogen and lipids. The nuclei are round to oval with prominent nucleoli.

Ancillary Tools

IHC [9]: Molecular/cytogenetics description [10]:

PAX8: ~100%, nuclear; PAX2 is similar but less sensitive.

CAIX: 75–100%, diffuse membranous (box-like), diminished expression in high-grade regions

CD10 (82–94%, membranous) and RCC (72–84%, cytoplasmic and membranous): proximal tubular brush border antigens, also present in normal cells

Epithelial markers: AE1/AE3, CAM 5.2, EMA

Vimentin (cytoplasm and membranous)

Somatic:

- 3p loss or biallelic alteration (mutation or hypermethylation of promoter region) in VHL tumor suppressor gene (3p25-26) in 80–98%
- 3p locus harbors at least 4 other clear cell RCC tumor suppressor genes: KD-M6A (also called UTX), KDM5C (also called JARID1C), SETD2, and PBRM1.
- Poor prognosis: allelic losses on chromosome 14q (40–60%), loss of 4p and 9p, loss of function mutations in the BAP1 gene; PBRM1 is also commonly mutated in clear cell RCC.
- Progression of clear cells in RCC can eventually lead to polyploid karyotype and further losses or gains of genetic material.

Familial:

- Von Hippel–Lindau familial cancer syndrome:
  70% lifetime risk of developing renal tumors, autosomal dominant, early onset; 35–45% of patients develop bilateral multifocal clear cell RCC; as many as 1100 cysts; and 600 microscopic clear cell RCCs.
- Patients are born with a germline defect in one of the two alleles of the VHL gene.
  Loss of the second allele results in clinical disease expression
- Families segregating constitutional chromosome 3 translocations

Renal Cell Carcinoma—Papillary Type

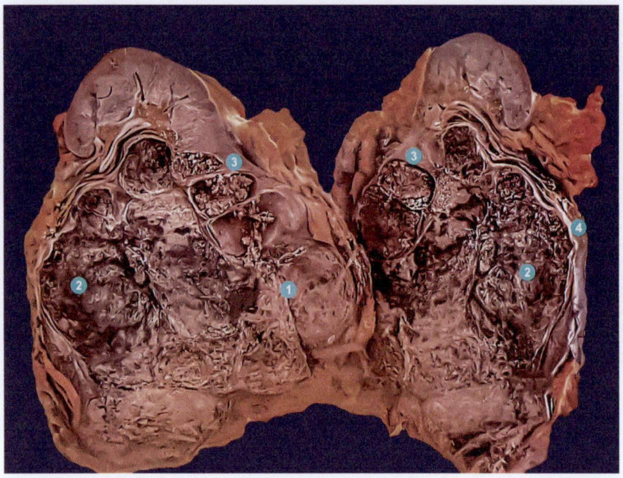

A kidney bisected longitudinally is mounted.

1. Well-circumscribed, large, globular, and lobulated tumor mass with brown parenchyma.
2. Areas of hemorrhage and necrosis are prominent.
3. The cut surface is friable with the presence of small, nipple-like projections, giving it the characteristic “papillary” appearance.
4. The tumor is surrounded by a rim of dense fibrous tissue.

Microscopic Picture of Renal Cell Carcinoma—Papillary Type (a, b)

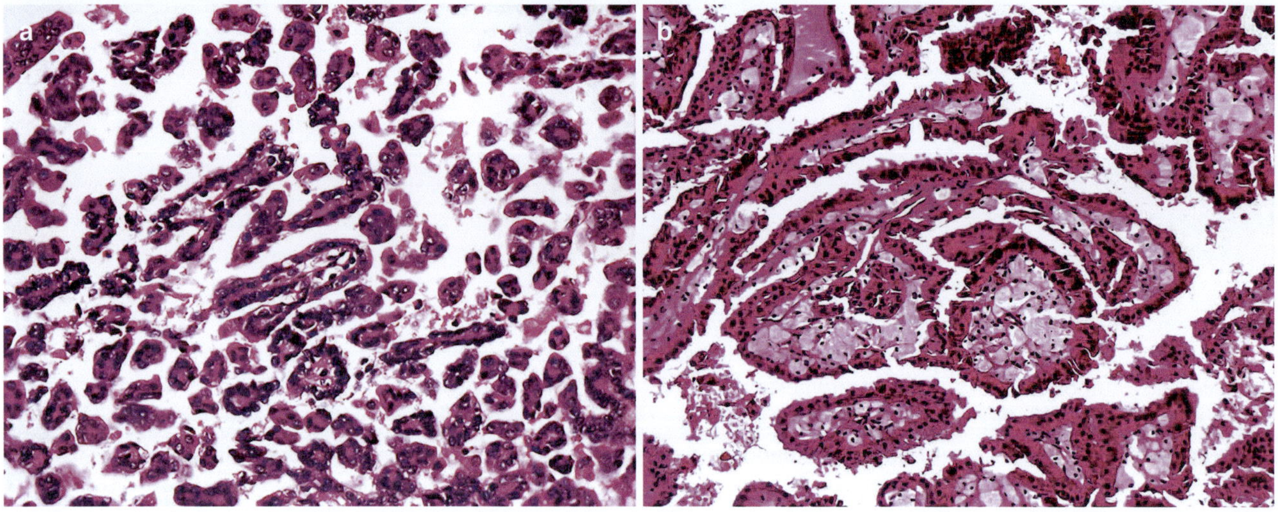

Sections show papillae lined by cuboidal or columnar cells. The tumor cells have eosinophilic cytoplasm and enlarged nuclei with prominent nucleoli. Papillary cores contain foamy macrophages.

Ancillary Tools

Molecular/cytogenetics description [11]:

No molecular markers specific for the diagnosis of PRCC

Chromosome 7 and 17 gains and loss of Y chromosome in low-grade tumors

MET mutations are seen in former type 1 and low-grade PRCC; CDKN2A mutation or promoter methylation in aggressive PRCC.

Exclude FH gene mutation and TFE3 rearrangements for high-grade PRCC.

Renal Cell Carcinoma—Cystic Type

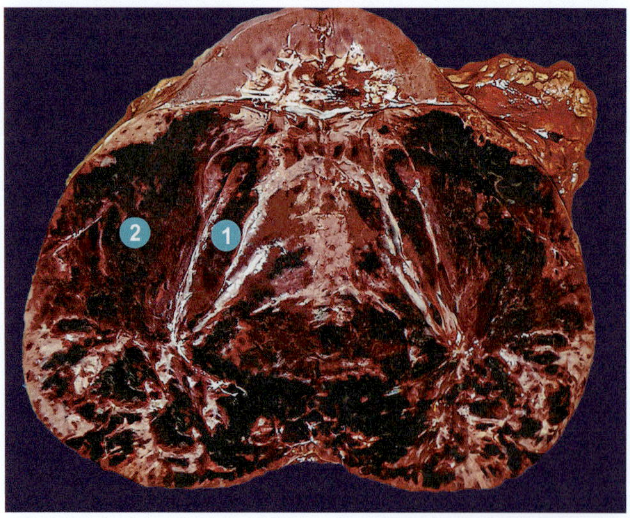

A kidney bisected longitudinally is mounted. The cut section shows:

1. A multilocular, large, cystic lesion separated by fibrous septa replacing most renal tissue.
2. Extensive hemorrhage.

Microscopic Picture of Renal Cell Carcinoma—Cystic Type (a–d)

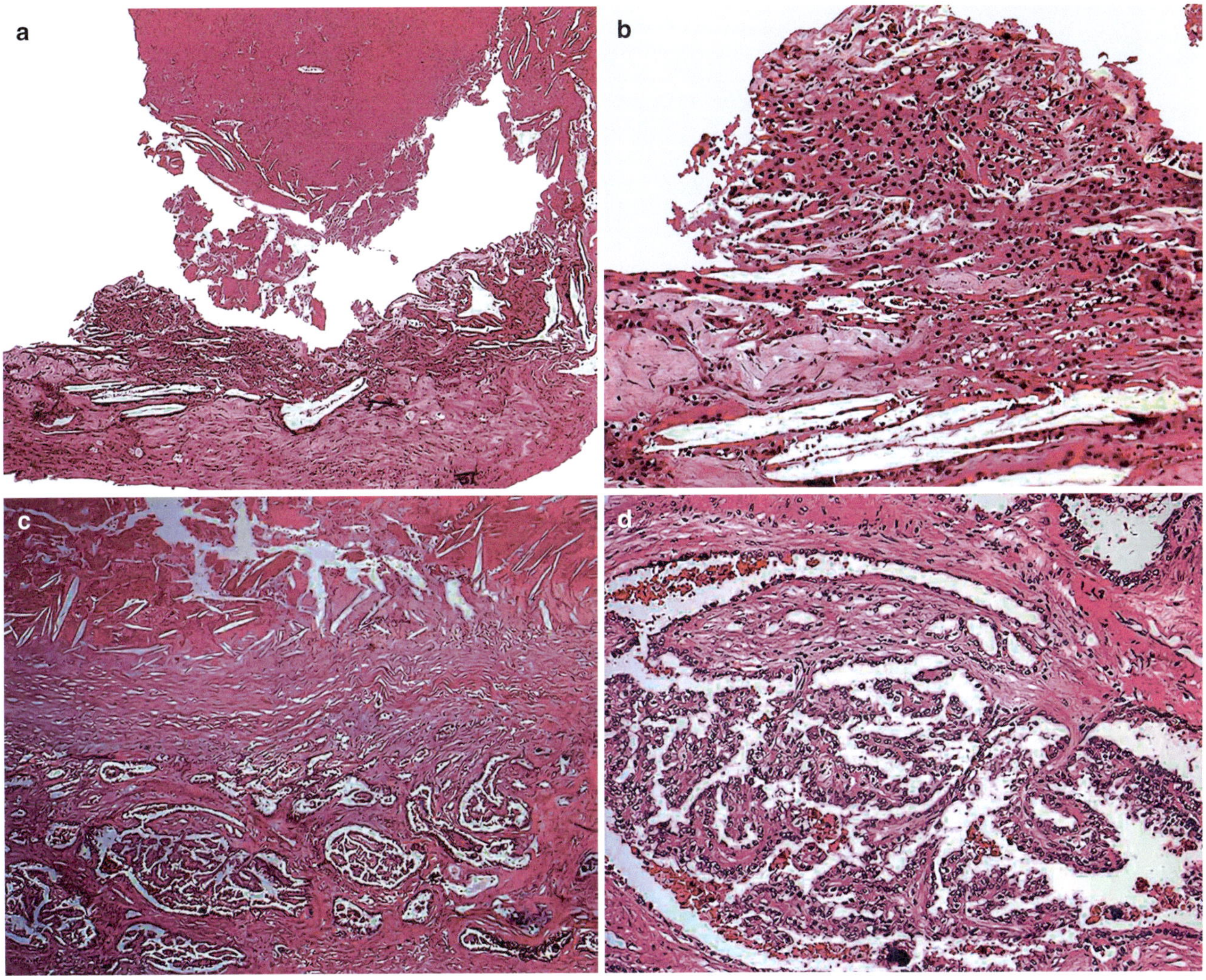

Sections show thin fibrous septa lined by tumor cells, which form multilayering focally with the formation of small intracystic papillae. The tumor cells have low-grade nuclei and eosinophilic cytoplasm. Extensive areas of hemorrhage are seen.

Chromophobe Renal Cell Carcinoma

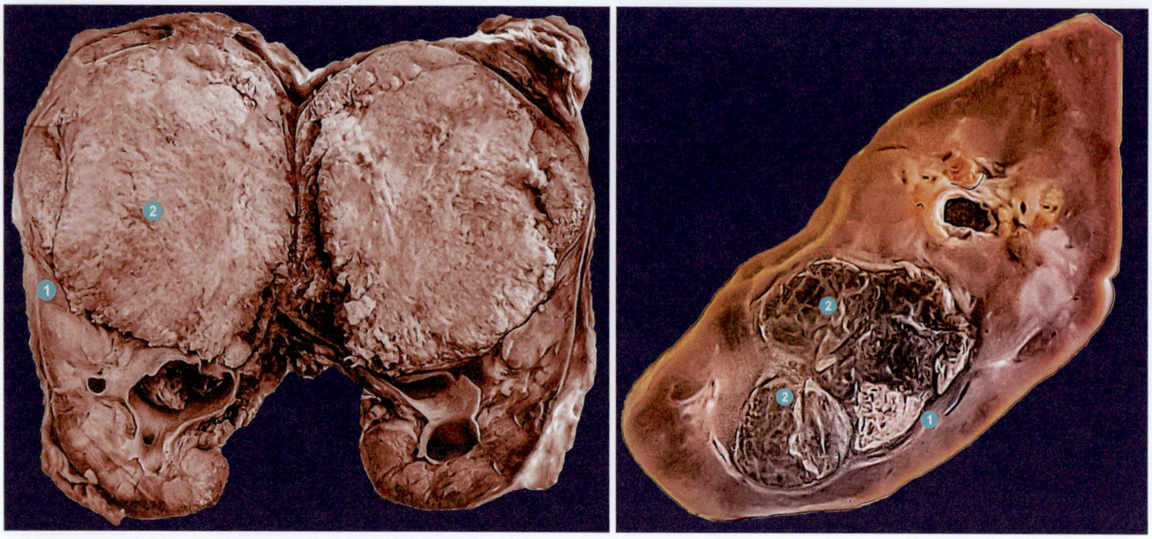

A kidney bisected longitudinally is mounted. The cut section shows:

1. Well-circumscribed, unencapsulated mass confined to the kidney.
2. The cut surface is reddish brown with areas of scarring.

Microscopic Picture of Chromophobe Renal Cell Carcinoma (a–d)

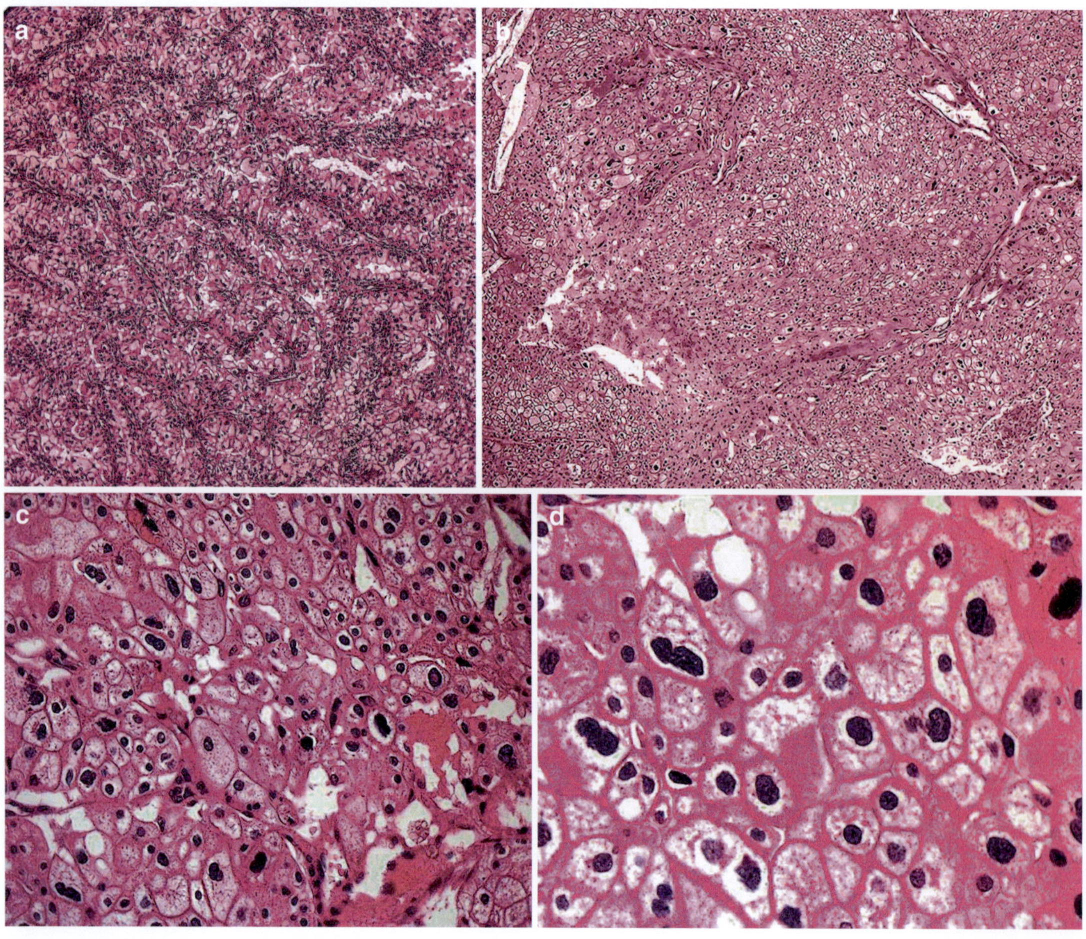

Sections show sheets of 2 types of malignant cells:

Type 1: large, polygonal cells with distinct, sharp plant-like cell borders (vegetable cells) and abundant cytoplasm

Type 2: smaller cells with finely granular eosinophilic cytoplasm.

There are marked variations in nuclear size and shape, irregularly shaped nuclear membranes, and perinuclear halos. Some nuclei have coarse chromatin, giving them a 'raisinoid' appearance. Some cells have two nuclei (binucleation), while others have no nuclei at all.

Ancillary Tools

Molecular/cytogenetics description [12]:

Multiple losses of whole chromosomes, most often 1, 2, 6, 10, 13, 17, 21, or Y (versus no loss in oncocytoma).

FISH and SNP arrays may be more helpful than karyotyping.

DNA rearrangement breakpoints within the TERT promoter region.

TP53 and PTEN mutated in 10–30% of cases (TCGA cohort)

NRAS, mTOR, and TSC1 / TSC2 in ~5% cases.

Mitochondrial (mt) mutations in DNA most commonly affect MT-ND5

Increased expression of genes encoding enzymes in the Krebs cycle (expression is suppressed in clear cell RCC).

Sarcomatoid tumors have different genetic abnormalities.

miRNA expression patterns may be associated with progression, recurrence-free survival, and overall survival.

Ancillary Tools

IHC [9]:

PAX8 and PAX2

CAIX: diffuse, membranous in 75–100% of clear cell RCC

Generally, CD10 (proximal tubular marker), RCC, vimentin, and epithelial markers, including AE1/AE3, CAM 5.2, and EMA

IHC panels

	Hale	KIT	CK7	S100A1	VIM	CAIX	AMACR	SDH	TFE3
Chromophobe RCC	+++	+++	+++	–	–	–	–	+++	–
Clear cell RCC	–	–	–	–	+++	+++	–	+++	–
Oncocytoma	–	+++	Rare	+++	–	–	–	+++	–
Papillary RCC	–	–	+++	–	+++	–	+++	+++	–
Translocation RCC	–	–	–	–	–	–	++	+++	+++
SDH deficient RCC	–	–	–	–	–	–	–	–	–

Metastatic Tumor in Kidney (a, b)

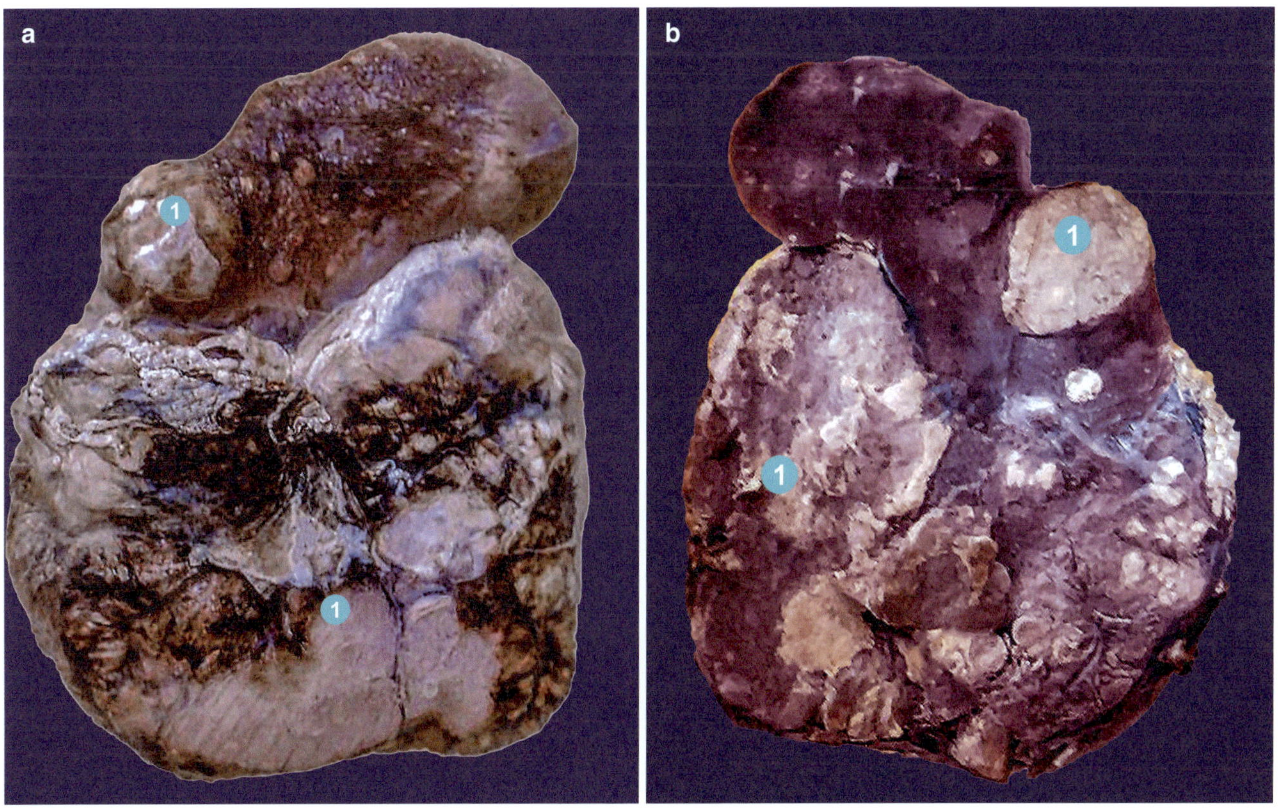

A kidney is mounted.

1. It is infiltrated by irregular, fleshy, and pink-yellow masses projecting on the surface.

6.2 Urinary Bladder

6.2.1 Neoplastic Lesions

Fungating Carcinoma of Urinary Bladder

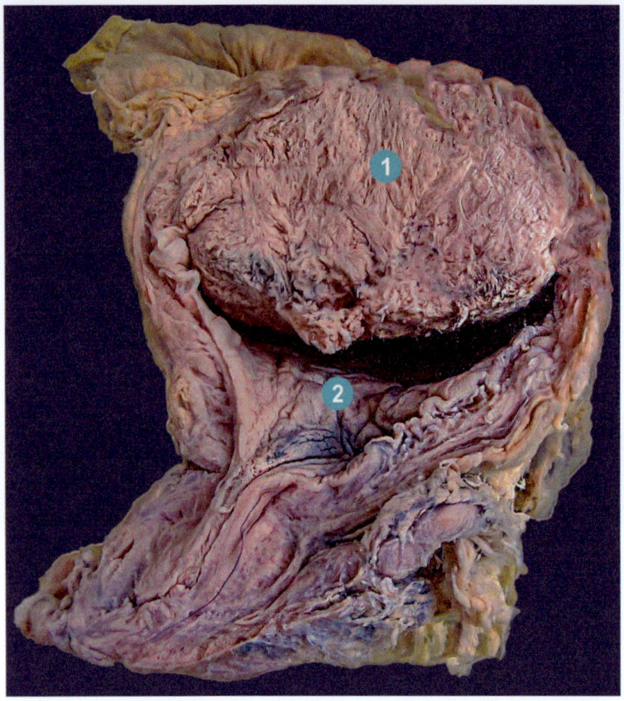

The sectioned urinary bladder is mounted.

1. The bladder cavity is nearly filled by a large fungating, fleshy, pale pink tumor mass infiltrating the bladder wall.
2. The rest of the bladder mucosa is dirty yellow, denoting chronic cystitis.

Fungating Carcinoma of Urinary Bladder

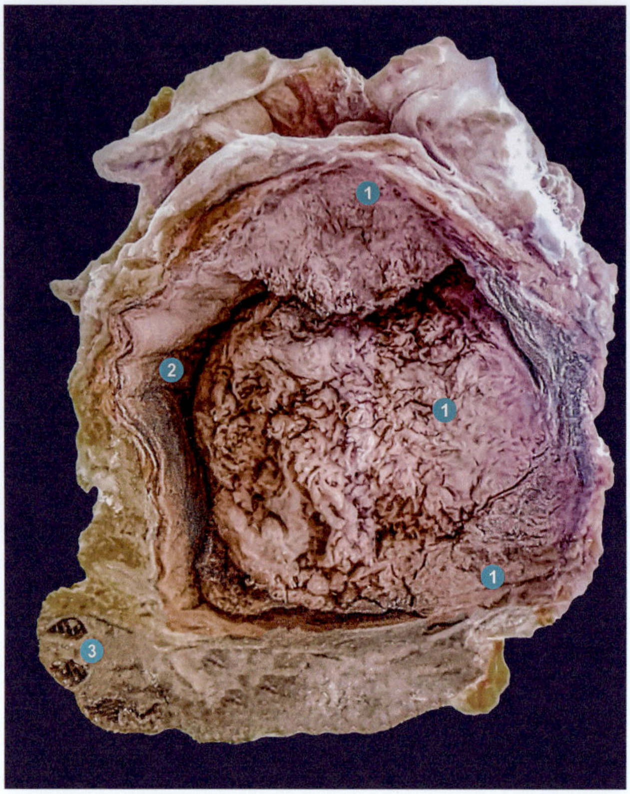

Sectioned urinary bladder and seminal vesicle are mounted.

1. The bladder cavity is nearly filled by a large fungating, fleshy, pale pink tumor mass infiltrating the bladder wall.
2. The rest of the bladder mucosa is dirty yellow, denoting chronic cystitis.
3. Seminal vesicles are enlarged with areas of fibrosis (proved microscopically to be calcified bilharzial ova).

Microscopic Picture of Well Differentiated Squamous Cell Carcinoma of Urinary Bladder and Chronic Bilharzial Cystitis (a–f)

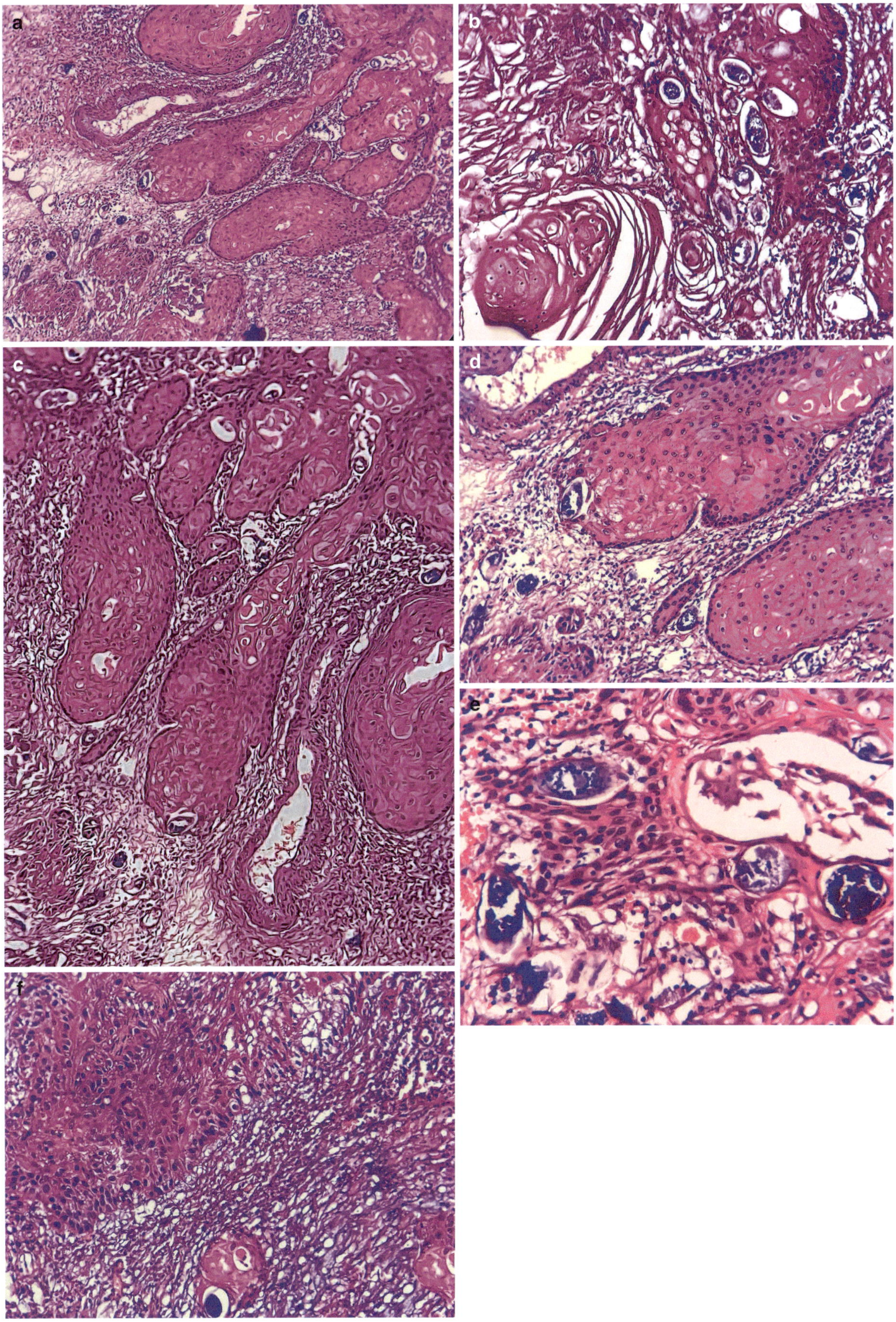

Sections show ulcerated urothelium. Clusters of malignant squamous cells with eosinophilic cytoplasm and areas of keratinization and horn pearl formation infiltrating the corium. The tumor cells are associated with a lot of calcified bilharzial ova with surrounding chronic inflammatory cellular infiltrate.

Ancillary Tools
IHC:

Positive for squamous markers CK5/6, p63, p40, CK14, and desmoglein 3

CK7 variable

Molecular/cytogenetics description [13]:

- HPV DNA in situ hybridization is negative; HPV positivity may be seen in association with condyloma or chronic injury.
- Basal/squamous molecular subgroup of muscle-invasive bladder cancer show frequent mutations in TP53 and RB.

Fungating Carcinoma of Urinary Bladder

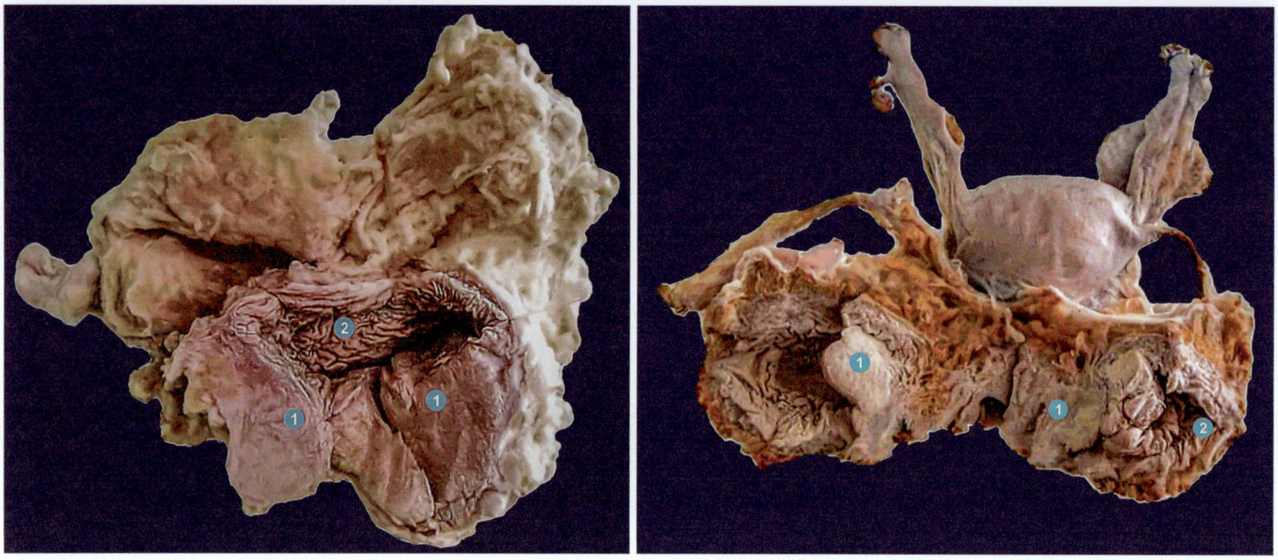

Sectioned urinary bladder, vagina, uterus, fallopian tubes, and ovaries are mounted.

1. The bladder cavity is nearly filled by a large fungating, fleshy, pale pink tumor mass infiltrating the bladder wall and vaginal wall.
2. The rest of the bladder mucosa is dirty yellow, denoting chronic cystitis.

Microscopic Picture of Urothelial Carcinoma—Noninvasive Papillary Urothelial Carcinoma, Low Grade (a, b)

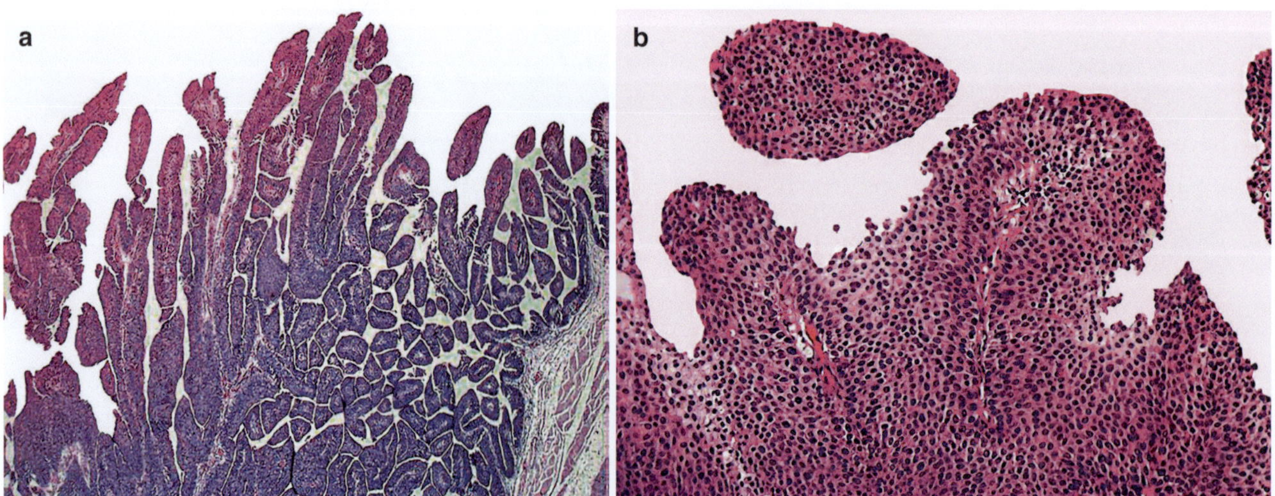

Sections show neoplastic urothelium lining fibrovascular cores. Urothelium is thrown into long, slender papillae with minimal fusing or branching. Orderly architecture at low magnification, some loss of polarity, and mild pleomorphism at medium magnification. Cells are generally uniform in size, may have slight variation but no significant nuclear pleomorphism or nucleomegaly, occasional slight irregularities in nuclear contour

Microscopic Picture of Urothelial Carcinoma—Invasive Papillary Urothelial Carcinoma, High Grade (c–g)

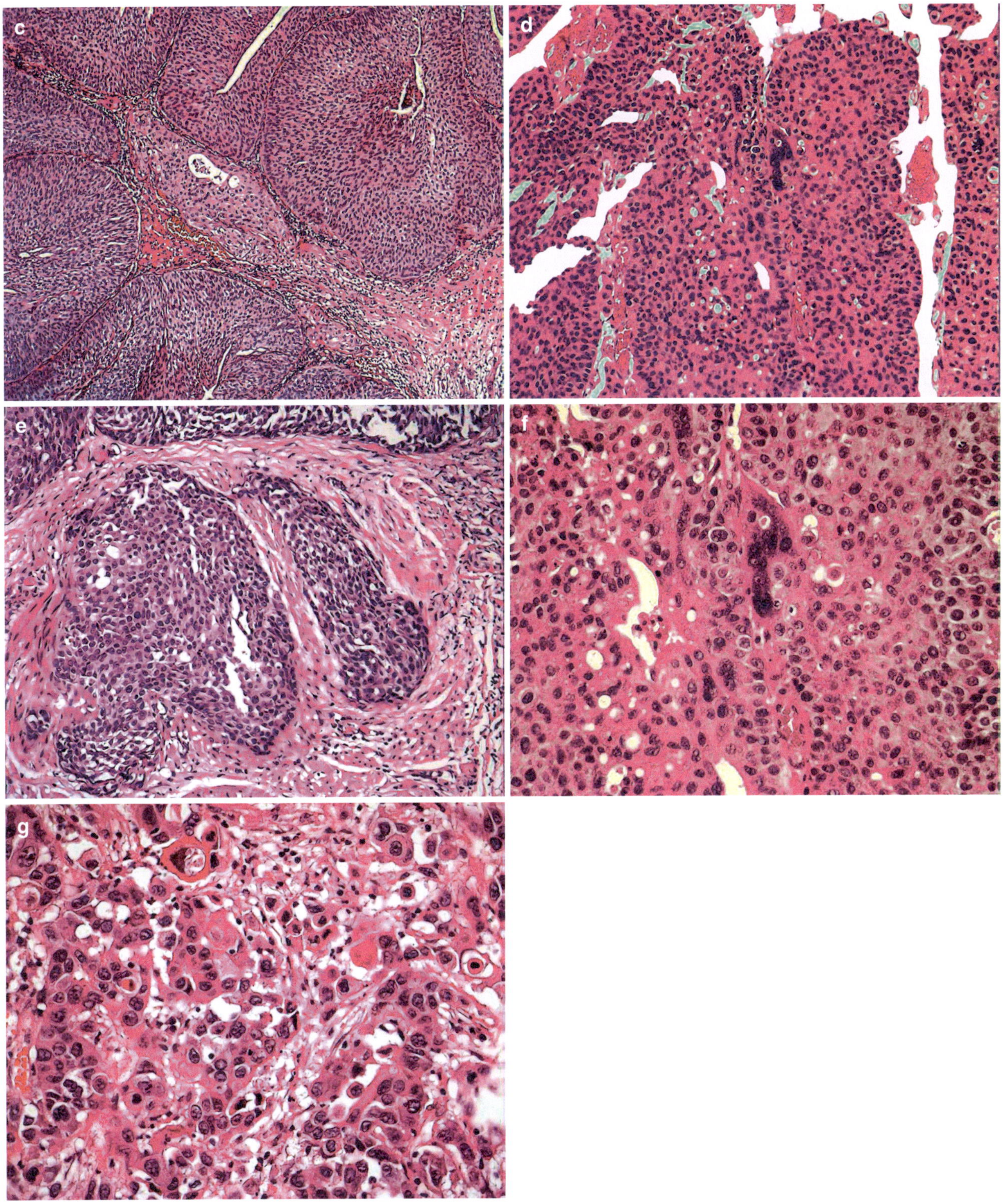

Sections show neoplastic cells arranged in irregular nests or single cells invading the lamina propria and muscularis propria. Retraction artifact is often seen and can mimic vascular invasion. High grade nuclear features: nuclear pleomorphism, hyperchromasia, high N/C ratio with frequent mitotic figures.

Ancillary Tools

IHC [14]:

GATA3, CK7, CK20, p63, p40, uroplakins II and III, HMWCK, thrombomodulin

Immunostaining can distinguish luminal and basal phenotypes:

Luminal: CK20, GATA3, FOXA1, XBP1, CD24

Basal: HMWCK (CK5, CK6, and CK14), CDH3, CD44

Molecular/cytogenetics description [15, 16]

Most commonly mutated genes are associated with cell cycle progression, including TP53, PIK3CA, RB1, and FGFR3.

UroVysion is an FDA-approved fluorescent in situ hybridization (FISH) that detects aneuploidy in chromosomes 3, 7, and 17 and loss of the 9p21 locus (72% sensitivity and 83% specificity).

Nuclear matrix proteins (NMP22): group of proteins produced by cancerous cells.

The NMP22 BladderChek test is an FDA-approved qualitative assay for surveillance and detection of bladder cancer (50% sensitivity and 87% specificity).

Bladder tumor antigen (BTA): antigen produced by cancerous cells.

BTA Trak (quantitative) and BTA Stat (qualitative) are FDA approved assays for surveillance (68–77.5% sensitivity and 50–75% specificity).

References

1. Prasad A.K. et al. (2013). Polycystic horseshoe kidney Indian J Nephrol. 23(5): 387. doi: https://doi.org/10.4103/0971-4065.116337. PMCID: PMC3764720.
2. Kundu R. et al. (2019). Clinicopathological Spectrum of Xanthogranulomatous Pyelonephritis. Indian J Nephrol. 29(2):111-115. doi: https://doi.org/10.4103/ijn.IJN_50_18. PMID: 30983751; PMCID: PMC6440323.
3. Torricelli F.C.M. and Monga M.(2020). Staghorn renal stones: what the urologist needs to know. Int Braz J Urol.46(6): 927–933. doi: https://doi.org/10.1590/S1677-5538.IBJU.2020.99.07. PMCID: PMC7527092.
4. Picken M.M. (2020). The Pathology of Amyloidosis in Classification: A Review. Acta Haematol. 143(4):322-334. doi: https://doi.org/10.1159/000506696. PMID: 32392555.
5. Fenoglio R. et al. (2022). Renal Involvement in Transthyretin Amyloidosis: The Double Presentation of Transthyretin Amyloidosis Deposition Disease. Nephron.146(5):481-488. doi: https://doi.org/10.1159/000522370. PMID: 35307708.
6. Isharwal S. et al. (2019). Genomic landscape of inverted urothelial papilloma and urothelial papilloma of the bladder. J Pathol.248(3):260-265. doi: https://doi.org/10.1002/path.5261. PMID: 30838648.
7. Ooms AHAG. et al (2020).Renal Tumors of Childhood-A Histopathologic Pattern-Based Diagnostic Approach. Cancers (Basel). 12(3):729. doi: https://doi.org/10.3390/cancers12030729. PMID: 32204536; PMCID: PMC7140051.
8. Treger TD. et al. (2019). The genetic changes of Wilms tumor. Nat Rev Nephrol.15(4):240-251. doi: https://doi.org/10.1038/s41581-019-0112-0. PMID: 30705419.
9. Zhao W. et al. (2015). DOG1, cyclin D1, CK7, CD117, and vimentin are useful immunohistochemical markers in distinguishing chromophobe renal cell carcinoma from clear cell renal cell carcinoma and renal oncocytoma. Pathol Res Pract.211(4):303-7. doi: https://doi.org/10.1016/j.prp.2014.12.014. PMID: 25596994.
10. Cancer Genome Atlas Research Network. (2013). Comprehensive molecular characterization of clear cell renal cell carcinoma. Nature. 499(7456):43-9. doi: https://doi.org/10.1038/nature12222. PMID: 23792563; PMCID: PMC3771322.
11. Cancer Genome Atlas Research Network. (2016).Comprehensive Molecular Characterization of Papillary Renal-Cell Carcinoma. N Engl J Med.374(2):135-45. doi: https://doi.org/10.1056/NEJMoa1505917. PMID: 26536169; PMCID: PMC4775252.
12. Davis CF. et al. (2014).The somatic genomic landscape of chromophobe renal cell carcinoma. Cancer Cell. 26(3):319-330. doi: https://doi.org/10.1016/j.ccr.2014.07.014. PMID: 25155756; PMCID: PMC4160352.
13. Samarska IV, Epstein JI. (2019). Condyloma Acuminatum of Urinary Bladder: Relation to Squamous Cell Carcinoma. Am J Surg Pathol. 43(11):1547-1553. doi: https://doi.org/10.1097/PAS.0000000000001339. PMID: 31368913.
14. Guo CC. et al. (2020). Assessment of Luminal and Basal Phenotypes in Bladder Cancer. Sci Rep. 10(1):9743. doi: https://doi.org/10.1038/s41598-020-66747-7. PMID: 32546765; PMCID: PMC7298008.
15. Cancer Genome Atlas Research Network. (2014). Comprehensive molecular characterization of urothelial bladder carcinoma. Nature. 507(7492):315-22. doi: https://doi.org/10.1038/nature12965. PMID: 24476821; PMCID: PMC3962515.
16. Bhat A, Ritch CR. (2019). Urinary biomarkers in bladder cancer: where do we stand? Curr Opin Urol. 29(3):203-209. doi: https://doi.org/10.1097/MOU.0000000000000605. PMID: 30855372.

7 Diseases of the Male Reproductive Tract

The male genital system is an intricate, complex arrangement of organs and structures that participate in vital functions including reproduction and hormone regulation. This chapter delves into the gross and microscopic pathology of this system. Disease conditions may result in significant changes to the structure of these organs, leading to changes in function, and ultimately to various symptoms and clinical findings. A variety of disease processes can affect the male genital system, including infections, inflammation, trauma, congenital abnormalities, and neoplastic diseases.

This chapter will serve as a resource for medical students, pathology residents, urologists, and any health professionals who are interested in expanding their knowledge of the male genital system from a pathological perspective.

The diseases studied in this chapter will be arranged in this manner:

1. Diseases of Tunica Vaginalis
   (a) Pyocele
   (b) Hematocele
2. Inflammation of Testis
   (a) Elephantiasis (Filariasis) of the Scrotum
   (b) Tuberculous epididymo-orchitis
3. Tumors of Testis
   (a) Seminoma
   (b) Testicular Teratoma
4. Diseases of Prostate
   (a) Nodular Hyperplasia
   (b) Prostatic Carcinoma
5. Diseases of Penis
   (a) Penile Carcinoma

G. Dawood, *Color Atlas of Human Gross and Microscopic Pathology*, https://doi.org/10.1007/978-3-031-76007-5_7

7.1 Diseases of Tunica Vaginalis

Pyocele (a, b)

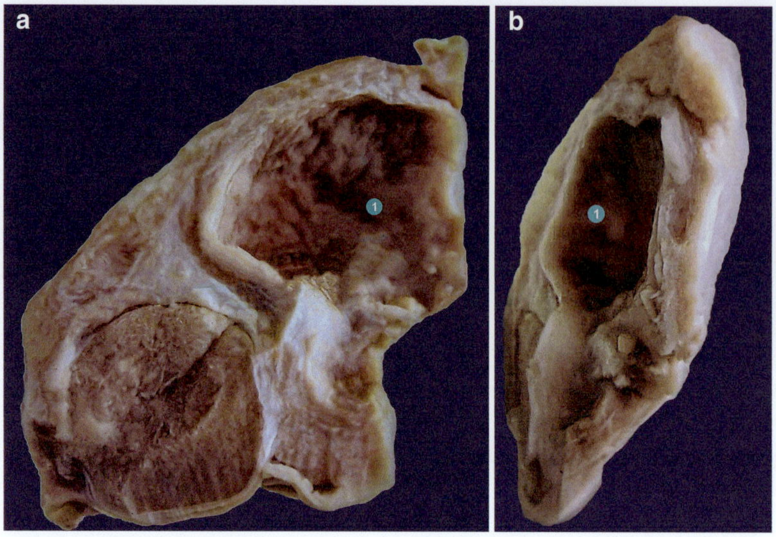

The testis with opened tunica vaginalis is mounted.

1. The inner surface of the tunica is dull yellow and shaggy.

Hematocele

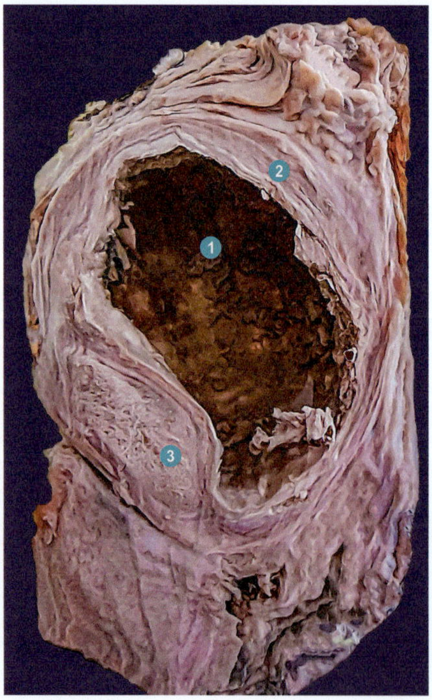

The testis and opened tunica vaginalis are mounted.

1. The tunica is dilated and filled with clotted blood.
2. The tunica has markedly thickened white fibrous wall.
3. The testis appears atrophic and compressed to one side of the tunica.

7.2 Inflammation of Testis

Elephantiasis (Filariasis) of the Scrotum and Testis (a, b)

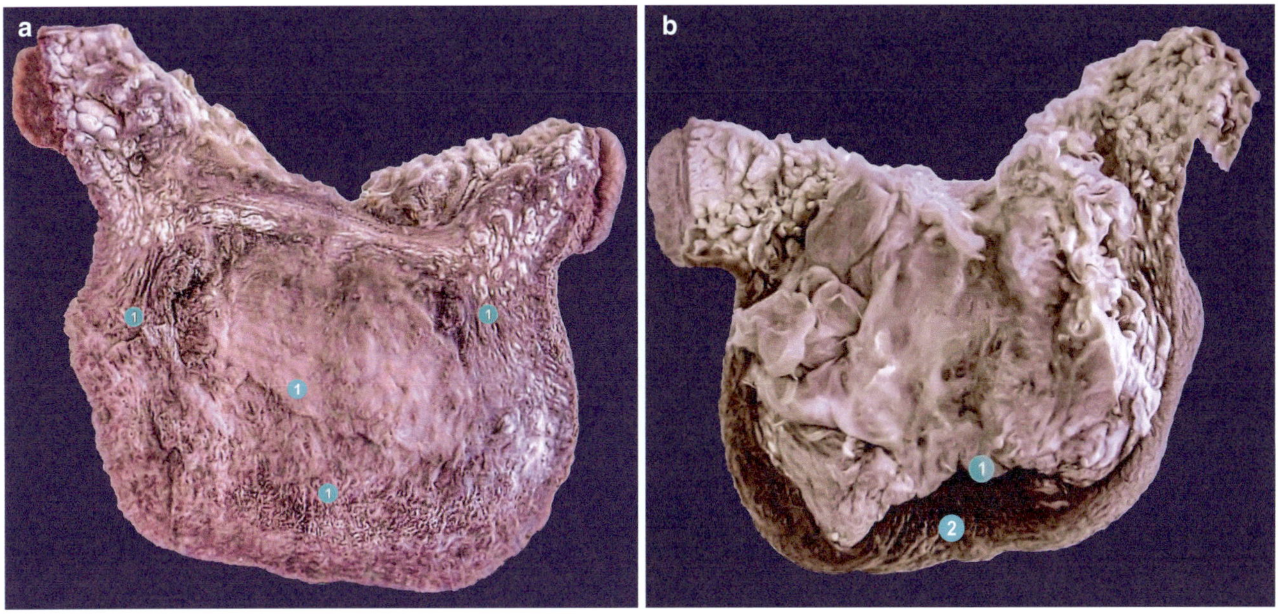

An opened scrotum is mounted.

1. The testis and tunica albuginea are masked by extensive fibrous tissue.
2. The skin is rough and nodular, with increased skin markings and subcutaneous tissue.

Tuberculous Epididymo-Orchitis

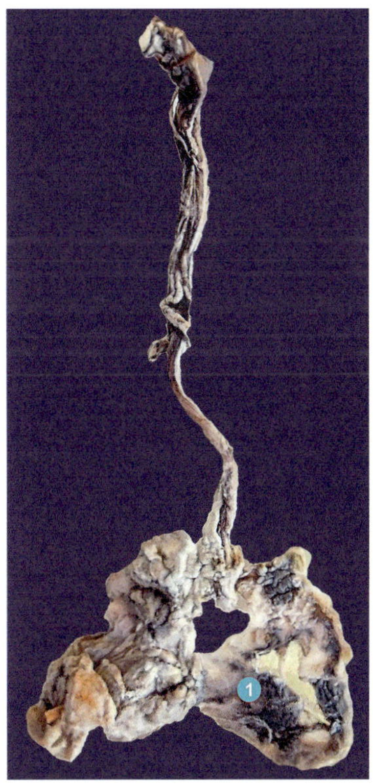

The testis, epididymis, and vas deferens are mounted.

1. The cut section of the testis and epididymis shows opaque yellow caseous areas surrounded by fibrosis.

Microscopic Picture of Tuberculous Epididymo-Orchitis (a, b)

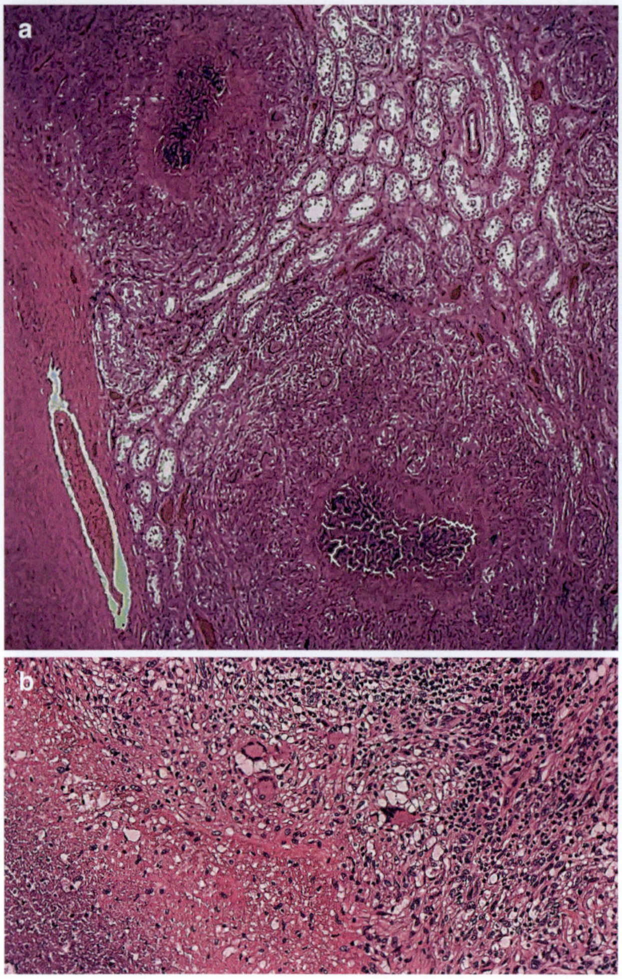

Sections showing multiple caseating epithelioid granulomas infiltrating epididymis and in-between seminiferous tubules. The granulomas are formed of epithelioid cells, Langhans giant cells, and lymphocytes.

7.3 Testicular Neoplasms

Seminoma of Testis

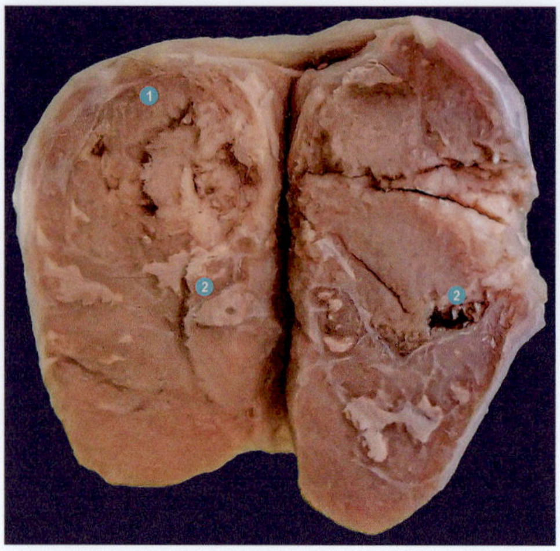

The bisected testis is mounted.

1. It is enlarged and replaced by fleshy, homogeneous, lobulated, pink-yellow tumor tissue.
2. Focal areas of necrosis, hemorrhage, and cystic cavitation are seen.

Seminoma of Testis

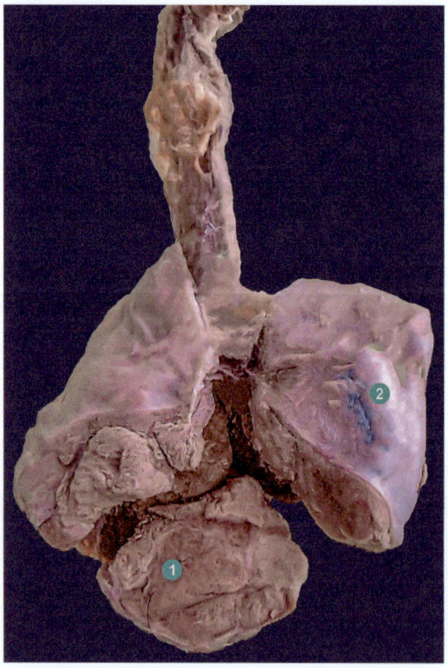

Bisected testis and spermatic cord are mounted.

1. It is enlarged and replaced by fleshy, homogeneous, lobulated, pink-yellow tumor tissue with focal areas of necrosis, hemorrhage, and cystic cavitation.
2. Tunica shows dilated veins.

Seminoma of Testis

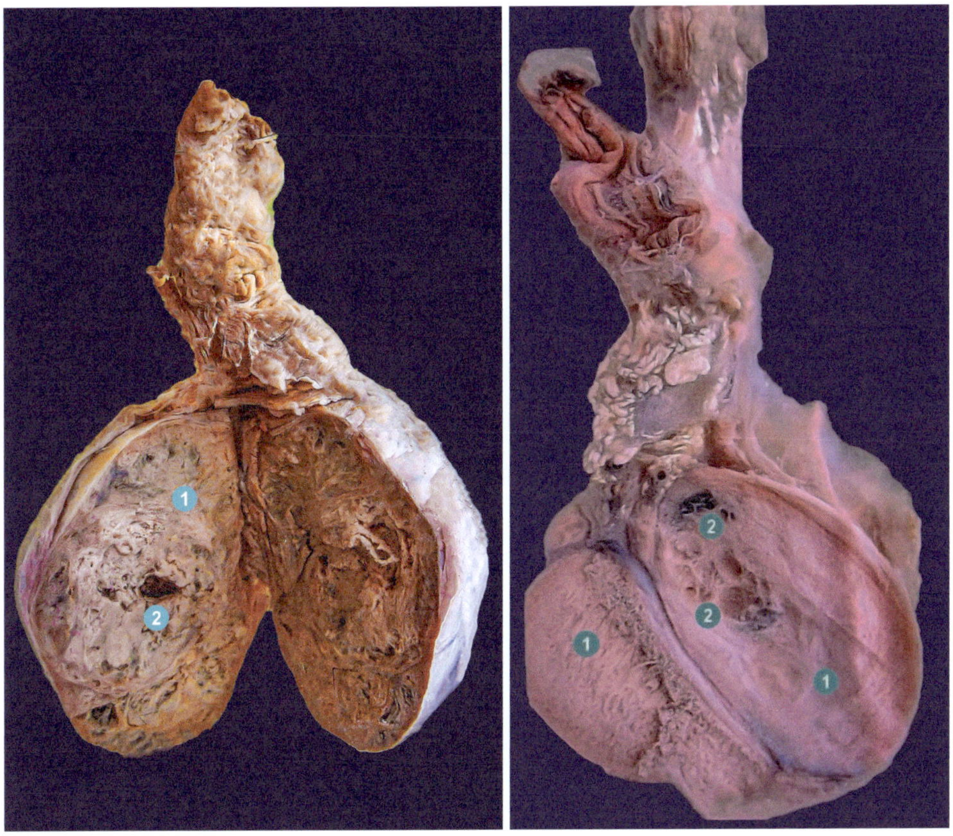

Bisected testis and spermatic cord are mounted.

1. It is enlarged and replaced by fleshy, homogeneous, lobulated, pink-yellow tumor tissue.
2. Focal areas of necrosis, hemorrhage, and cystic cavitation are seen.

Microscopic Picture of Seminoma (a–d)

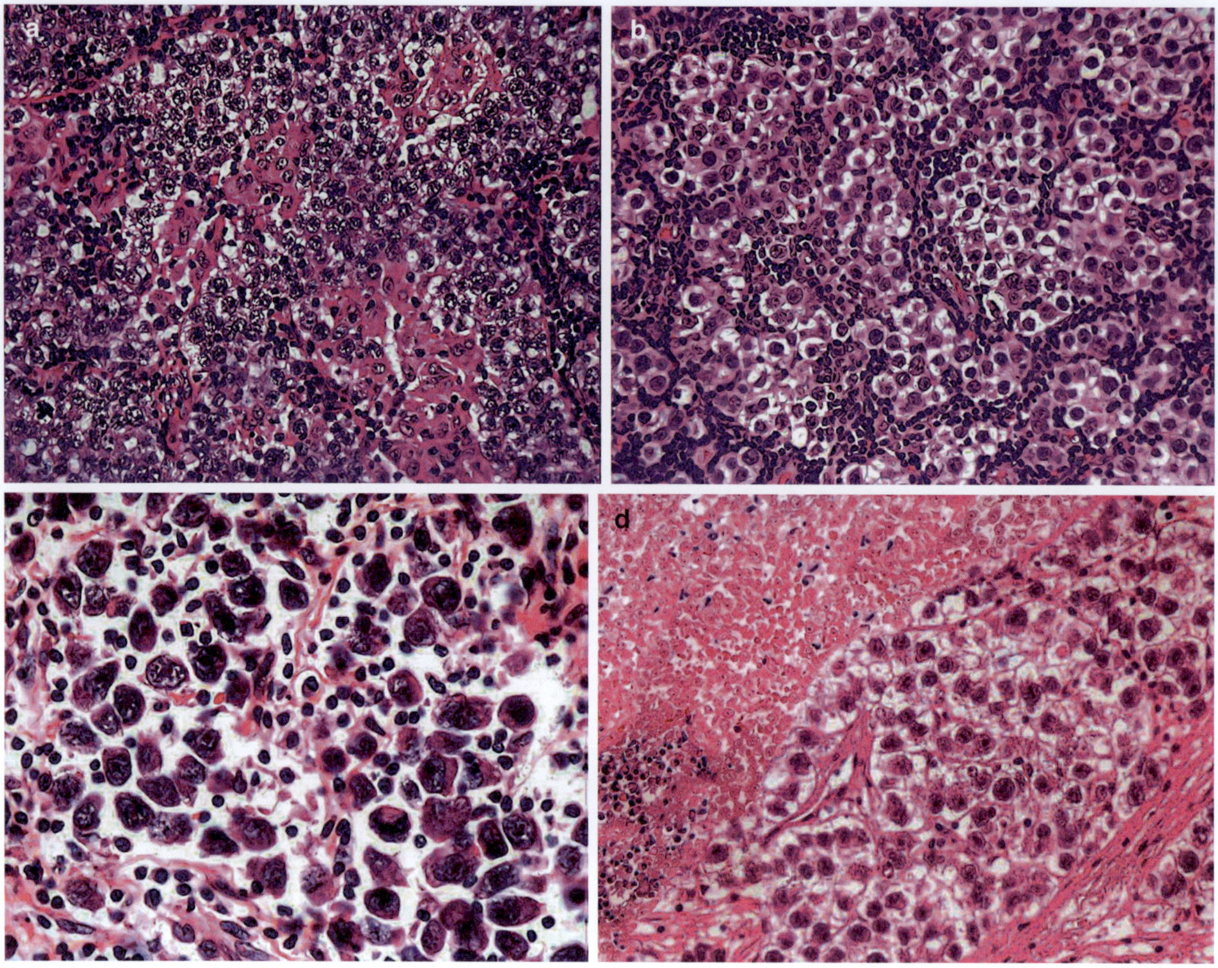

Sections show sheets of solid, lobulated masses of uniform, large, round, or polygonal cells, with well-defined cell borders, that are separated by a fibrous stroma infiltrated with lymphocytic infiltrates with areas of granulomatous formations. The cells have a clear or pale cytoplasm, and their nuclei are centrally located and often contain one or more prominent nucleoli. Areas of coagulative necrosis are observed.

Ancillary Tools

IHC [1]:

OCT 3/4, CD117, D2–40, PLAP, SALL4, SOX17

Molecular/cytogenetics description [2]:

Isochromosome from the short arm of chromosome 12, i(12p) present

KIT mutations

Pearls

The criteria adopted to define anaplasia are unclear and poorly reproducible. The anaplastic variant has been removed from the WHO 2016 edition, and the use of such a definition is no longer recommended [3].

Postpubertal Testicular Teratoma

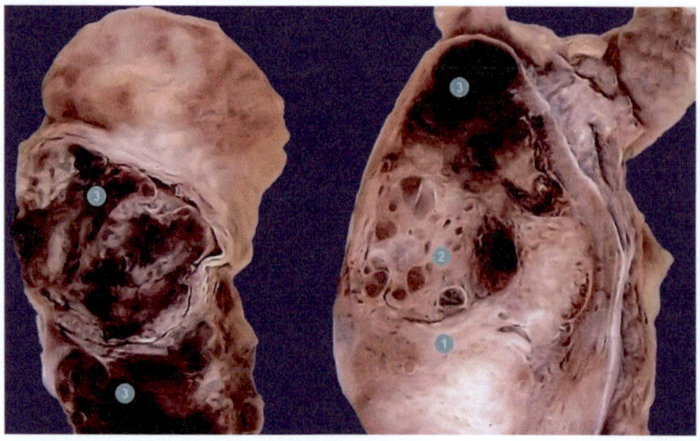

The orchiectomy specimen is mounted.

1. Testicular tissue is replaced by tumor tissue.
2. The tumor is multinodular and heterogenous with solid and cystic areas.
3. Areas of hemorrhage and necrosis.

Microscopic Picture of Testicular Teratoma (a–h)

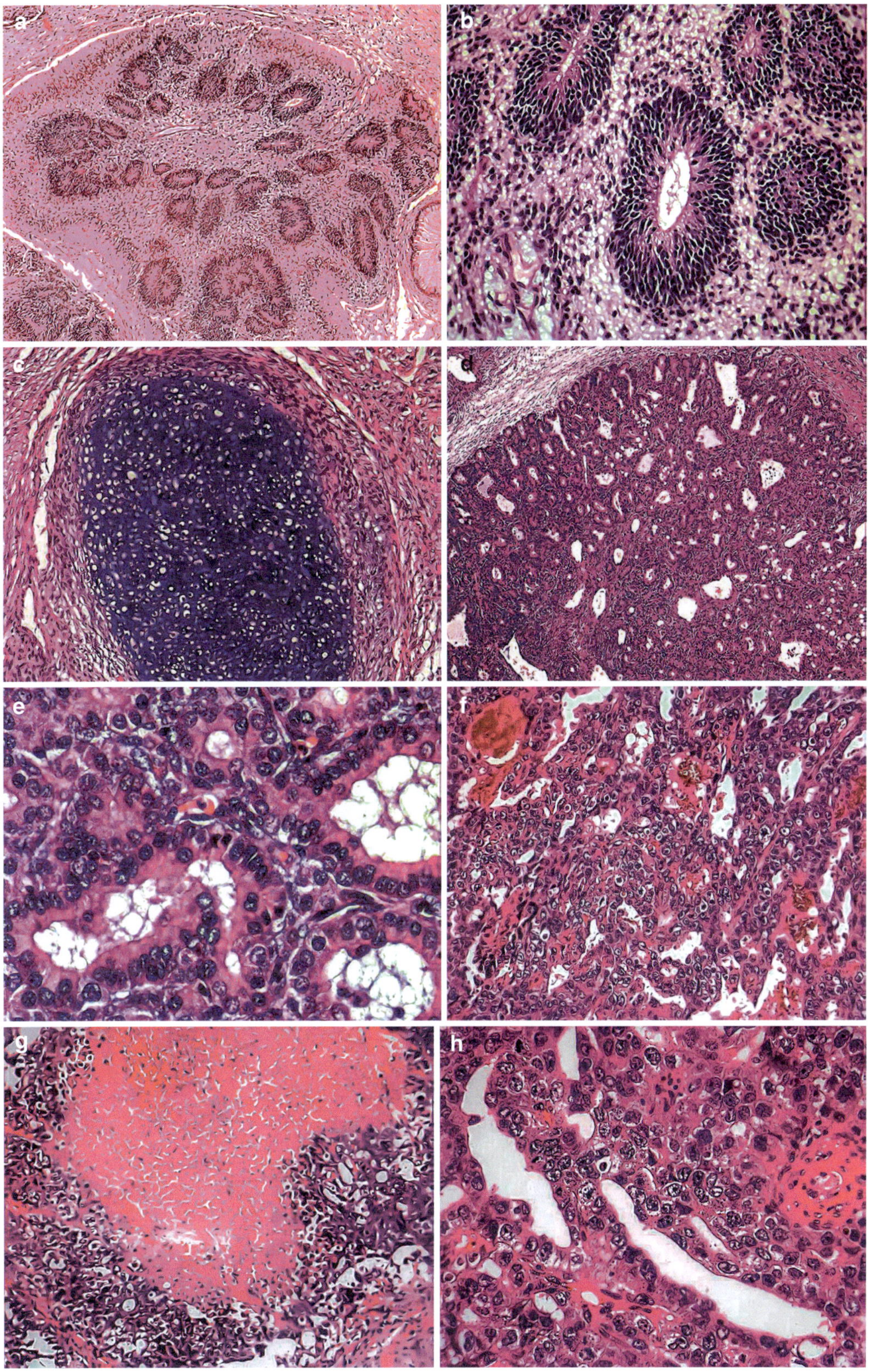

Sections show a mixed germ cell tumor. The tumor is formed mostly of immature neuroepithelium, cartilage, and glands. An area of embryonal carcinoma is observed formed of solid sheets of crowded, polygonal, and pleomorphic cells with indistinct cell borders with extensive necrosis.

Ancillary Tools

Molecular/cytogenetics description:

12p amplification present in postpubertal teratomas and teratomas with somatic type malignancy [4].

7.4 Diseases of Prostate

Nodular Hyperplasia of the Prostate

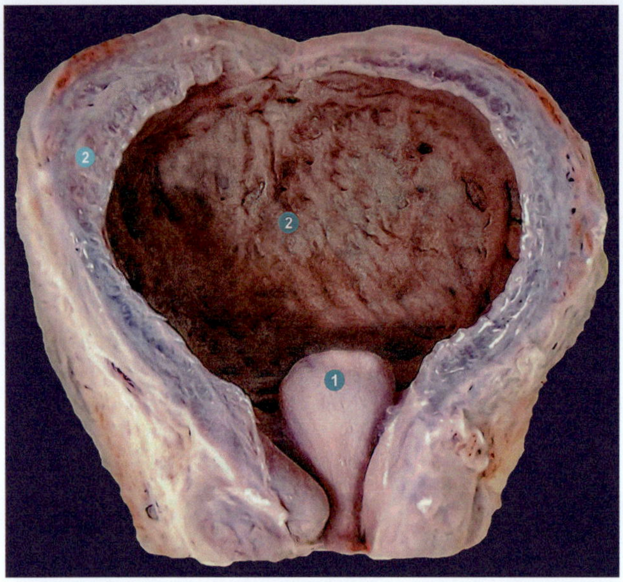

Urinary bladder and prostate are mounted.

1. The middle lobe of the prostate is enlarged and projected upwards into the lumen of the urinary bladder.
2. The urinary bladder has thickened walls and dark brown thickened mucosa with marked trabeculation.

Nodular Hyperplasia of the Prostate

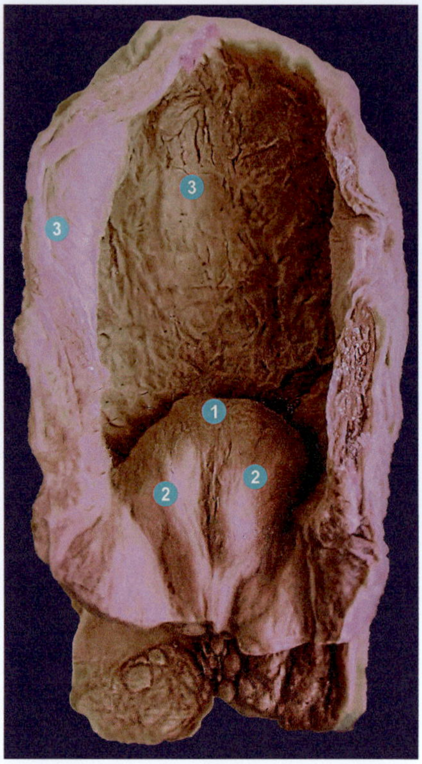

Urinary bladder and prostate are mounted.

1. The middle lobe of the prostate is enlarged and projected upwards into the lumen of the urinary bladder.
2. The two lateral lobes are enlarged and show multiple nodules separated by fibrous tissue.
3. The urinary bladder has thickened walls and dark brown mucosa.

Nodular Hyperplasia of the Prostate, Diverticulosis of the Urinary Bladder, and Multiple Stones

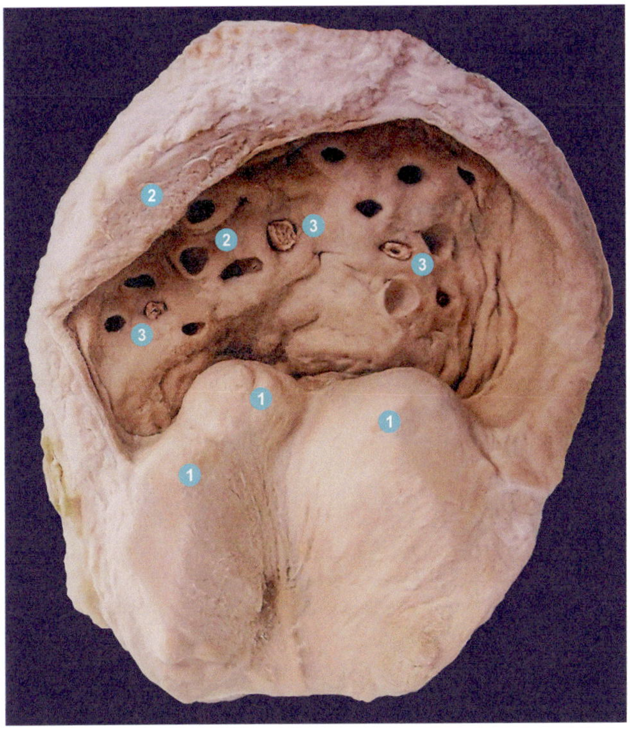

Urinary bladder and prostate are mounted.

1. The middle and lateral lobes of the prostate are nodular, enlarged, and projected upwards into the lumen of the urinary bladder.
2. The urinary bladder has thickened walls, dark brown mucosa, and diverticulae.
3. Some diverticulae contain small yellow stones formed because of urinary stasis and secondary bacterial infection.

Nodular Hyperplasia of the Prostate

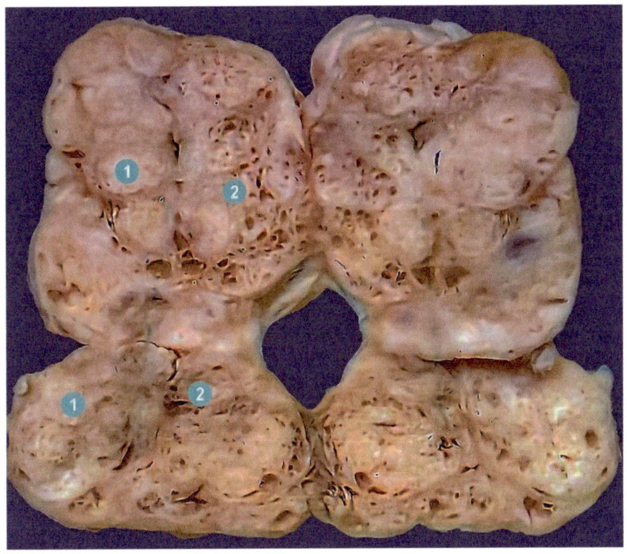

The prostate sectioned longitudinally is mounted.

1. The cut section is multinodular with nodules separated by fibrous septa.
2. Each nodule is formed of prostatic acini embedded in a fibrous stroma.

Microscopic Picture of Nodular Hyperplasia of Prostate (a–c)

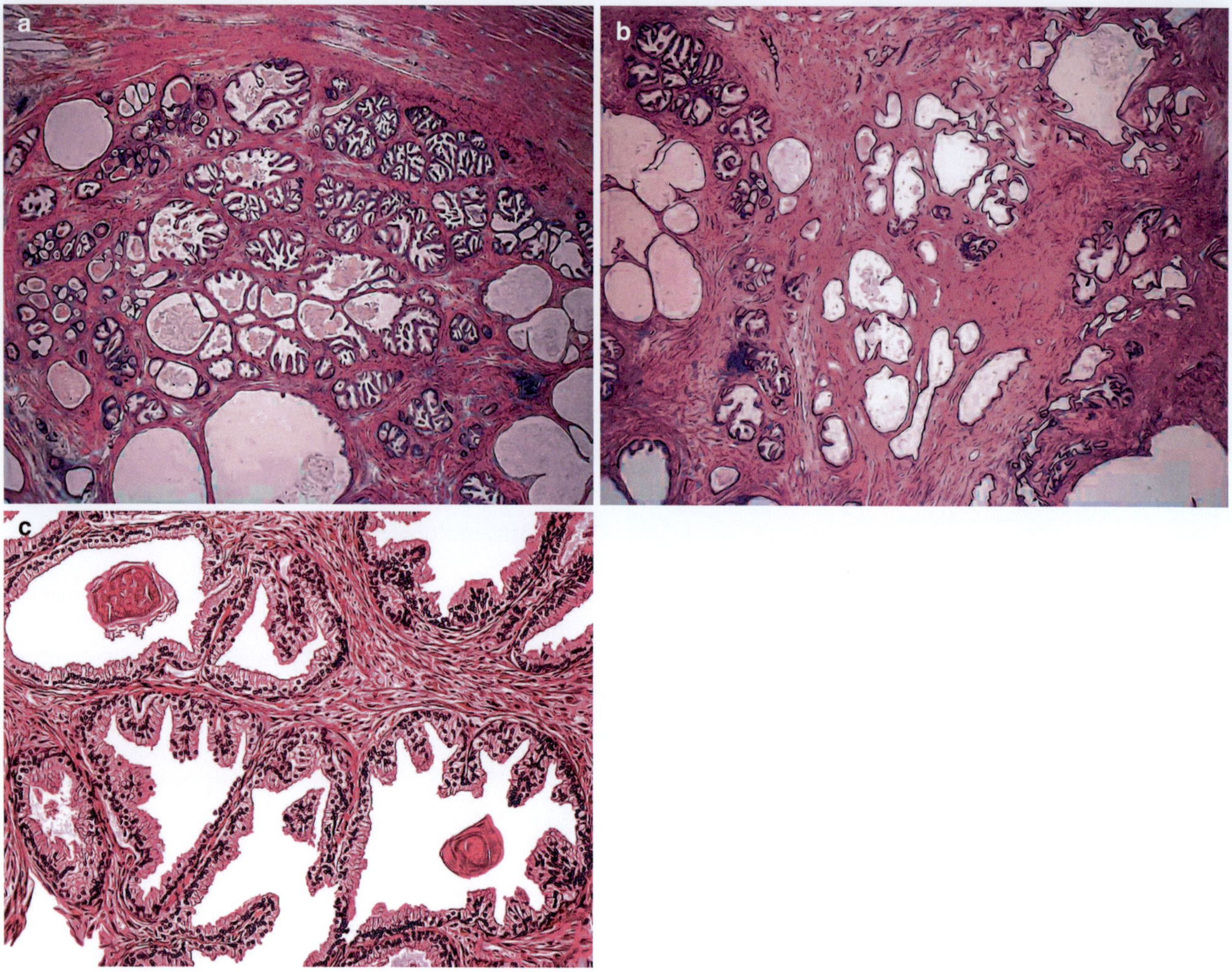

Sections show an increase in the number of both glandular and stromal cells, leading to the formation of multiple nodules that vary greatly in size. The glandular acini appear compressed or cystically dilated and contain luminal corpora amylecia, with a varying degree of hyperplasia and infoldings of the epithelial lining. The stromal component is a mix of muscle and fibrous tissue and is infiltrated by variable chronic inflammatory cellular infiltrate.

Microscopic Picture of Basal Cell Hyperplasia (d–h)

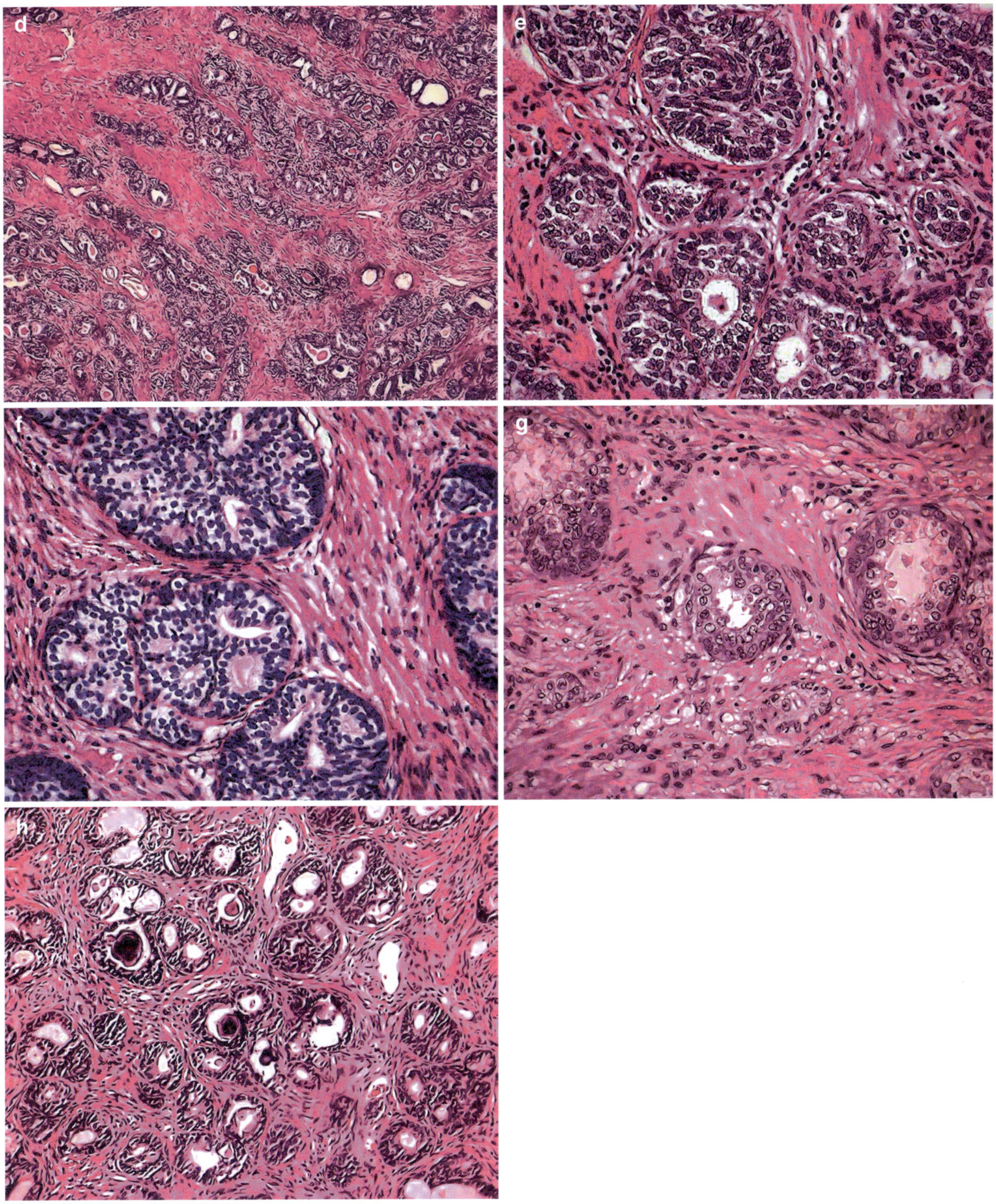

Sections show basophilic nodular solid nests and back-to-back proliferating, uniform, and small glands arranged in a pseudo-cribriform pattern (which differs from the true cribriform pattern in which there is a solid nest of cells with punched-out lumina) lined with a benign-appearing round to elongated to polygonal acinar epithelial cells having clear to eosinophilic scant cytoplasm with stratified crowded nuclei. Some BCH may show prominent nucleoli. Some glandular lumina contain psammomatous calcifications. The surrounding stroma is unremarkable.

Ancillary Tools

IHC [5]:

Immunostains are typically not needed.

Basal cells

- High molecular weight cytokeratin (e.g., 34 beta E12, CK5/6, CK14)
- p63

Secretory (luminal) cells

- PSA, PSAP, NKX3.1

Stromal cells

- CD34, smooth muscle actin (SMA)
- Desmin variable

Pearls

The incidence of basal cell hyperplasia in the setting of usual nodular hyperplasia has been reported to range from 3.1 to 8.9%. Basal cell hyperplasia is not exclusively a transition zone process associated with nodular hyperplasia (benign prostatic hyperplasia) but rather may also be identified in tissue samples from the peripheral zone of the prostate, including 10% of needle core biopsy samples from the peripheral zone. This finding has diagnostic implications because basal cell hyperplasia, particularly basal cell hyperplasia with prominent nucleoli or atypical basal cell hyperplasia, may be misdiagnosed under the light microscope as high-grade prostatic intraepithelial neoplasia or adenocarcinoma [6].

Prostatic Carcinoma

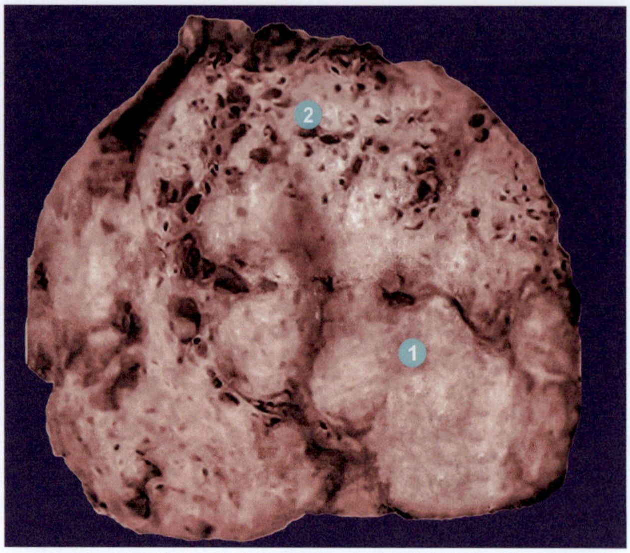

A transverse section of prostatectomy is mounted.

1. An ill-defined, irregular, pale, and variegated mass
2. Areas of benign prostatic hyperplasia are present at the periphery of the main tumor mass.

Microscopic Picture of Prostatic Acinar Adenocarcinoma (a–p)

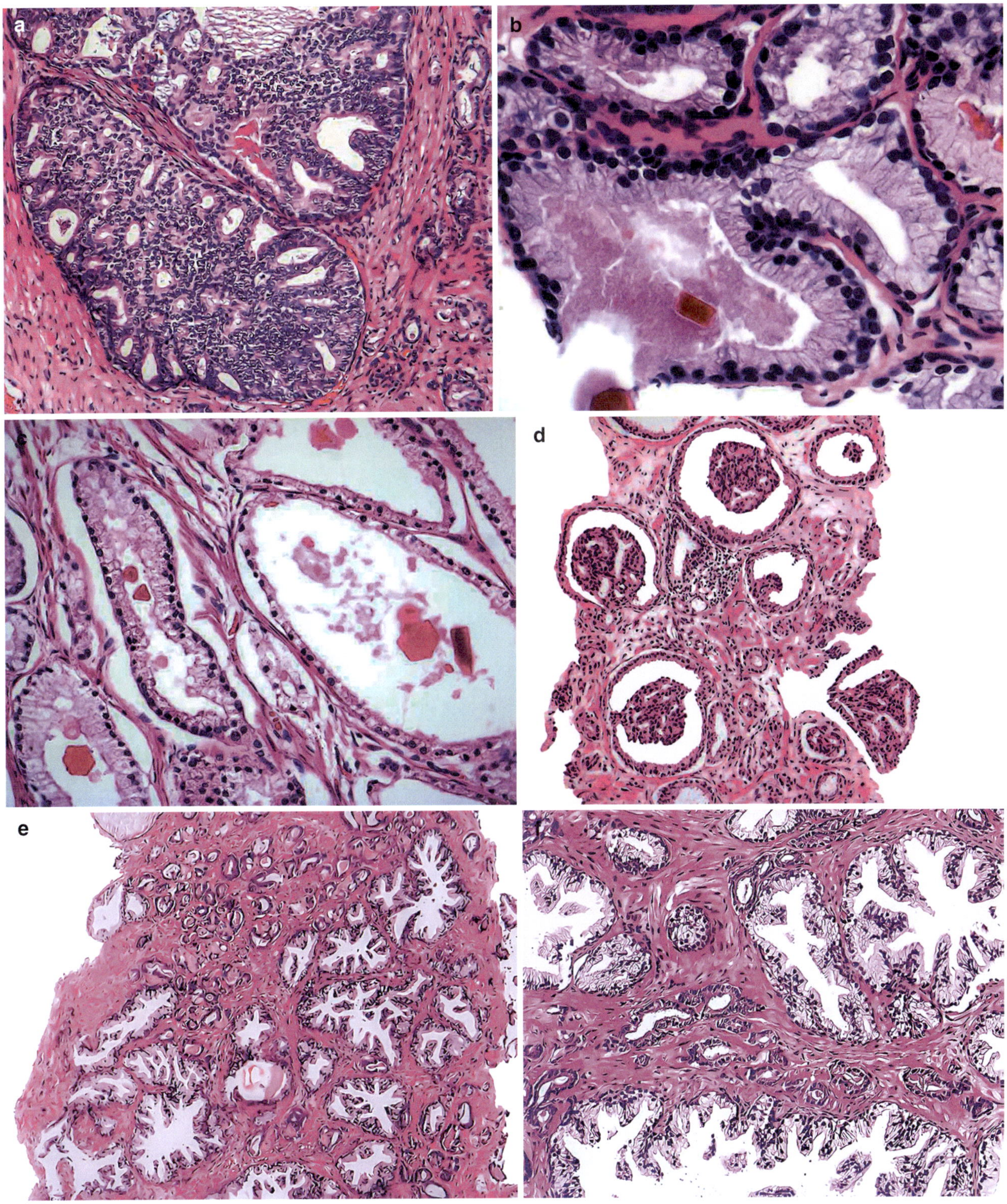

Sections show an abnormal architectural glandular pattern with effacement of normal prostatic microanatomy. The malignant glands are single, separate, or well-formed. They may be crowded and nodular, or maybe haphazardly arranged and infiltrative into the stroma. The malignant acini show absent basal cells with the presence of nuclear atypia, in the form of nuclear and nucleolar enlargement and increased mitoses, especially in high-grade Gleason pattern 5, and amphophilic cytoplasm. Their lumina may contain wispy blue mucin, pink amorphous secretions, or brightly eosinophilic crystalloids (b and c). The luminal border of gland-forming cells, although often flat, can be ruffled with bleb or snout formation. The stroma is desmoplastic. Perineural invasion is a hallmark of prostatic carcinoma.

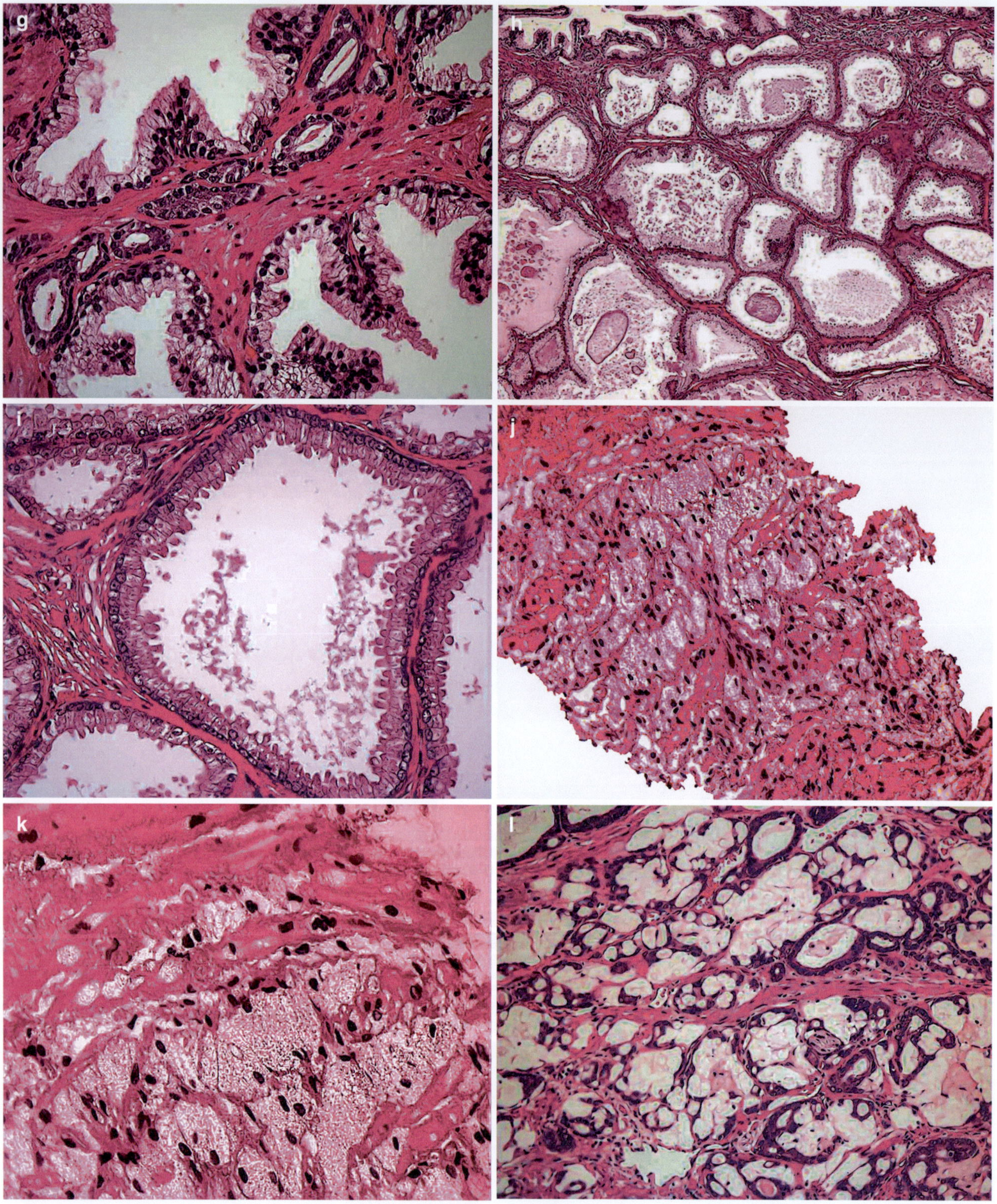

Other patterns of prostatic acinar adenocarcinoma, shown here, include:

- **(d) Glomeruloid structures, or glomerulations**, are renal glomerulus-like epithelial aggregates within the acini of prostatic adenocarcinoma. This pattern of intraluminal epithelial growth is thought to be specific for carcinoma. It is characterized by rounded to ball-like tufts or buds into small to medium-sized malignant glands. The glomeruloid bodies typically comprise only a minority of the carcinoma. They represent a high-grade Gleason pattern 4.
- **(e–g) Pseudohyperplastic** can simulate the appearance of usual epithelial hyperplasia with papillary infoldings, luminal undulations, branching, and cystic dilatation, and no basal cells are found in the glands of concern.

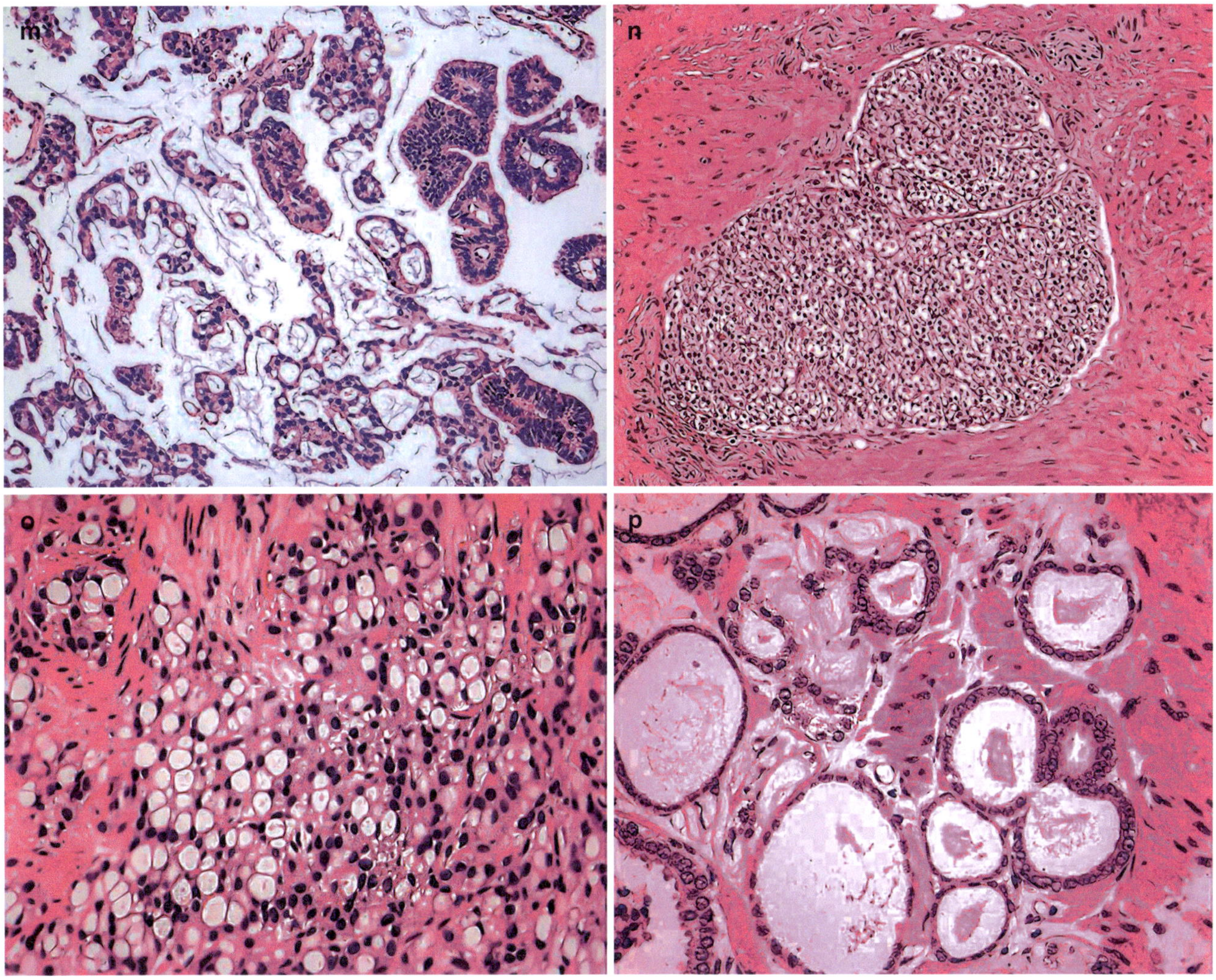

- **(h, i) Microcystic**: the expansion of the luminal spaces generates a rounded profile, and the luminal cell-lining layer is flat with or without atrophic changes. Intraluminal crystalloids and blue mucin are uniformly present.
- **(j, k) Foamy glands**: characterized by abundant foamy or xanthomatous-type cytoplasm with pyknotic nuclei. It is usually observed admixed with the usual acinar adenocarcinoma.
- **(l, m) Mucinous (colloid)**: at least 25% of the tumor comprised of tumor cells "floating" or embedded within prominent pools of mucin
- **(n, o) Signet ring-like cell**: rare and is microscopically characterized by carcinoma cells with nuclear displacement and indentation by clear cytoplasmic vacuoles.
- **(p) Adenocarcinoma with atrophic features**: characterized by round acini, often dilated and distorted, and lined by flattened attenuated epithelium with scant cytoplasm and infiltrative growth pattern. Nuclear enlargement and prominent nucleoli are present.

Ancillary Tools

IHC [7]:

CK7, CK20, high molecular weight cytokeratins (34 beta E12, CK5, CK5/6)

p63

CDX2

GATA3

TTF1

Molecular/cytogenetics description [8]:

Prostate cancer is a heritable disease.

Family history of a first-degree relative with prostate cancer increases the risk of developing prostate cancer by two-fold.

30–40% of familial risk is due to genetic factors.

Highly penetrant variants occur in BRCA2 and HOXB13.

Over 280 SNPs have been identified as prostate cancer risk factors.

Somatic mutations occur in genes such as ERG, ETV1/4, FLI1, SPOP, FOXA1, IDH1, PTEN, TP53, MYC, and CDH1.

The most common somatic genomic rearrangement is the fusion of the androgen-regulated gene TMPRSS2 with a member of the ETS transcription family.

Somatic mutation profiles of prostate cancer are associated with clinical and pathological outcomes.

There are 7 major subtypes, which are defined by either specific gene fusions of ETS transcription family members (ERG, ETV1, ETV4, and FLI1) or mutations (SPOP, FOXA1, IDH1).

Pearls

In the Gleason system, the histologic patterns are categorized into five basic grade patterns at relatively low magnification (using a 4× or 10× objective) by the extent of glandular differentiation and the pattern of growth of the tumor in the prostatic stroma. These five basic grade patterns are used to generate a histologic score, which can range from 2 to 10, by adding the primary grade patterns and the secondary grade pattern. The primary pattern is the one that is predominant in the area on simple visual inspection. The secondary pattern is the second most common pattern. If only one grade is in the tissue sample, then that grade is multiplied by two to give the score. The number of grades assigned depends on the tumor sample size and the size of the tumor in the whole gland [7].

Some prostate cancers are comprised of more than two grades. While the majority of so-called "tertiary" grading reported in the literature refers to a higher grade—typically pattern 5—the term has been used variably regarding the extent, ranging from a more limited, minor, or <5% higher grade carcinoma component in initial publications (3, 4) to a third most common pattern of any percentage. The accepted method for reporting "tertiary" patterns also differs between needle biopsy and radical prostatectomy (RP). For RP specimens bearing three grading patterns, since the pathologist may assess the entire tumor, the "tertiary" terminology has been recommended. The latter recommendation is based on an array of studies showing that cancers with a tertiary higher-grade pattern (TP) are associated with increased stage and/or biochemical recurrence following RP [9].

Penile Carcinoma

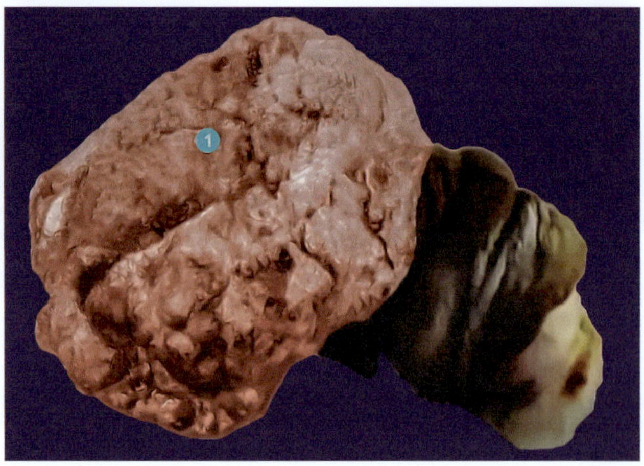

A penectomy specimen is mounted.

1. Broad-based white to gray exophytic neoplasm with a verruciform pattern of growth destroying the penile structures.

Microscopic Picture of Penile HPV-Independent Well-Differentiated Squamous Cell Carcinoma—Usual Type (a, b)

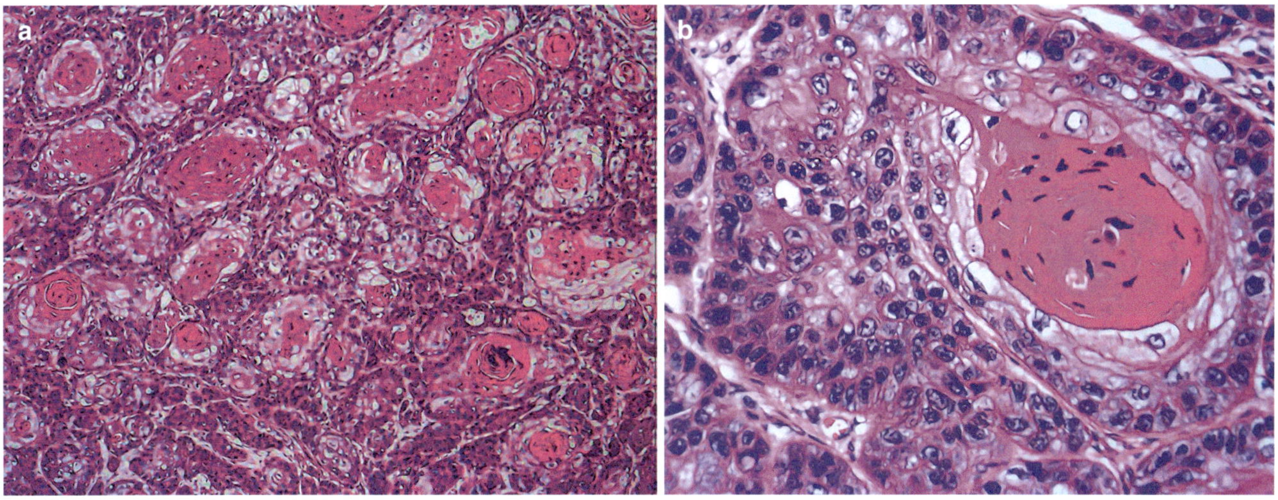

Sections show multiple nests formed of malignant squamous cells with central keratinization. The stroma is fibrous and infiltrated with chronic inflammatory cells.

Ancillary Tools

IHC:

EGFR [10]

Molecular/cytogenetics description [11]:

Mutations in PIK3CA, HRAS, or KRAS genes

Epigenetic silencing (by methylation) of the FHIT gene

References

1. Ulbright TM. et al. (2014). Best practices recommendations in the application of immunohistochemistry in testicular tumors: report from the International Society of Urological Pathology consensus conference. Am J Surg Pathol.38(8):e50-9. doi: https://doi.org/10.1097/PAS.0000000000000233. PMID: 24832161.
2. McIntyre A. et al. (2005). Amplification and overexpression of the KIT gene is associated with progression in the seminoma subtype of testicular germ cell tumors of adolescents and adults. Cancer Res. 65(18):8085-9. doi: https://doi.org/10.1158/0008-5472.CAN-05-0471. PMID: 16166280.
3. Ronchi A. et al. (2019). Testicular germ cell tumors: the changing role of the pathologist. Ann. Transl. Med.7(Suppl 6): S204. doi: https://doi.org/10.21037/atm.2019.07.01. PMCID: PMC6789349.
4. Ye H, Ulbright TM. (2012). Difficult differential diagnoses in testicular pathology. Arch Pathol Lab Med.136(4):435-46. doi: https://doi.org/10.5858/arpa.2011-0475-RA. PMID: 22458906.
5. McNeal JE. (1988). Normal histology of the prostate. Am J Surg Pathol.12(8):619-33. doi: https://doi.org/10.1097/00000478-198808000-00003. PMID: 2456702.
6. Thorson P. et al. (2003). Basal Cell Hyperplasia in the Peripheral Zone of the Prostate. Mod Pathol 16, 598–606. https://doi.org/10.1097/01.MP.0000073526.59270.6E.
7. Humphrey PA. (2017). Histopathology of Prostate Cancer. Cold Spring Harb Perspect Med. 7(10):a030411. doi: https://doi.org/10.1101/cshperspect.a030411. PMID: 28389514; PMCID: PMC5629988.
8. Faisal FA, Lotan TL. The Genomic and Molecular Pathology of Prostate Cancer: Clinical Implications for Diagnosis, Prognosis, and Therapy. Adv Anat Pathol. 27(1):11-19. doi: https://doi.org/10.1097/PAP.0000000000000245. PMID: 31503032.
9. Fine SW. et al. (2020). Practice Patterns in Reporting Tertiary Grades at Radical Prostatectomy: Survey of a Large Group of Experienced Urologic Pathologists. Arch Pathol Lab Med. 144(3):356-360. doi: https://doi.org/10.5858/arpa.2019-0224-OA. PMID: 31584841; PMCID: PMC7480272.
10. Lavens N, Gupta R, Wood LA. (2010). EGFR overexpression in squamous cell carcinoma of the penis. Curr Oncol.17(1):4-6. doi: https://doi.org/10.3747/co.v17i1.471. PMID: 20179797; PMCID: PMC2826775.
11. Yanagawa N. et al. (2008). Frequent epigenetic silencing of the FHIT gene in penile squamous cell carcinomas. Virchows Arch. 452(4):377-82. doi: https://doi.org/10.1007/s00428-008-0597-6. PMID: 18299890.

8 Diseases of the Female Reproductive Tract

The female genital system is susceptible to various pathological conditions due to a variety of factors.

Gross and histopathology play a critical role in understanding, diagnosing, and treating these conditions by providing insights into the structural changes brought about by these diseases and establishing a foundation for understanding the potential mechanisms and pathways of disease progression.

This chapter aims to provide a comprehensive overview of the gross and microscopic pathological changes that occur in various diseases of the female genital system, focusing on each organ or part of the female genital system and providing detailed descriptions of common pathological conditions and their clinical implications.

By the end of this chapter, readers should have a solid understanding of the pathological aspects of the female genital system, which should facilitate a more comprehensive approach to diagnosing and managing diseases of the female reproductive tract.

This chapter will be organized in the following order:

1. **Vulva**
   (a) **Inflammatory Lesions**
   - Elephantiasis (Filariasis) of the Vulva

   (b) **Neoplastic Lesions**
   - Bartholin's Gland Carcinoma
   - Ulcerative carcinoma of vulva
2. **Cervix**
   (a) **Neoplastic Lesions**
   - **Cervical Carcinoma**
3. **Uterus**
   (a) **Congenital Lesions**
   - Bicornuate uterus

   (b) **Inflammatory Lesions**
   - Puerperal sepsis

   (c) **Adenomyosis**
   (d) **Tumor-Like Lesions**
   - Endometrial polyp

   (e) **Endometrial Epithelial Tumors and Precursors**
   - Endometrial hyperplasia without atypia
   - Atypical hyperplasia of the endometrium
   - Endometrioid Adenocarcinoma NOS

   (f) **Mesenchymal Tumors Specific to the Uterus**
   - Leiomyoma
   - Leiomyosarcoma
   - Endometrial stroma sarcoma
4. **Fallopian Tubes**
   (a) Hydrosalpinx
   (b) Tuberculous salpingitis
5. **Ovary**
   (a) **Primary Tumors**
   - **Surface Epithelial Tumors**
     - Serous tumors
       Serous cystadenoma
       Serous cystadenocarcinoma
     - Mucinous tumors
       Mucinous cystadenoma
       Mucinous cystadenocarcinoma
     - Brenner Tumor
     - Clear cell carcinoma
   - **Germ Cell Tumors**
     - Teratoma
     - Yolk sac (endodermal sinus) tumor
     - Dysgerminoma
   - **Sex Cord-Stromal Tumors**
     - Fibroma
     - Granulosa cell tumor
     - Granulosa-theca cell tumor

   (b) **Metastatic Tumors**
   - Krukenberg tumor

G. Dawood, *Color Atlas of Human Gross and Microscopic Pathology*, https://doi.org/10.1007/978-3-031-76007-5_8

6. **Disorders of Pregnancy**
   (a) **Ectopic Tubal Pregnancy**
   (b) **Gestational Trophoblastic Disease**
   - Molar Pregnancy
     - Partial mole
     - Complete mole

   (c) **Gestational Trophoblastic Tumor**
   - Choriocarcinoma NOS

8.1 Vulva

8.1.1 Inflammatory Lesions

Elephantiasis (Filariasis) of Vulva

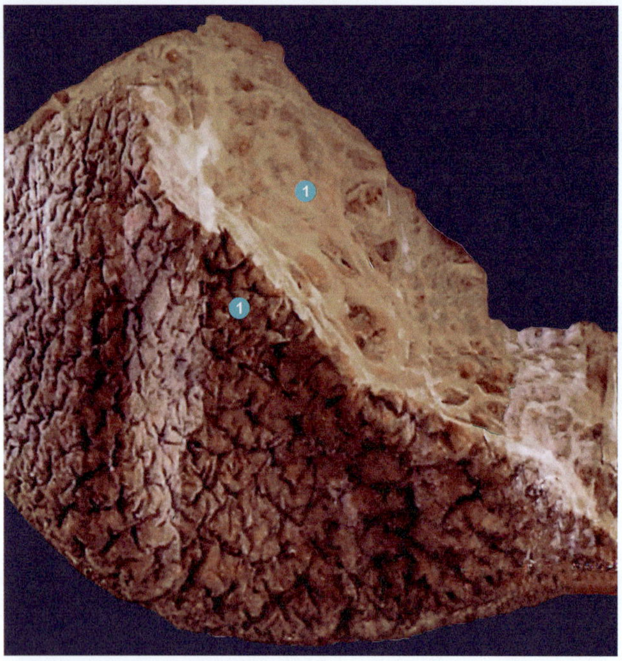

A labium majus is mounted.

1. The skin is rough and nodular, with increased skin markings and subcutaneous tissue.

8.1.2 Neoplastic Lesions

Bartholin's Gland Carcinoma

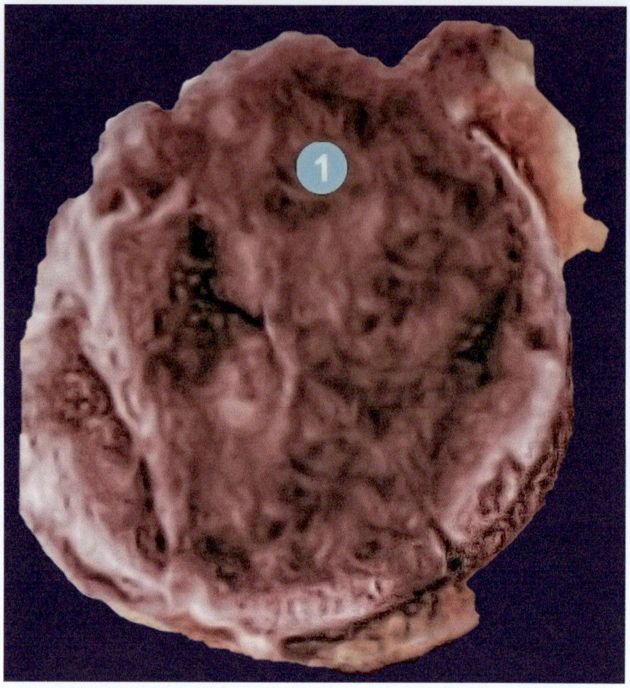

A vulvectomy specimen is mounted.

1. A round, disk-shaped, and exophytic mass is seen on the inner surface of the labia minora with a brown-cut section and areas of necrosis.

Ulcerative Carcinoma of Vulva

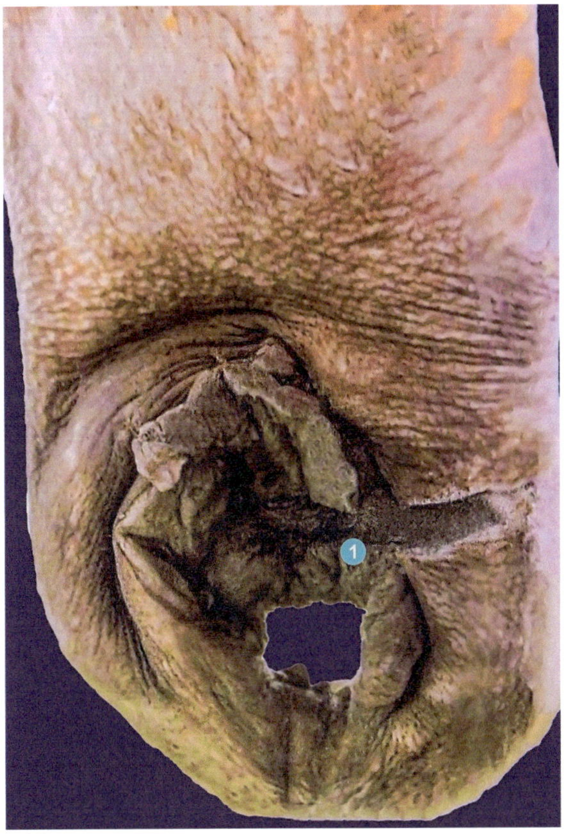

Vulvectomy specimen with the surrounding skin.

1. The anterior half shows a malignant ulcer with a raised everted edge and necrotic floor.

Microscopic Picture of Well-Differentiated Squamous Cell Carcinoma of Vulva (a)

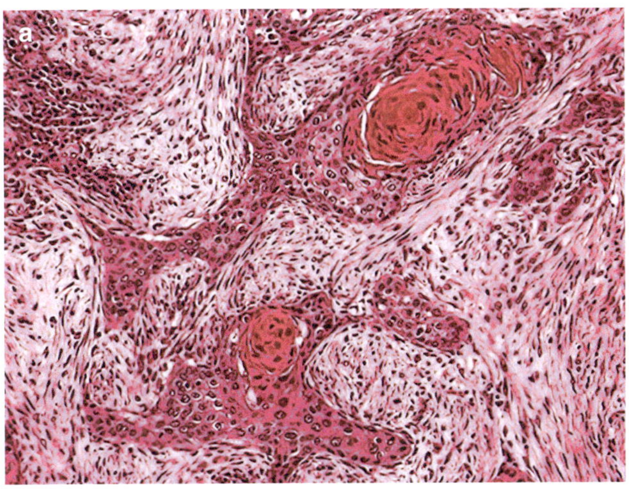

The section shows clusters of malignant squamous cells with eosinophilic cytoplasm and with areas of keratinization and horn pearl formation.

8.2 Cervix

8.2.1 Neoplastic Lesions

Infiltrative Carcinoma of Cervix

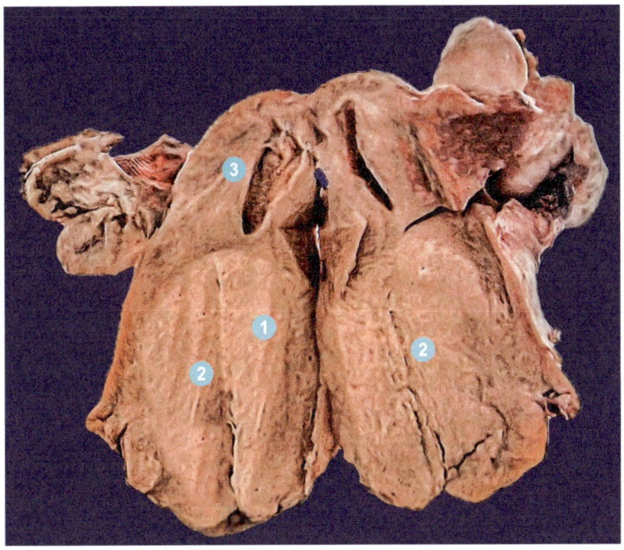

The uterus and cervix are bisected longitudinally.

1. The cervix appears to be infiltrated by a large mass of neoplastic tissue, which infiltrates and destroys the muscle layer.
2. The cervical canal is obstructed by infiltrating growth.
3. The uterine cavity is dilated and lined by a pyogenic membrane (pyometra).

Ulcerative Carcinoma of Cervix

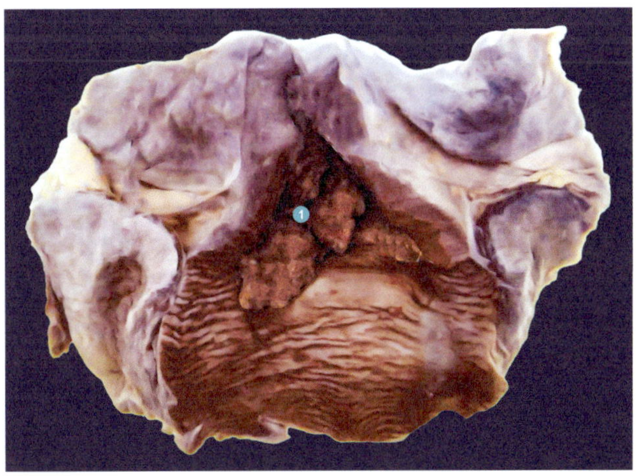

The specimen is formed of a small-sized (senile) uterus and an opened vagina.

1. The cervix is destroyed and replaced by white-brown nodular ulcerated growth infiltrating the upper vagina.

Low-Grade Squamous Intraepithelial Lesion (LGSIL) (CIN I) (a, b)

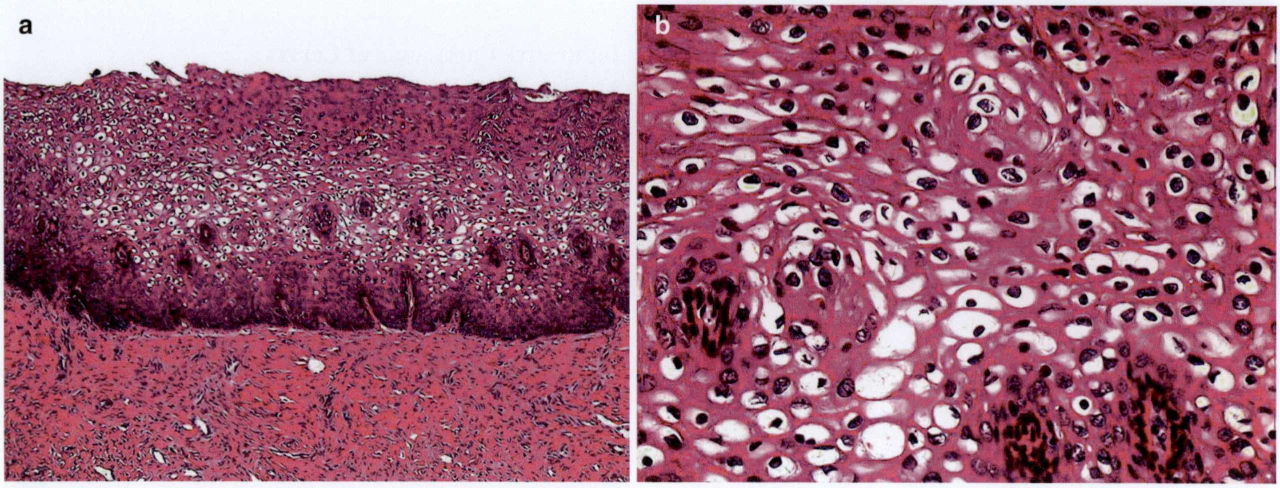

Sections show preserved maturation of squamous epithelium with preserved polarity of basal cell layer and loss of polarity of intermediate and superficial cells. Nuclei in the superficial layer are large, hyperchromatic, and irregular with perinuclear halos (koilocytosis / koilocytotic atypia).

High-Grade Squamous Intraepithelial Lesion (HGSIL) (CIN III) (a–h)

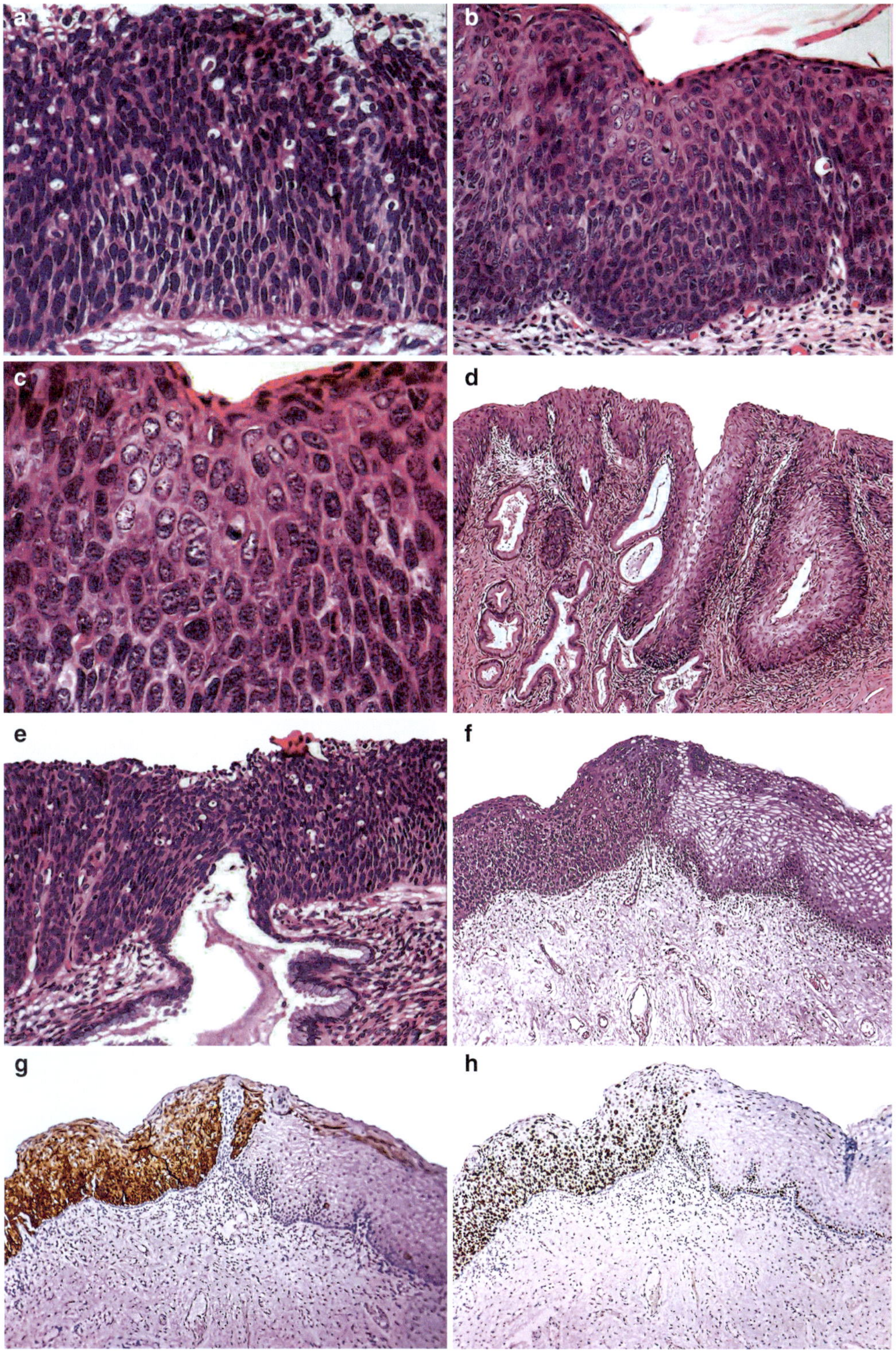

Sections show full-thickness basal/parabasal type with a lack of maturation of cells throughout the epithelial layers and an absence of maturation difference across layers. Cytologically, the cells have hyperchromatic nuclei with coarse chromatin and irregular nuclear contours and inconspicuous nucleoli with a high nuclear-to-cytoplasmic ratio (N/C ratio). There is increased mitotic activity with the presence of abnormal mitoses.

The atypical cells have infiltrated the underlying endocervical glands. These glands have smooth, round borders and lack a desmoplastic stromal reaction. The epithelial cells stained positively with p16 (g) and Ki67 (h).

Microscopic Picture of Keratinizing, Well-Differentiated Squamous Cell Carcinoma of Cervix (a)

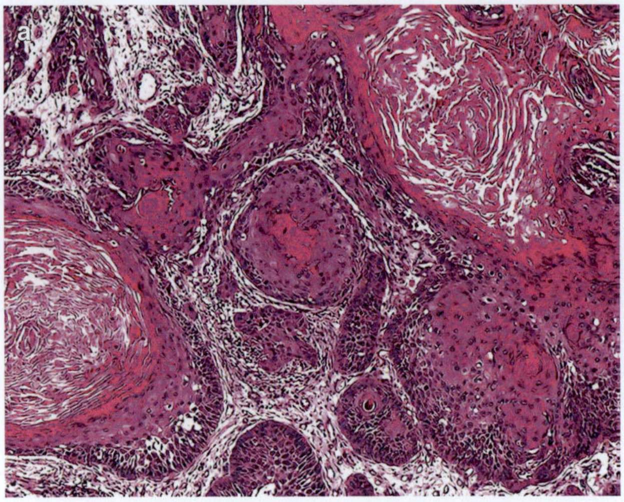

The section shows clusters of malignant squamous cells with eosinophilic cytoplasm and with areas of keratinization and horn pearl formation.

Microscopic Picture of Non-keratinizing, Poorly Differentiated Squamous Cell Carcinoma of Cervix (a, b)

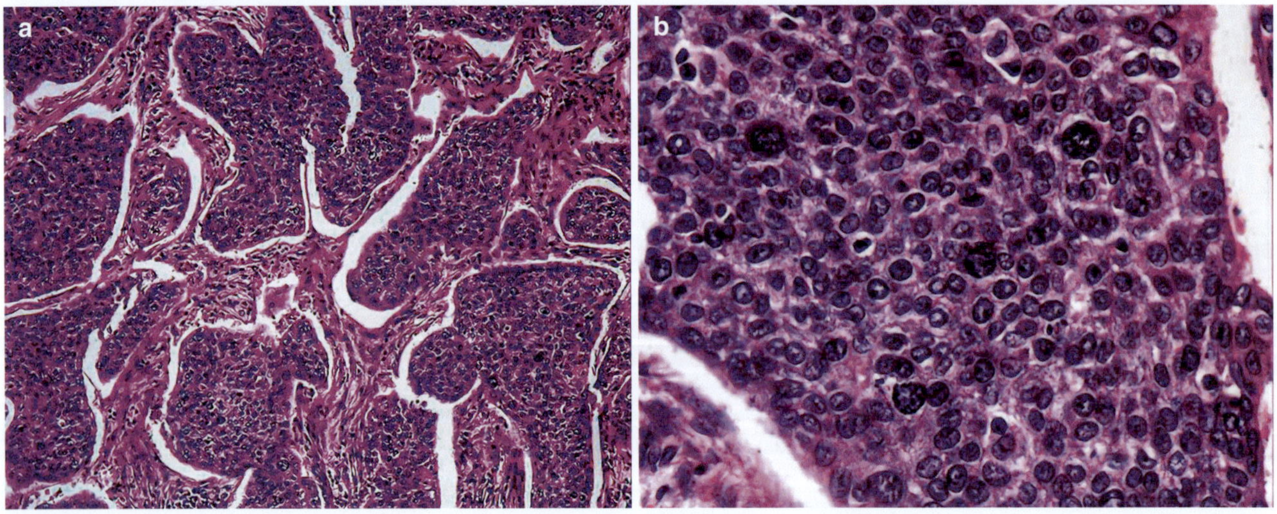

Sections show invasive, irregularly-shaped clusters and sheets of highly malignant tumor cells with an increased number of mitotic figures, many of which are atypical. Tumor cells do not show any evidence of glandular formation or keratin production, as evidenced by the absence of eosinophilic cytoplasmic keratinization.

Microscopic Picture of Basaloid Squamous Cell Carcinoma (a, b)

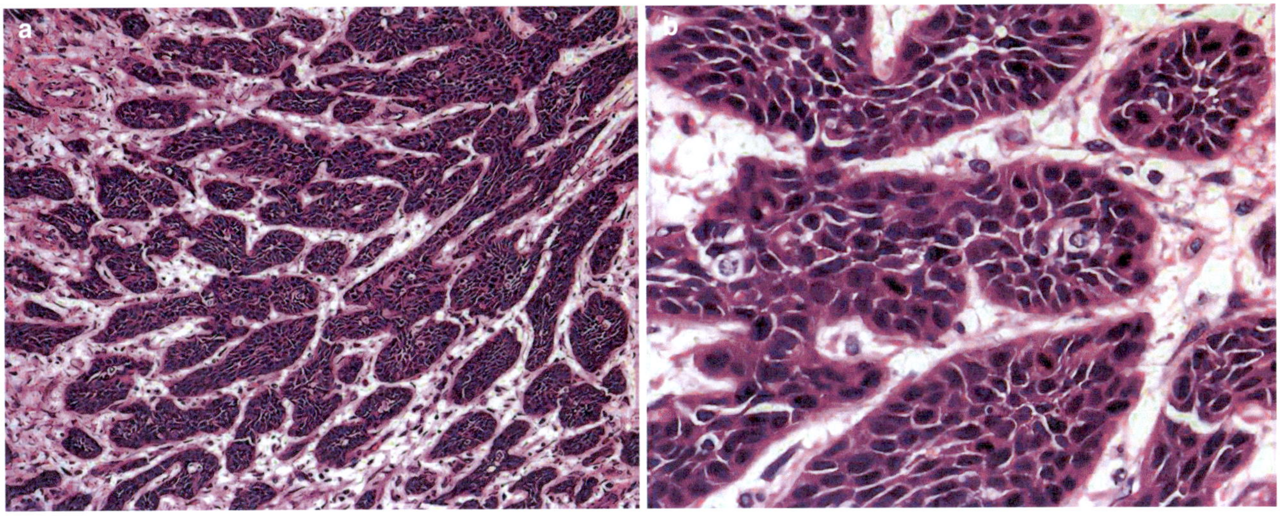

Sections show nests or cords of immature small basaloid squamous cells; prominent peripheral palisading of cells in the tumor cell nests; and the absence of significant stromal reaction. Tumor cells have hyperchromatic nuclei with high nucleus-to-cytoplasm ratios.

Microscopic Picture of Adenoid Basal Carcinoma (a–c)

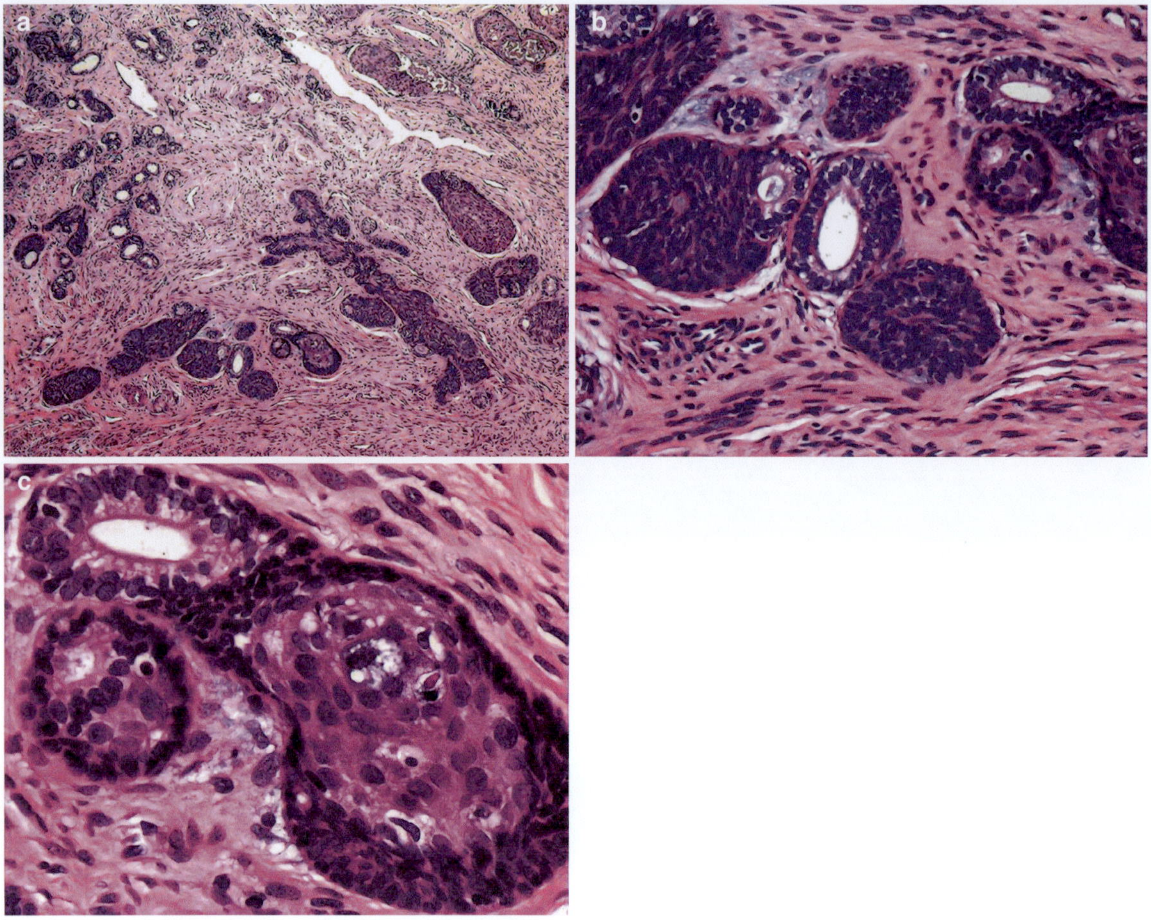

Sections show scattered basaloid cellular proliferations arranged in nests with peripheral palisading and microcyst formation with columnar cell differentiation. Focal areas of the squamous component with basal cells at the periphery and maturation at the center are observed. The tumor cells are uniform, round to oval cells with scant cytoplasm, small hyperchromatic nuclei with inconspicuous nucleoli, and minimal nuclear atypia.

Microscopic Picture of Carcinosarcoma of Cervix (a, b)

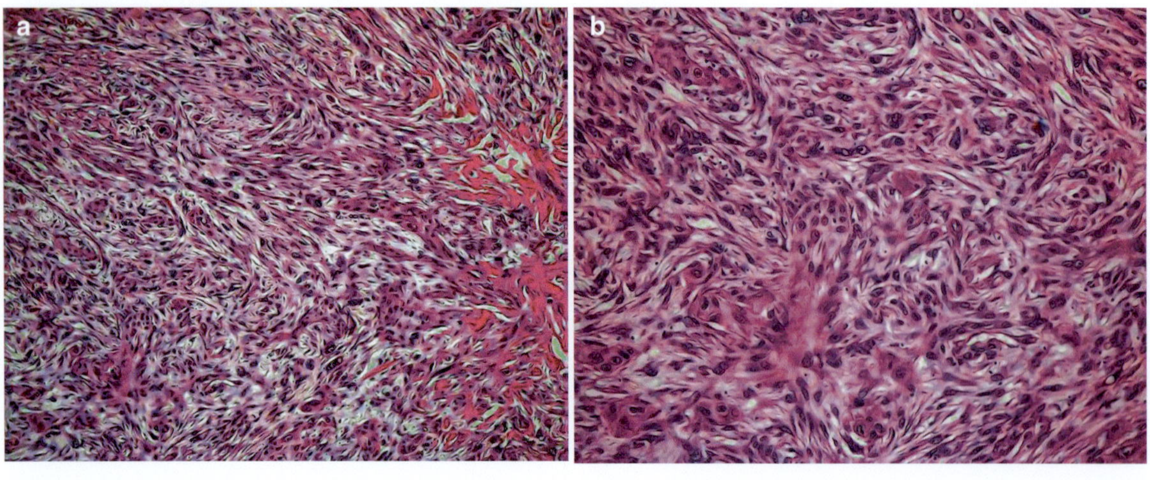

Sections show neoplastic epithelial and mesenchymal components. The invasive epithelial component is the keratinizing squamous cell. Sarcomatous component is homologous, resembling fibrosarcoma.

Microscopic Picture of Adenocarcinoma in Situ (AIS): HPV-Related (a–c)

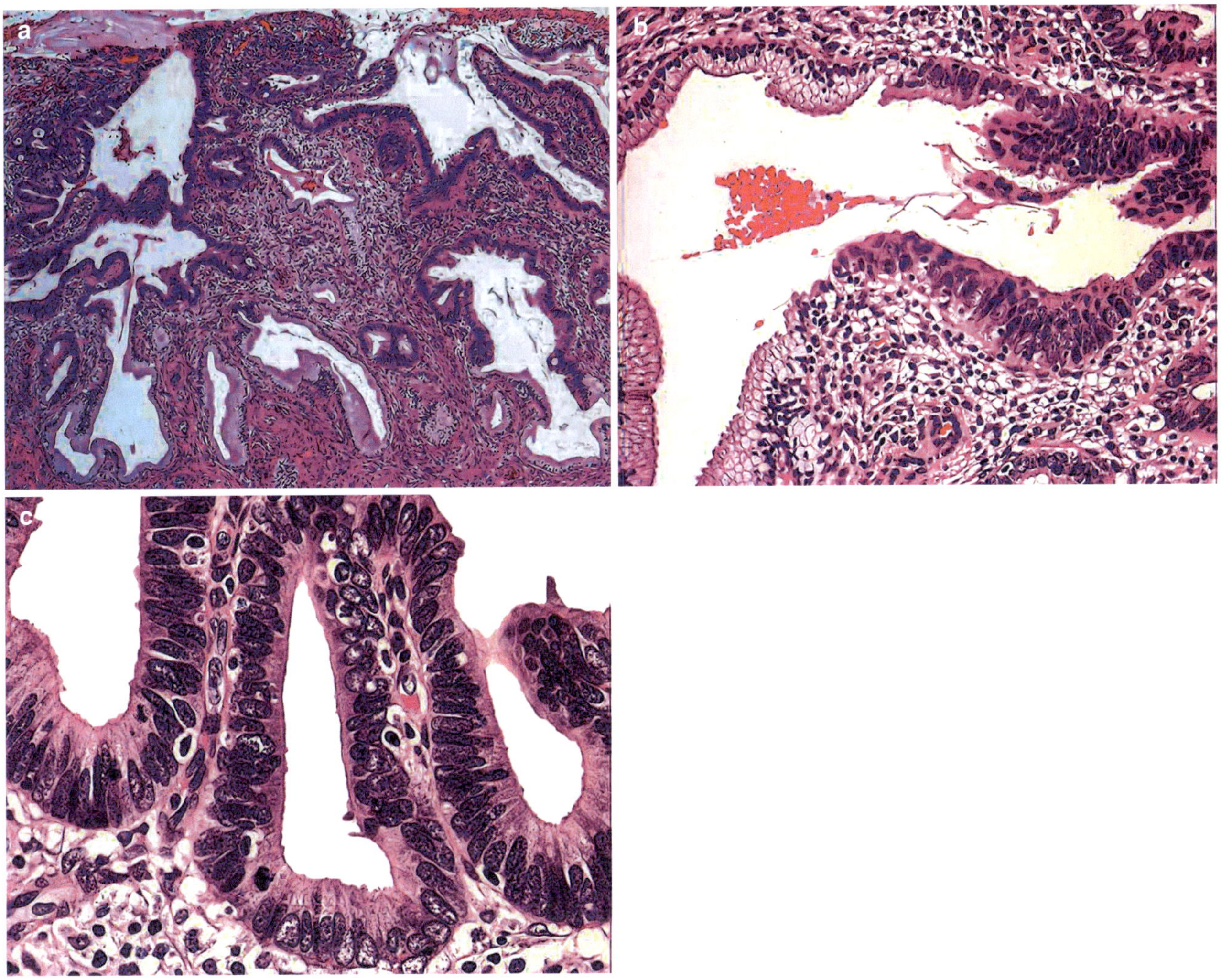

Sections show partial replacement of the normal endocervical epithelium on the surface and within pre-existing glands, but with a largely preserved overall architecture of the endocervix. There is an abrupt transition from normal to dysplastic epithelium, both between glands and even within individual glands (intralesional heterogeneity). Skip lesions, areas of normal epithelium interspersed with dysplastic regions, are also present. The dysplastic cells exhibit pseudostratified, enlarged, fusiform, and hyperchromatic nuclei, prominent nucleoli, and frequent mitotic figures. The cytoplasm varies, ranging from eosinophilic to mucinous. The stroma is mildly infiltrated with chronic inflammatory cells without evidence of significant desmoplasia.

Microscopic Picture of Endocervical Adenocarcinoma, Usual Type (a, b)

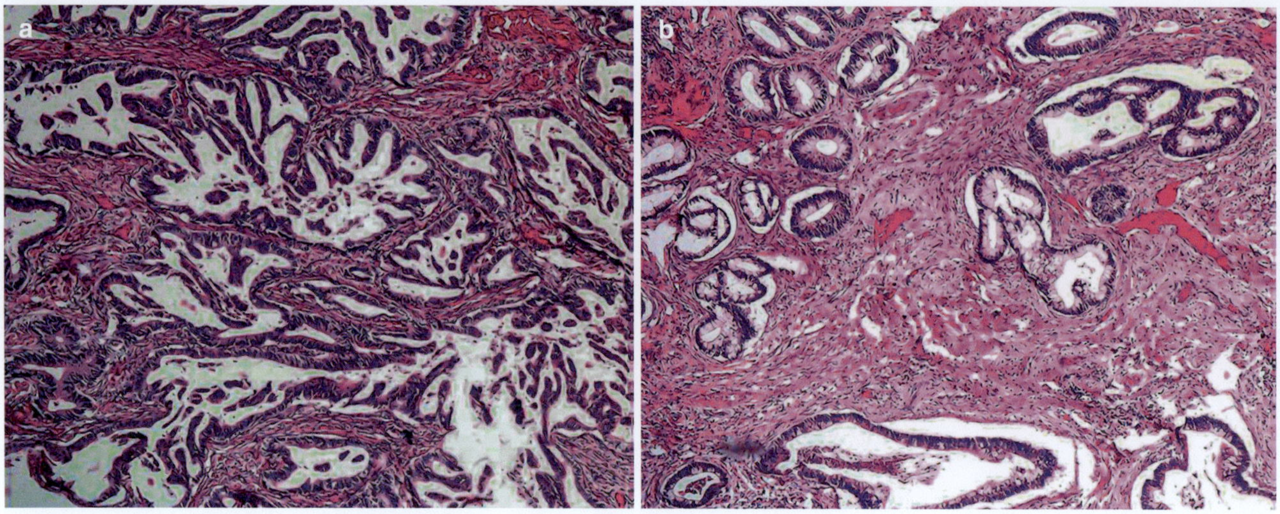

Sections show mucin-depleted epithelium, i.e., mucinous cells comprise <50% of the tumor volume. Most of the population has columnar, non-mucinous, indistinct cytoplasm.

Tumor cells are columnar with elongated, enlarged, and hyperchromatic nuclei with coarse chromatin. This is accompanied by loss of polarity and nuclear overlapping.

Microscopic Picture of Endocervical Adenocarcinoma, Mucinous Type (a)

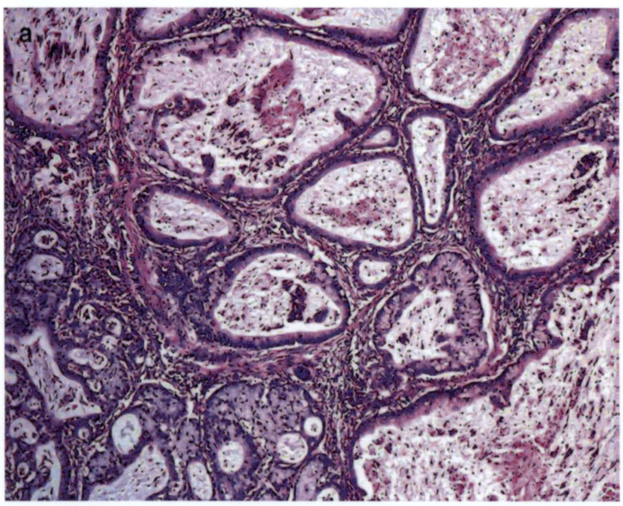

The section shows dense, crowded, dilated, and complex malignant acini, compared to the normal endocervix. The glands are lined with endocervical-type mucinous epithelium, forming 50% or more of the tumor volume (usually represents the majority of the lesion).

Microscopic Picture of Endocervical Adenosquamous Carcinoma (a)

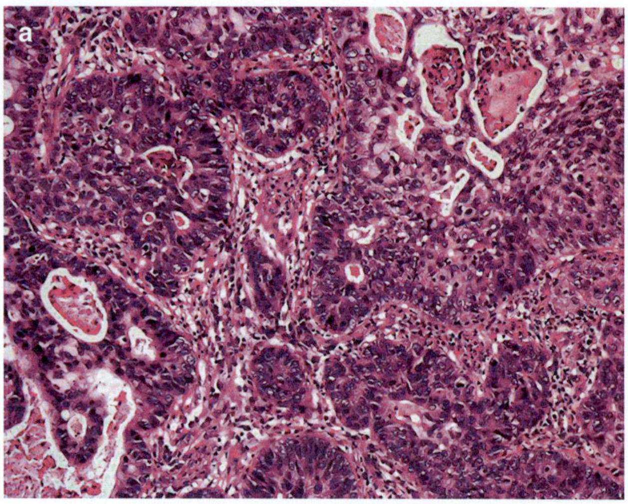

The section shows malignant, moderately to poorly differentiated glandular and squamous components. The glandular component is endocervical and has cytoplasmic vacuoles or luminal mucin.

Ancillary Tools

For HPV-associated cervical squamous cell carcinoma

- IHC [1]:
- Pancytokeratin
- p63
- p40
- CK5/6

EMA

p16 (**g**): diffuse, block-like staining (except verrucous variant)

PDL1: positive in ~80% of cases; reported as combined positive score (CPS) = (number of positive tumor cells, lymphocytes, and macrophages/total number of tumor cells) × 100; the cutoff point for positivity is ≥1%.

CEA

CK7 (in 66–87% of cases)

RNA in situ hybridization for high-risk human papillomavirus

Molecular/cytogenetics description [2]:

Mutations in PIK3CA are most frequent (37%); low frequency of KRAS mutations

TP53 mutations in 16% of cases

Loss of heterozygosity (LOH) in multiple loci (1q, 3p, 3q, 6p, 6q, 11q, 17p, 18q)

For HPV-associated adenocarcinoma (usual type and variants)

IHC [1]:

p16: overexpressed in >95% of cases (diffuse, strong nuclear and cytoplasmic staining)

mCEA: 100% (any degree of staining)

CK7

Molecular/cytogenetics description [2]

Associated with HPV 16 and HPV 18 in 85–95% of cases

Frequent KRAS and PIK3CA mutations, particularly in tumors with destructive stromal invasion

HPV-related adenocarcinomas have lower mutational burdens compared with HPV-independent adenocarcinomas.

Pearls

High-risk HPV acts via E6 and E7 oncogenes. E6 binds to tumor suppressor p53, causing its proteolytic degradation and inactivation, p53-mediated DNA damage, and apoptosis.

E7 binds to the retinoblastoma gene (Rb), displacing transcription factors normally bound by Rb and the inactivating Rb-mediated cell cycle regulation pathway.

Rb inactivation leads to overexpression of p16, a tumor suppressor gene involved in cell cycle regulation by inhibition of cyclin-dependent kinases [3].

8.3 Uterus

8.3.1 Congenital Lesions

Bicornuate Uterus

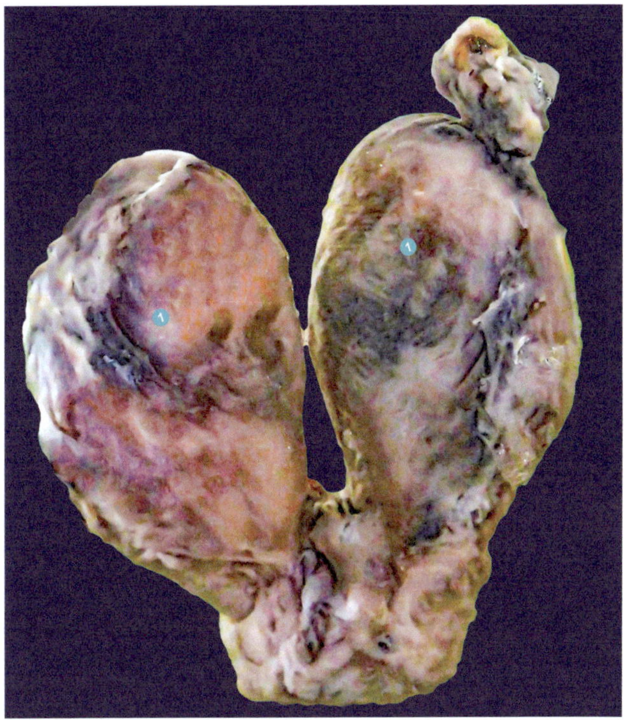

1. The specimen shows two normal-looking uteri that converge on a single cervical canal.

Bicornuate Uterus with Pregnancy in One Horn

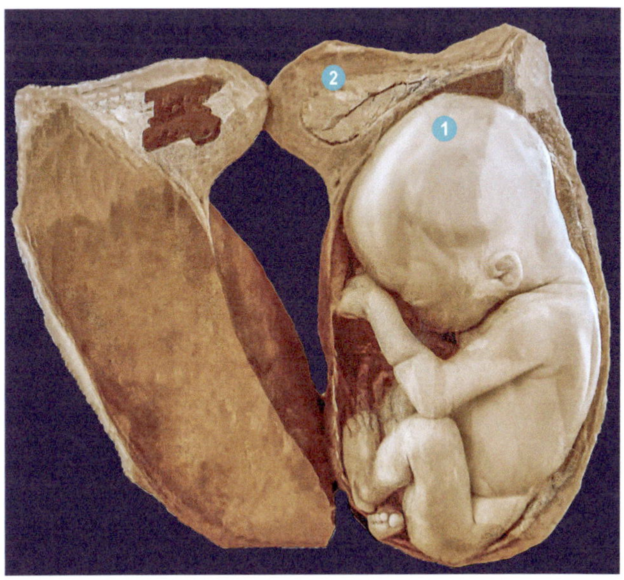

1. A 5-month-fetus in one horn
2. Decidual reaction.

8.3.2 Inflammatory Lesions

Puerperal Sepsis

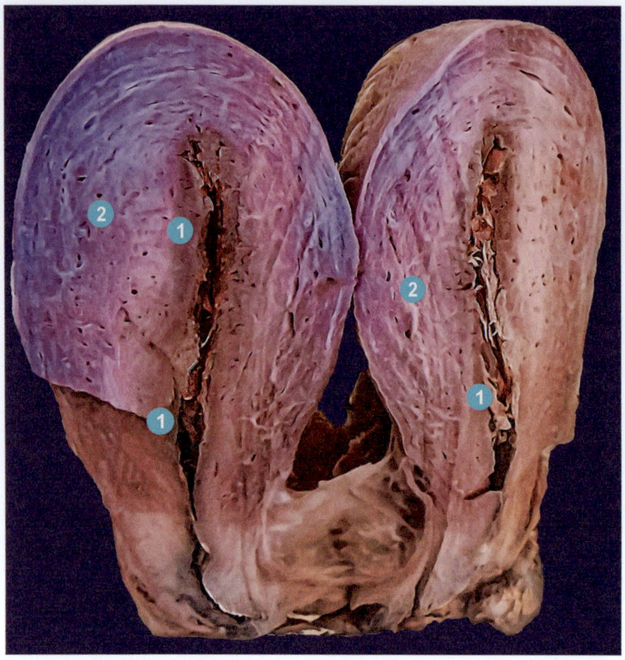

A pregnant, enlarged uterus is mounted.

1. The endometrial cavity is lined by a dirty, purulent, yellow-brown irregular, and shreddy membrane extending down to the upper part of the vagina.
2. The uterine wall is thickened and shows dilated blood vessels filled with thrombi.

8.3.3 Adenomyosis

Adenomyosis

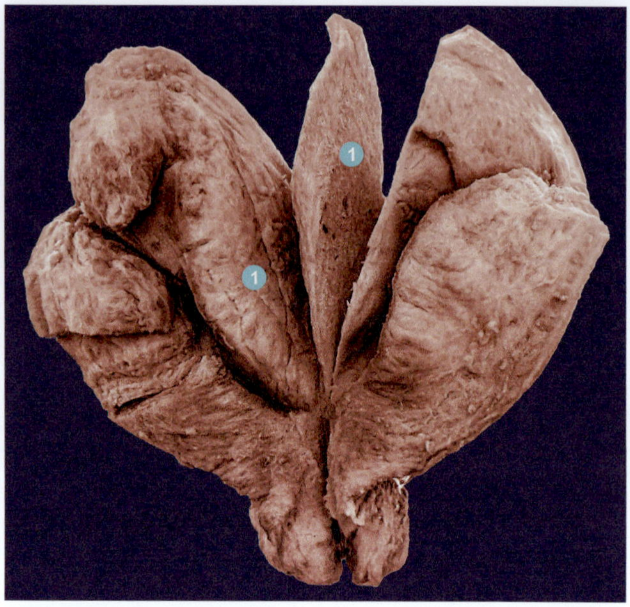

The uterus is sectioned longitudinally into several slices.

1. The cut sections show diffuse and uniform thickening with some cystic spaces and focal hemorrhage.

Microscopic Picture of Adenomyosis (a–d)

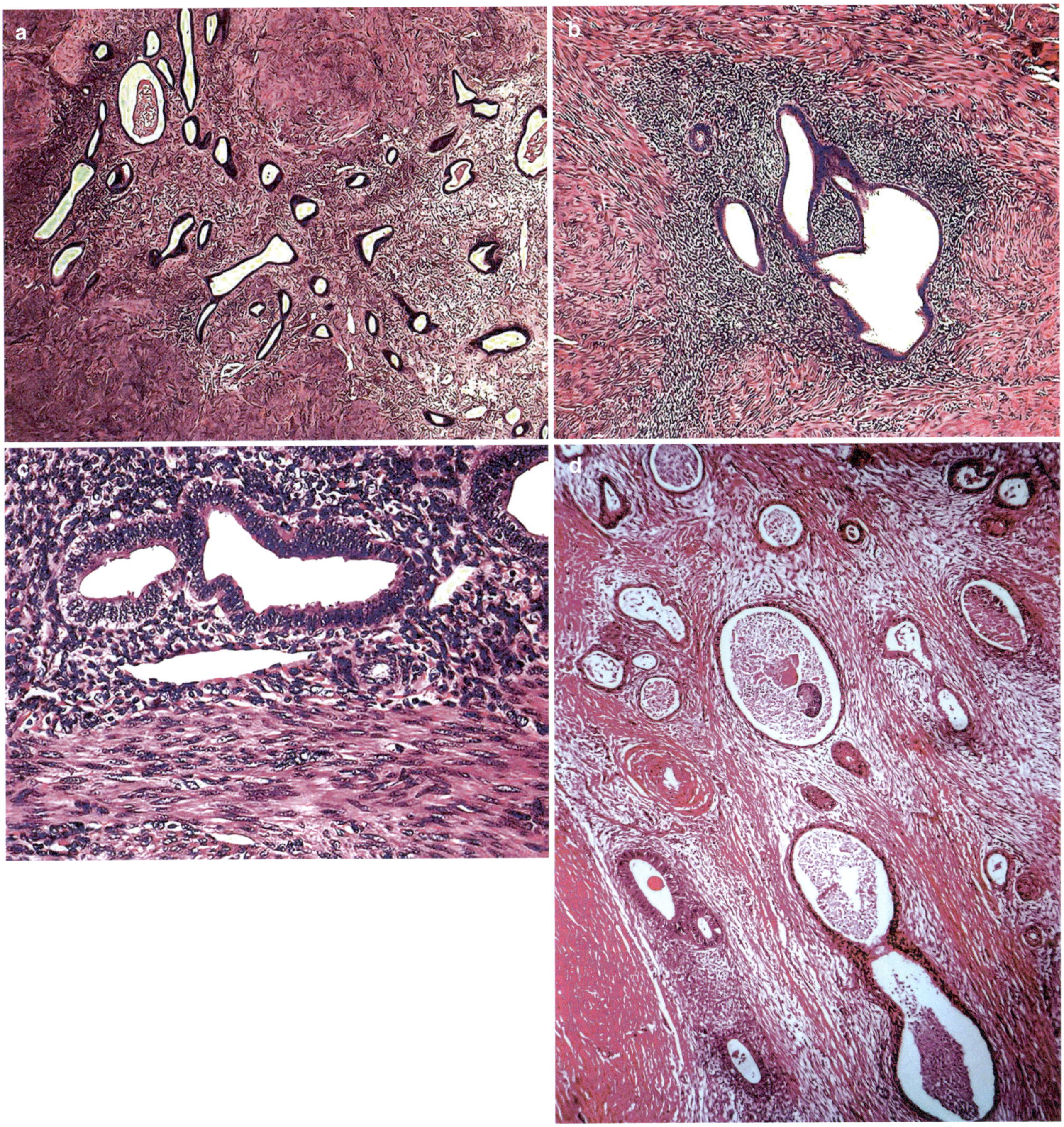

Sections show islands of endometrial glands and stroma enmeshed between and surrounded by irregular bundles of myometrium. Other areas show endometrial glands surrounded by fibrous tissue. Adenomyotic cysts are observed within the myometrium. These cysts are lined by endometrial epithelium and contain blood.

Localized Adenomyosis

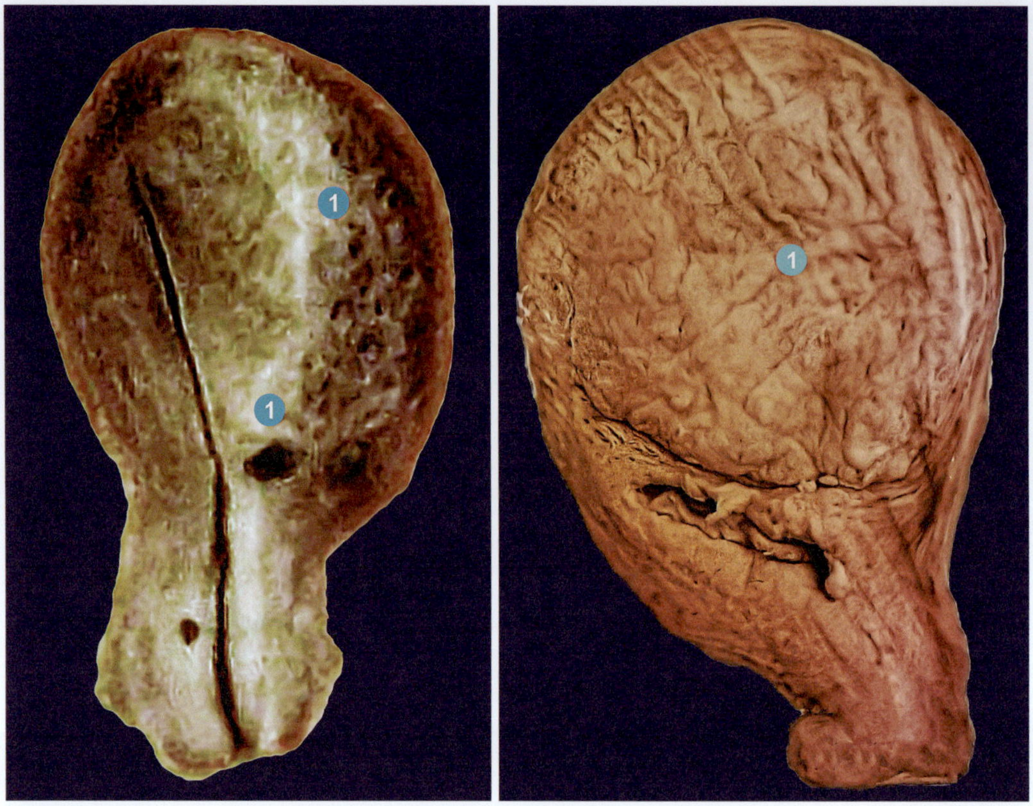

A sagittal section through the uterus is mounted.

1. A well-circumscribed, whorled mass in the anterior wall, within which there are hemorrhagic and yellowish areas.

Adenomyosis and Ovarian Endometriosis

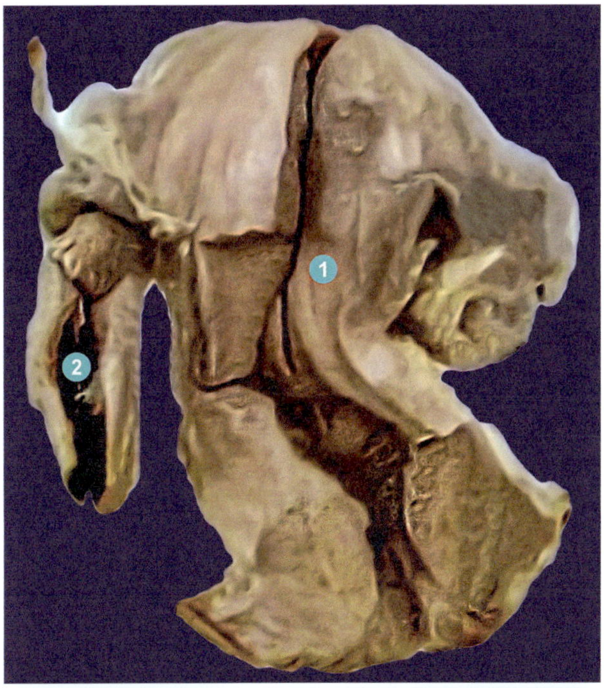

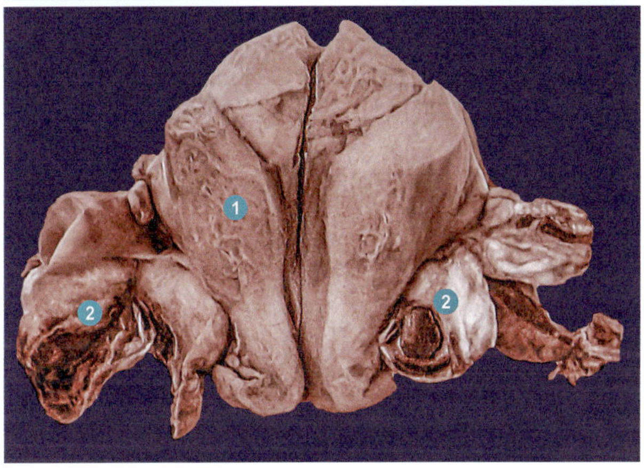

The uterus, both tubes and ovaries are mounted.

1. The uterus shows diffuse and uniform thickening with some cystic spaces and focal hemorrhage.
2. The ovaries are enlarged and contain brown hemorrhagic cysts.

Microscopic Picture of Ovarian Endometriosis (a)

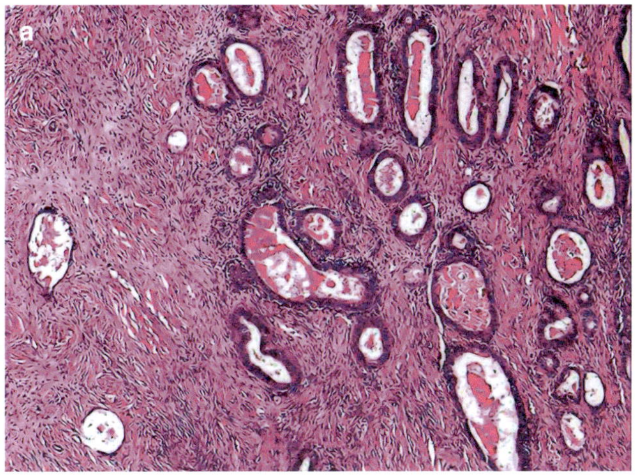

The section shows endometrial glands within the ovarian tissue. The glands appear as small, round structures lined by columnar epithelial cells and filled with blood. The glands are embedded in a fibrous stroma mildly infiltrated by chronic inflammatory cells.

8.3.4 Endometrial Tumor-Like Lesions

Endometrial Polyps

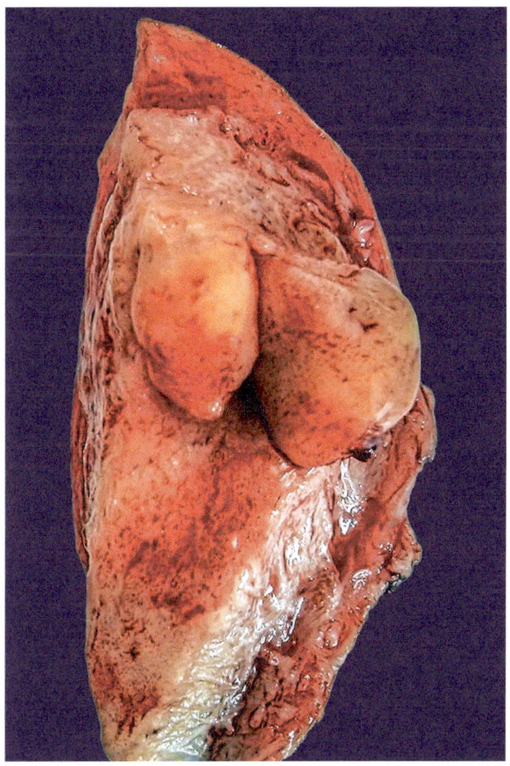

Two pink, well-circumscribed, pedunculated, and fleshy masses with smooth surfaces.

Microscopic Picture of Endometrial Polyps (a–c)

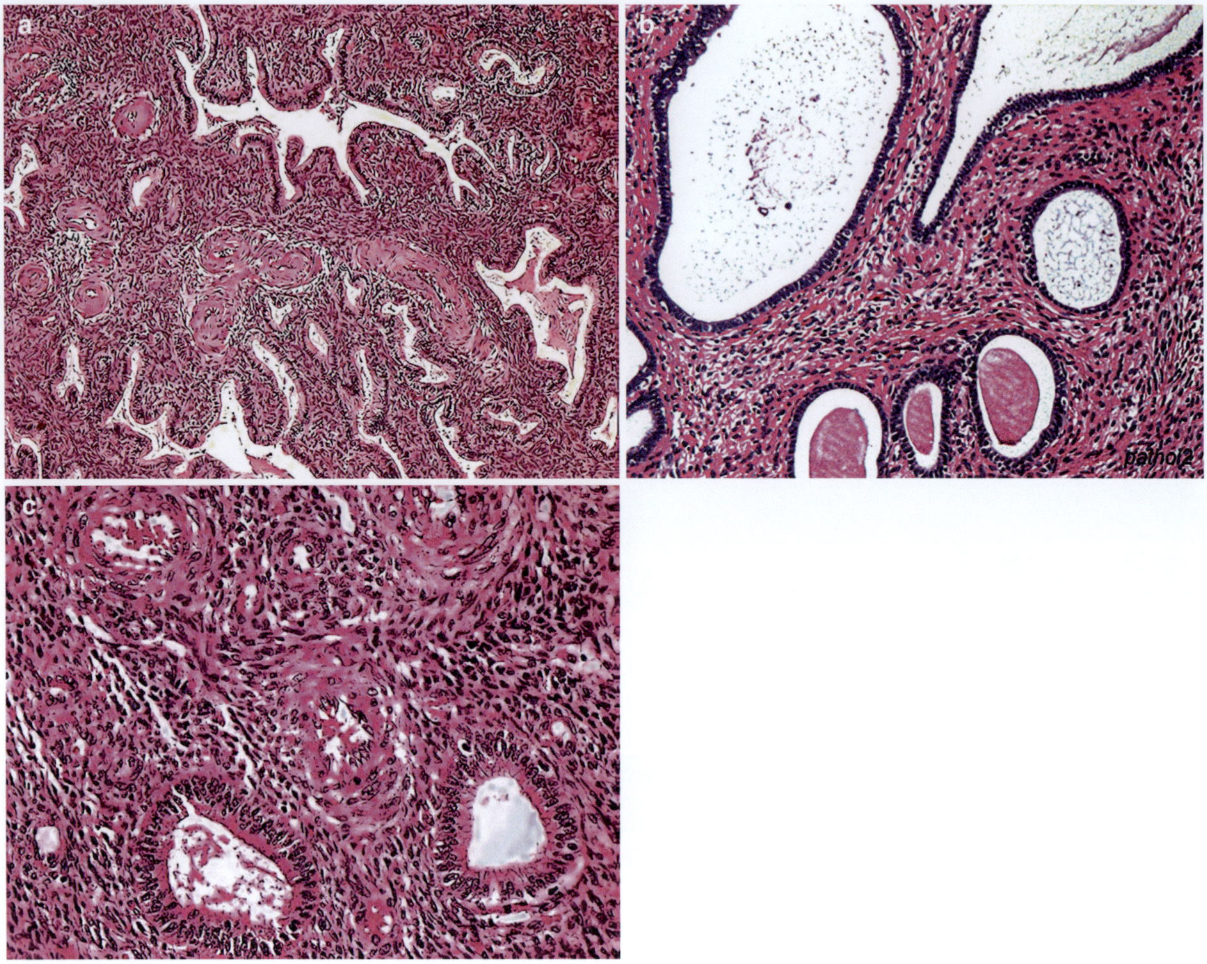

Sections show proliferative, irregularly-shaped, and cystically dilated endometrial glands lined with columnar epithelium. The stroma is cellular with areas of fibrosis. The stroma contains large, thick-walled muscular blood vessels.

Ancillary Tools

IHC [4]:

In glands: pankeratin, cytokeratin 7, PAX8, ER, PR

In stroma: ER, PR, smooth muscle actin (in smooth muscle), p16 (usually peri-glandular)

Increased expression of TGFβ1 and VEGF

Can express p63, P450 arom, and SF1

Molecular/cytogenetics description [5]:

Clonal translocations involving 6p21-22, 12q13-15, or 7q22

6p21 aberrations are characteristically seen only in the stromal component, whereas the epithelial cells are diploid.

8.3.5 Endometrial Epithelial Tumors and Precursors

8.3.5.1 Endometrial Hyperplasia

Endometrial Hyperplasia

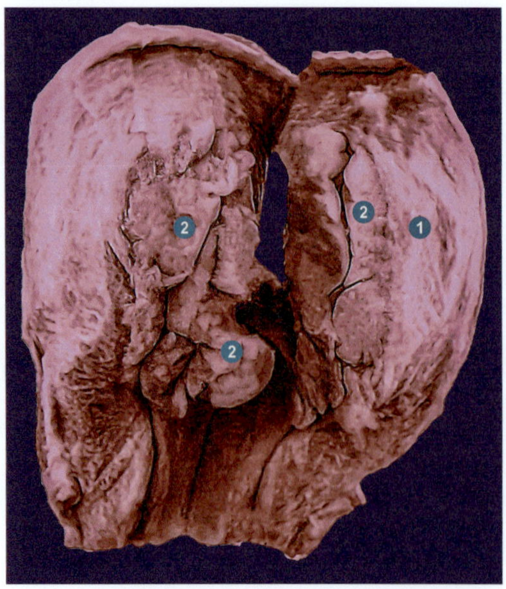

An open uterus is mounted.

1. The uterus is enlarged and irregular in shape.
2. The endometrium is thickened and thrown into polypoid projections without necrosis or evidence of muscle invasion.

Microscopic Picture of Endometrial Hyperplasia without Atypia (a–d)

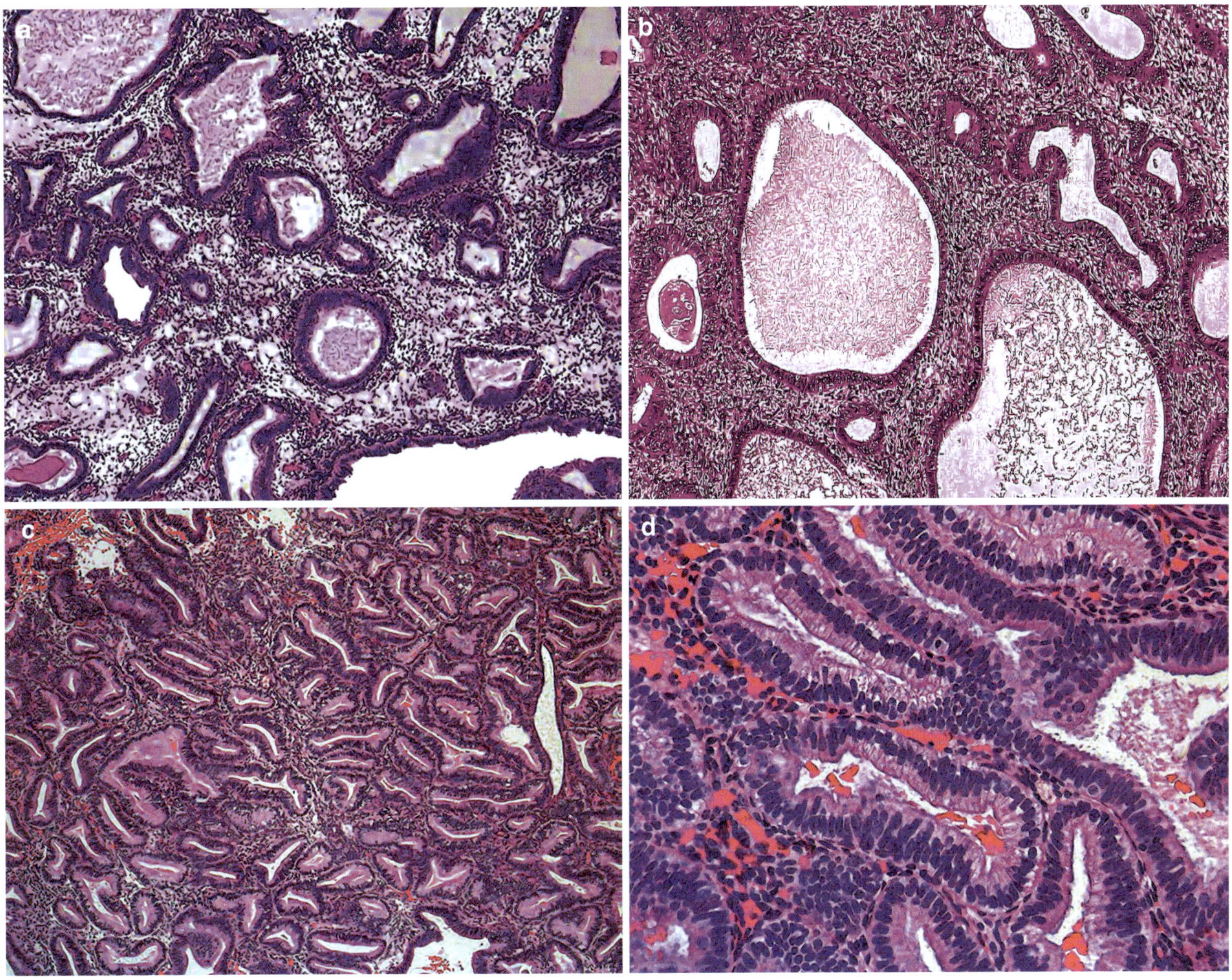

Sections show hyperplastic, irregularly shaped, and crowded endometrial glands with an increased gland/stroma ratio. The glands are variable in size and shape, cystically dilated, and with irregular luminal contours. The glandular epithelium is reminiscent of normal proliferative endometrium with pseudostratified, mitotically active, elongated columnar cells that show mild cellular enlargement but retain smooth nuclear contours without distinct nucleoli. The endometrial stroma is hypercellular.

Microscopic Picture of Atypical Endometrial Hyperplasia (e– i)

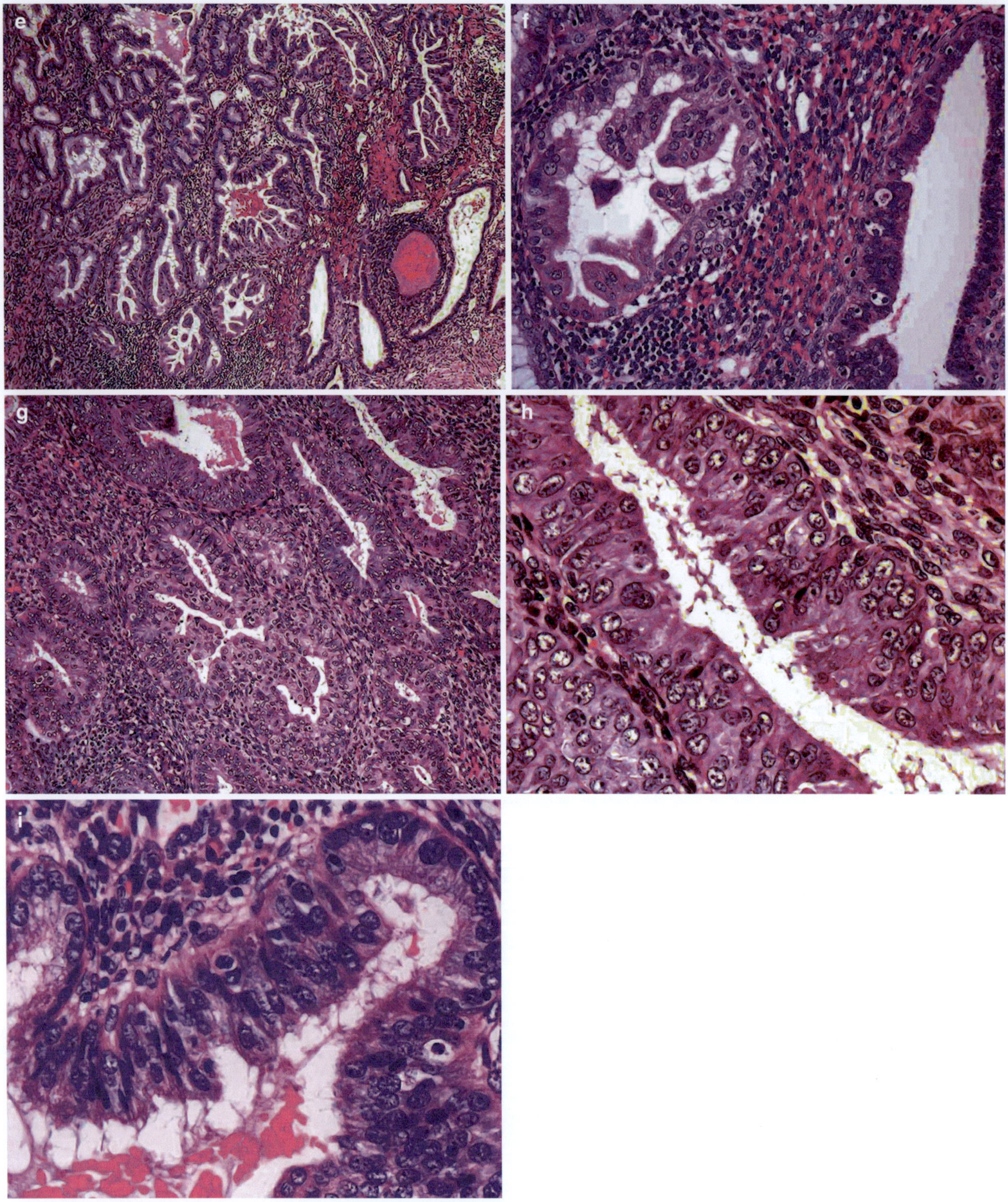

Sections show an architecture similar to that of endometrial hyperplasia without atypia. The glandular epithelium shows enlarged, rounded, and irregular nuclear contours and prominent, enlarged nucleoli with coarse and vesicular chromatin. Occasionally, cytoplasmic eosinophilia imparts a distinct low-power appearance. Stratified cells demonstrate loss of polarity in relation to the basement membrane.

Endometrial Carcinoma

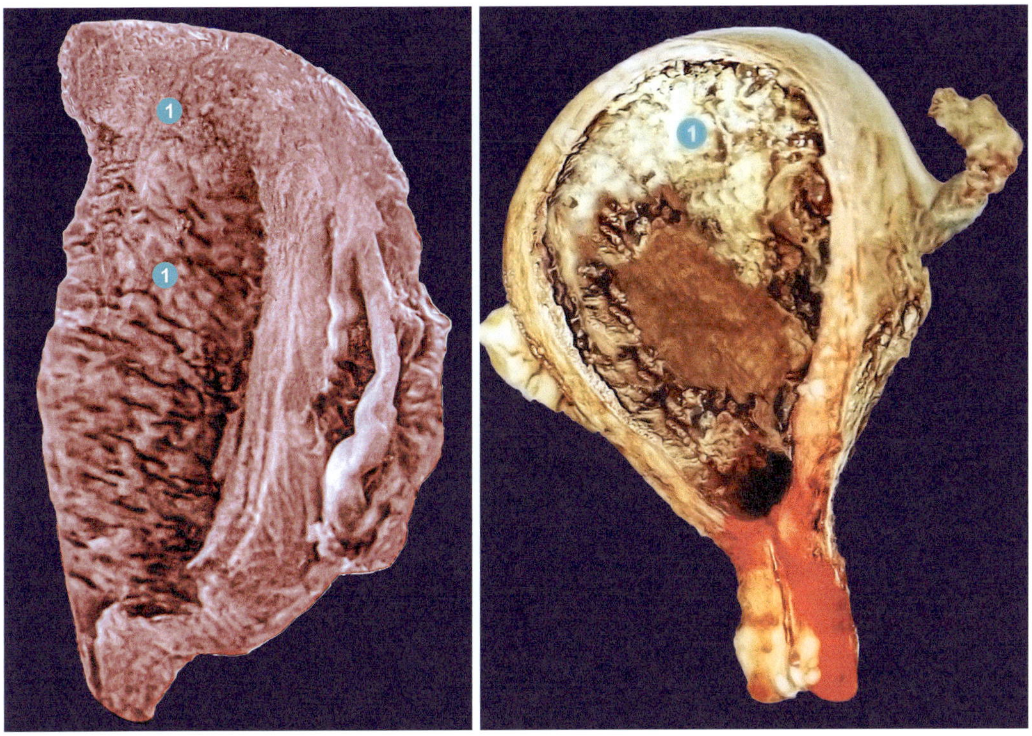

An open uterus is mounted.

1. The endometrium is replaced by a hemorrhagic, necrotic tumor mass filling the uterine cavity.

Endometrial Carcinoma-Polypoid Carcinoma

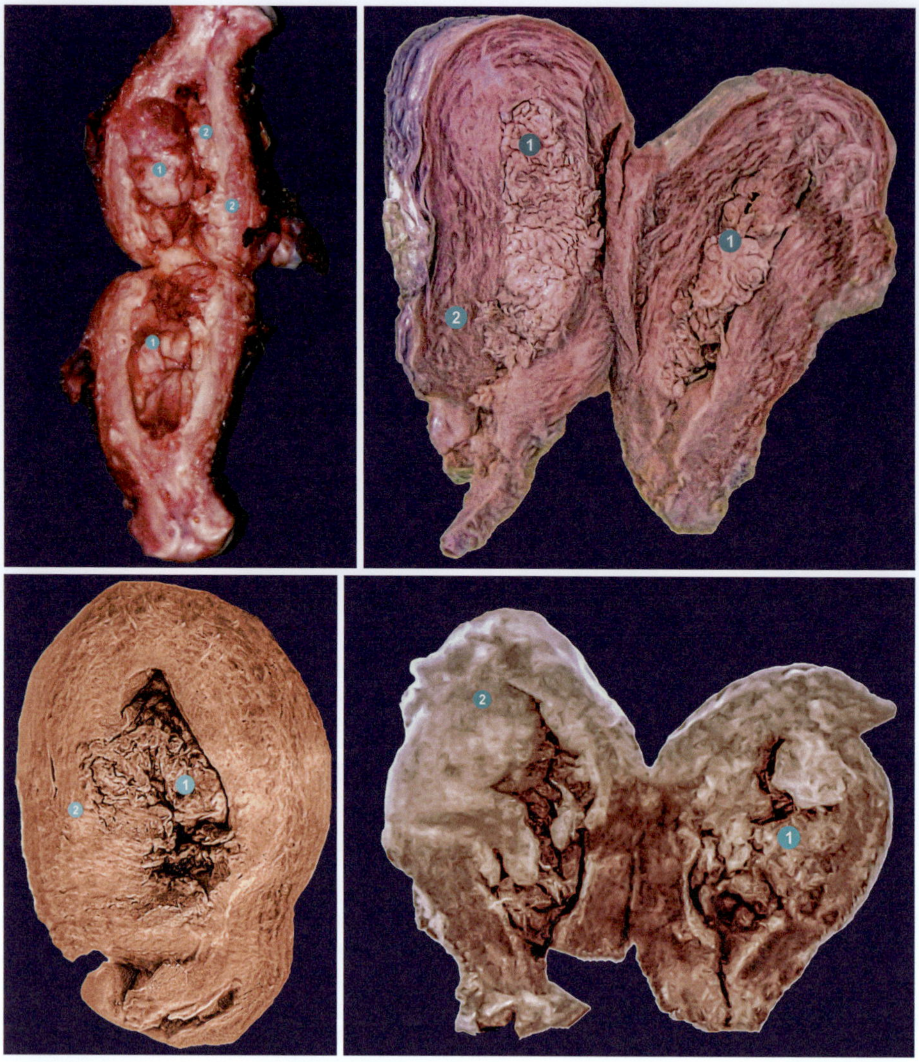

An open uterus is mounted.

1. Exophytic, friable red-tan mass with a nodular surface, located primarily in the fundus and extending down to fill the endometrial cavity.
2. Focal muscle infiltration.

Microscopic Picture of Endometrioid Adenocarcinoma (a–o)

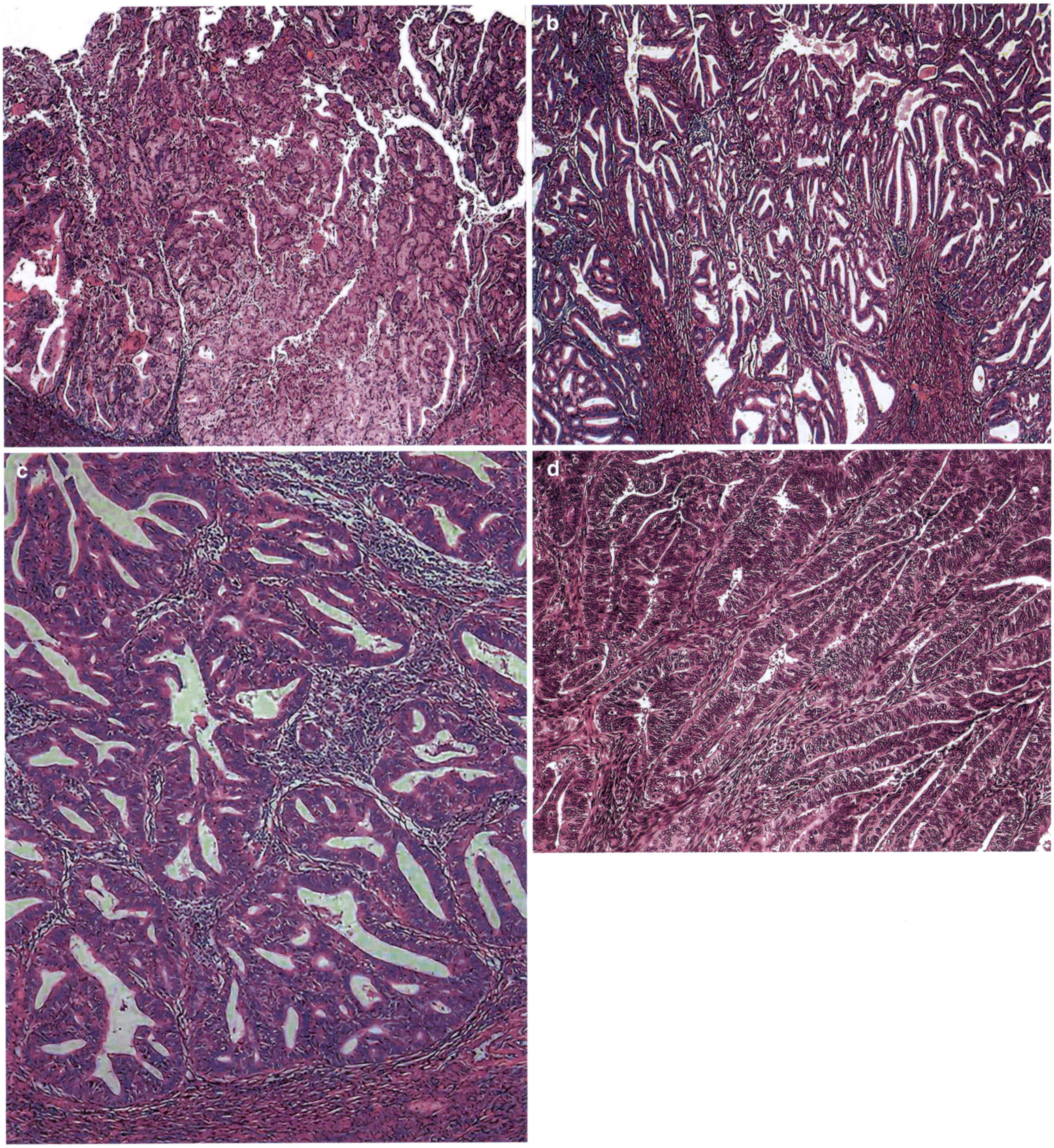

Sections show **endometrioid-type carcinoma** in the form of:

(a–i): confluent or back-to-back glands lacking intervening stroma with areas of complex papillary, acinar, and microacinar configurations. The lining epithelial cells show cellular/nuclear enlargement, nuclear rounding (rather than elongation) with large nucleoli, loss of polarity, and pseudostratification.

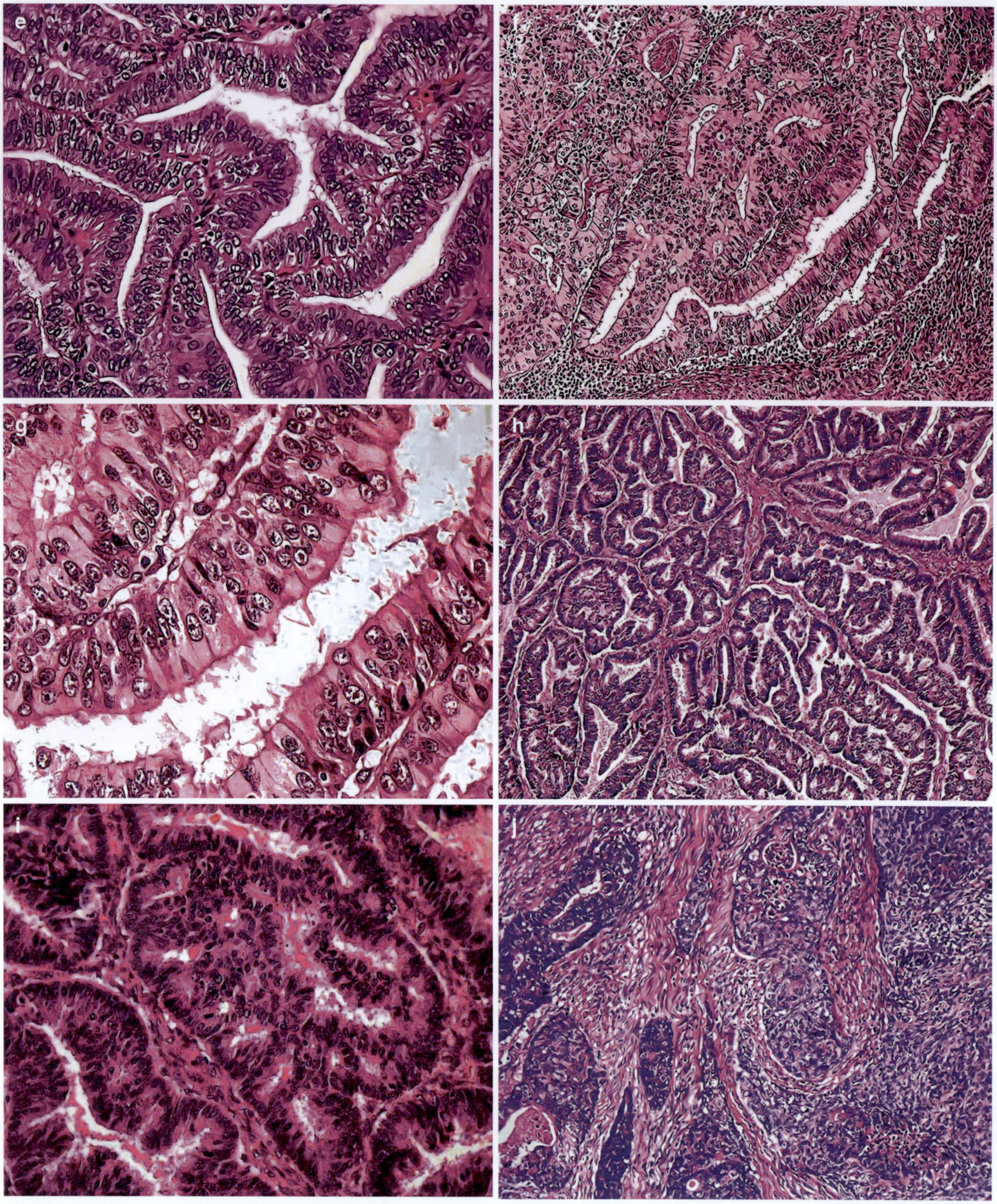

(j, k) **Adenosquamous carcinoma**-type tumor shows cytoplasmic eosinophilia and In areas of cytologically malignant squamous differentiation.

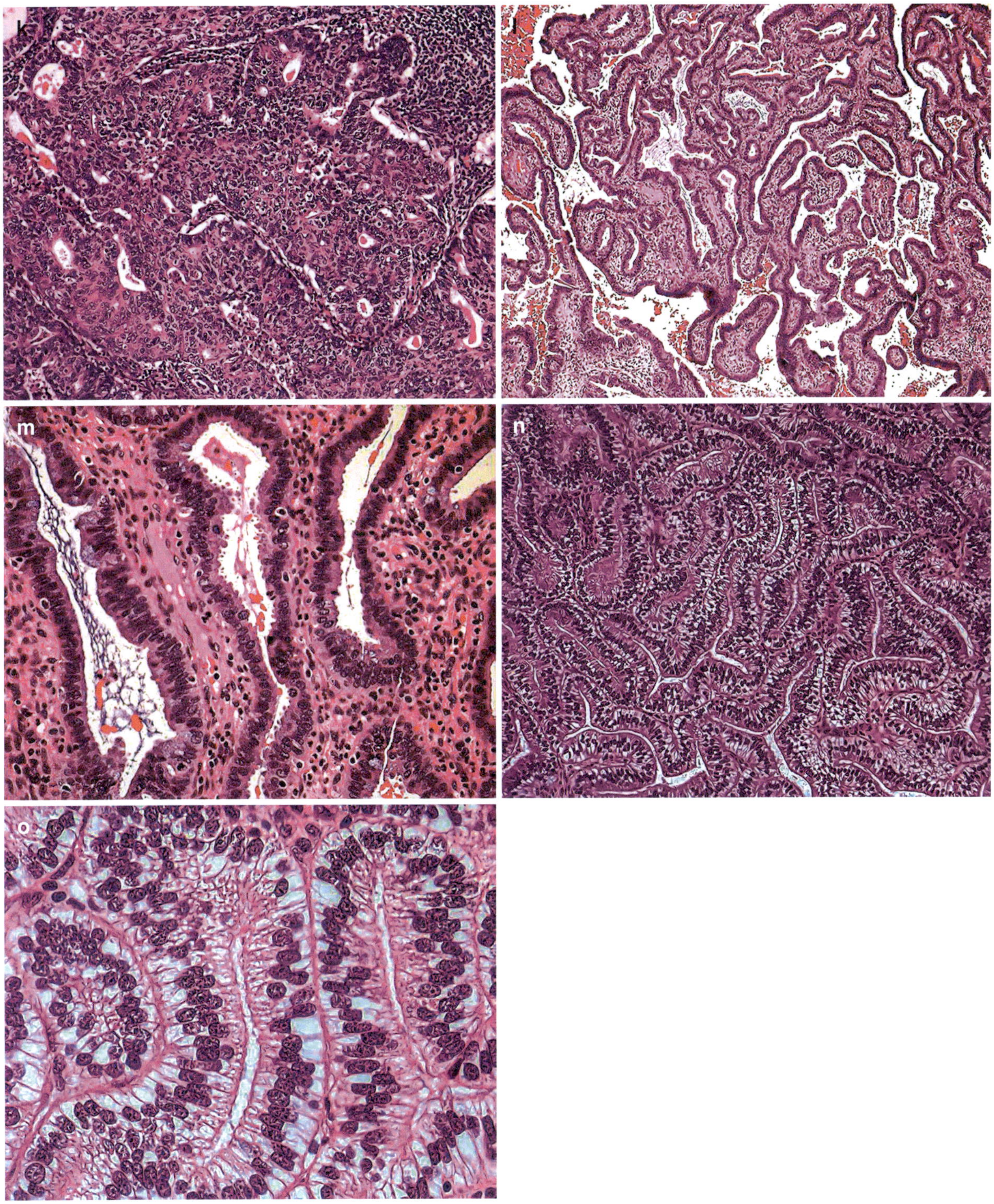

(l, m) **Villoglandular-type** tumors may show finger-like projections lined by tall columnar cells with bland nuclei.

(n, o) **Secretory features** in which there is a well-differentiated adenocarcinoma in which the neoplastic glands have tall columnar epithelial cells showing mild-to-moderate pleomorphism and having small, vesicular, and uniform nuclei with fine nuclear chromatin. The cytoplasm of these cells is clear and exhibits a severe degree of supra-nuclear and subnuclear vacuolization.

Ancillary Tools

IHC [6]:

CK7, CK8/18, CK19.

Also, vimentin (65%), CEA (areas of squamous metaplasia), CA-125, ER, PR, and PTEN (80%), cyclin D1 (40%).

IFITM1, another endometrial stroma marker, has superior specificity in this differential.

Molecular/cytogenetics description [7]:

Molecular subtypes of Endometrial Carcinoma:

The Cancer Genome Atlas (TCGA) project identified four distinct POLEmuts: Characterized by mutations in the POLE gene, responsible for DNA proofreading, leading to hypermutation and microsatellite instability.

- MMR deficient (dMMR): Harboring defects in the mismatch repair (MMR) machinery, resulting in the accumulation of mutations throughout the genome.
- p53 mutated (p53mut): Associated with mutations in the TP53 tumor suppressor gene, involved in cell cycle regulation and apoptosis.
- No specific molecular profile (NSMP): Lacking any of the defining alterations of the other three groups, representing the most heterogeneous category.

Cytogenetic Abnormalities:

Hyperdiploidy: The most frequent abnormality, observed in two-thirds of ECs, characterized by an increased number of chromosomes compared to the normal diploid karyotype.

Numerical aberrations: Gains or losses of specific chromosomes, frequently involving chromosomes 1, 3, 7, and 10.

Structural rearrangements: Translocations, deletions, and inversions involving various chromosomes, contributing to gene activation or inactivation.

The specific molecular and cytogenetic alterations influence the clinical course of EC. For instance, POLEmut and MMR-deficient tumors tend to have a favorable prognosis, while p53mut and NSMP ECs are often associated with aggressive behavior and poorer outcomes.

8.3.5.2 Mesenchymal Tumors Specific to the Uterus

Uterine Submucous Leiomyoma

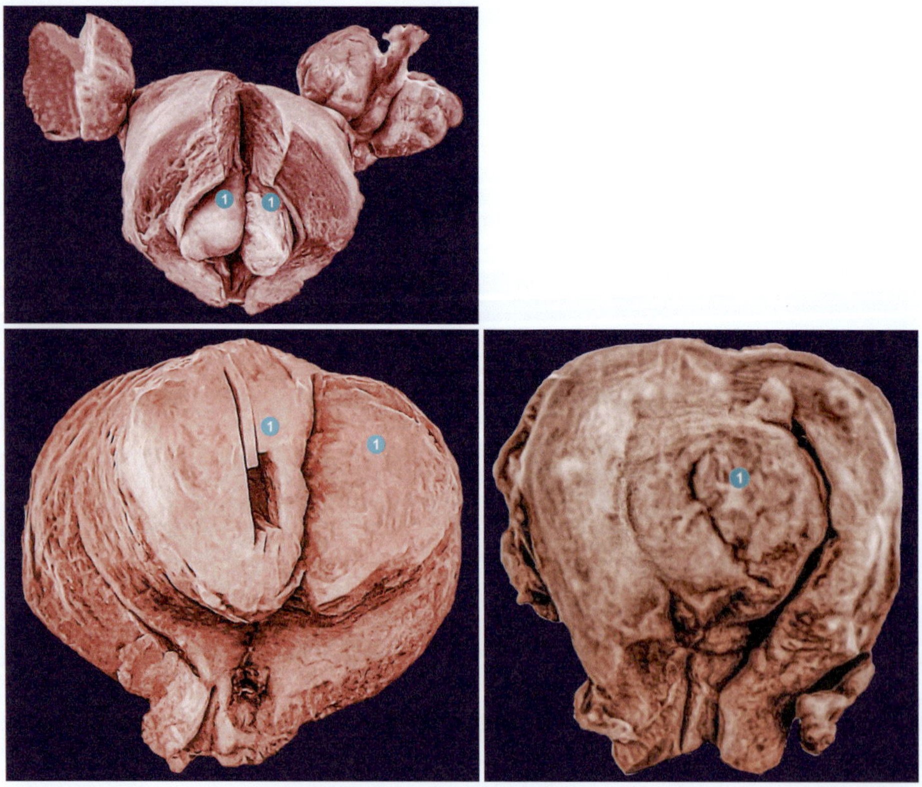

An open uterus is mounted.

1. The uterine cavity is opened to show a well-circumscribed, uncapsulated, globular mass covered with endometrium.

Multiple Leiomyomas (Interstitial and Subserous)

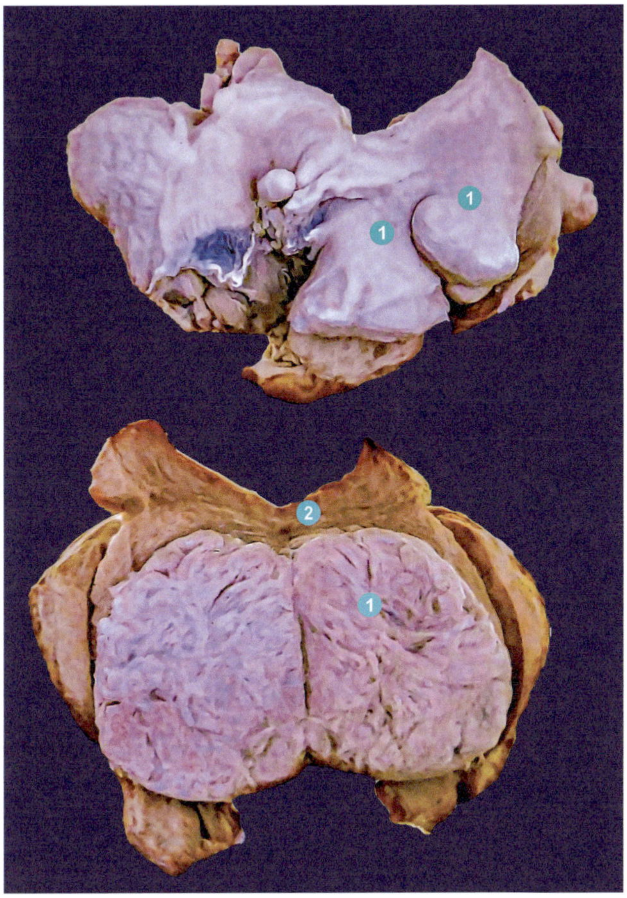

Two uteri are mounted.

1. They have an irregular nodular surface with multiple subserous fibroids with interlacing bundles of smooth muscle and fibrous tissue seen in the cut sections.
2. The surrounding muscle is compressed into a thin layer, forming a false capsule.

Microscopic Picture of Leiomyoma (a–c)

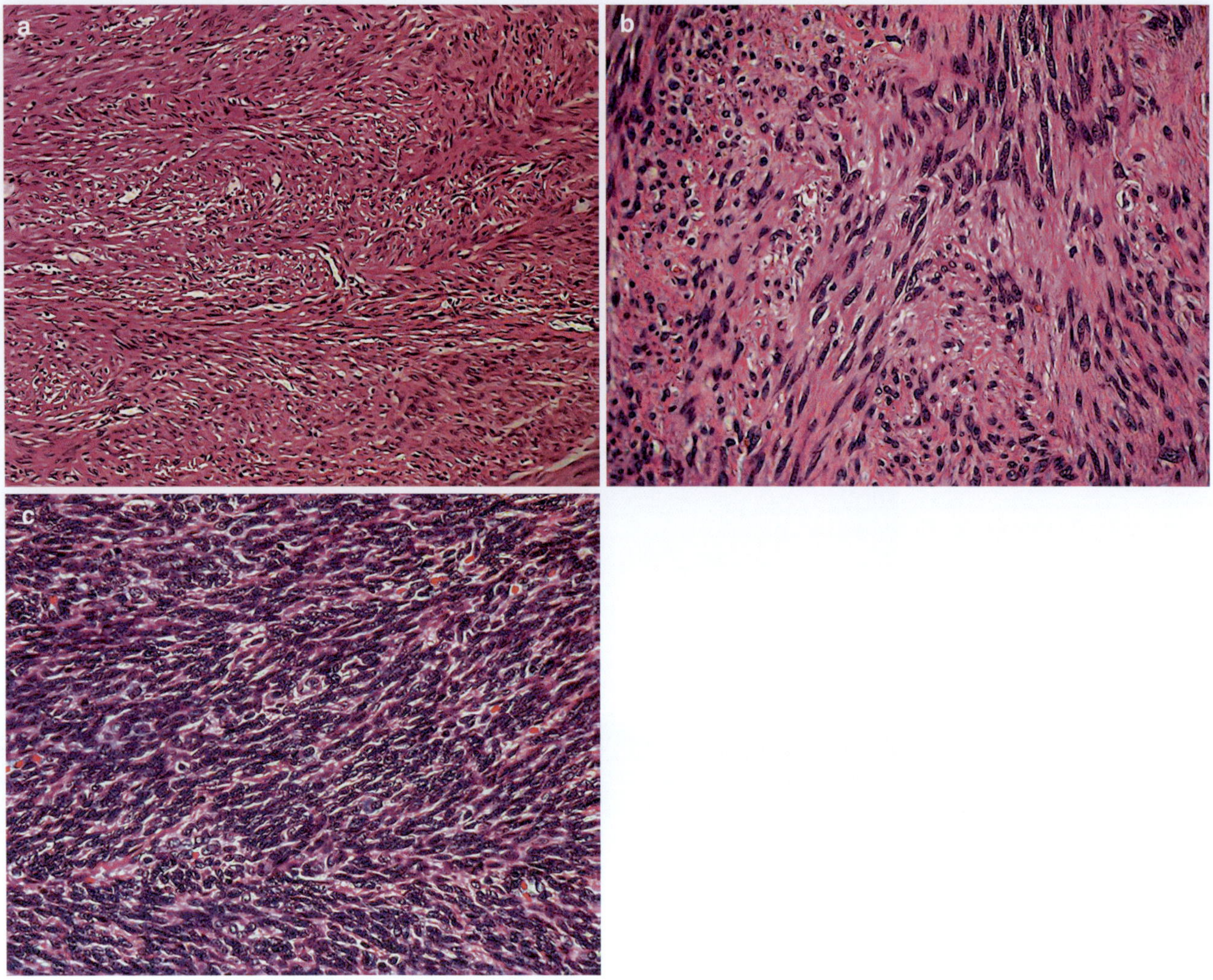

Sections show intersecting bundles of smooth muscle cells interspersed by fibrovascular stroma. Smooth muscle cells have tapered ends and cigar-shaped nuclei, while fibroblasts are spindle-shaped cells with tapered-end nuclei. Cellular leiomyoma in (c) is more cellular than the normal myometrium but lacks nuclear atypia, tumor cell necrosis, or increased mitotic activity.

Ancillary Tools

IHC [8]:

Desmin

h-caldesmon

Smooth muscle actin

Transgelin

Smooth muscle markers can be weak in epithelioid and myxoid leiomyomas.

Estrogen and progesterone receptors.

WT1

Up to 40% of leiomyomas are CD10 positive (especially cellular leiomyomas).

Molecular/cytogenetics description [9]:

About 70% of conventional leiomyomas harbor MED12 mutations and nearly 40% HMGA2/HMGA1 rearrangements, COL4A5/COL4A6 deletions, or FH mutations.

Other less frequent alterations include 7q22 deletion involving CUX1 gene, 22q deletion with DEPDC5 gene, and 1p deletion with NPHP4 gene.

Leiomyomatous Polyp

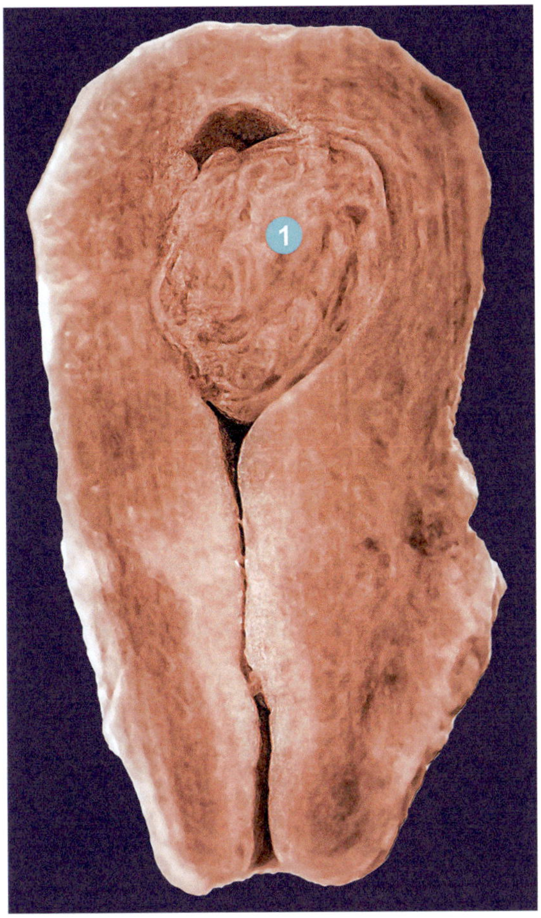

An open uterus is mounted.

1. A globular, well-circumscribed, uncapsulated mass with a whorl-like cut section is seen attached to the fundus.

Fibroid Uterus with Endometrial Hyperplasia (a, b)

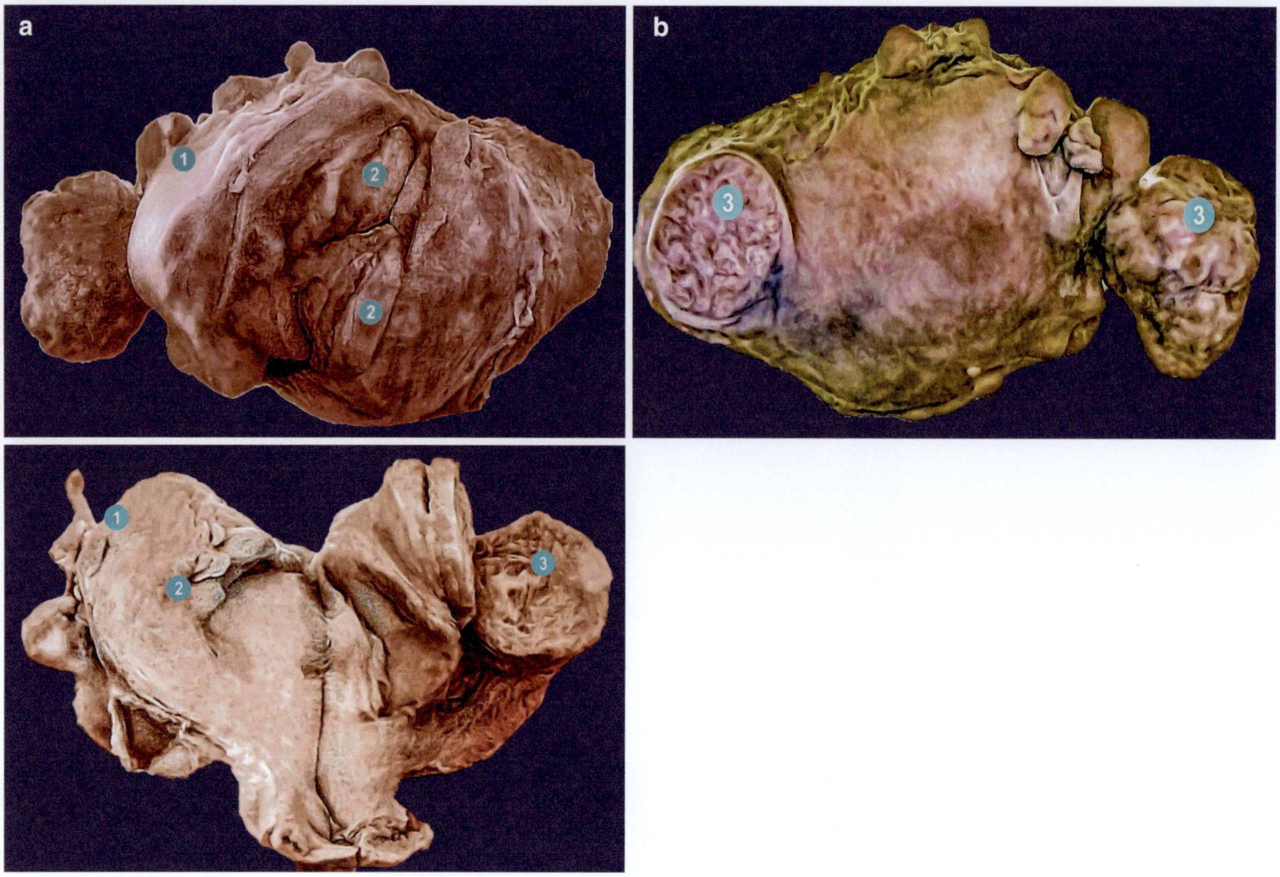

An open uterus is mounted.

1. The uterus is enlarged and irregular in shape.
2. A large tumor mass projects from the lumen covered by thickened endometrium, which is thrown into polypoid projections without necrosis or evidence of muscle invasion.
3. Multiple subserous fibroids project from the back and the upper end of the uterus with a whorl-like cut section.

Uterine Leiomyoma with Hyaline Degeneration

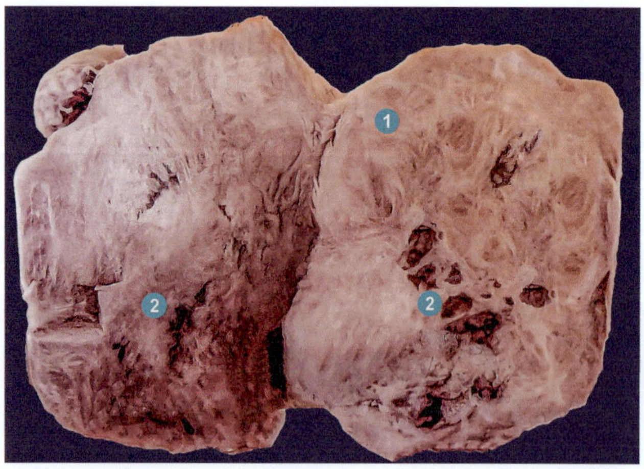

Two globular masses are mounted.

1. They are well-defined, uncapsulated, with whorl-like cut sections formed by interlacing brown smooth muscle fibers and intersecting fibrous tissue.
2. Irregular cavities are seen resulting from the falling of degenerated hyaline material.

Leiomyoma with Red Degeneration

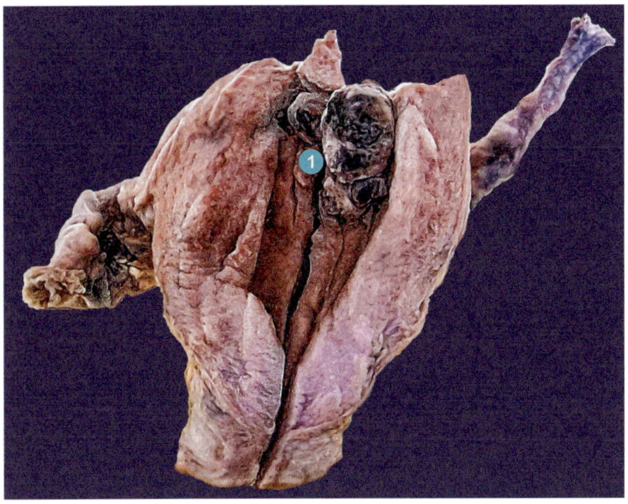

An open uterus is mounted.

1. A mass is seen attached to the fundus. It is dark red with a whorl-like cut section in areas and focal necrosis and hemorrhage.

Uterine Leiomyosarcoma

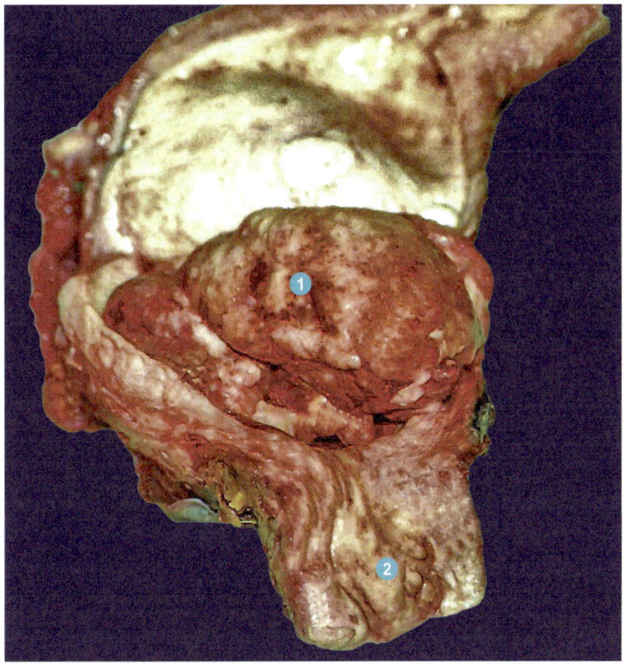

The uterus, opened laterally, is mounted.

1. There is a large, bulky, irregular, and fleshy tumor with focal areas of hemorrhage and necrosis protruding from the myometrium into the endometrial cavity.
2. The cervix looks normal.

Microscopic Picture of Conventional/Spindle Cell Uterine Leiomyosarcoma (a–d)

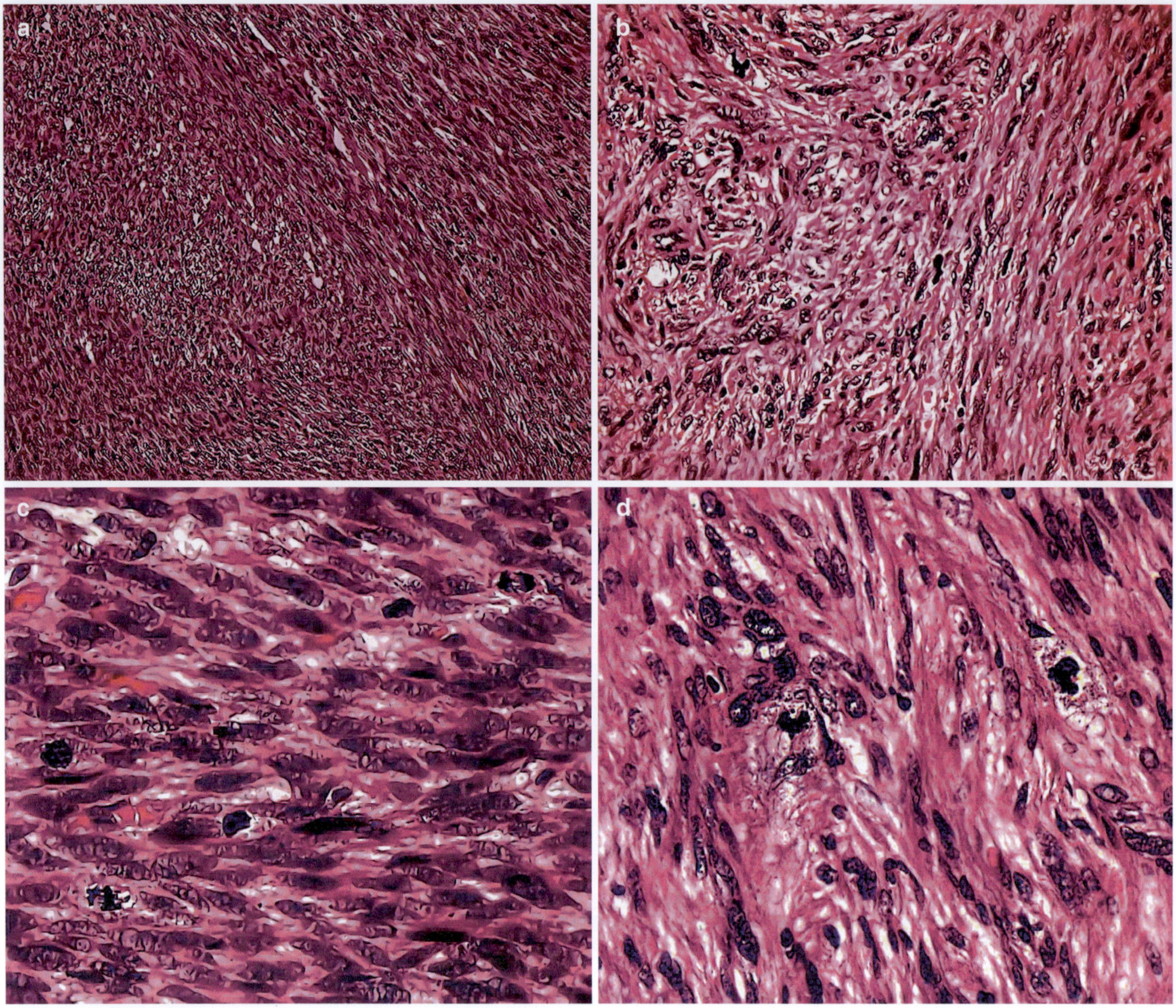

Sections show a hypercellular tumor formed of haphazardly arranged fascicles of malignant spindle cells with eosinophilic cytoplasm and hyperchromatic nuclei with an increased number of mitotic figures; many are atypical.

Ancillary Tools

IHC [10]:

Smooth muscle markers, including h-caldesmon (more specific), desmin, and SMA:

May be weak or patchy, especially in myxoid leiomyosarcoma.

p53 may show aberrant expression.

p16 often shows diffuse expression.

ER/PR

WT1, keratins, EMA, and CD10 are often positive.

A high Ki67 proliferation index (>10% nuclear staining) can be helpful unless differentiating it from a leiomyoma with bizarre nuclei.

Molecular/cytogenetics description [11]:

No specific diagnostic/pathognomonic molecular alterations.

Substantial mutational heterogeneity, widespread DNA copy number alterations, including chromothripsis, and frequent whole genome duplication.

Hallmarks of "BRCAness," including alterations in homologous recombination DNA repair genes, multiple structural rearrangements, and enrichment of specific mutational signatures.

Alternative telomere lengthening (78%)

Somatic mutations

TP53 (30–60%)

ATRX (24–30%)

RB1 (27–61%)

MED12 (~20%)

PTEN (~31–57%)

C-MYC (18%) and TERT (26%) amplifications

Endometrial Stromal Sarcoma

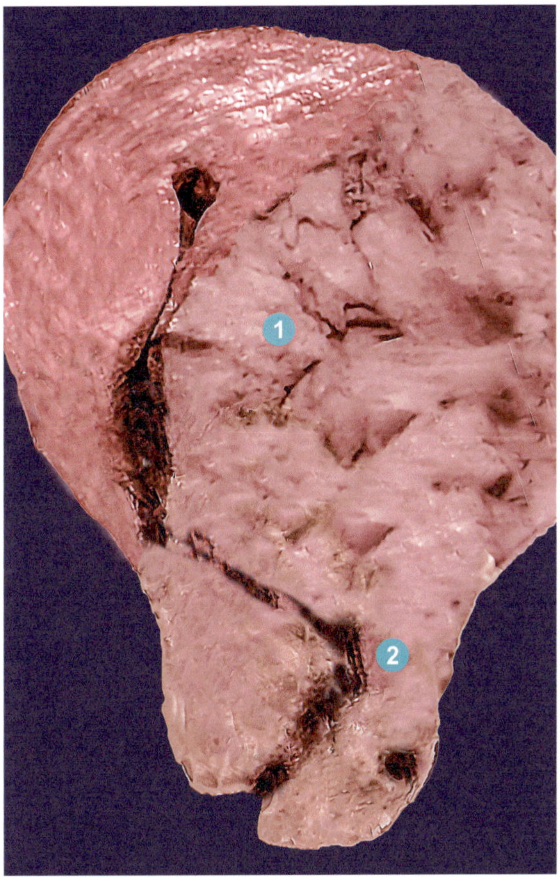

The uterus bisected longitudinally is mounted.

1. A large polypoid hemorrhagic mass is seen infiltrating the uterine wall and endometrium.
2. The mass infiltrates the lower uterine segment and uterine serosa with the presence of areas of hemorrhage and necrosis.

Microscopic Picture of High-Grade Endometrial Stromal Sarcoma (a–f)

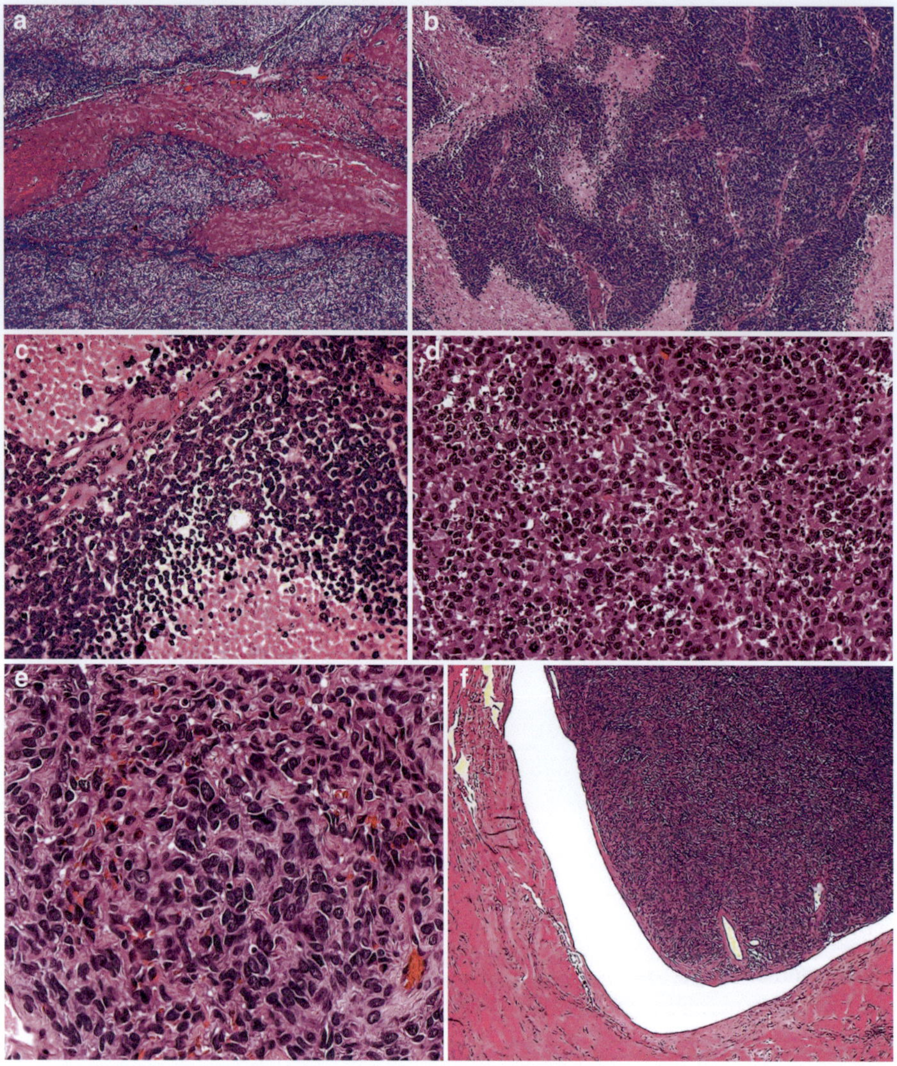

Sections show permeative and infiltrative islands of malignant tumor cells composed of small round blue cells with scant to moderate eosinophilic cytoplasm and nuclear atypia and increased mitoses; many are atypical. Tumor cell necrosis and lymphovascular invasion are seen.

The patient was an elderly postmenopausal female who presented with a large swelling in her leg. FNA was performed and revealed pleomorphic sarcoma cells. TAH + BSO was performed and revealed this high-grade endometrial stromal sarcoma. The patient died shortly after the operation.

Ancillary Tools

IHC [12]:

YWHAE::NUTM2A/B fusions (Pathology 2018;50:162, Int J Gynecol Pathol 2019;38:528):

High-grade component:
Cyclin D1 (>70% of cells)
BCOR
CD117/KIT
Pan-TRK
CD56
CD99
Low-grade component:
CD10
ER
PR
BCOR rearranged
CD10
Cyclin D1 (>70% of cells)
Pan-TRK
BCOR (~50%)

BCOR ITD
BCOR (both high- and low-grade components)
Cyclin D1 (both high- and low-grade components)
Pan-TRK
High-grade transformation of low-grade endometrial stromal sarcoma
High-grade component:
CD10 (50%)
ER (50%)
PR (56%)
Molecular/cytogenetics description [12]:
YWHAE::NUTM2A/B fusions

t(10;17)(q22;p13)
Produces the 14-3-3 oncoprotein

BCOR rearranged

ZC3H7B is the most common gene partner; t(X;22)(p11;q13)

Less frequent partners include L3MBTL2, EP300, NUTM2G, RALGPS1, MAP7D2, RGAG1, ING3, NUGGC, KMT2D, and CREBBP.
MDM2 amplification (45–100%)
FRS2 amplification (40%)
CDK4 amplification (38–60%)
Homozygous deletion of CDKN2A (20–28%) and CDKN2B (18%)

BCOR ITD

Internal tandem duplications of different lengths involving exon 15
CDKN2A/2B homozygous deletion (20%)
No MDM2 or CDK4 amplifications

High-grade transformation of low-grade endometrial stromal sarcoma

JAZF1::SUZ12 fusions most common

8.4 Fallopian Tubes

Hydrosalpinx (a, b)

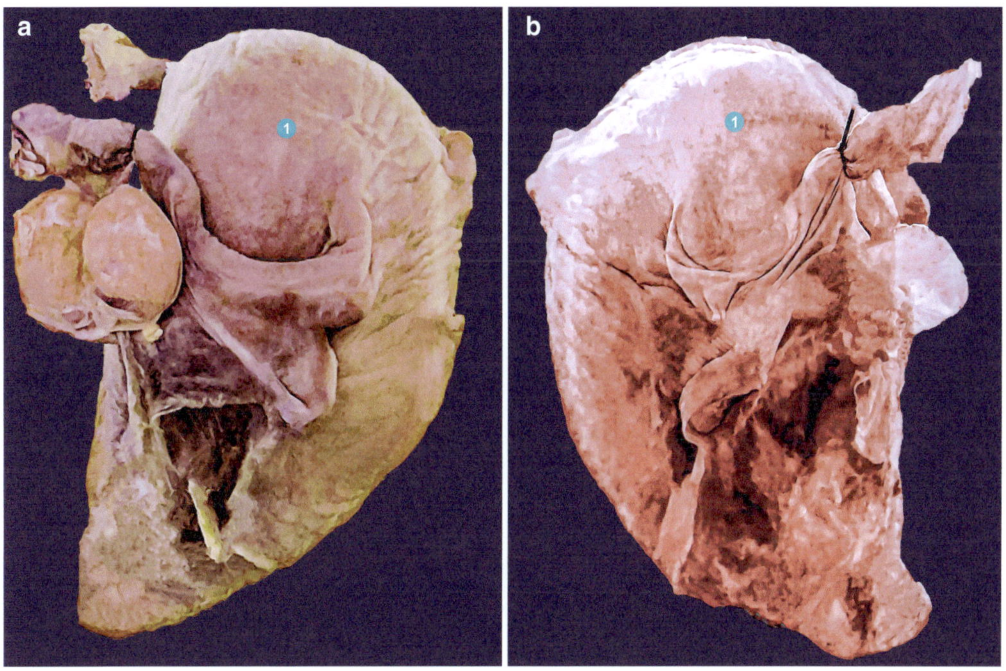

Both Fallopian tubes are mounted.

1. Both are markedly distended with clear fluid and have a thin wall.

Microscopic Picture of Tuberculous Salpingitis (c–e)

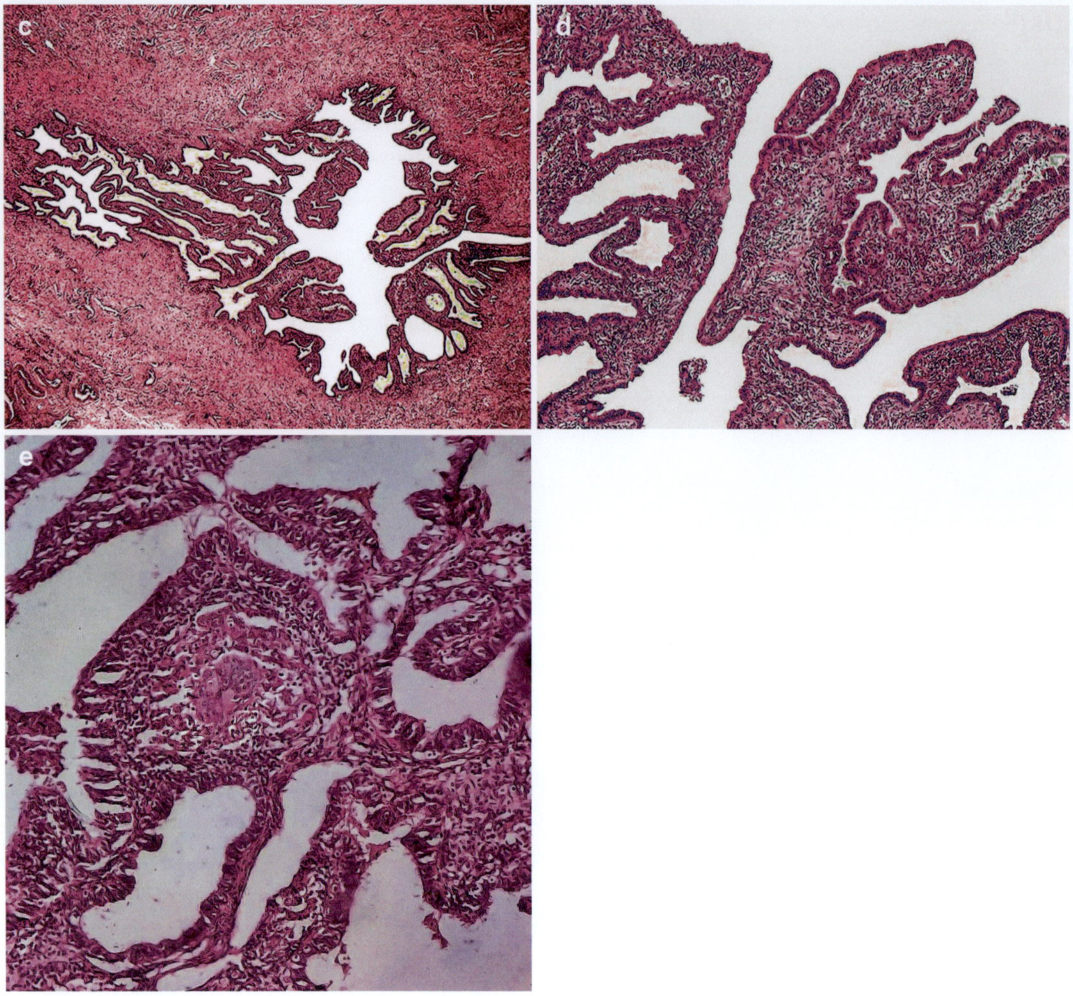

Sections show thickened and fused plicae, mimicking a pattern of thyroid follicles, with thick fibrous stroma infiltrated by tuberculoid infiltrate formed of lymphocytes, histiocytes, and Langhans giant cells. Plicae are lined with hyperplastic tubal epithelium.

8.5 Ovary

8.5.1 Surface Epithelial Tumors

Serous Cystadenoma of Ovary

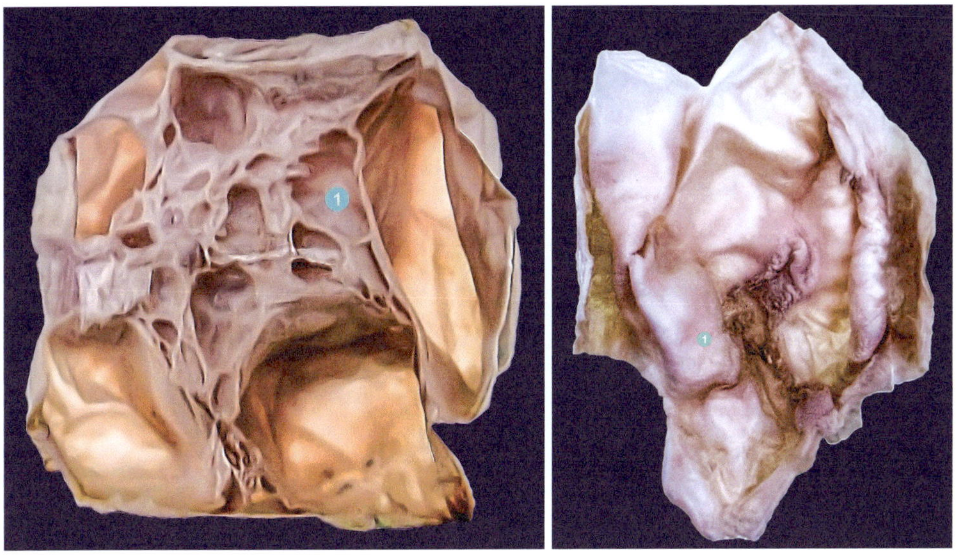

An ovarian cyst is mounted.

1. The cyst is multilocular with thin, smooth walls.

Papillary Serous Cystadenoma of Ovary

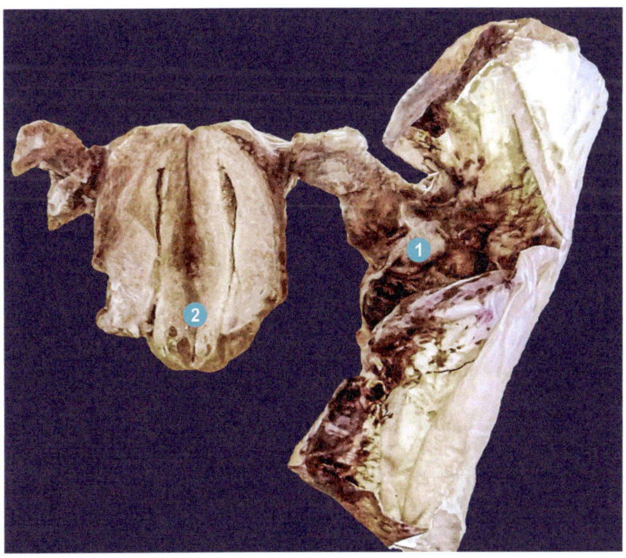

An ovarian cyst is mounted.

1. The ovary is replaced by a thin-walled cyst with some fine papillary processes.
2. The cervix shows Nabothian cysts indicative of chronic cervicitis.

Papillary Serous Cystadenoma of Ovary

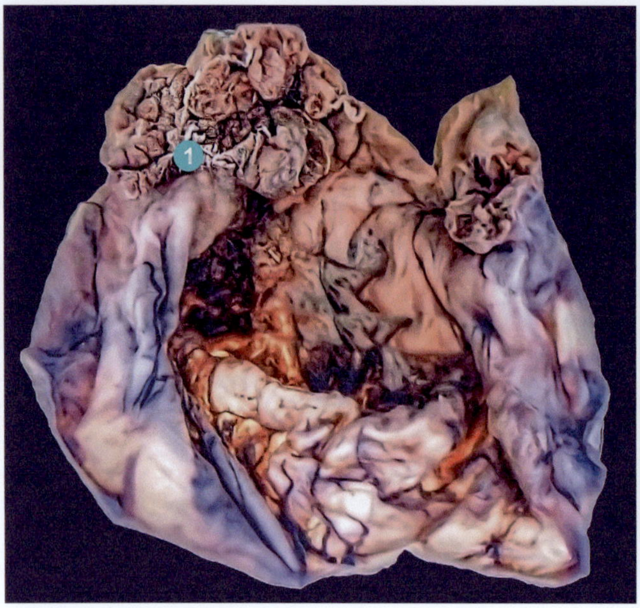

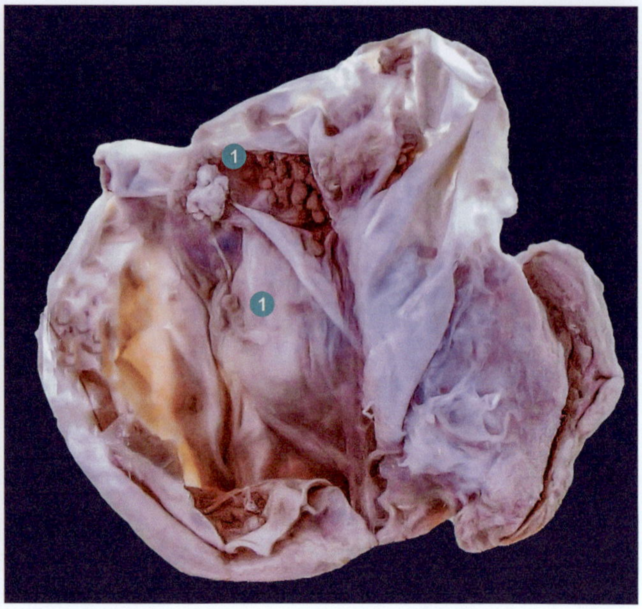

An ovarian cyst is mounted.

1. The ovary is replaced by a thin-walled cyst with some papillary processes in an area.

Microscopic Picture of Serous Cystadenoma of Ovary (a, b)

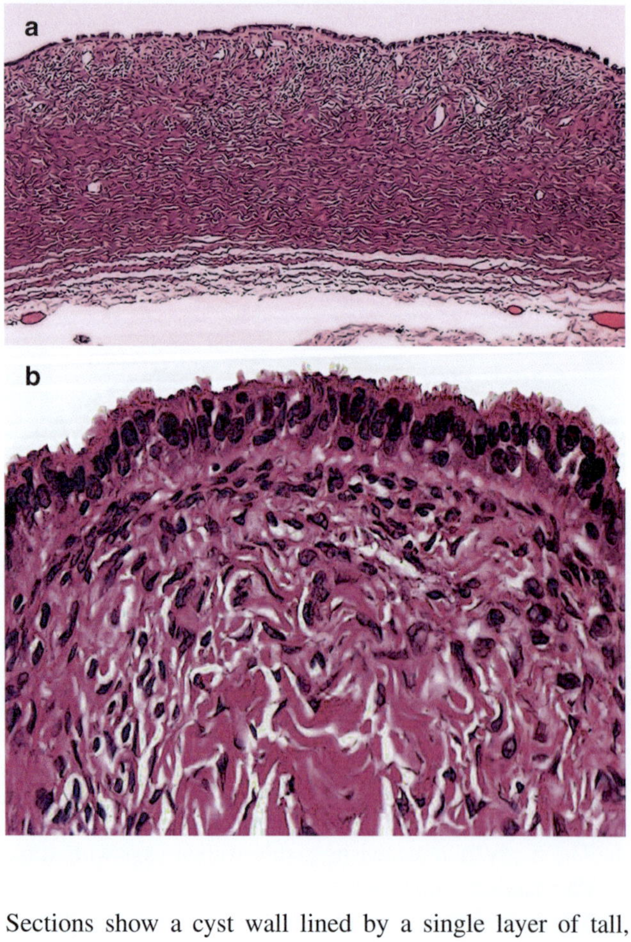

Sections show a cyst wall lined by a single layer of tall, columnar, ciliated cells resembling normal tubal epithelium. Stroma contains spindle fibroblasts.

Papillary Serous Cystadenocarcinoma of Ovary (a, b)

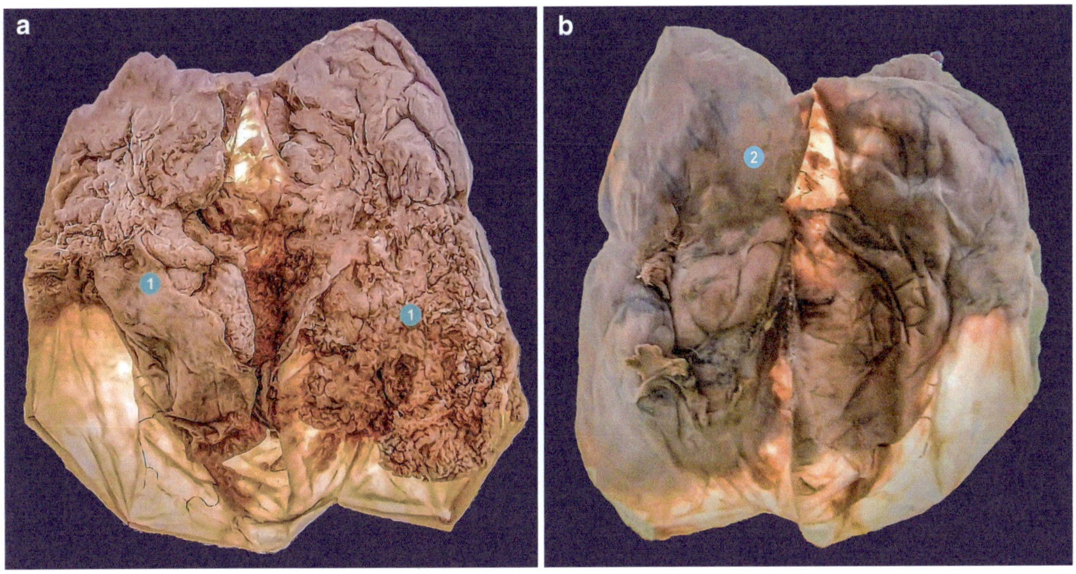

An ovarian tumor is mounted.

1. A unilocular cyst filled with a tumor mass composed of compound sessile papillae with solid areas and a bossy surface.
2. The tumor has a smooth outer surface.

Microscopic Picture of Invasive Papillary Serous Cystadenocarcinoma of Ovary (c–g)

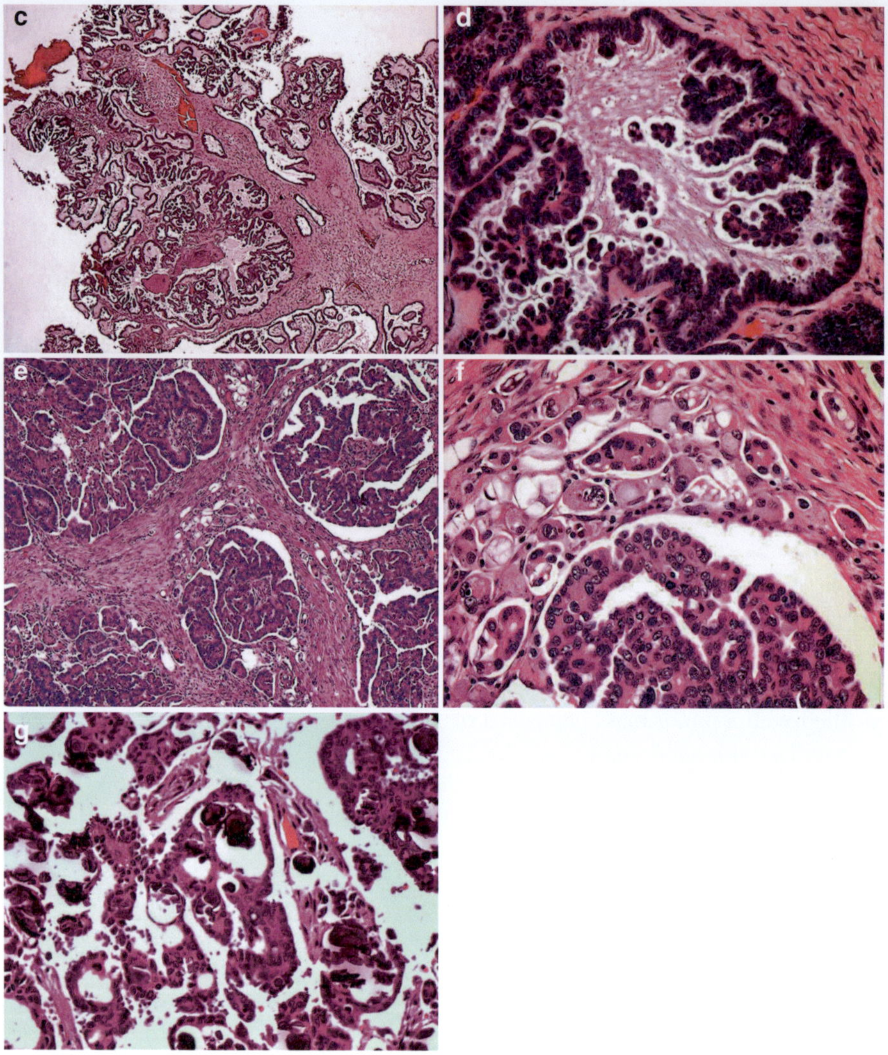

Sections show complex papillary tumors infiltrating the ovarian stroma. The papillae have fibrovascular cores and are lined with columnar to cuboidal cells with eosinophilic cytoplasm. The cells are pleomorphic with large irregular and hyperchromatic nuclei and prominent nucleoli. Areas of psammomatous calcification are observed.

Ancillary Tools

IHC [13]:

CK7, PAX8, WT1, ER (95%), PR (50%)

Ki67 proliferation index

Molecular/cytogenetics description [14]:

KRAS and BRAF mutations in 50–60% of cases

NRAS mutations

Few chromosomal abnormalities: 1p36 loss is the most significant copy number alteration.

BRAF mutations are rare in advanced-stage disease.

Mucinous Cystadenoma of Ovary

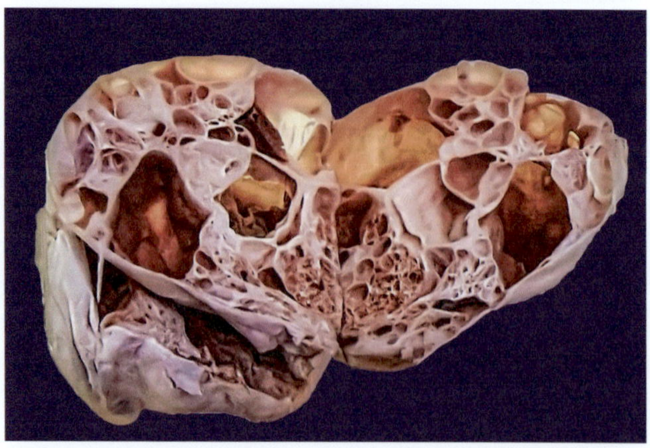

A sectioned ovarian tumor.

1. The tumor is a multilocular cystic mass with a smooth inner lining. Some loci are filled with mucin.

Microscopic Picture of Mucinous Cystadenoma of Ovary (a–c)

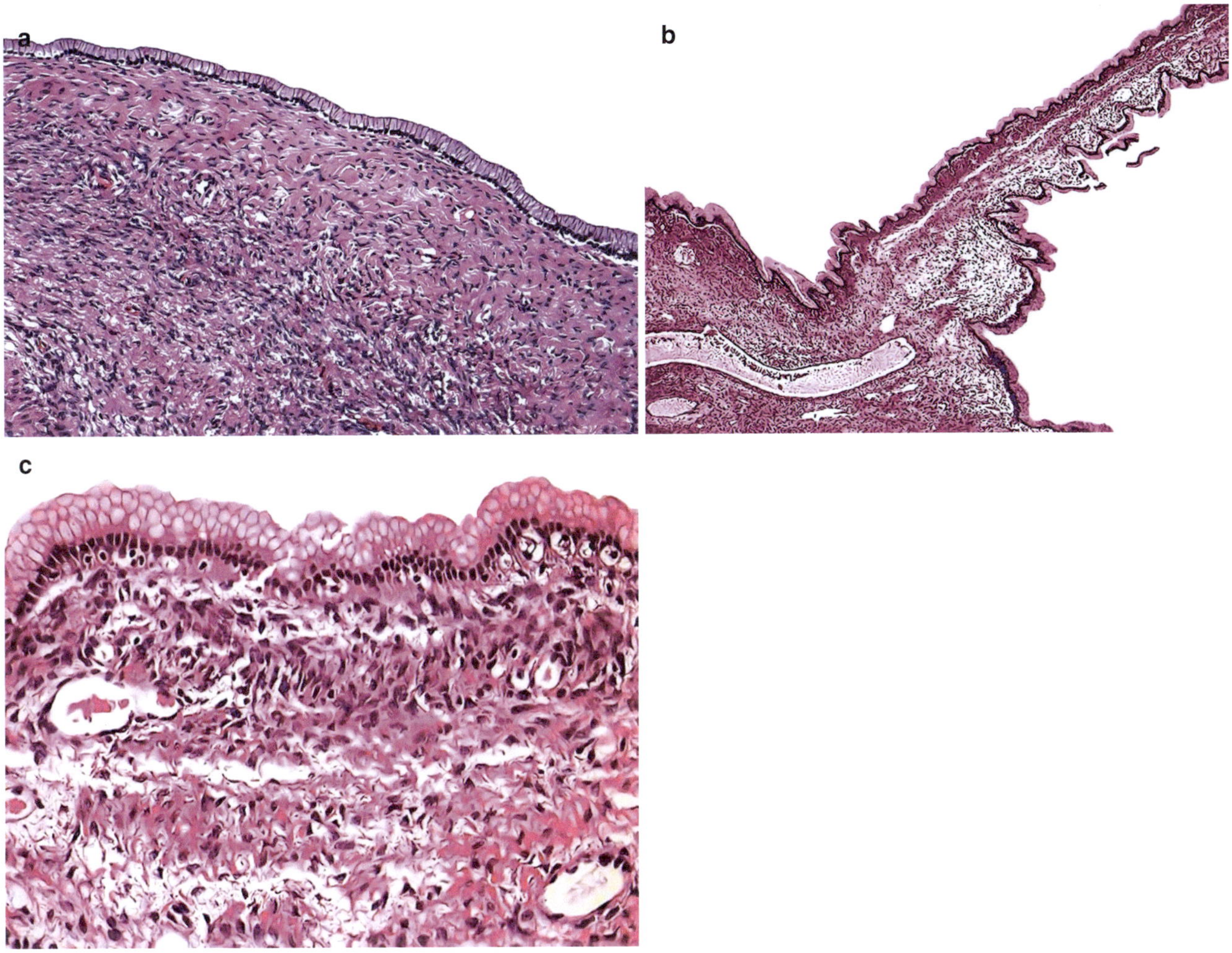

Sections show a cyst lined with a single layer of bland columnar mucinous epithelium with basal nuclei.

Mucinous Cystadenocarcinoma of Ovary

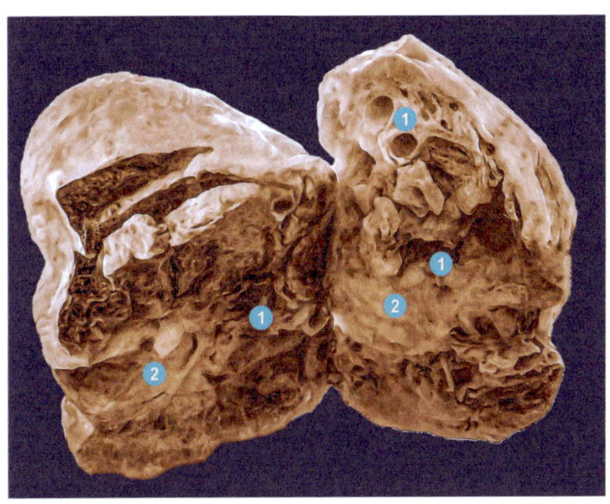

A sectioned ovarian tumor.

1. A multilocular cystic mass filled with thick mucin.
2. A solid area of the tumor

Microscopic Picture of Mucinous Cystadenocarcinoma of Ovary (a–f)

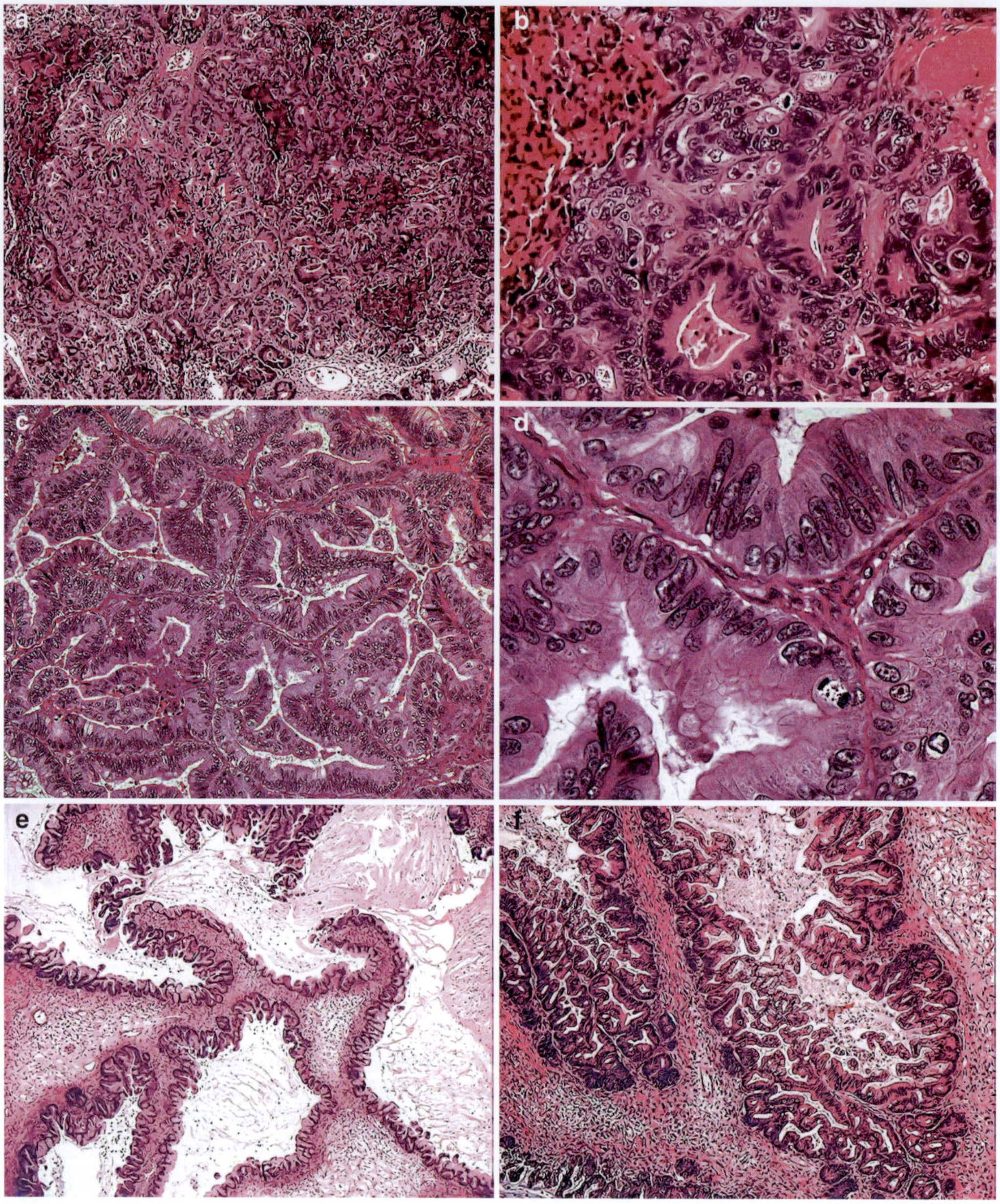

Sections show complex glandular structures lined with malignant intestinal-type epithelium and filled with mucin. Other areas show solid growth within the tumor, where the tumor cells form solid sheets, nests, and papillae instead of glandular structures. The tumor cells lining these glands are columnar, have abundant cytoplasm, and show nuclear atypia.

(a–d) **The expansile subtype** has no destructive stromal invasion but exhibits confluent or complex malignant glands (back to back glands) with or without minimal intervening stroma.

(e, f) **The infiltrative type** has stromal invasion in the form of glands, cell clusters, or individual cells, unsystematically infiltrating the stroma and often associated with a desmoplastic stromal reaction.

Ancillary Tools

IHC [15]:

CEA, CK7, CK20, CA125 (weak).

Molecular/cytogenetics description [16]:

K-ras mutations are a key early event for ovarian mucinous tumors. Oncogenic RAS has been linked to genomic instability through several mechanisms, including replication stress and shortened G2.

Bilateral Brenner Tumor of Ovaries (a, b)

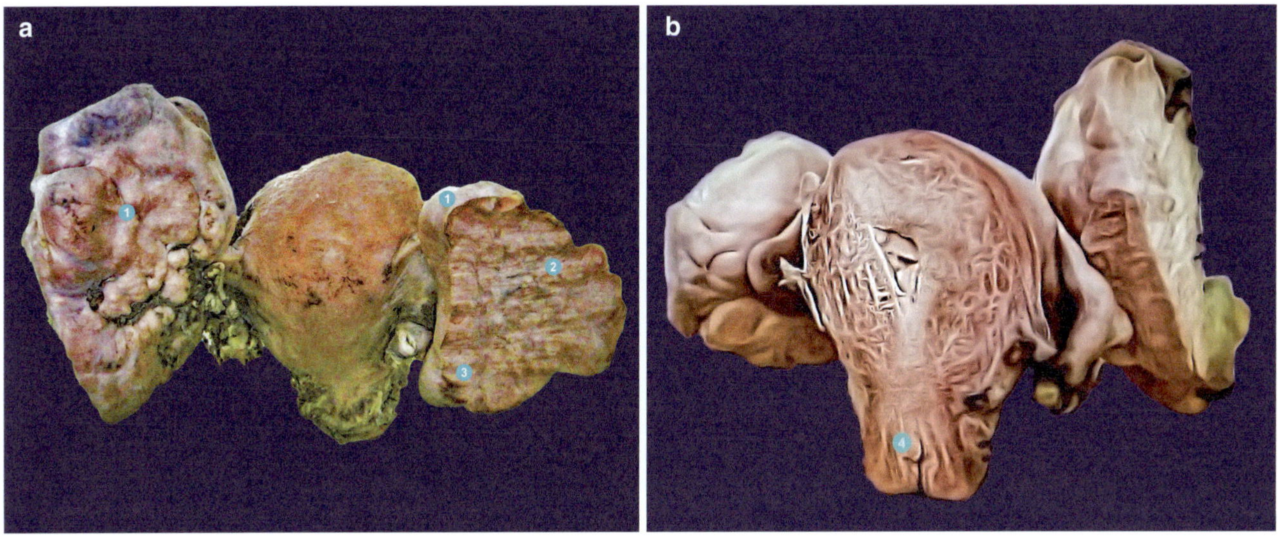

Hysterectomy with bilateral oophorectomy specimen is mounted

1. Bilateral solid, sharply demarcated, and firm ovarian tumors.
2. The cut-sectioned surfaces are yellow-white, lobulated, and have a fibroma-like appearance.
3. Small cystic spaces are seen in an area.
4. A small submucous fibroid is seen at the upper end of the cervical canal.

Microscopic Picture of Brenner Tumor of Ovaries (c–k)

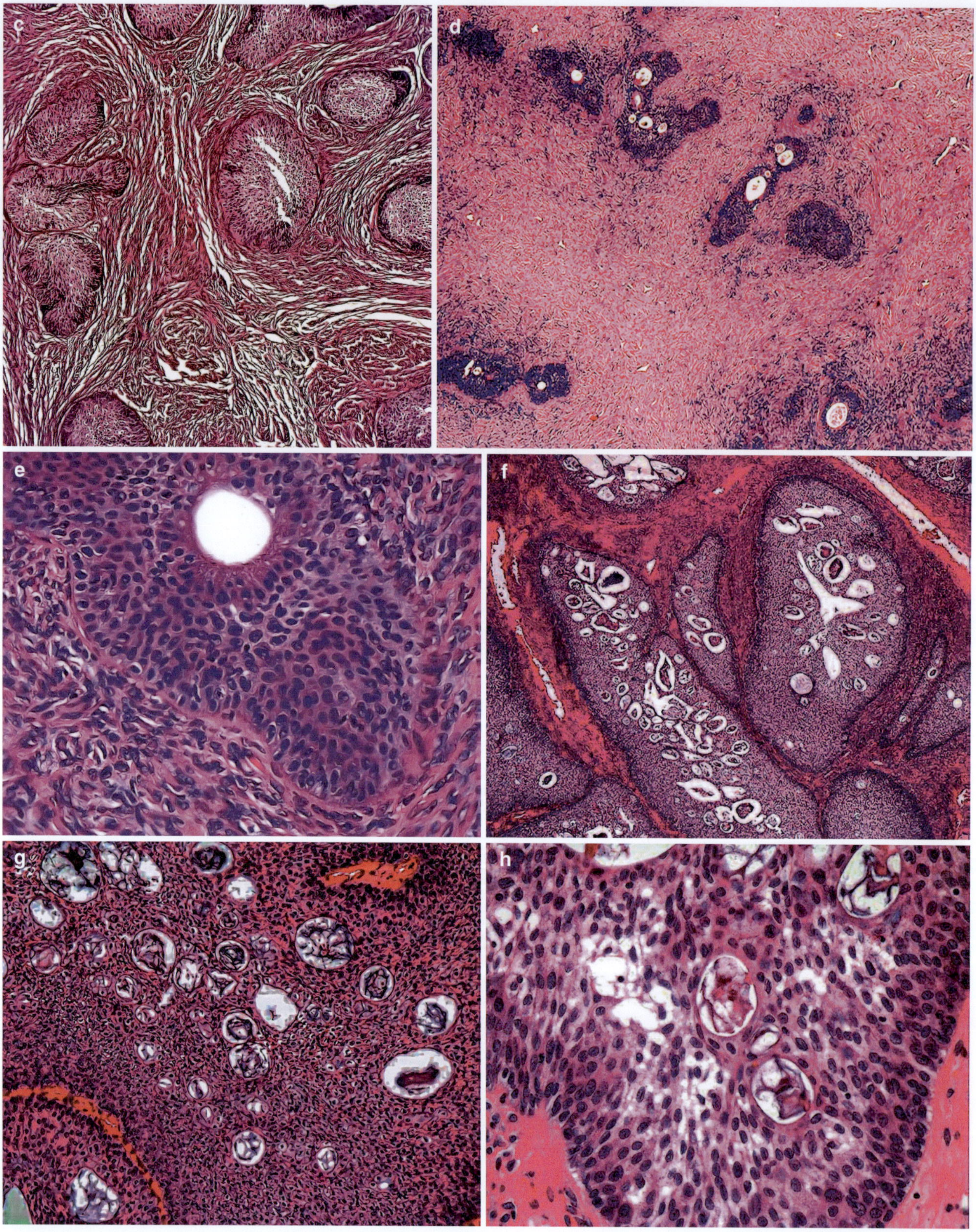

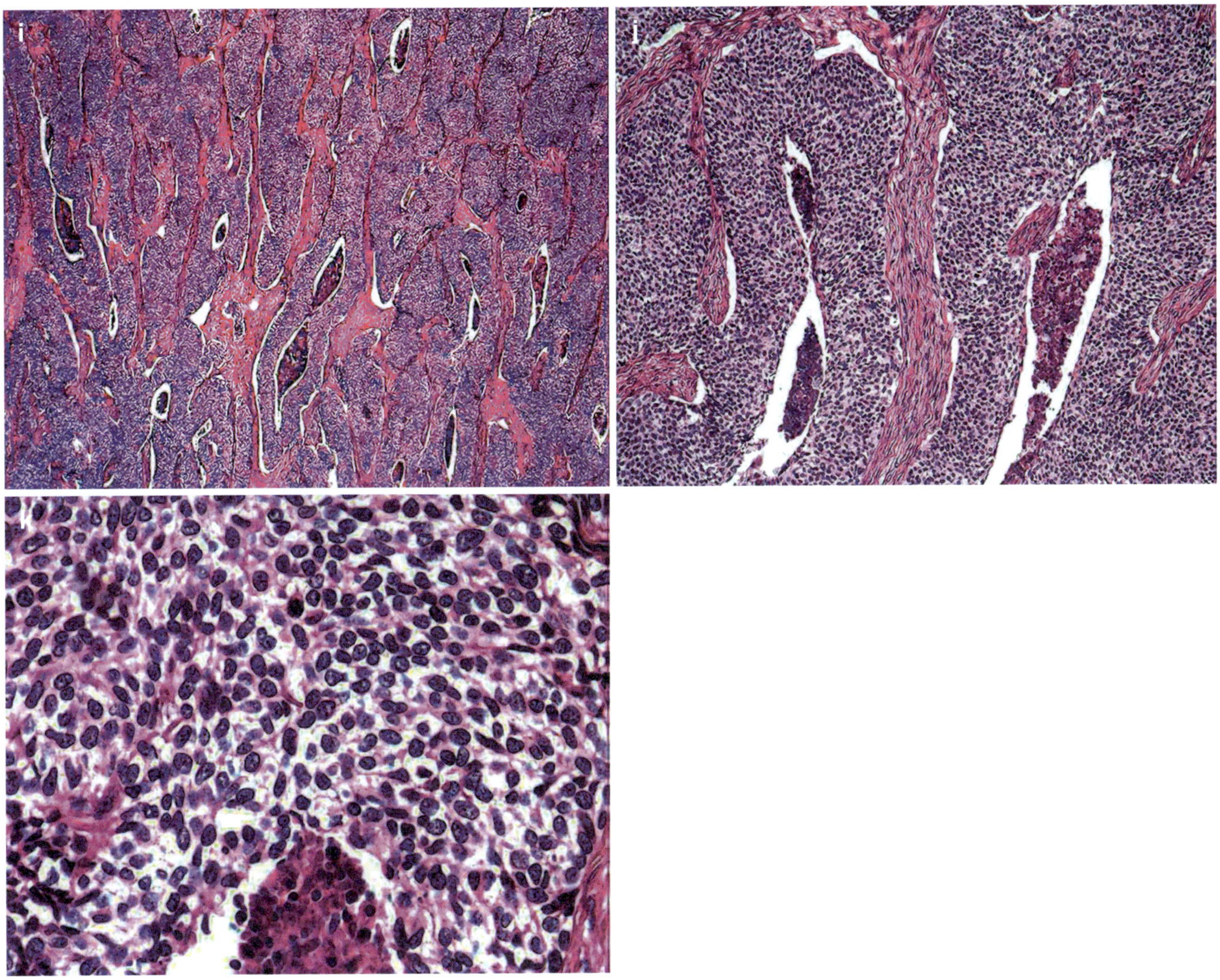

Sections show:

(c–e) **Benign Brenner Tumor:** Tumor cells are arranged in sharply defined solid clusters, nests, and trabeculae within a dense stromal component, which resembles ovarian fibroma or thecoma. In some areas, it becomes hyalinized. The transitional cells have pale eosinophilic or clear cytoplasm, uniform round or ovoid nuclei, which may have grooves, fine chromatin, and punctate nucleoli. Some of the nests show central cystic spaces containing mucin or eosinophilic secretions. The cystic spaces are lined by transitional, flattened, or columnar epithelium. There is no cytologic atypia, and mitotic activity is not increased.

(f–h) **Borderline Brenner Tumor**: Complex glandular and papillary formation. Squamous metaplasia and prominent mucinous change are seen within some nests. Nuclear atypia including hyperchromatic nuclei, coarse chromatin clumping, prominent nucleoli, and increased mitotic activity may be observed.

(i–k) **Malignant Brenner Tumor:** Stromal invasion by carcinoma with transitional cell features, with irregular nests of cells and single cells in an infiltrative pattern

Squamous or mucinous differentiation and focal areas of necrosis may be observed.

Ancillary Tools

IHC [17]:

GATA3, p63, CK7, S100, AR, Uroplakin, Thrombomodulin.

Clear Cell Carcinoma of the Ovary

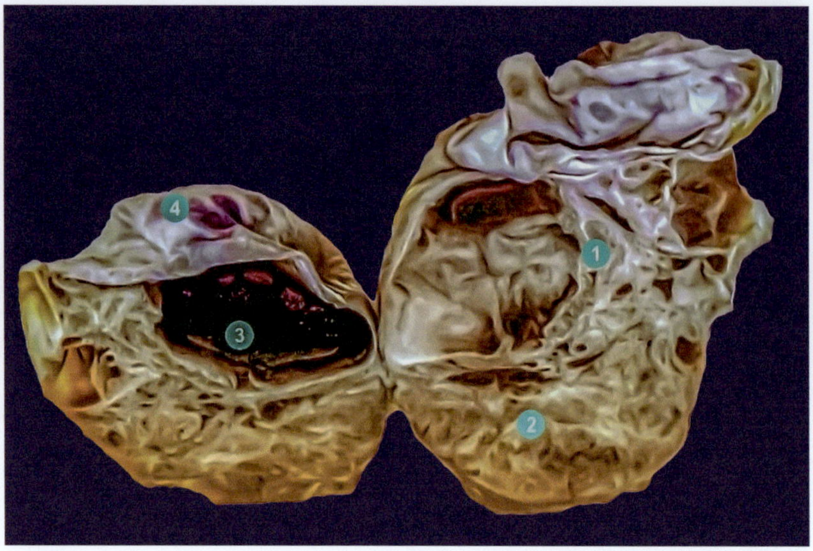

An ovarian tumor is mounted.

1. Pale yellow to brown appearance
2. The cut section is mainly cystic, with fleshy nodules protruding into the cyst lumen.
3. Cyst contains chocolate brown fluid.
4. An area of hemorrhage

Microscopic Picture of Clear Cell Carcinoma of Ovary (a–e)

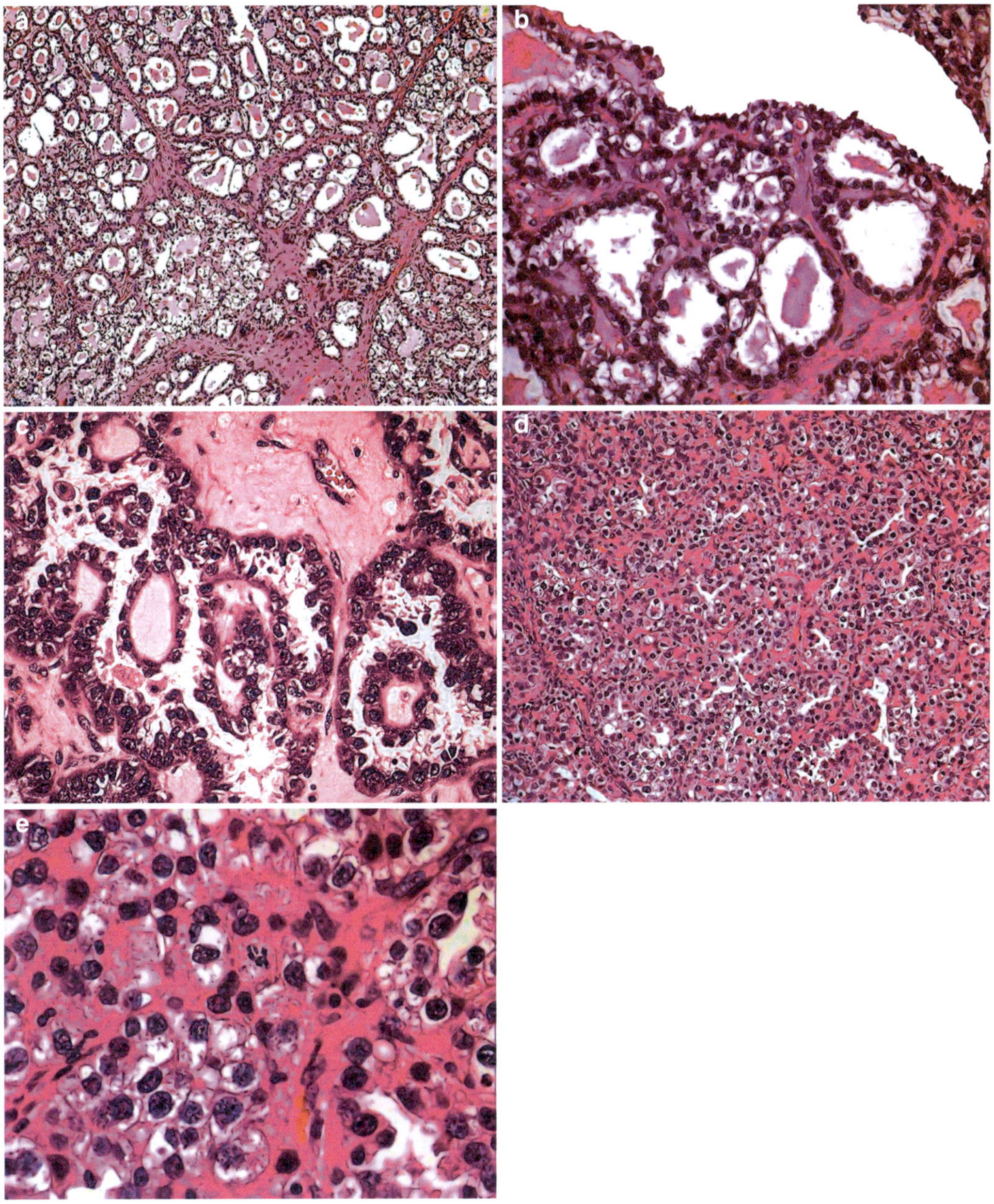

Sections show a mixture of tubulocystic, papillary, and solid growth patterns.

(a, b) The **tubulocystic pattern** is formed of variably sized tubules and cysts, with or without intraluminal dense eosinophilic secretions and outpouchings lined by a single layer of hobnail, cuboidal, or flattened cells.

(c) **Papillary/micropapillary pattern** is formed of edematous stroma and is lined by 1–2 layers of cuboidal tumor cells with uniformly atypical nuclei and clear to pale eosinophilic cytoplasm with the presence of hobnail cells and micropapillary tufts.

(d, e) A s**olid pattern** is composed of tumor cells with uniformly atypical nuclei and clear to pale eosinophilic cytoplasm.

Ancillary Tools

IHC [18]:

CK7

EMA

PAX8

HNF1β: sensitive but not specific

Napsin A: specific with intermediate sensitivity

AMACR: specific but not sensitive

p53: aberrant in 7–24% of cases

PAS-positive diastase-sensitive material (glycogen) in clear cells, diastase-resistant intracytoplasmic material in targetoid cells.

Molecular/cytogenetics description [19]:

Loss of function mutations in ARID1A, a tumor suppressor gene from the SWI/SNF chromatin remodeling complex (50%)

PIK3CA mutations (40%), often associated with ARID1A mutations

TERT promoter mutations (16%)

KRAS mutations (10%)

8.5.2 Germ Cell Tumors

Mature Cystic Teratoma (Dermoid Cyst) of Ovary

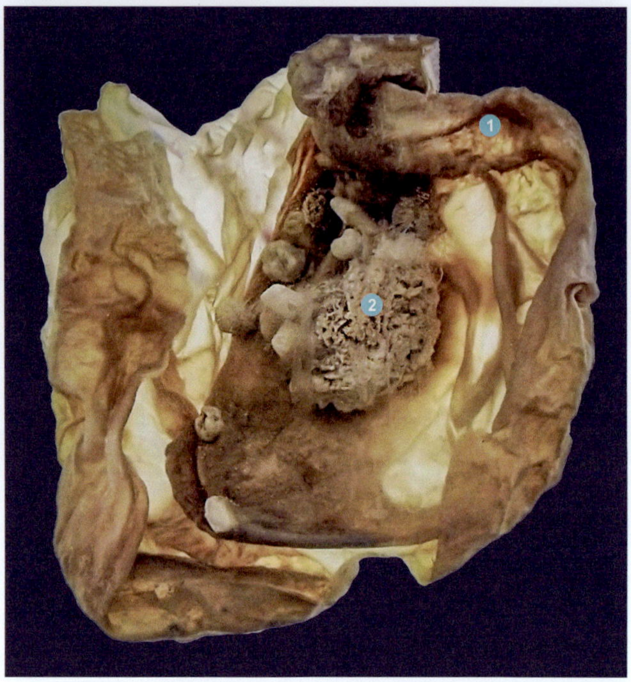

An opened ovarian tumor is mounted.

1. A unilocular, thin-walled cystic mass.
2. A solid area (genital ridge) to which many teeth-like structures are attached is seen in the center.

Microscopic Picture of Mature Cystic Teratoma (Dermoid Cyst) of Ovary (a–d)

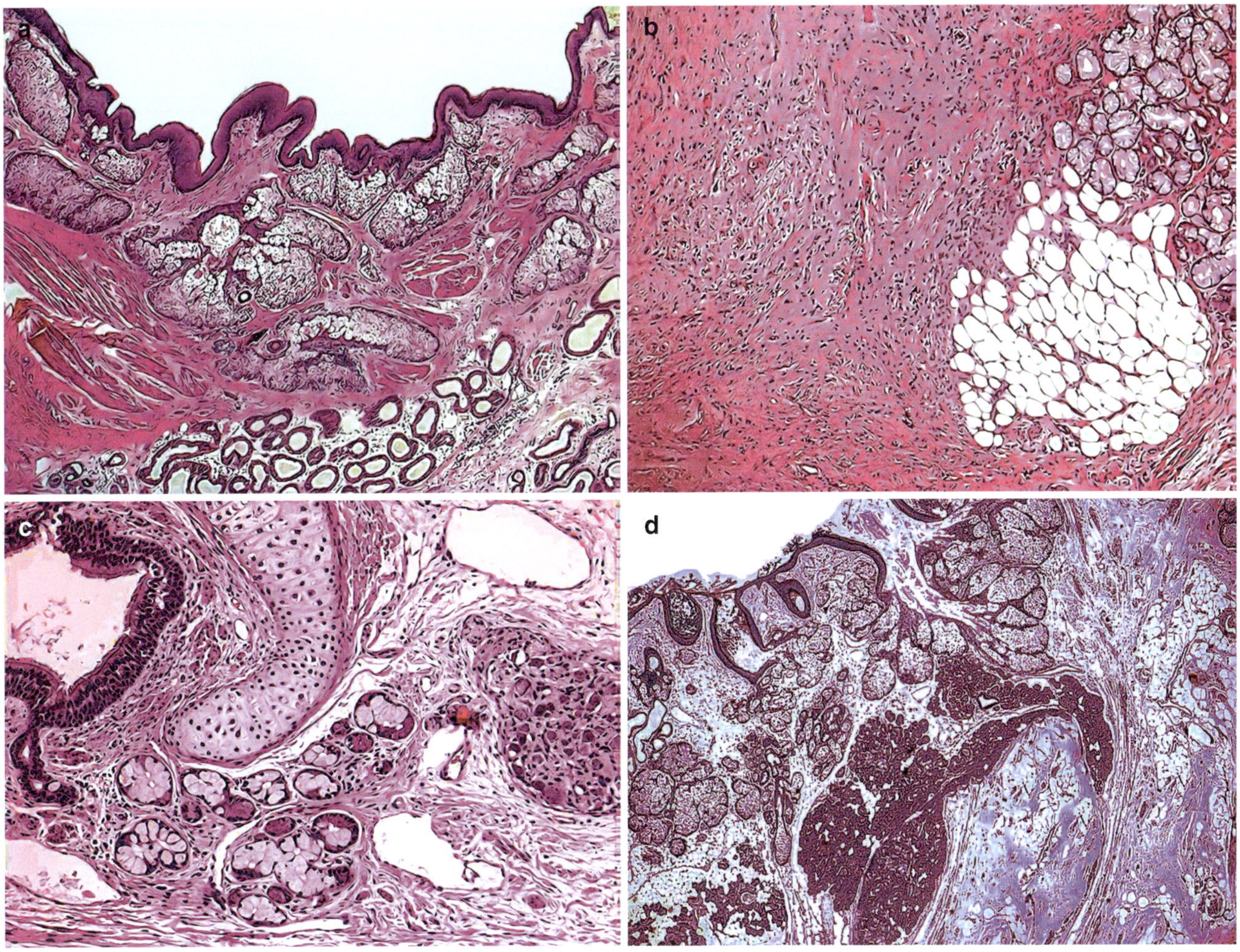

Sections show variable mature benign structures representing the 3 germ layers: ectoderm as squamous epithelium, sebaceous glands, hair follicles, and mature neural tissue; mesoderm as cartilage and fibro-adipose tissue; and endoderm as respiratory epithelium and salivary glands.

Mature Cystic Teratoma (Dermoid Cyst) of Ovary

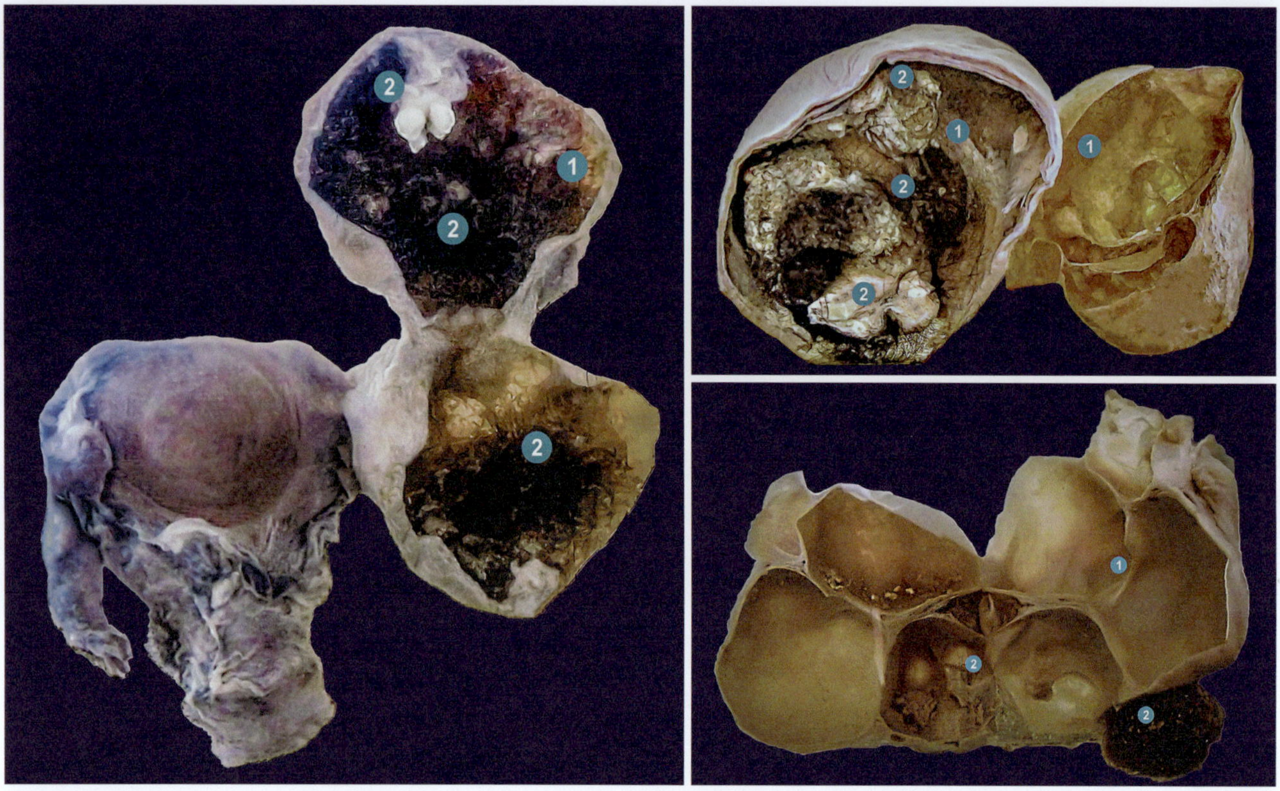

An opened ovarian tumor is mounted.

1. A multilocular, thin-walled cystic mass.
2. A solid area (genital ridge) in one locus and a tuft of hairs in another one are observed.

Yolk Sac (Endodermal Sinus) Tumor

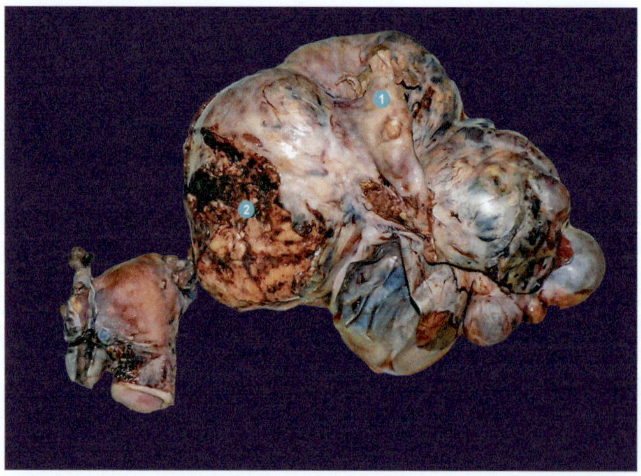

The uterus and one ovary are mounted.

1. A large, well-encapsulated mass with a smooth glistening and nodular external surface.
2. The sectioned surface is solid and cystic and shows soft, gray-to-yellow tissue with extensive areas of hemorrhage and necrosis.

Microscopic Picture of Yolk Sac (Endodermal Sinus) Tumor (a–f)

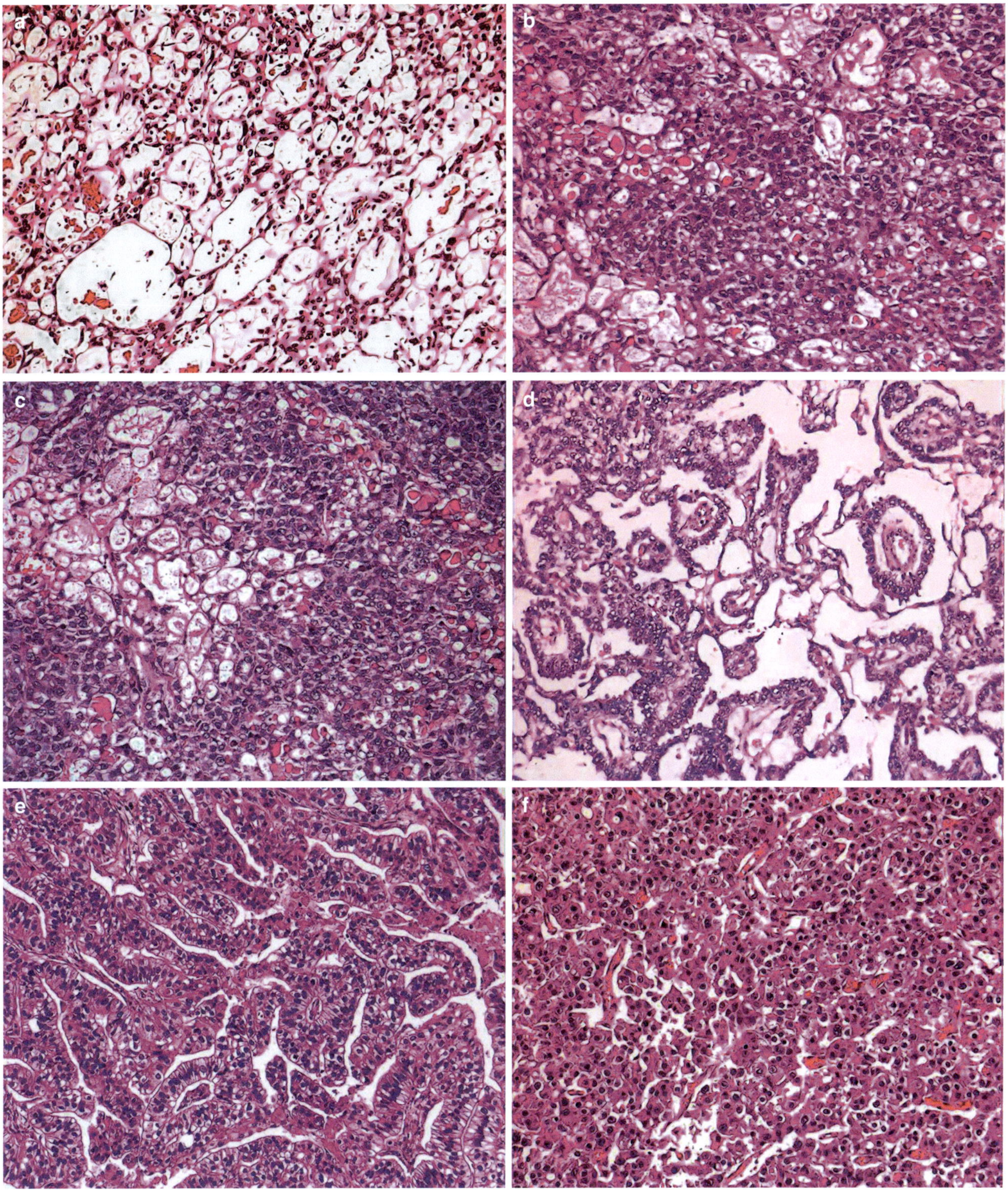

Sections show multiple histologic patterns.

(a-c) Reticular/microcystic pattern formed of a loose meshwork of anastomosing channels and variably sized cysts (macro or micro cysts) lined by primitive tumor cells with varying amounts of clear to eosinophilic cytoplasm. Cysts contain eosinophilic hyaline globules and amorphous, eosinophilic acellular basement membrane-like material.

(d) Endodermal sinus pattern formed of an anastomosing network of labyrinthine-like spaces lined by tumor cells. Formation of vaguely glomeruloid perivascular structures (Schiller-Duval bodies) is the hallmark of yolk sac tumors (but their absence does not rule out the diagnosis). They are rounded to elongated papillary structures containing a central fibrovascular core with a single central vessel, surrounded by tumor cells projecting into a cystic/sinusoidal space (resembling immature glomeruli).

(e) Papillary pattern: Papillae containing fibrovascular cores lined by pleomorphic tumor cells with brisk mitoses Fibrovascular cores may be hyalinized

(f) Hepatoid pattern: It is composed of cells with eosinophilic, uniform, or granular cytoplasm, showing a solid pattern and considerable resemblance to hepatocytes.

Ancillary Tools

IHC [20]:

SALL4: a marker of primitive germ cell differentiation

AFP: highly specific but 60% sensitive, often patchy/focal and weak

Glypican 3: less specific but stronger expression

HNF1β

Pancytokeratin

GATA3: positive in reticular/microcystic, papillary, and polyvesicular vitelline patterns but not in the glandular pattern

HepPar1: positive in glandular and hepatoid patterns

CEA, albumin: positive in hepatoid pattern

TTF1: positive in foregut/respiratory pattern

CDX2: positive in glandular intestinal type pattern

Villin: positive in reticular/microcystic and glandular intestinal type patterns.

Dysgerminoma of the Ovary (a, b)

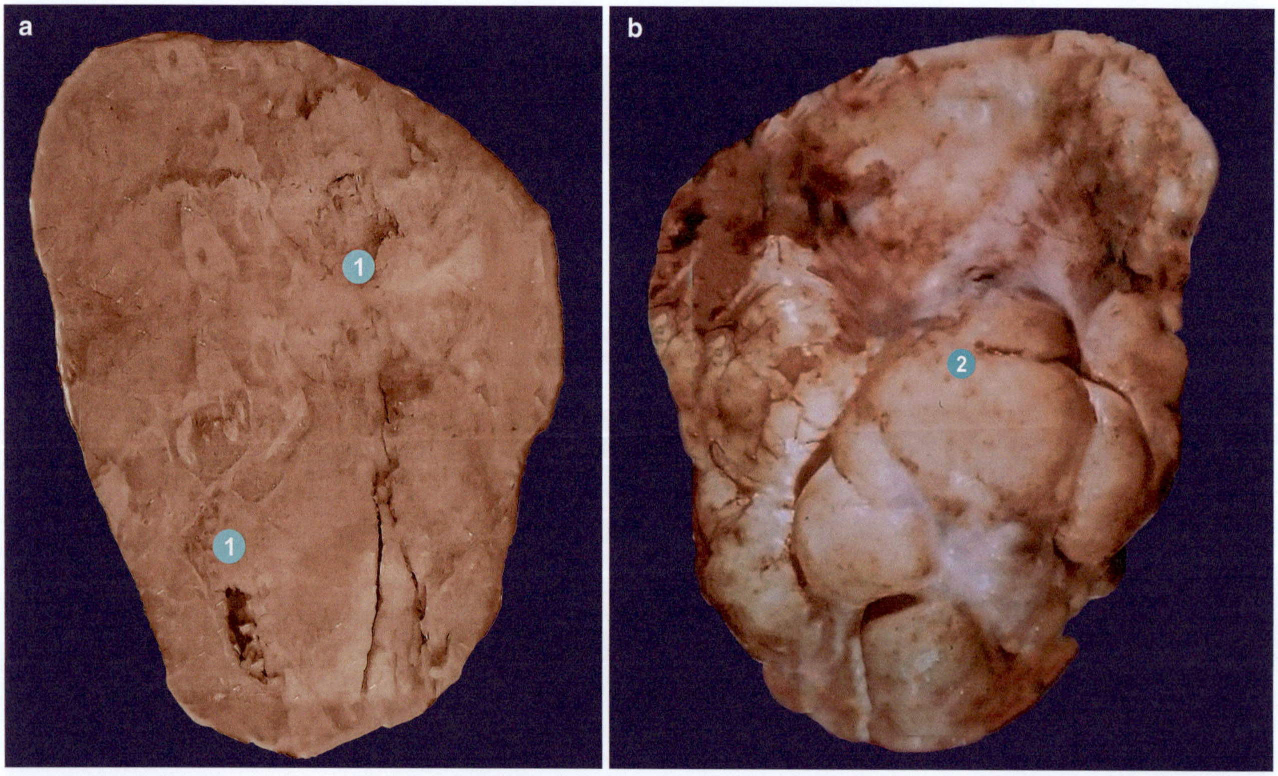

An ovarian tumor is mounted.

1. Half of a large tumor with solid consistency and a yellow-tan or cream color appearance with focal areas of necrosis.
2. The capsule is thick with surface lobulation.

Microscopic Picture of Dysgerminoma of Ovary (c)

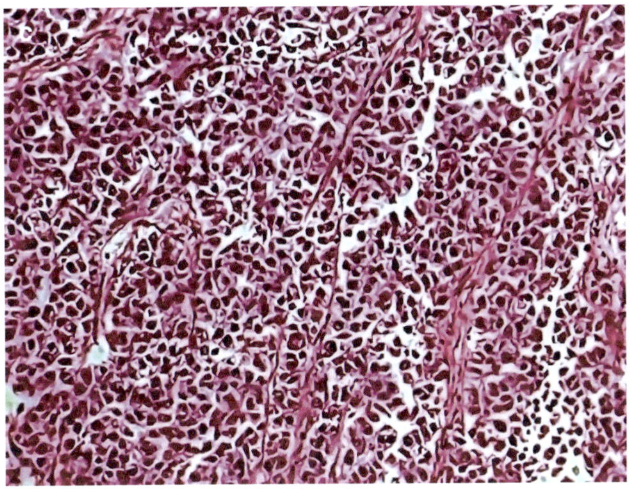

The section shows a picture that resembles seminomas. The tumor is composed of monomorphic tumor cells arranged in trabeculae, cords, or nests separated by delicate fibrous septa.

Ancillary Tools

IHC [20]:

OCT3/4 (nuclear), CD117 (KIT; membranous), D2-40 (membranous and cytoplasmic)

NANOG (nuclear) and SALL4 (nuclear) stem cell markers

PLAP (membranous and cytoplasmic)

May focally express keratins with cytoplasmic dots or rim-like staining: CAM 5.2 (positive in up to 10% of tumor cells in <50% of dysgerminomas); AE1/AE3 and CK7 (positive in up to 10% of tumor cells in <25% of dysgerminomas).

hCG, inhibin, glypican 3, and CK7 can highlight syncytiotrophoblastic giant cells; they can search for these cells in patients with moderate serum hCG elevation.

Molecular/cytogenetics description [21]:

Isochromosome 12p in 81%

KIT mutations in exon 17 codon 816 or KIT amplification were detected in approximately 33% of cases and associated with advanced-stage presentation.

8.5.3 Sex Cord-Stromal Tumors

Ovarian Fibroma (a, b)

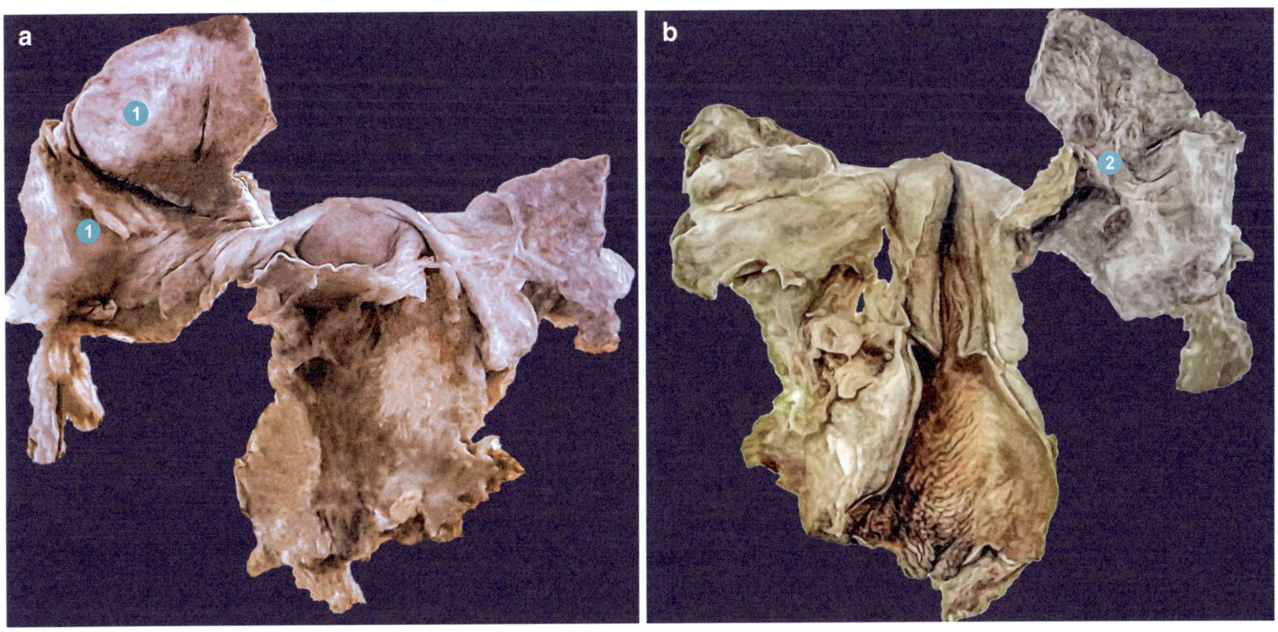

The uterus and one ovary are mounted.

1. The ovary is replaced by a large, pale, solid, and encapsulated tumor.
2. The cut section is lobulated, whorl-like, and gray-white.

Microscopic Picture of Ovarian Fibroma (c–e)

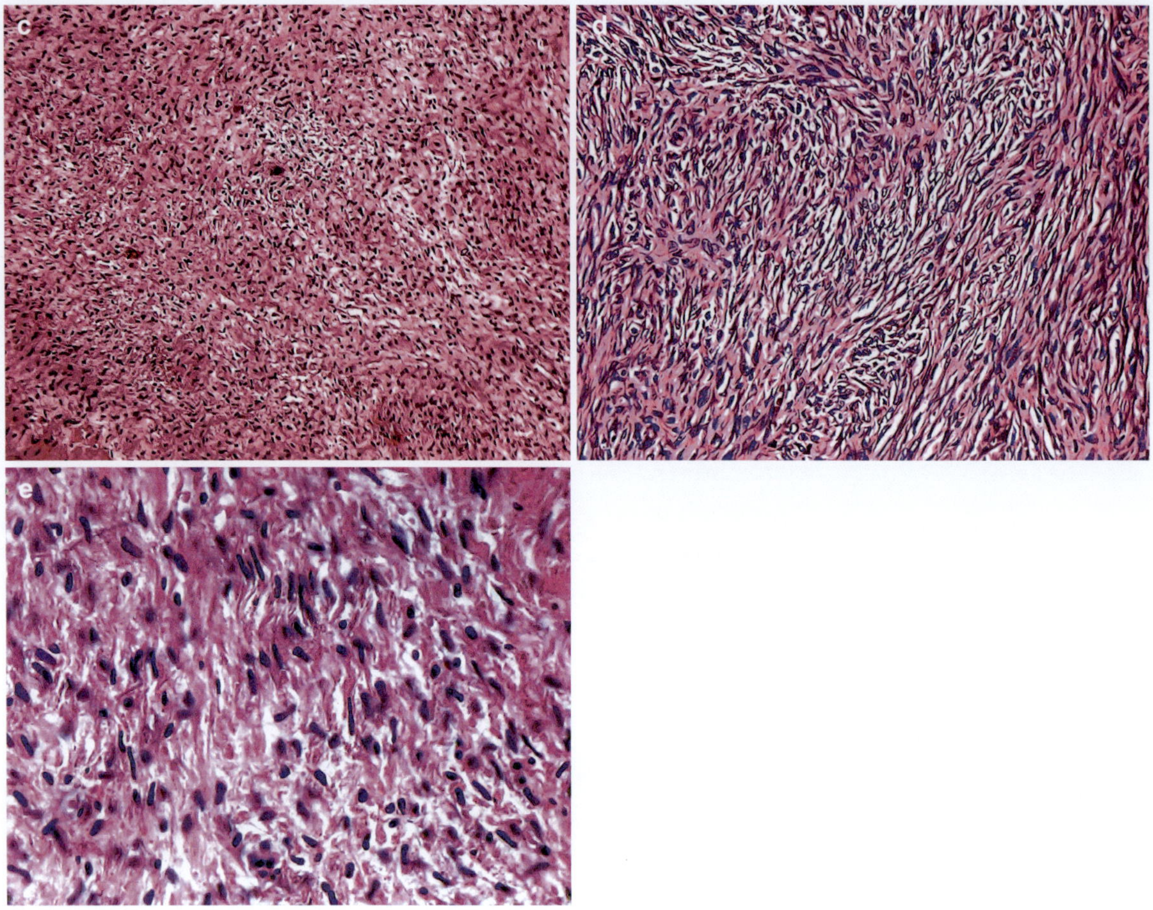

Sections show densely cellular fascicular growth of tumor cells with little intercellular collagen. The cells have bland spindled to ovoid nuclei with pointy ends and scant eosinophilic cytoplasm blending with surrounding stroma.

Ancillary Tools

IHC [22]:

- WT1
- SF1
- FOXL2
- Inhibin: 50% of cases, often focal or weak
- Vimentin
- CD56
- ER beta
- PR
- SMA

Special Stain:

Reticulin: differentiates fibroma (individual pericellular reticulin staining pattern) from a diffuse type of adult granulosa cell tumor (nested reticulin staining pattern).

Adult Granulosa Cell Tumor of Ovary

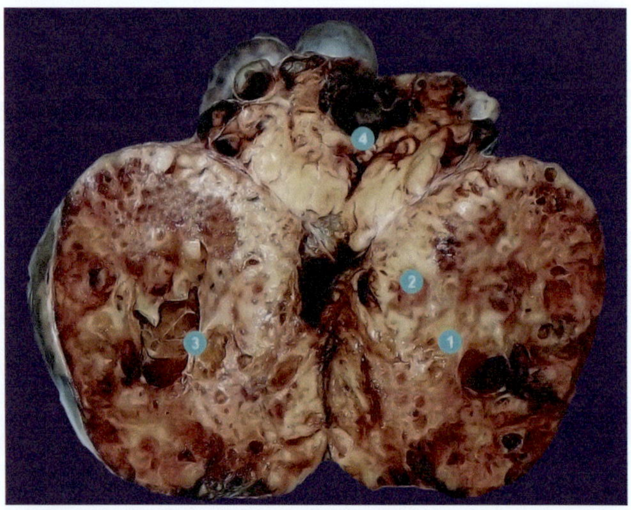

An opened, encapsulated, large ovarian tumor is mounted.

1. The cut section is mainly solid with cystic areas.
2. The solid areas are yellow.
3. The cystic areas are hemorrhagic.
4. Focal areas of hemorrhage and necrosis are seen.

Microscopic Picture of Adult Granulosa Cell Tumor of Ovary (a–h)

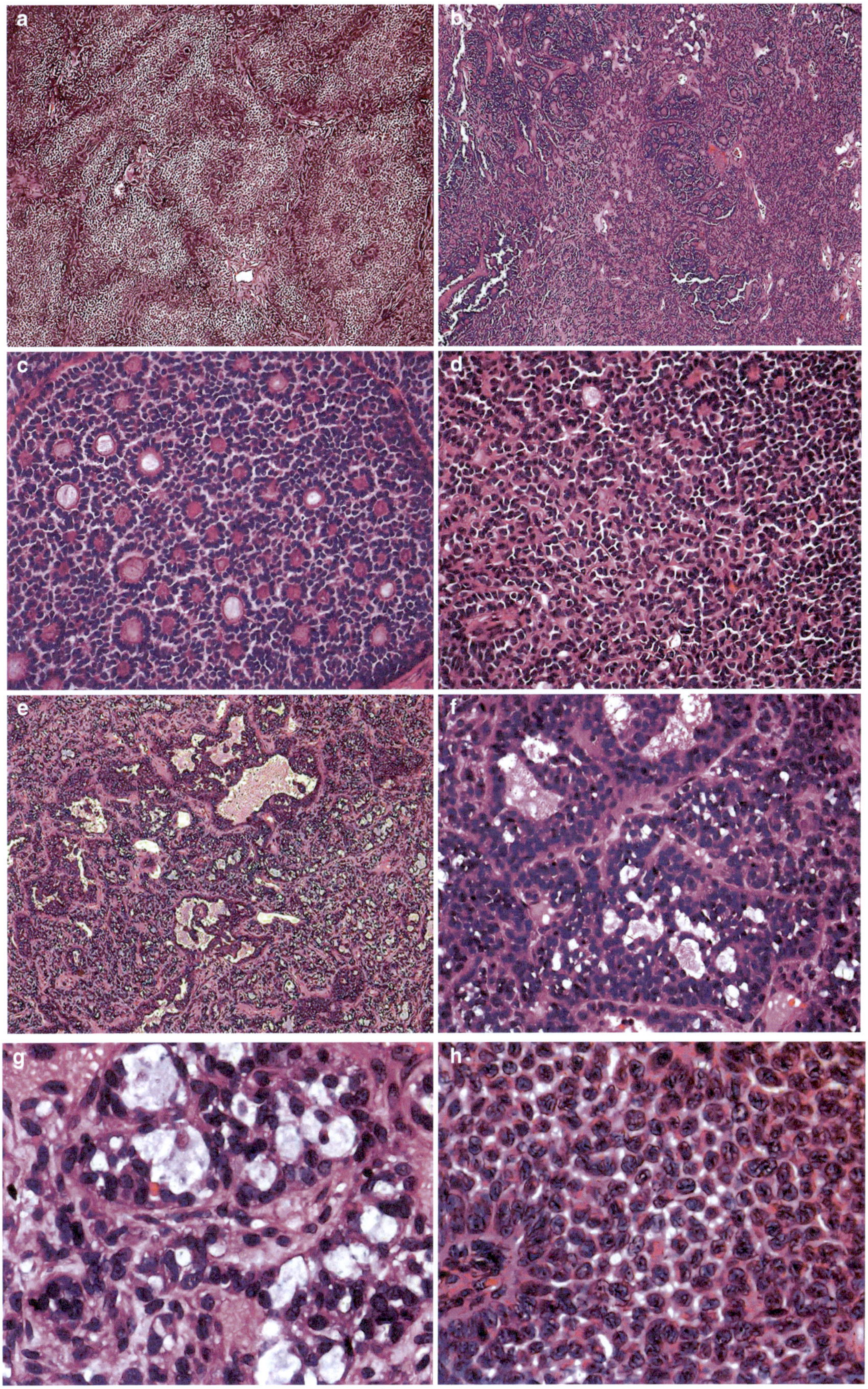

Sections show a mixed growth pattern formed of:

(a) **Diffuse pattern** (the most common

(b–d) **Microfollicular pattern:** (resembling Call-Exner bodies of the Graafian follicles: small follicle-like structures filled with eosinophilic material)

(e–g) A s**olid pattern** of cells is punctured by oval to round follicles differing in size and containing basophilic fluid.

Other patterns include trabecular and macrofollicular (the least common). Luteinized adult type (such as during pregnancy): rare (1%) if extensive (>50%), plump cells with moderate to abundant eosinophilic cytoplasm, conspicuous nucleoli, no nuclear grooves, myxoid, or edematous stroma.

(h) The tumor cells are small, bland, cuboidal to polygonal cells with scant cytoplasm and pale, uniform angulated, and usually grooved nuclei (coffee bean). Stroma is hypervascular with variable amounts of fibroblasts.

Ancillary Tools

IHC [23]:

FOXL2 immunostaining is a sensitive (80%) and specific (99%) marker for sex cord-stromal tumors (SCST), superior to α-inhibin and calretinin, and is positive in almost all SCST (98%).

SF1: a most sensitive marker for this as well as the most common sex cord stromal tumors.

Inhibin A: a more specific marker

Calretinin

Low molecular weight cytokeratin (CAM5.2, AE1/AE3): 30–60%, usually dot-like or globoid perinuclear pattern

S100: 50%

CD99: 70%

EGFR: 65% of primary and 85% of recurrent

Vimentin, WT1, CD56, and SMA

Special Stain:

Reticulin: shows lack of pericellular staining and highlights nests or large groups of granulosa cells and vessels; helps differentiate diffuse patterns from fibrothecoma.

Molecular/cytogenetics description [23]:

FOXL2 402C → G (C134W) somatic mutation is highly sensitive and specific for the diagnosis of adult GCT.

More than half of cases show chromosomal imbalances.

The most common chromosomal abnormalities are trisomy 12, trisomy 14, monosomy 16/16q deletion, and monosomy 22.

Ovarian Sex-Cord Stromal Tumor with Annular Tubules

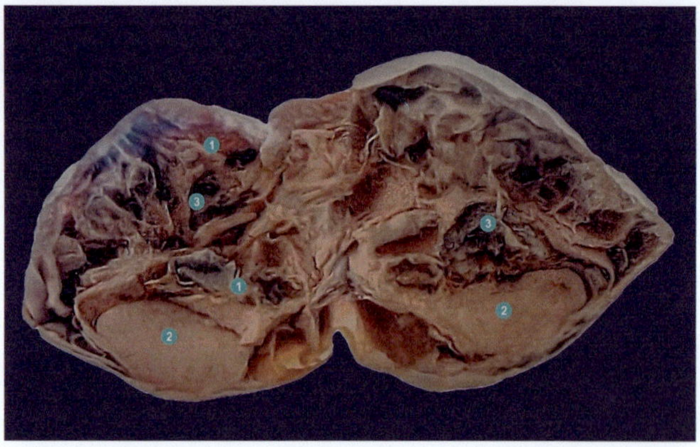

An opened ovarian tumor is mounted.

1. The cut section is solid with cystic areas.
2. The solid area is yellow-tan.
3. A focal area of hemorrhage and necrosis is observed.

Microscopic Picture of Ovarian Sex-Cord Stromal Tumor with Annular Tubules (a–c)

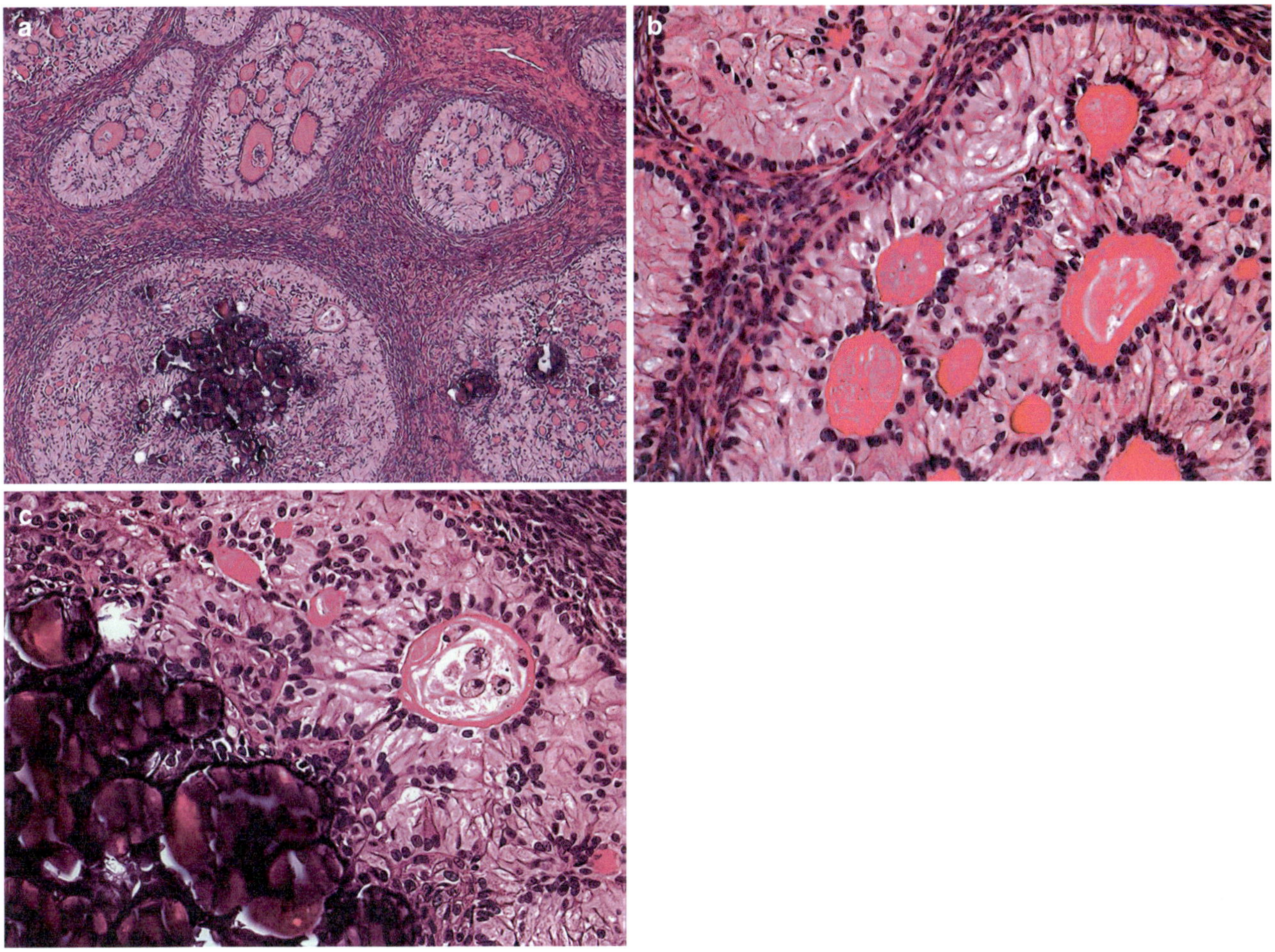

Sections show variably sized round nests of sharply delineated simple and complex tubules containing basement membrane-like material, which may also be present around the tubules. Sertoliform tubules are classified as annular by their arrangement as small concentric secondary ring-shaped acini peripherally arranged around the circumference of a larger tubule. Tall cells with an ample amount of pale cytoplasm and basally located round nuclei often with antipodal nuclear distribution within the tubules. Tumors associated with Peutz–Jeghers syndrome show calcifications within the tubules.

Ancillary Tools

IHC [24]:

- Calretinin
- WT1
- Inhibin
- SF1
- FOXL2
- CD56

Molecular/cytogenetics description [25]:

If syndromic, associated with a germline STK11 gene mutation on chromosome 19p13.3

8.5.4 Metastatic Tumors

Bilateral Krukenberg's Tumor of Ovaries (a, b)

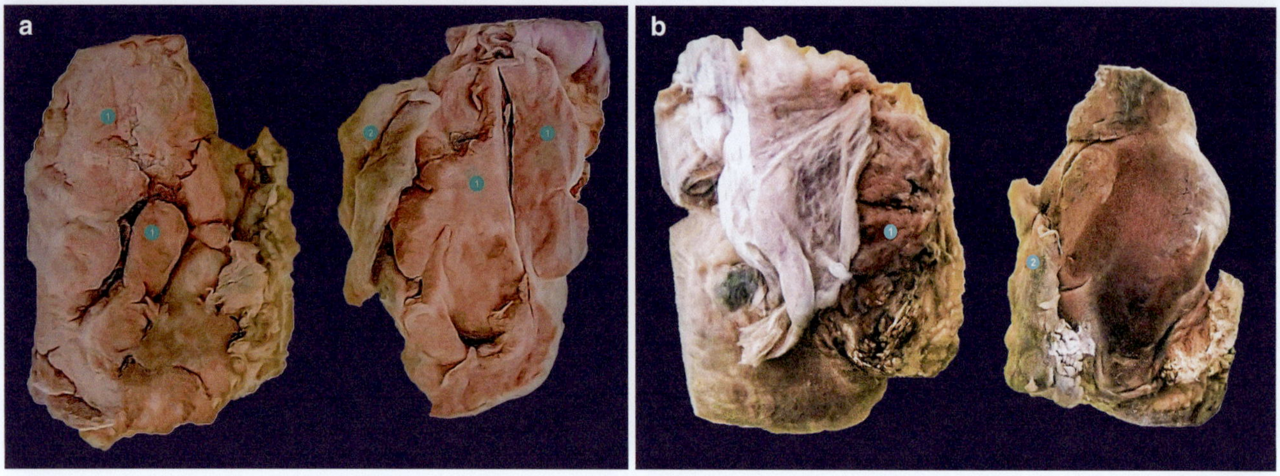

Both ovaries are mounted.

1. They are enlarged and solid, with an irregular bossy surface.
2. A loop of the intestine is adherent to one of them.

Microscopic Picture of Krukenberg's Tumor of Ovaries (c–e)

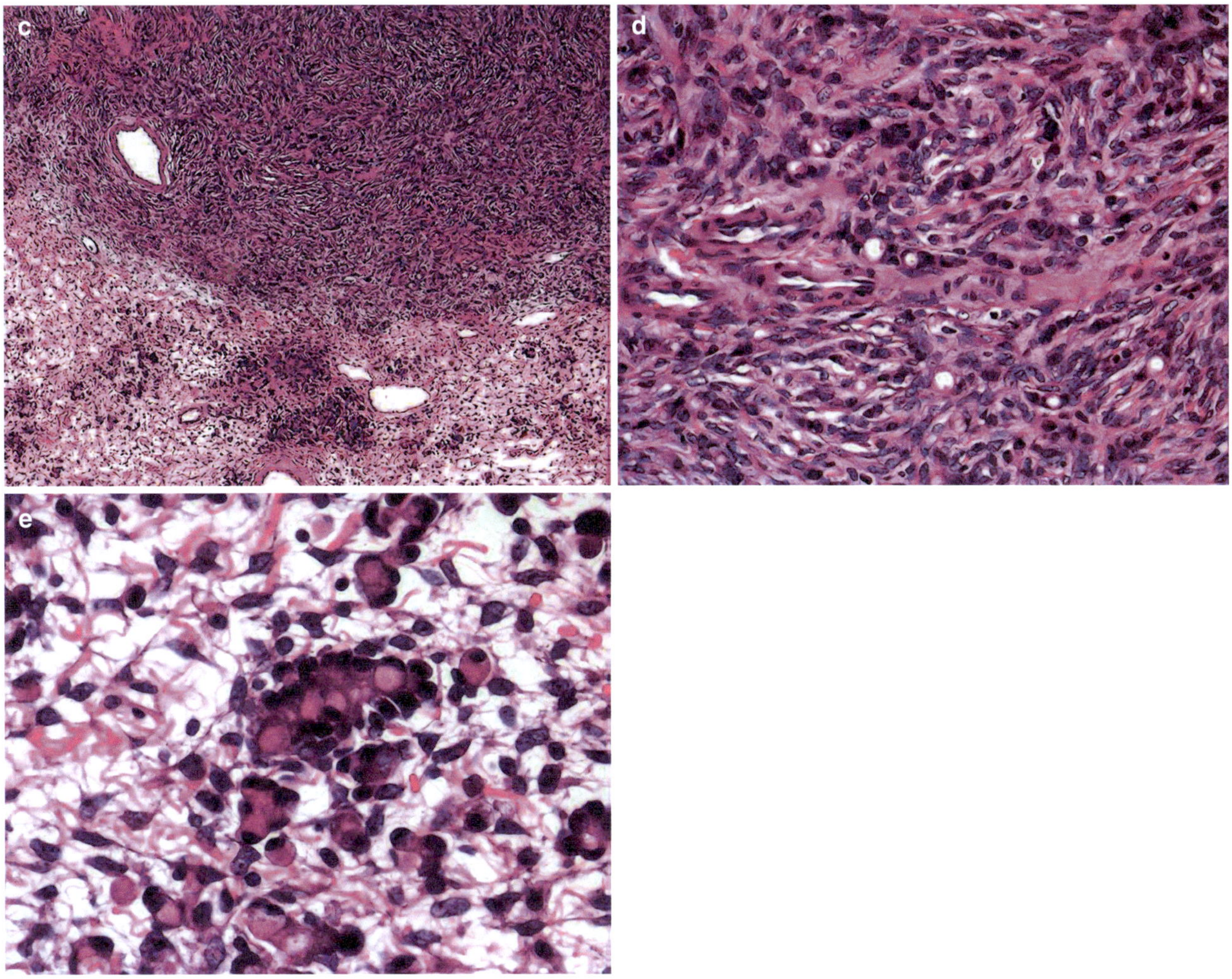

Sections show the involvement of the ovarian surface and superficial cortex with an infiltrative growth pattern and stromal desmoplasia with the presence of hypercellular and hypocellular (edematous) regions in which malignant signet ring cells are seen in clusters.

8.6 Disorders of Pregnancy

8.6.1 Ectopic Tubal Pregnancy

Ectopic Tubal Pregnancy

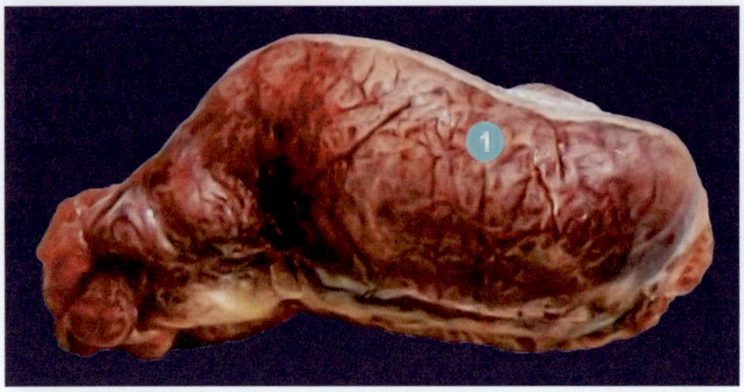

A salpingectomy specimen is mounted

1. The mid and distal ends of the tube are dilated and sausage-shaped. The outer surface is congested.

Microscopic Picture of Ectopic Pregnancy (a, b)

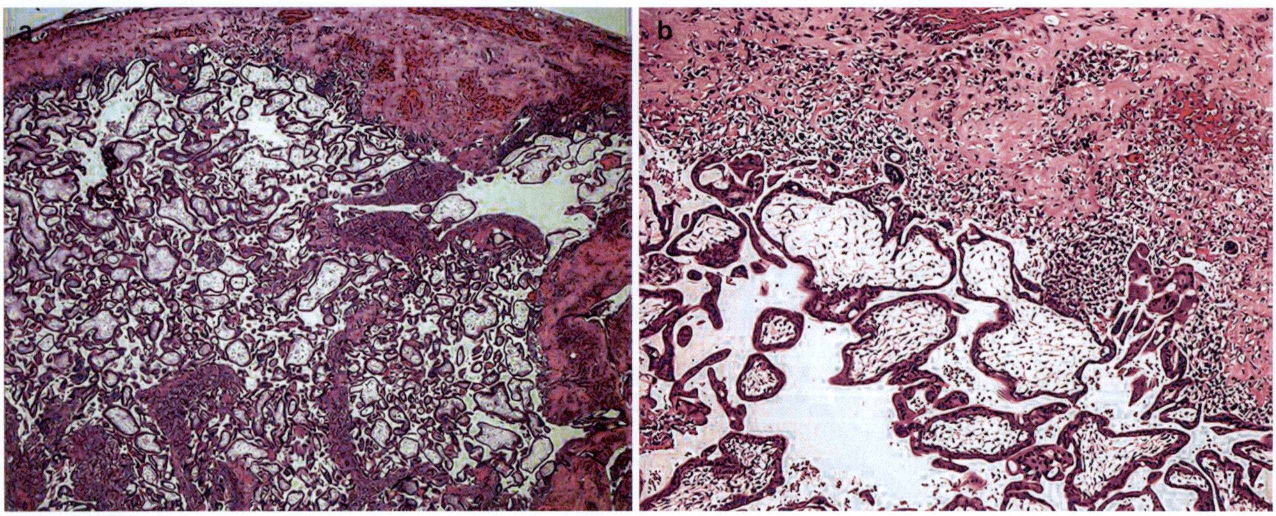

Sections show extrauterine chorionic villi and extra-villous trophoblastic cells. There is reactive mesothelial proliferation on the surface of the fallopian tube associated with dilated congested vessels, edema, and mild inflammatory infiltrate.

8.6.2 Gestational Trophoblastic Disease

8.6.2.1 Molar Pregnancy

Partial Vesicular Mole

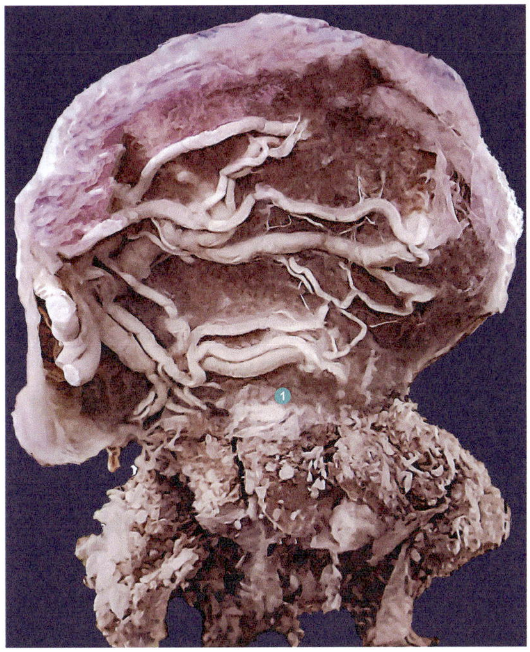

Placenta is mounted

1. Immature placental tissue admixed with vesicles that are smaller and less numerous than those of a complete mole

Microscopic Picture of Partial Vesicular Mole (a–g)

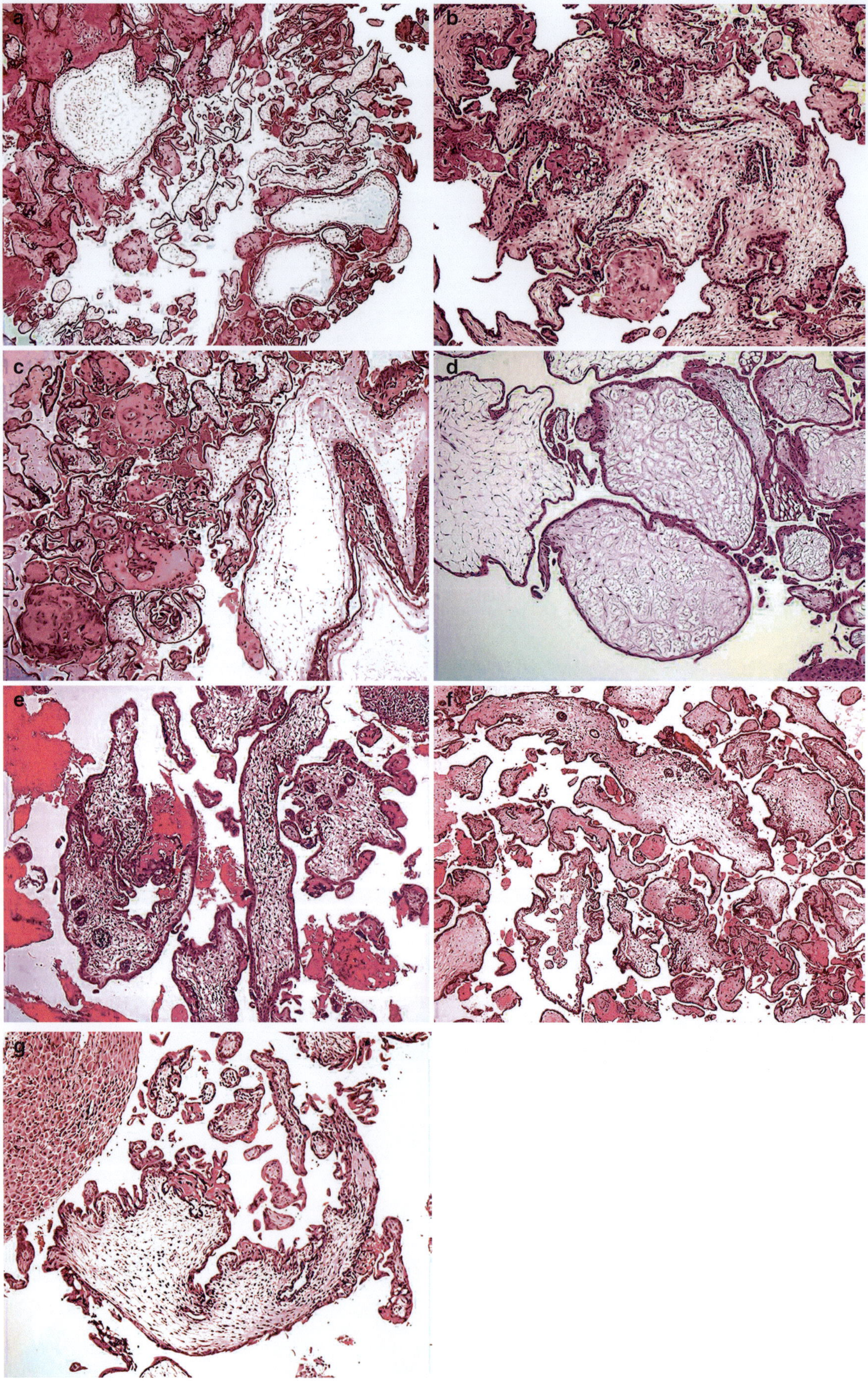

Sections show heterogeneity in villous size with 2 discrete populations (large, hydropic villi and small, fibrotic villi). Enlarged villi are irregularly shaped with scalloped borders and secondary trophoblastic pseudoinclusions. Cistern formation can be seen in enlarged villi. Mild circumferential trophoblastic hyperplasia. Fetal parts and nucleated red blood cells are present.

Complete Vesicular Mole

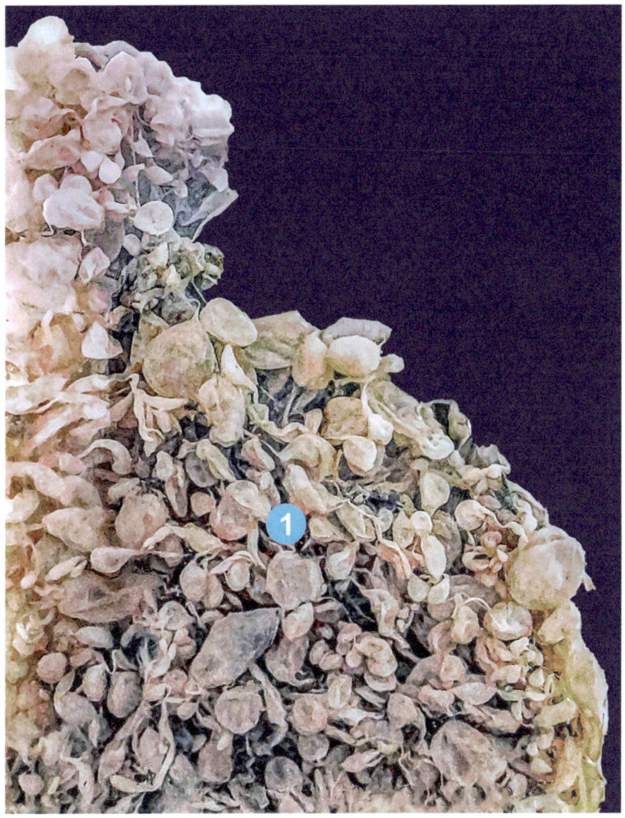

A sample of vesicular mole.

1. The vesicles are small and clear and attached together to form the grapes. No fetal parts or placental tissue is observed.

Molar Pregnancy

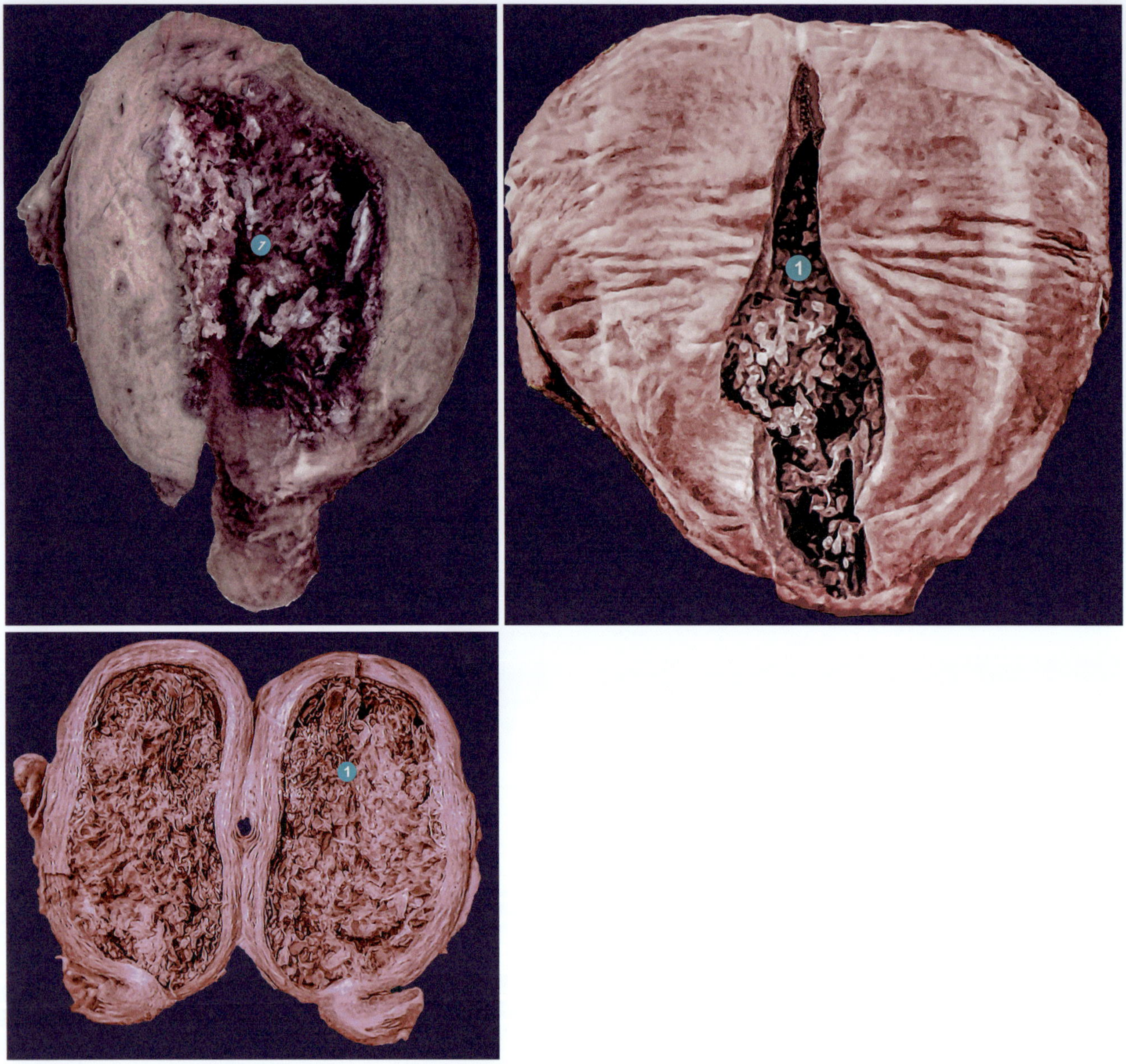

An opened, enlarged pregnant uterus is mounted.

1. The uterus shows the absence of fetal parts and placenta, which is replaced by multiple tiny translucent vesicles attached in a grape-like pattern.

Microscopic Picture of Complete Vesicular Mole (a–d)

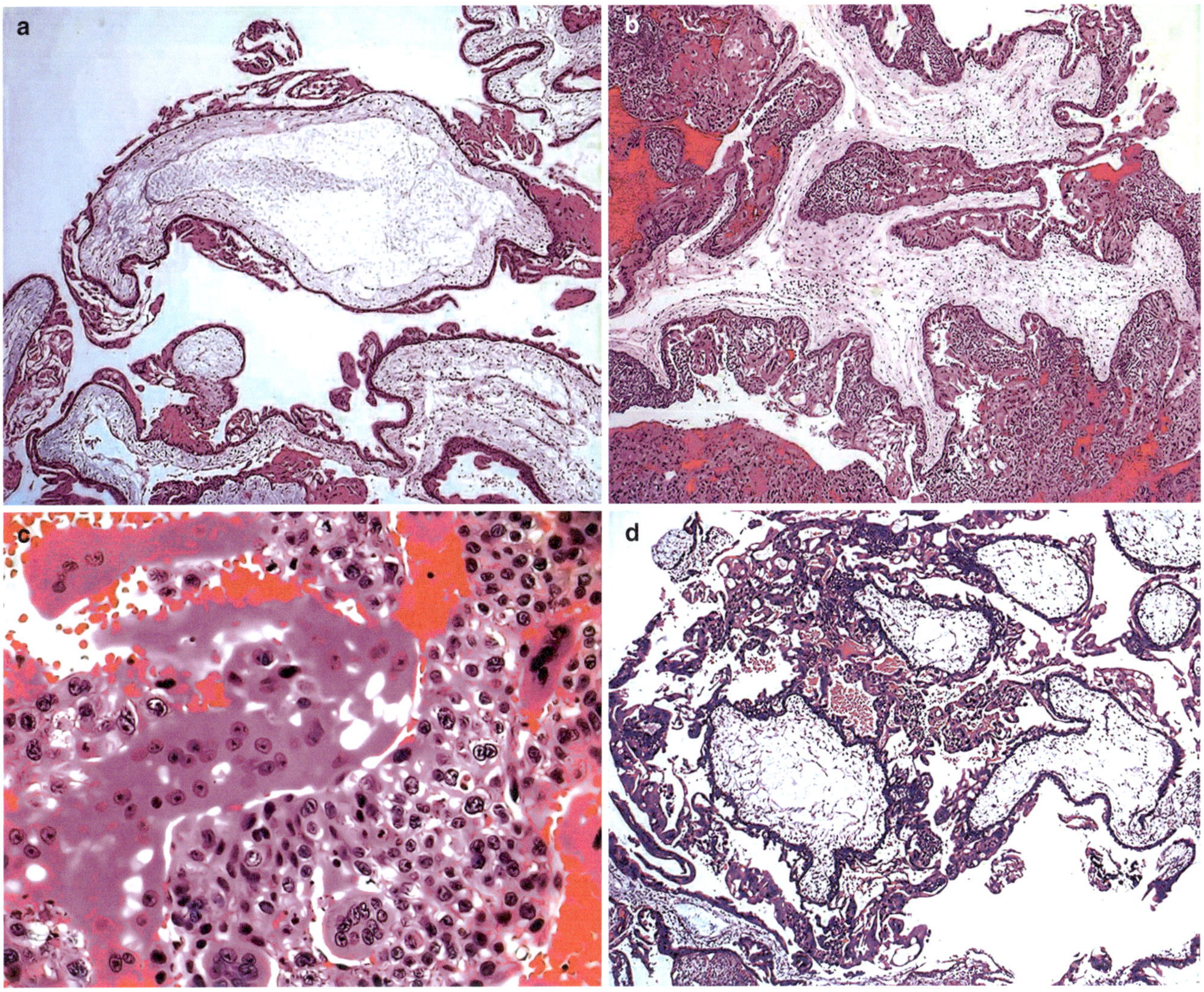

Sections show diffuse, villous enlargement with marked hydropic changes, cistern formation, and marked trophoblastic hyperplasia, usually in a circumferential pattern.

Remarkable cytologic atypia is almost always present with mitoses. Stromal changes of molar villi, which include stromal mucin and stromal nuclear debris (apoptosis), appear very early and represent a diagnostic clue. Fetal blood vessels are absent.

Ancillary Tools

IHC [26]:

Intact nuclear expression of p57 in the villous cytotrophoblast and villous stromal cells in partial hydatidiform mole

hCG, HPL, PLAP

Molecular/cytogenetics description [26]:

Short tandem repeat (STR) DNA genotyping

- Complete mole shows absence of maternal genetic contribution.
- Partial mole shows diandric triploidy.

8.6.3 Gestational Trophoblastic Tumor

Uterine Choriocarcinoma NOS

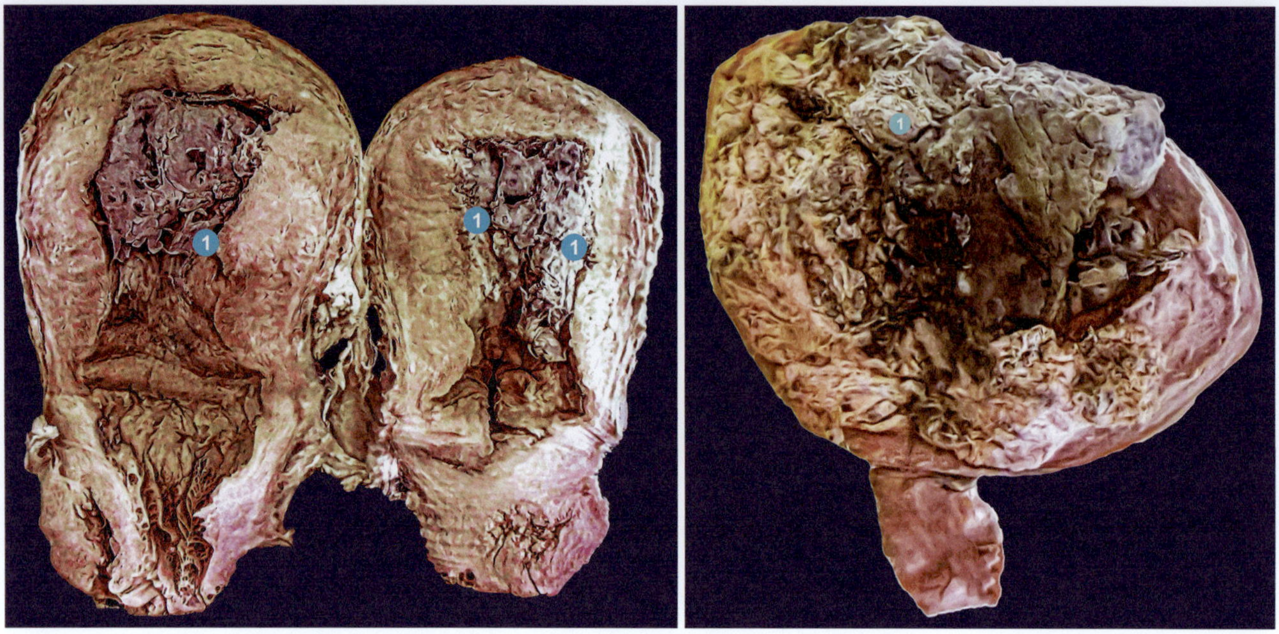

An enlarged puerperal uterus is mounted.

1. The cavity is dilated and shows a mass adherent to the uterine wall, which has large, hemorrhagic, friable, and pale necrotic areas.

Uterine Choriocarcinoma

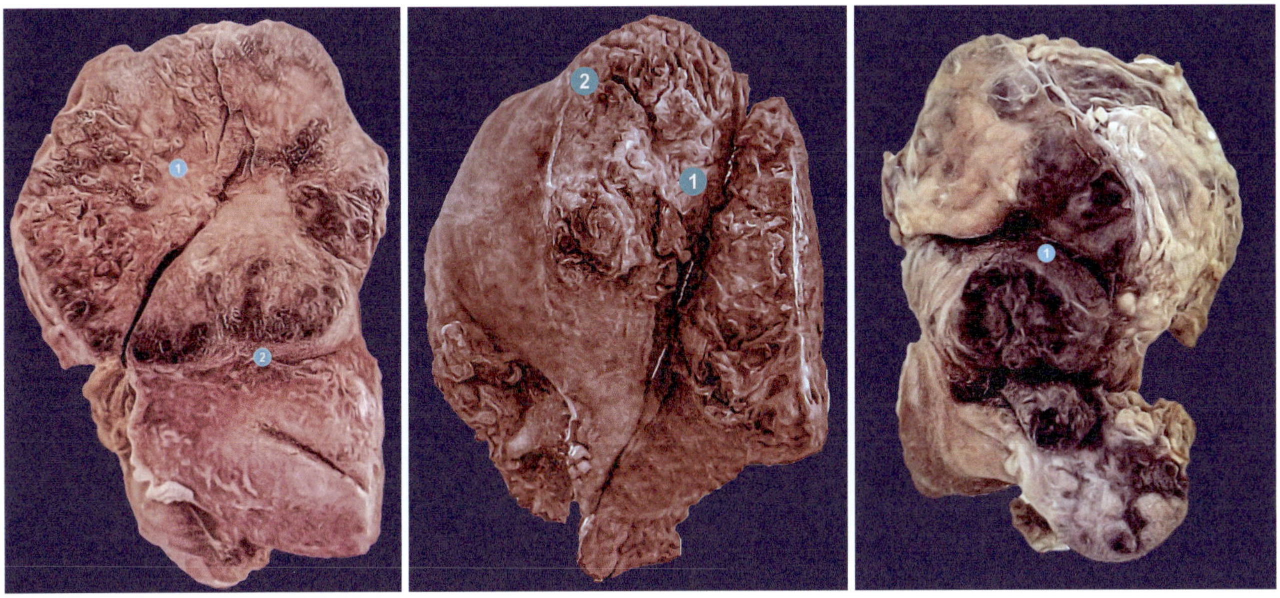

An enlarged puerperal uterus is mounted.

1. It shows a mass adherent to the uterine wall, which has large, hemorrhagic, friable, and pale necrotic areas.
2. The mass invades and destroys the uterine wall in some areas.

Microscopic Picture of Uterine Choriocarcinoma (a–d)

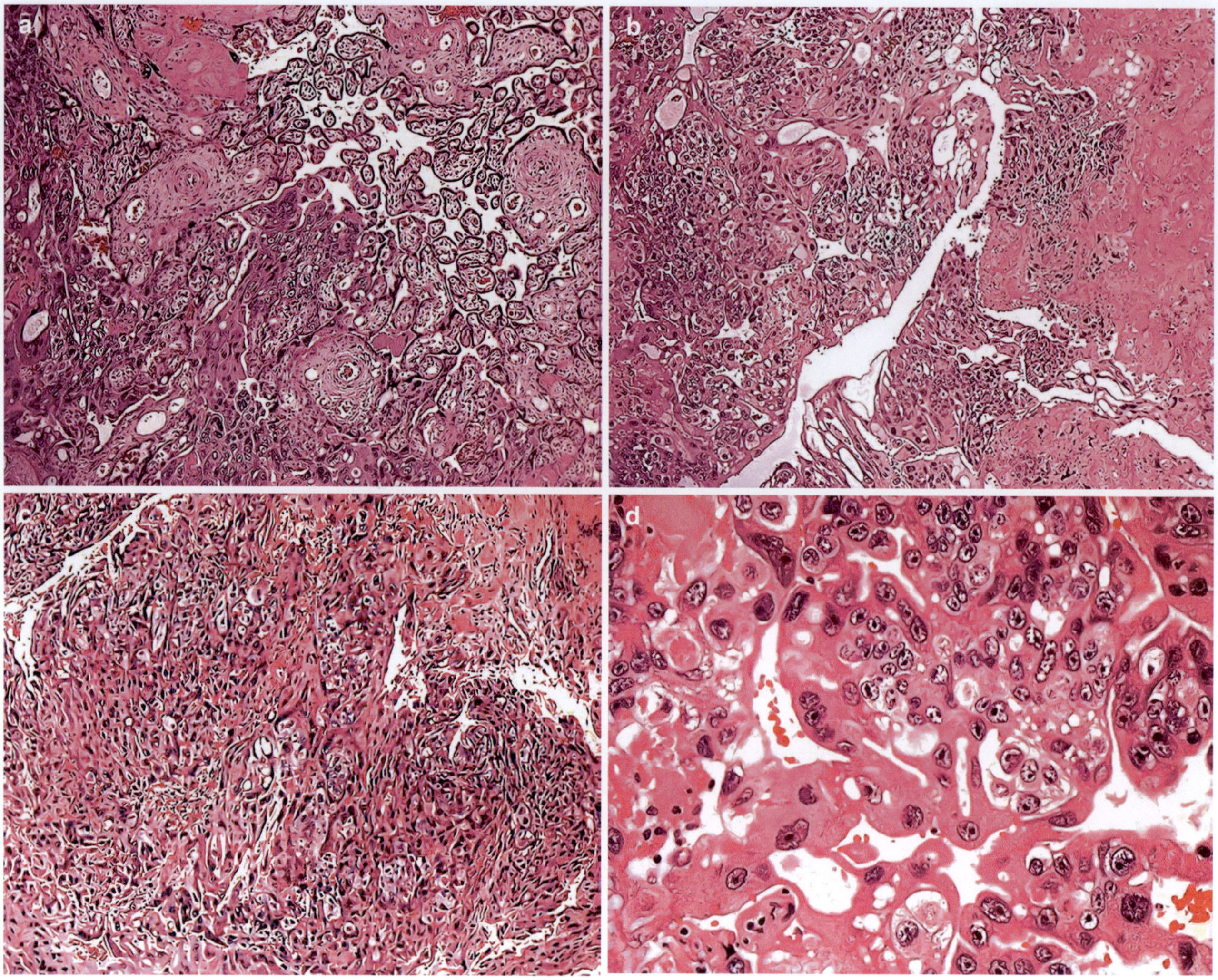

Sections show Infiltrative and destructive solid sheets of trophoblastic cells without chorionic villi in a background of hemorrhage and necrosis with the presence of malignant syncytiotrophoblast, cytotrophoblast, and intermediate trophoblast. The tumor cells are atypical trophoblastic cells with increased mitotic activity.

Ancillary Tools

IHC [27]:

All cells: AE1/AE3, cytokeratin 7, Ki67 > 90%

Syncytiotrophoblast: hCG, inhibin, HSD3B

Cytotrophoblast: SALL4, nuclear beta-catenin, GATA3

Intermediate trophoblast: p63 (focal), human placental lactogen (hPL), HLA-G, Mel-CAM (CD146), MUC4, inhibin, HSD3B1, GATA3

Molecular/cytogenetics description [28]:

Cytogenetics: the majority has XX sex chromosomes and complex karyotypes.

References

1. Li H. et al. (2020). A combination of cytokeratin 5/6, p63, p40, and MUC5AC are useful for distinguishing squamous cell carcinoma from adenocarcinoma of the cervix. Diagn Pathol. 15(1):104. doi: https://doi.org/10.1186/s13000-020-01018-7. PMID: 32843061; PMCID: PMC7448498.
2. Wright AA. et al. (2013). Oncogenic mutations in cervical cancer: genomic differences between adenocarcinomas and squamous cell carcinomas of the cervix. Cancer. 119(21):3776-83. doi: https://doi.org/10.1002/cncr.28288. PMID: 24037752; PMCID: PMC3972000.
3. Ramirez N. et al. (2015). Expressions of E2 and E7-HPV16 proteins in pre-malignant and malignant lesions of the uterine cervix. Biotech Histochem.90(8):573-80. doi:https://doi.org/10.3109/10520295.2015.1047794. PMID: 26052817.
4. Xuebing P. et al. (2011).Is endometrial polyp formation associated with increased expression of vascular endothelial growth factor and transforming growth factor-beta1? Eur J Obstet Gynecol Reprod Biol.159(1):198-203. doi: https://doi.org/10.1016/j.ejogrb.2011.06.036. PMID: 21726930.

5. Fletcher JA. (1992). Clonal 6p21 rearrangement is restricted to the mesenchymal component of an endometrial polyp. Genes Chromosomes Cancer. 5(3):260-3. doi: https://doi.org/10.1002/gcc.2870050315. PMID: 1384681.
6. Ioachin E. (2005). Immunohistochemical tumour markers in endometrial carcinoma. Eur J Gynaecol Oncol.26(4):363-71. PMID: 16122180.
7. Cancer Genome Atlas Research Network; Kandoth C. et al. (2013). Integrated genomic characterization of endometrial carcinoma. Nature. 497(7447):67-73. doi: https://doi.org/10.1038/nature12113. Erratum in: Nature. (2013). 500(7461):242. PMID: 23636398; PMCID: PMC3704730.
8. Oliva E. et al. (2002). An immunohistochemical analysis of endometrial stromal and smooth muscle tumors of the uterus: a study of 54 cases emphasizing the importance of using a panel because of overlap in immunoreactivity for individual antibodies. Am J Surg Pathol. 26(4):403-12. doi: https://doi.org/10.1097/00000478-200204000-00001. PMID: 11914617.
9. Mäkinen N. et al. (2017). Characterization of MED12, HMGA2, and FH alterations reveals molecular variability in uterine smooth muscle tumors. Mol Cancer. 16(1):101. doi: https://doi.org/10.1186/s12943-017-0672-1. PMID: 28592321; PMCID: PMC5463371.
10. Schaefer IM. et al. (2017). Abnormal p53 and p16 staining patterns distinguish uterine leiomyosarcoma from inflammatory myofibroblastic tumour. Histopathology.70(7):1138-1146. doi: https://doi.org/10.1111/his.13176. PMID: 28130839.
11. An Y. et al. (2017). Distinct molecular subtypes of uterine leiomyosarcoma respond differently to chemotherapy treatment. BMC Cancer. 17(1):639. doi: https://doi.org/10.1186/s12885-017-3568-y. PMID: 28893210; PMCID: PMC5594508.
12. Subbaraya S, Murthy SS, Devi G S. (2020). Immunohistochemical and Molecular Characterization of Endometrial Stromal Sarcomas. Clin Pathol. 13:2632010X20916736. doi: https://doi.org/10.1177/2632010X20916736. PMID: 32524088; PMCID: PMC7236392.
13. Manu V, Hein TA, Boruah D, Srinivas V. (2020). Serous ovarian tumors: Immunohistochemical profiling as an aid to grading and understanding tumorigenesis. Med J Armed Forces India. 76(1):30-36. doi: https://doi.org/10.1016/j.mjafi.2018.06.014. PMID: 32020965.
14. Murali R. et al. (2019). Somatic genetic alterations in synchronous and metachronous low-grade serous tumours and high-grade carcinomas of the adnexa. Histopathology.74(4):638-650. doi: https://doi.org/10.1111/his.13796. PMID: 30565721; PMCID: PMC6626549.
15. Babaier, A., Ghatage P. (2020). Mucinous Cancer of the Ovary: Overview and Current Status" Diagnostics 10(1): 52. https://doi.org/10.3390/diagnostics10010052.
16. Cheasley D. et al. (2019).The molecular origin and taxonomy of mucinous ovarian carcinoma. Nat Commun.10(1):3935. doi: https://doi.org/10.1038/s41467-019-11862-x. PMID: 31477716; PMCID: PMC6718426.
17. Alloush F. et al. (2023). Brenner Tumor of the Ovary: A 10-Year Single Institution Experience and Comprehensive Review of the Literature. Med Sci (Basel). 11(1):18. doi: https://doi.org/10.3390/medsci11010018. PMID: 36810485; PMCID: PMC9944520.
18. Vang R. et al. (2001). Immunohistochemical analysis of clear cell carcinoma of the gynecologic tract. Int J Gynecol Pathol. 20(3):252-9. doi: https://doi.org/10.1097/00004347-200107000-00008. PMID: 11444201.
19. Mabuchi S, Sugiyama T, Kimura T. (2016).Clear cell carcinoma of the ovary: molecular insights and future therapeutic perspectives. J Gynecol Oncol. 27(3):e31. doi: https://doi.org/10.3802/jgo.2016.27.e31. PMID: 27029752; PMCID: PMC4823362.
20. Rabban JT, Zaloudek CJ. (2013). A practical approach to immunohistochemical diagnosis of ovarian germ cell tumours and sex cord-stromal tumours. Histopathology. 62(1):71-88. doi: https://doi.org/10.1111/his.12052. PMID: 23240671.
21. Cossu-Rocca P. et al. (2006). Chromosome 12p abnormalities in dysgerminoma of the ovary: a FISH analysis. Mod Pathol.19(4):611-5. doi: https://doi.org/10.1038/modpathol.3800576. PMID: 16554737.
22. Adad SJ. et al. (2012). Cellular fibroma of the ovary with multiloculated macroscopic characteristics: case report. Case Rep Med. 2012:283948. doi: https://doi.org/10.1155/2012/283948. PMID: 22567015; PMCID: PMC3332172.
23. Li X, Tian B, Liu M, Miao C, Wang D. (2022). Adult-type granulosa cell tumor of the ovary. Am J Cancer Res. 12(8):3495-3511. PMID: 36119817; PMCID: PMC9442026.
24. Yahaya JJ, Mshana D, Mremi A. (2020). Ovarian sex cord tumour with annular tubules in a 13-year-old female: a case report. Oxf Med Case Reports. 2020(4):omaa024. doi: https://doi.org/10.1093/omcr/omaa024. PMID: 32477574; PMCID: PMC7243713.
25. Tan H. et al. (2016). Three novel mutations of STK11 gene in Chinese patients with Peutz-Jeghers syndrome. BMC Med Genet. 17(1):77. doi: https://doi.org/10.1186/s12881-016-0339-6. PMID: 27821076; PMCID: PMC5100203.
26. Buza N, Hui P. (2014). Immunohistochemistry and other ancillary techniques in the diagnosis of gestational trophoblastic diseases. Semin Diagn Pathol. 31(3):223-32. doi: https://doi.org/10.1053/j.semdp.2014.03.004. PMID: 24907943.
27. Mao TL. et al. (2007). Immunohistochemistry of choriocarcinoma: an aid in differential diagnosis and in elucidating pathogenesis. Am J Surg Pathol. 31(11):1726-32. doi: https://doi.org/10.1097/PAS.0b013e318058a529. PMID: 18059230.
28. Bettio D. et al. (1993).Cytogenetic abnormalities detected by direct analysis in a case of choriocarcinoma. Cancer Genetics and Cytogenetics. 68 (2): 149-151. doi:https://doi.org/10.1016/0165-4608(93)90014-D.

9 Diseases of Breast

The human breast is a complex organ that is prone to a variety of diseases, including breast cancer. Pathological examination of the breast involves the macroscopic and microscopic examination of diseased breast tissue to identify and characterize different pathological conditions.

This chapter will provide an overview of the gross and microscopic pathology of the breast, focusing on specific pathological conditions, their unique manifestations, and how understanding these characteristics can help pathologists and clinicians make more accurate preliminary diagnoses, decide on subsequent steps for microscopic analysis, and plan an appropriate course of treatment.

The chapter will cover a wide range of breast diseases, from benign alterations such as fibrocystic changes and fibroadenomas to some types of invasive breast cancers. Using photographic illustrations and detailed descriptions, the chapter will outline the gross and microscopic characteristics of these conditions.

This chapter is intended to serve as a reference for healthcare professionals, particularly pathologists, oncologists, and students in the medical field.

The breast lesions studied in this chapter will be organized in the following order:

1. **Fibrocystic Changes**
   (a) Fibrocystic changes
2. **Fibroepithelial Tumors**
   (a) Fibroadenoma
   (b) Tubular Adenoma
   (c) Phyllodes Tumor
3. **Breast Carcinomas**
   (a) Duct Carcinoma in Situ (DCIS)
   (b) Infiltrating Ductal Carcinoma
   (c) Lobular Carcinoma in Situ (LCIS)
   (d) Classic Invasive Lobular Carcinoma
   (e) Invasive Tubular Carcinoma
   (f) Mucinous (Colloid) Carcinoma
   (g) Male Breast Carcinoma

G. Dawood, *Color Atlas of Human Gross and Microscopic Pathology*, https://doi.org/10.1007/978-3-031-76007-5_9

9.1 Fibrocystic Changes

Fibrocystic Changes

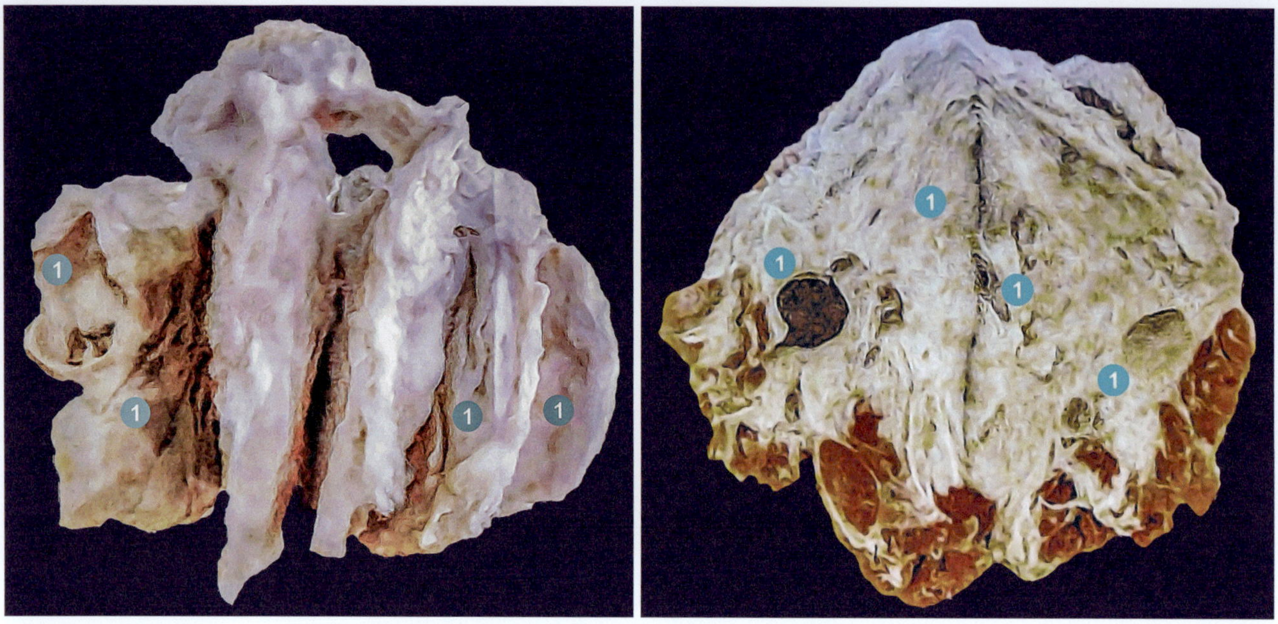

An irregularly sectioned piece of breast tissue is mounted.

1. It shows diffuse gray-white fibrous tissue with multiple and variably-sized cysts with smooth walls.

Microscopic Picture of Nonproliferative Fibrocystic Changes (a–f)

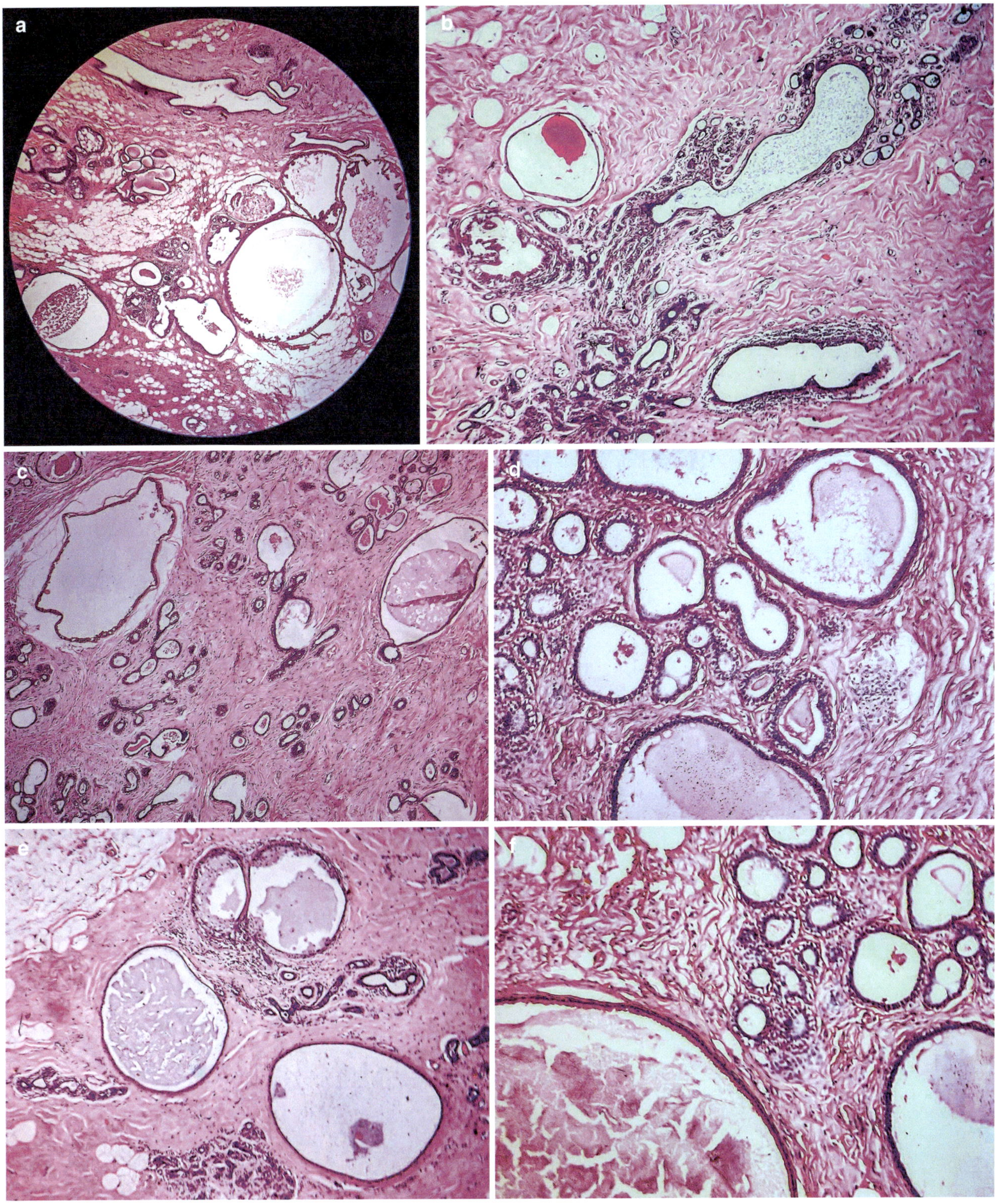

Sections show the three components of nonproliferative fibrocystic changes, namely:

adenosis: Increased number of acini per lobule. Acini are lined by columnar cells.

Stromal fibrosis

cyst formation: cystically dilated ducts or lobules containing eosinophilic secretions. The cysts are lined by cuboidal epithelium or may have apocrine metaplasia. The outer myoepithelial layer is present but attenuated.

Apocrine metaplasia: single or multilayered ductal epithelium with abundant granular eosinophilic cytoplasm, apical snouts, enlarged nuclei, and prominent nucleoli, and columnar cell change frequently with apical snouts.

9.2 Fibroepithelial Tumors

Fibroadenoma

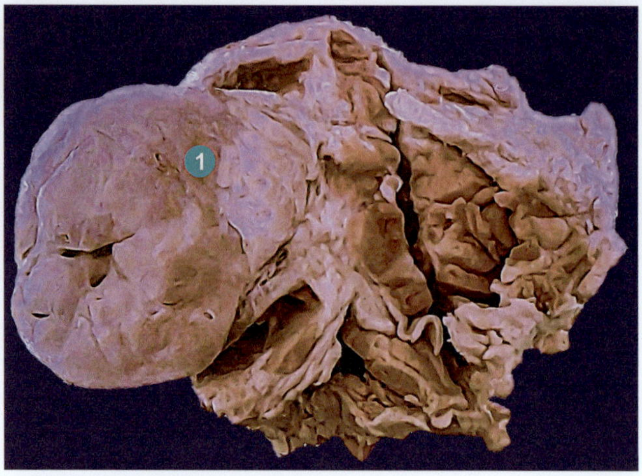

A specimen from the breast is mounted.

1. There is a rounded, well-defined, encapsulated, lobulated, gray-white mass surrounded by fatty tissue with a gray-white cut section.

Microscopic Picture of Fibroadenoma (a–d)

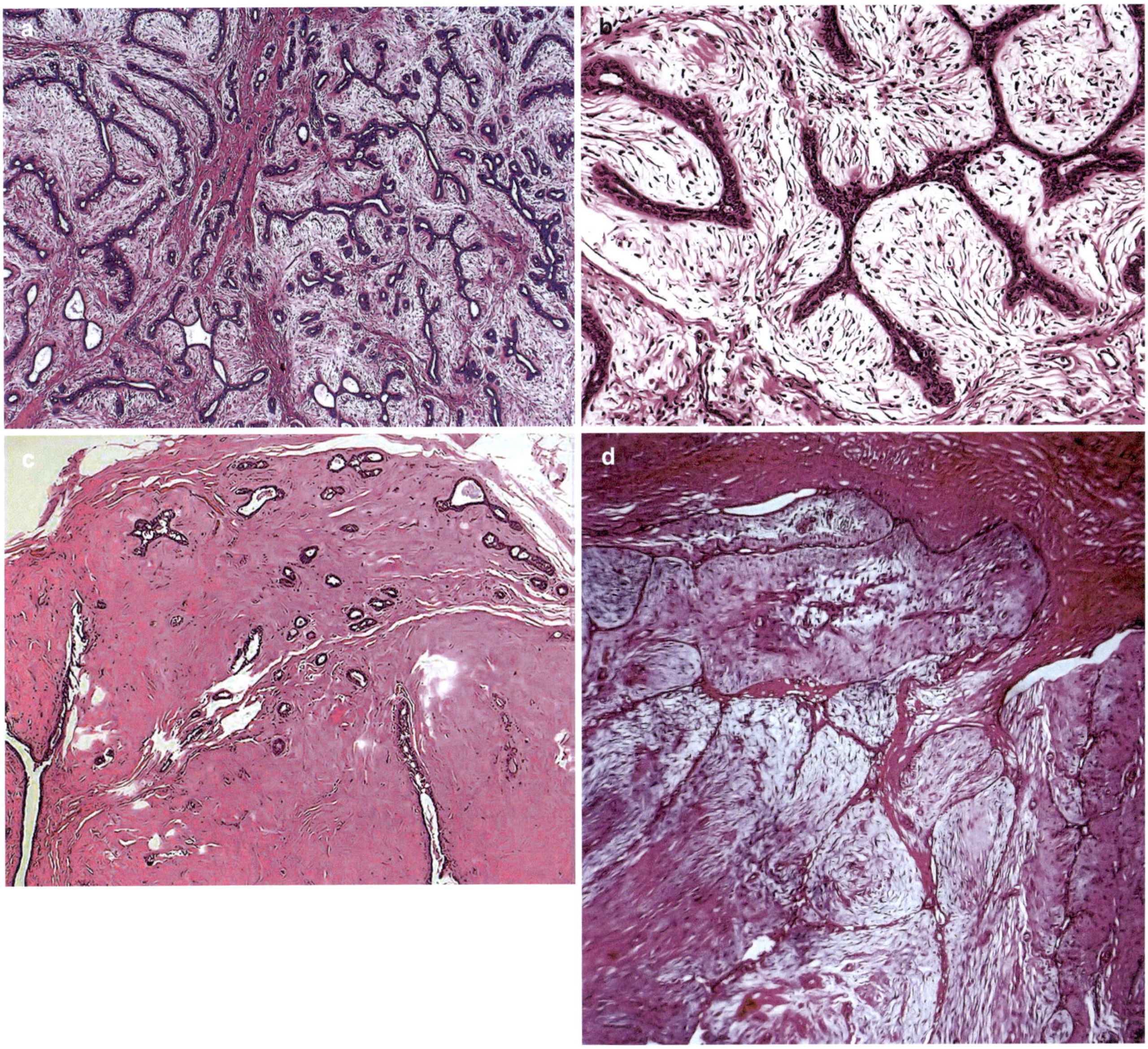

Sections show both glandular and stromal components of the tumor. The glandular component is formed of two recognized growth patterns (of no clinical significance; both patterns may occur within a single lesion): Intracanalicular glands are compressed into linear branching structures by proliferating stroma, and pericanalicular glands retain open lumens but are separated by expanded stroma. In both patterns, glandular elements have intact myoepithelial cell layers. The stromal component has uniform cellularity within a given lesion formed of collagen and bland spindle-shaped stromal cells with ovoid or elongated nuclei. Neither mitotic activity nor stromal atypia is observed. Stroma may show myxoid change.

Tubular Adenoma

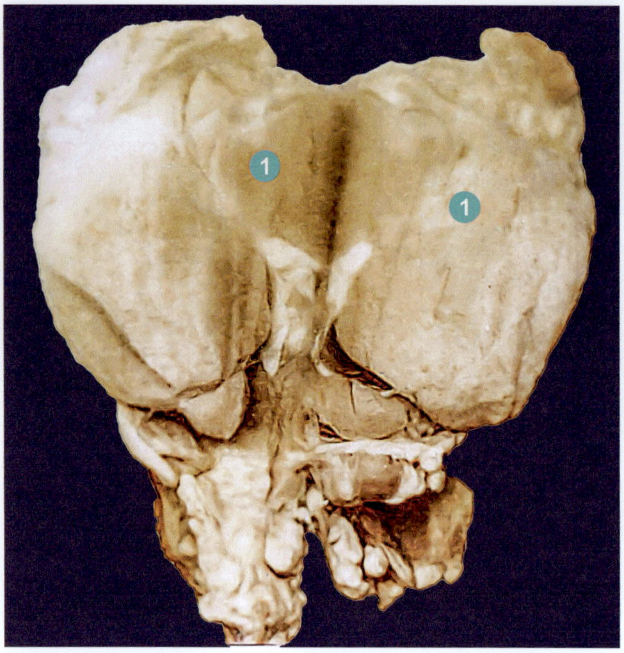

A mass resected from the breast is mounted.

1. A well-circumscribed, solid, white-yellow mass with a smooth cut surface.

Microscopic Picture of Tubular Adenoma (a, b)

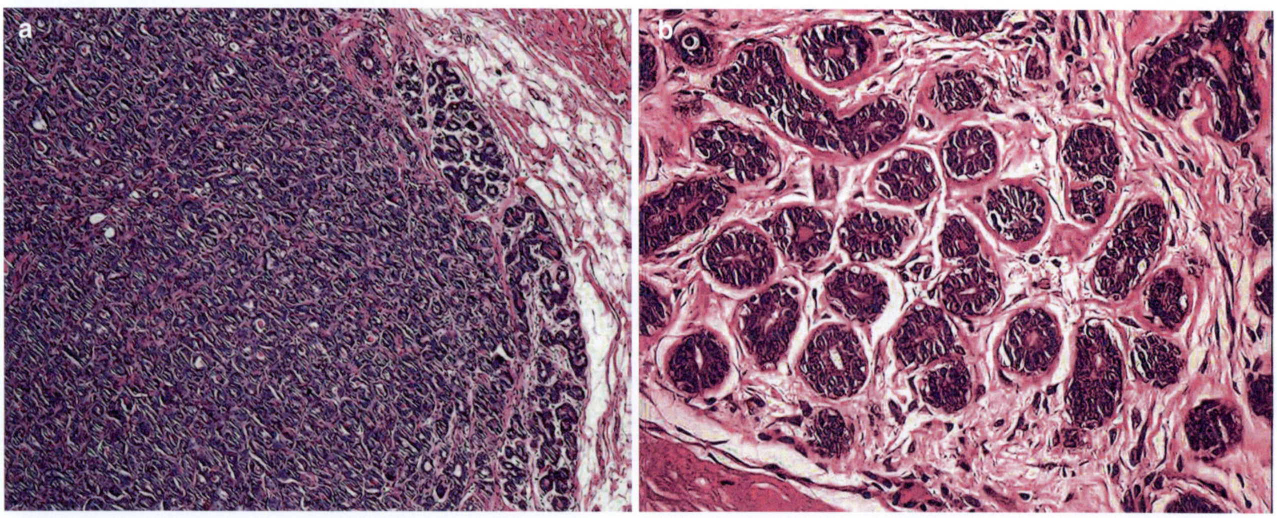

Sections show well-defined borders of the tumor. The tubules are small, uniform, closely packed, and round with a sparse intervening fibrovascular stroma. The tubules are lined by an inner layer of luminal epithelial cells and an outer layer of myoepithelial cells.

Ancillary Tools
IHC [1]:

Myoepithelial cells: CK5/6, p63, S100, SMA, and other myoepithelial markers.

Molecular/cytogenetics description [2]:

Next-generation sequencing demonstrated that tubular adenomas and fibroadenomas show different mutation profiles.

Phyllodes Tumor (a, b)

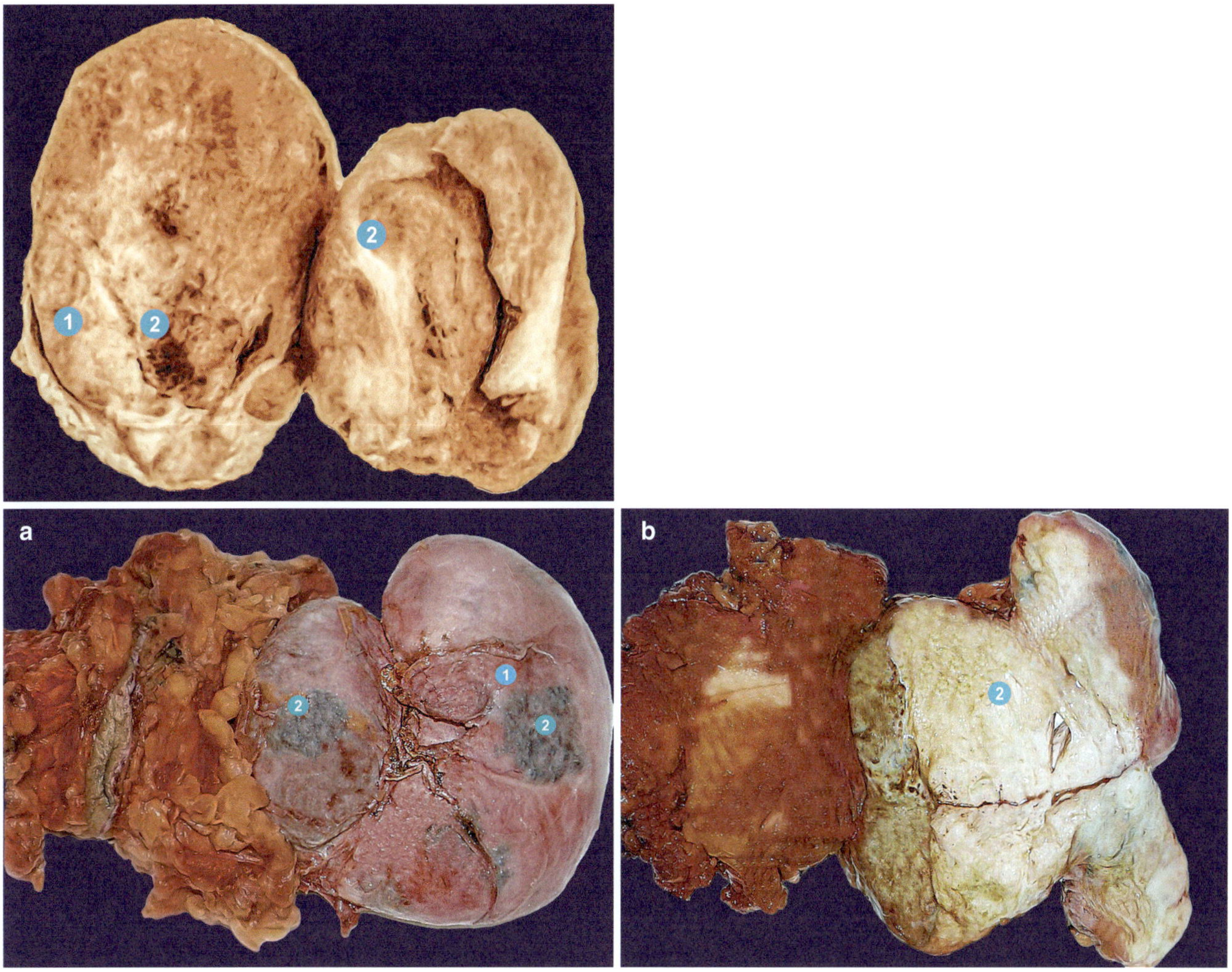

A specimen from the breast is mounted.

1. There is a large, round, well-defined, partially encapsulated, lobulated, gray-white mass.
2. The cut section shows transverse slits with the presence of focal areas of hemorrhage and necrosis.

Microscopic Picture of Benign Phylloides Tumor (c–h)

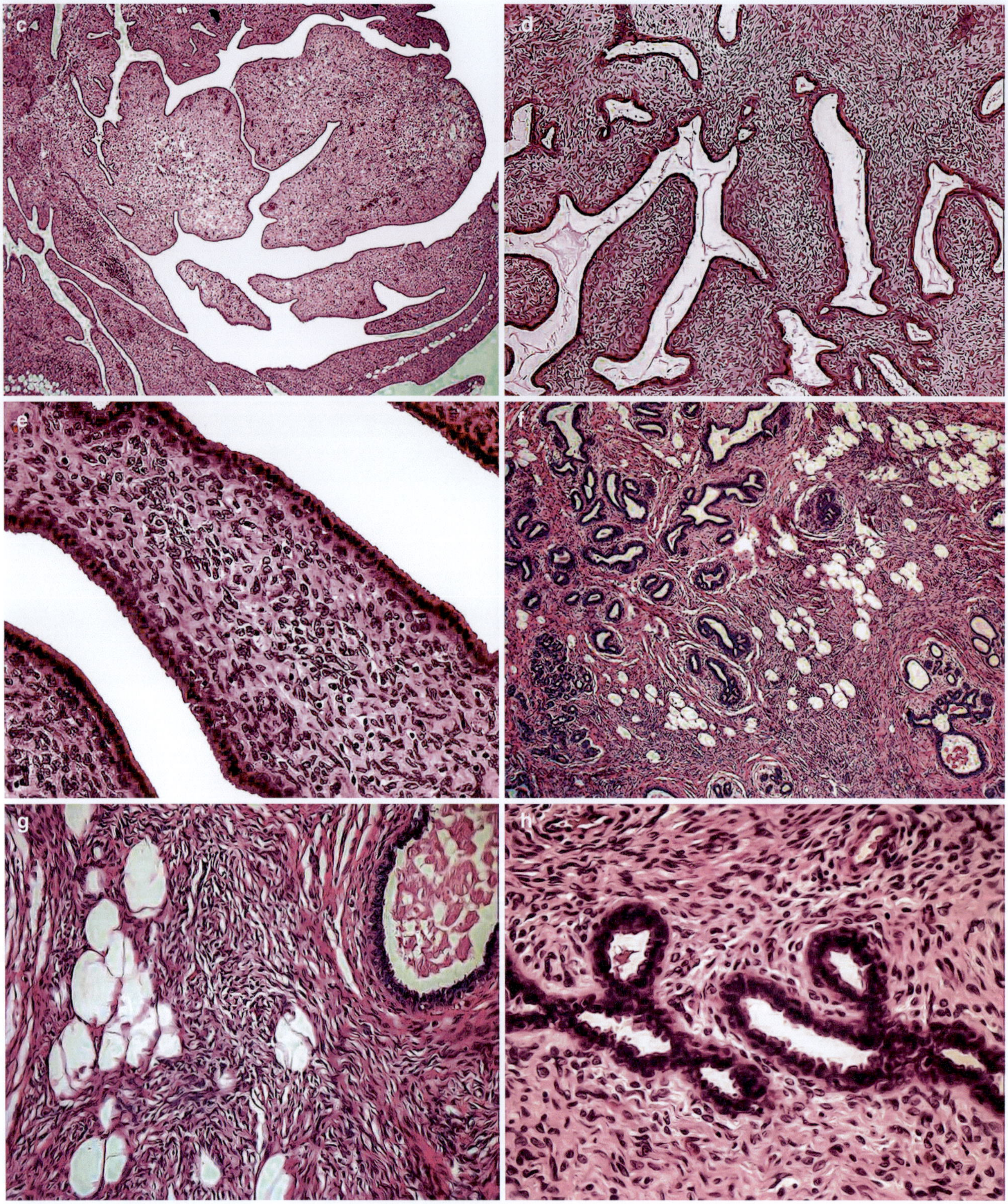

Sections show leaf-like (phyllodal) ducts lined by bland epithelium and attenuated myoepithelial cells. There is subepithelial condensation of the stroma with increased stromal cellularity adjacent to epithelium with a low stroma-to-epithelium ratio without stromal overgrowth.

Microscopic Picture of Malignant Phylloides Tumor (i–n)

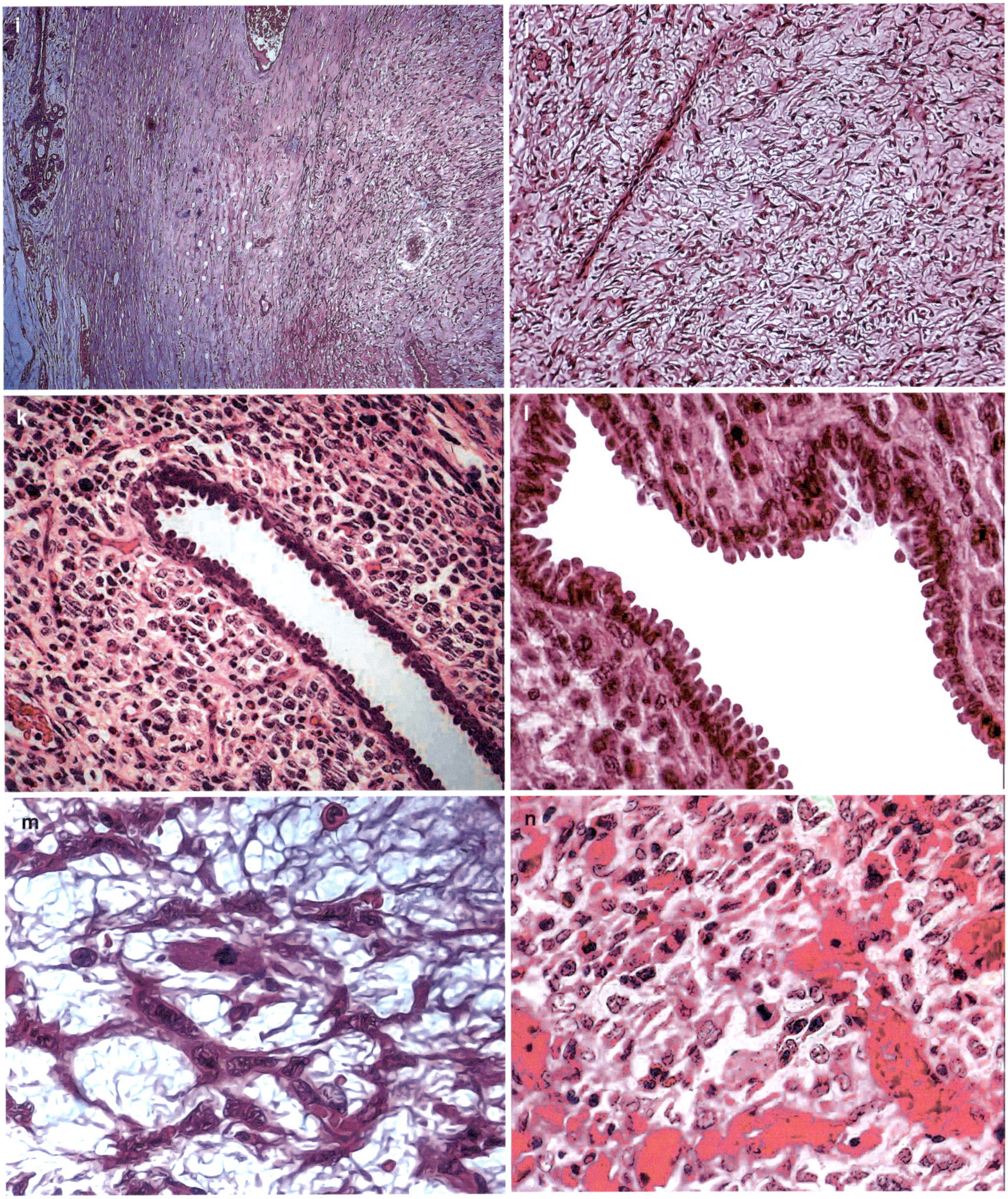

Sections show stromal overgrowth by markedly and diffusely increased cellularity and myxoid change. Stromal cells show marked atypia and increased mitotic figures (≥10/10 HPF), many of which are atypical.

Ancillary Tools

IHC [3]:

Epithelial cells: Cytokeratins, ER, PR, GCDFP-15

Stromal cells: Vimentin, CD34, BCL2, ER beta, Cytokeratins, and p63.

Molecular/cytogenetics description [4]:

Recurrent MED12 and RARA mutations in benign phyllodes tumors and fibroadenoma.

9.3 Breast Carcinomas

Infiltrating Carcinoma

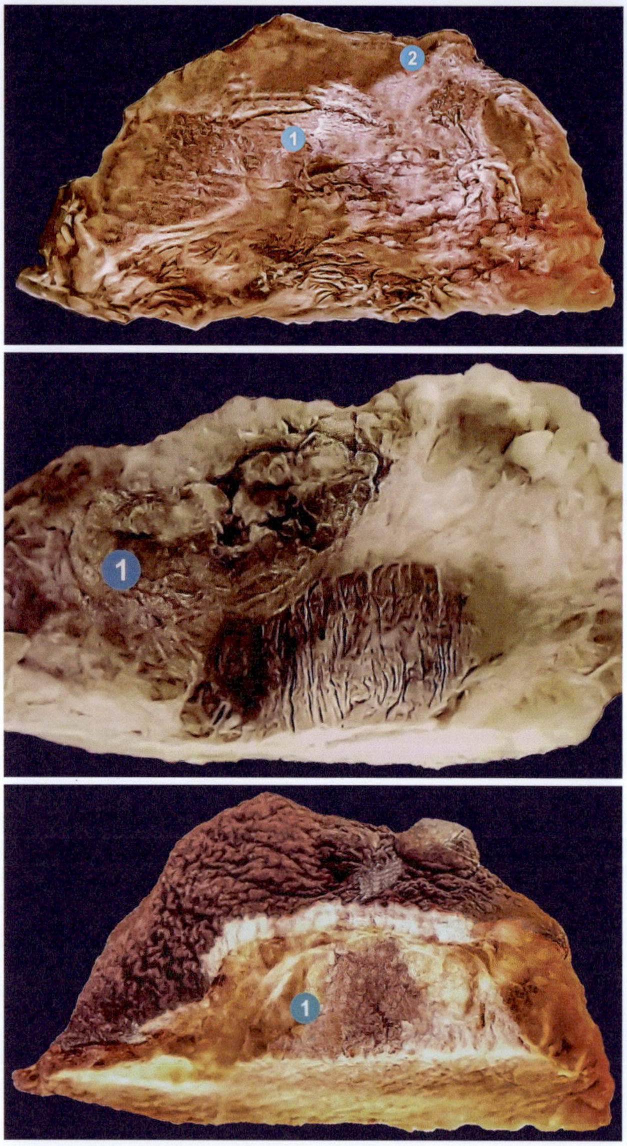

A specimen of the breast is mounted.

1. The cut section shows a gray-white, firm, irregular, and ill-defined mass.
2. The tumor mass is seen under the areola infiltrating the overlying skin.

Microscopic Picture of Duct Carcinoma in Situ (DCIS) (a–j)

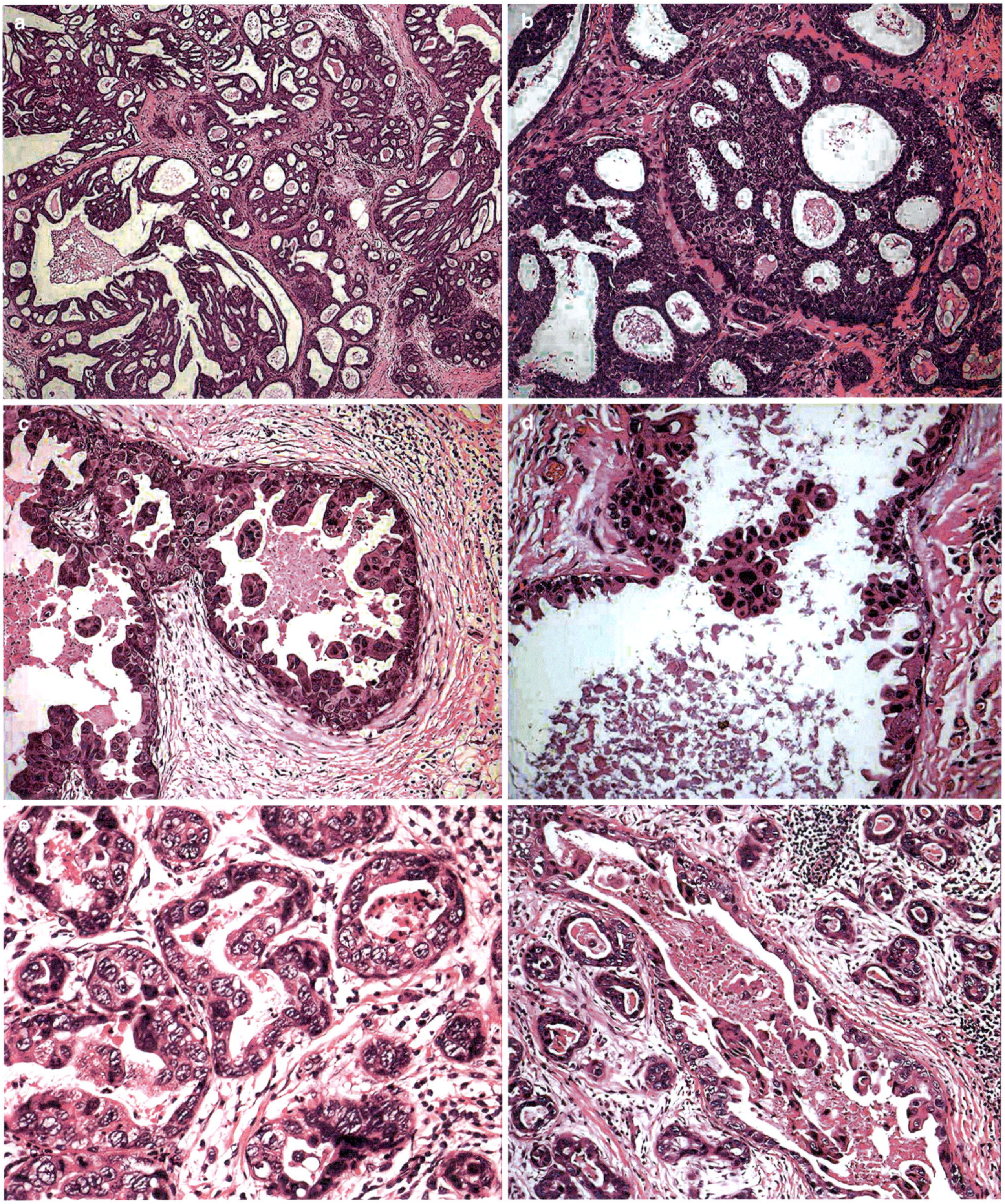

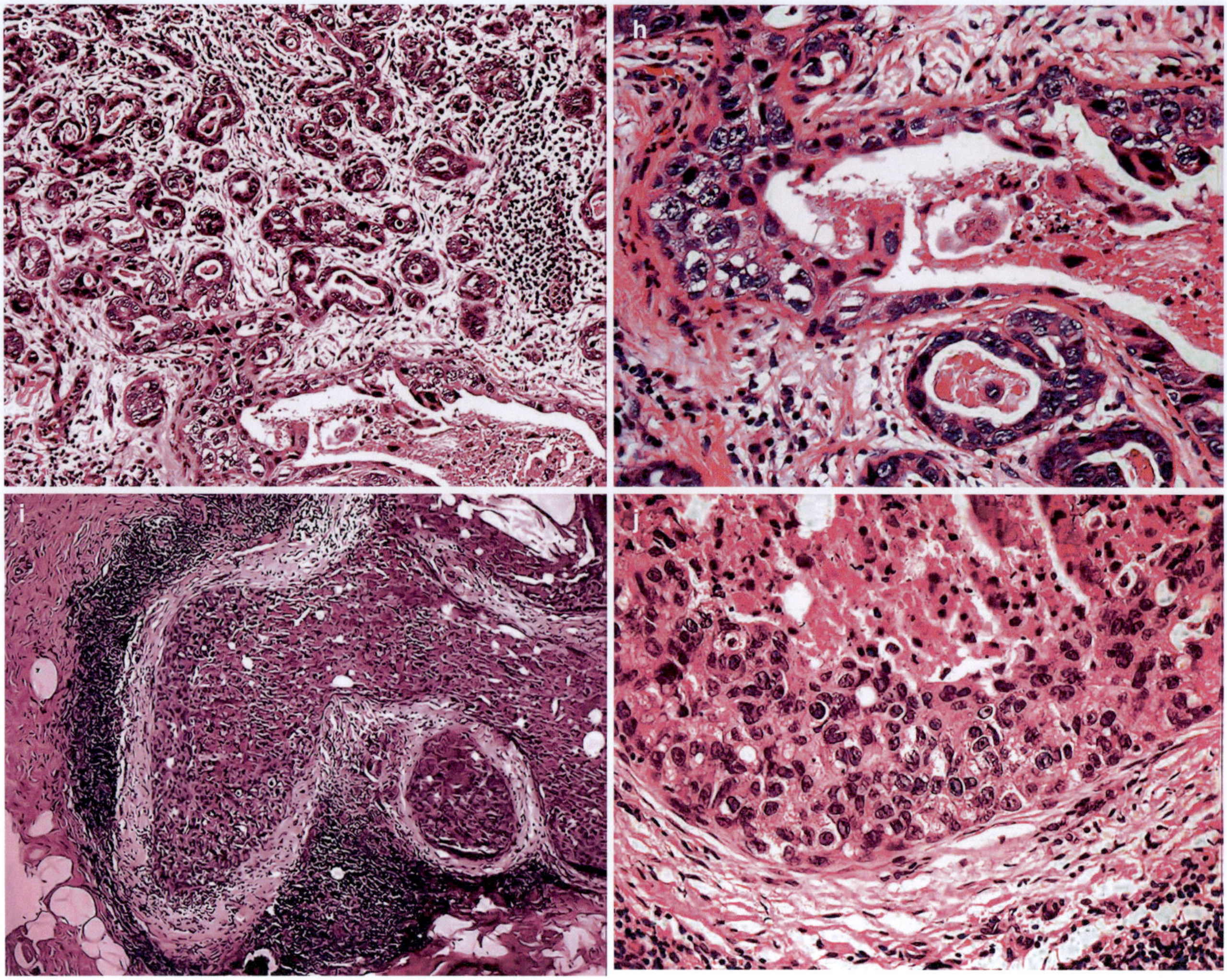

Sections show malignant mammary ductal epithelial cells confined within the ductal-lobular system without evidence of invasion through the basement membrane into the surrounding stroma. The tumor cells are arranged in one or more of the following patterns:

(a, b) **Cribriform pattern** in which there is fenestrated proliferation with multiple, round, rigid extracellular lumens with punched-out appearance.

(c, d) **Micropapillary pattern** in which papillary fronds and tufts lacking fibrovascular cores projecting into duct lumen are observed. Papillae often have club-shaped cells comprising the micropapillae that are uniform in appearance.

(e–h) **Flat pattern** in which there are 1–2 layers of generally high-grade malignant cells lining a gland with a large empty lumen.

(i, j) **Comedo pattern,** which shows central expansile necrosis containing cellular debris and is generally associated with high-grade DCIS.

Microscopic Picture of Infiltrating Duct Carcinoma NOS (a–h)

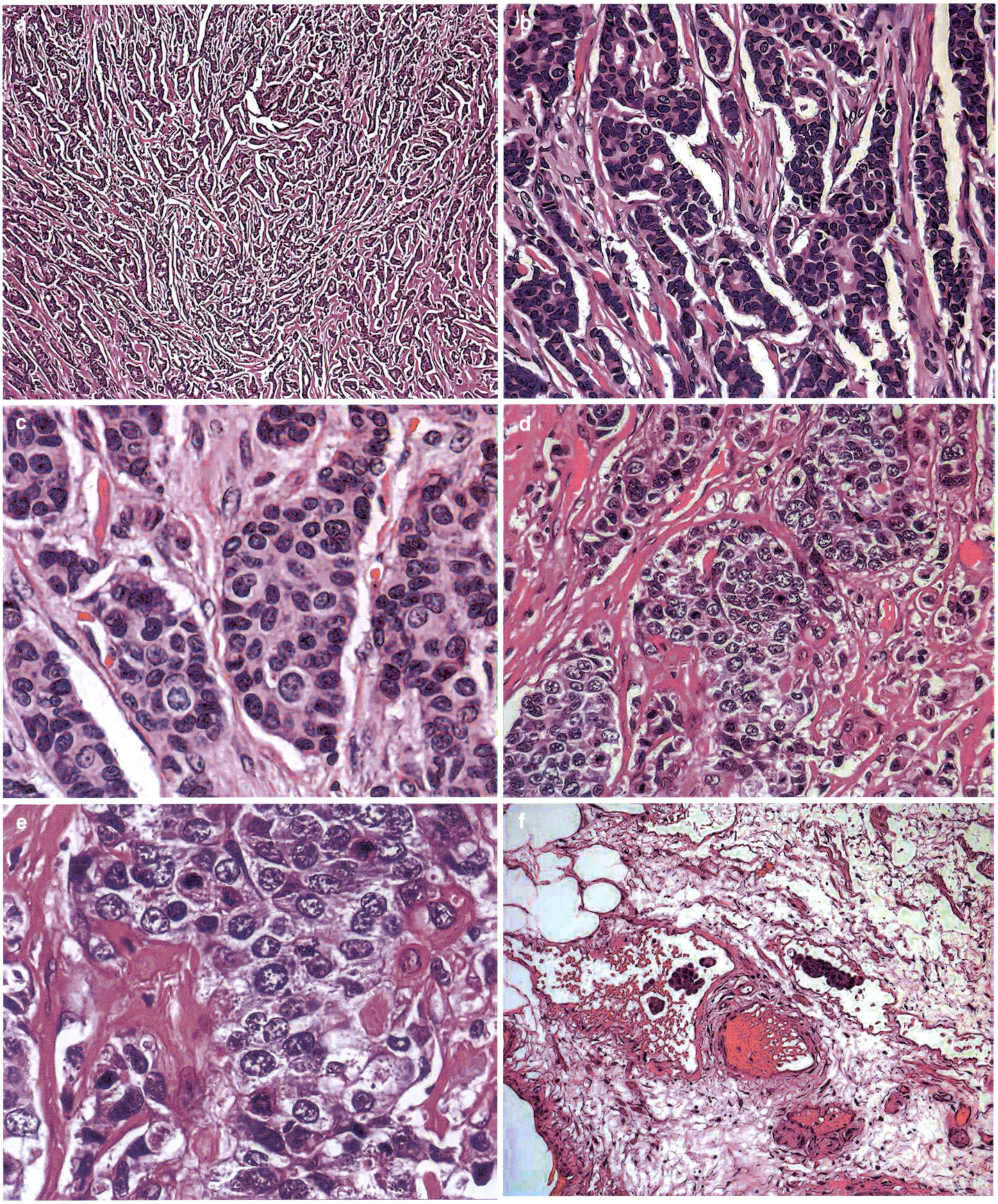

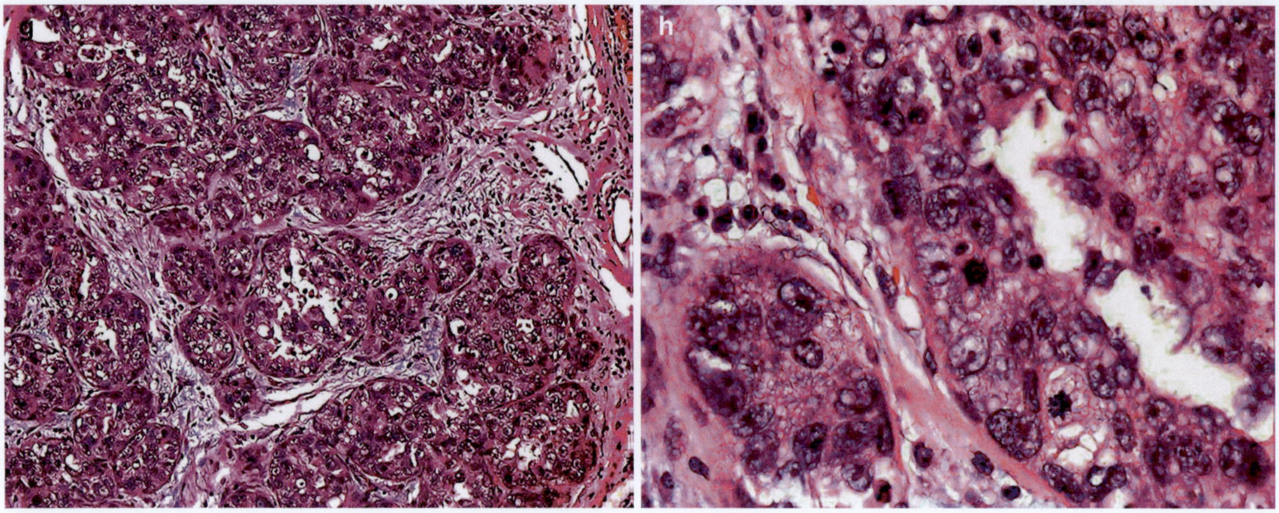

Sections show solid nests, clusters, and cords of malignant ductal epithelial cells with attempts at tubular formation. The cells have enlarged, pleomorphic hyperchromatic nuclei with prominent nucleoli and increased mitotic activity. Tumor formations are embedded in a desmoplastic stroma with the presence of areas of lymphovascular invasion.

Ancillary Tools

IHC [5]:

Luminal low molecular weight cytokeratins (CK8/18, CK19, and CK7) and pancytokeratins such as AE1/AE3, CAM 5.2, MNF-116, EMA, E-cadherin, p120, ER (60–80%), PR (50–70%), HER2 (15–20%)

GCDFP-15 (30–40%)

GATA3 (~91–100% of hormone receptor-positive breast cancers, ~43–66% in triple-negative breast cancer)

Also, mammaglobin, milk fat globule, lactalbumin, CEA, B72.3, BCA225

High molecular weight cytokeratins (CK5/6, CK14, and CK17) (10–30%)

Glycogen (60%), mucin (moderate/marked in 20%)

S100 (10–45%), RCC Ma (renal cell carcinoma marker)

CD5 clone 4C7

TRPS1

SOX10 (57–58% of triple-negative breast cancers)

Molecular/cytogenetics description [5, 6]:

ER+ pathway: characterized by gains of 1q, loss of 16q, sometimes amplification of 17q12

ER− pathway: characterized by loss of 13q, gain of 11q13, amplification of 17q12, p53 mutations common, increased expression of genes associated with cell proliferation

PI3KCA mutations associated with endocrine therapy resistance

p53 mutations in many basal-like tumors

HER2 gene amplification in approximately 15

Gene expression profiling stratifies breast cancers into several intrinsic molecular subtypes (e.g., luminal A, luminal B, HER2-enriched, basal-like, etc.)

5–10% of breast cancers are hereditary as a result of mutations in various genes, such as BRCA1, BRCA2, TP53, STK11, CD1, PTEN, MDM2, RB, and CHEK2

ESR1 mutations associated with resistance to endocrine therapy.

Microscopic Picture of Lobular Carcinoma in Situ (LCIS) (a–d)

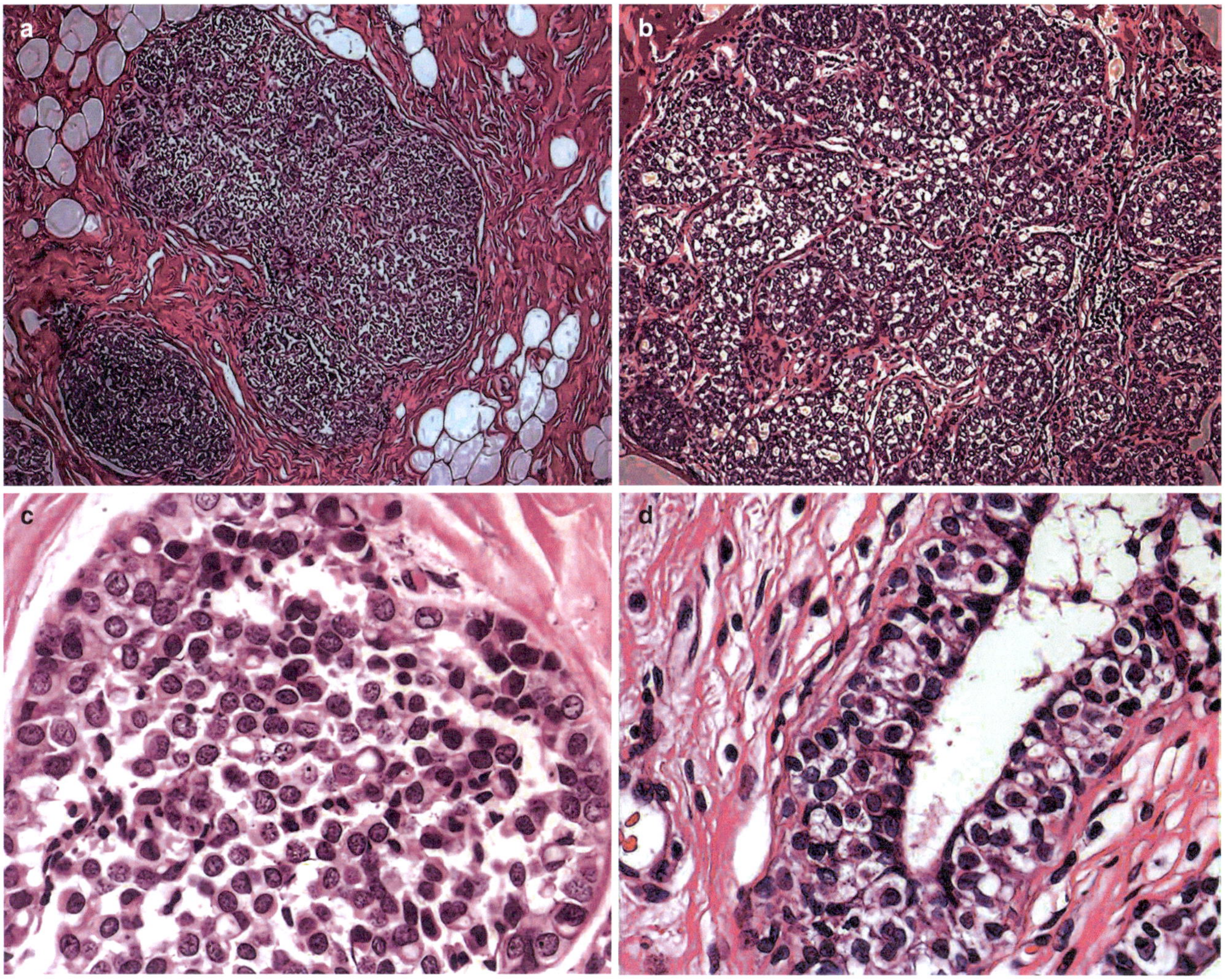

Sections show involvement of the terminal duct lobular unit (TDLU) by tumor cells filling and distending >50% of the acini in a TDLU (a and b). Pagetoid spread in ducts is the characteristic growth of cells between luminal and myoepithelial layers of a duct without destroying ductal epithelium or filling up ductal lumina (d). Cells are monomorphic, evenly spaced, loosely cohesive, and do not show polarization or gland formation. The nuclei are small to slightly enlarged (1–1.5× the size of a lymphocyte) with uniform round nuclei and inconspicuous nucleoli without nuclear pleomorphism or mitosis. The cytoplasm of LCIS cells is typically pale to lightly eosinophilic with indistinct cell borders.

Microscopic Picture of Classic Invasive Lobular Carcinoma (a–g)

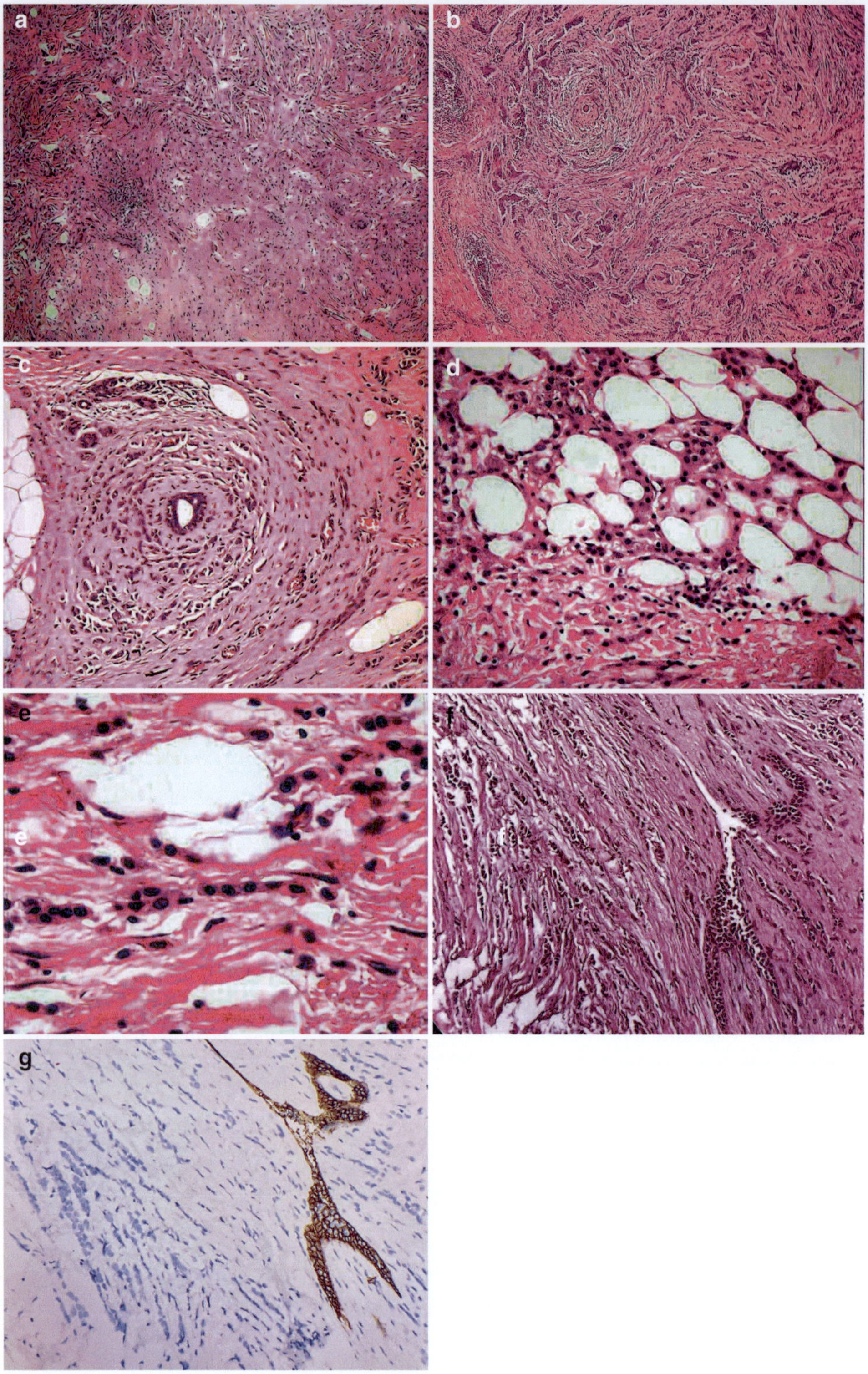

Sections show malignant tumor cells arranged in single files, cords, and single cells arranged in areas concentrically around normal ducts, giving a targetoid appearance (c). Tumor cells are discohesive, small, monomorphic, and lacking marked atypia. Round or notched ovoid nuclei, usually grade 1 or 2 nuclear score. Scant cytoplasm, occasionally with intracytoplasmic lumen.

Invasive lobular carcinoma (ILC) and lobular carcinoma in situ characteristically show loss of E-cadherin expression as in (g) which shows positively-stained benign ductal epithelium while the tumor cells are negative. Immunohistochemistry for E-cadherin is being increasingly used as a tool to differentiate between lobular and ductal lesions in challenging situations.

Ancillary Tools [7]

IHC:

Estrogen receptor (97%) and progesterone receptor (80%)

Androgen receptor (87%)

Abnormal expression of catenins

p120 (88%) (cytoplasmic)

Beta-catenin (42% nuclear and cytoplasmic; 23% retained membranous staining)

GATA3 (97–100%)

Mammaglobin (69%)

GCDFP-15 (52%) Mucicarmine (highlights intracellular mucin)

Molecular/cytogenetics description:

Mostly luminal A subtype by gene expression profiling

Followed by luminal B but rarely HER2-enriched or basal-like

1q gain, 16p gain, and 16q loss frequent

CDH1 gene located at 16q22.1

CDH1 (65%) and PIK3CA (48%) mutations common

CDH1 loss of function through truncating mutation or promoter hypermethylation combined with the loss of heterozygosity at chromosome 16, resulting in loss of protein

Microscopic Picture of Invasive Tubular Carcinoma (a–d)

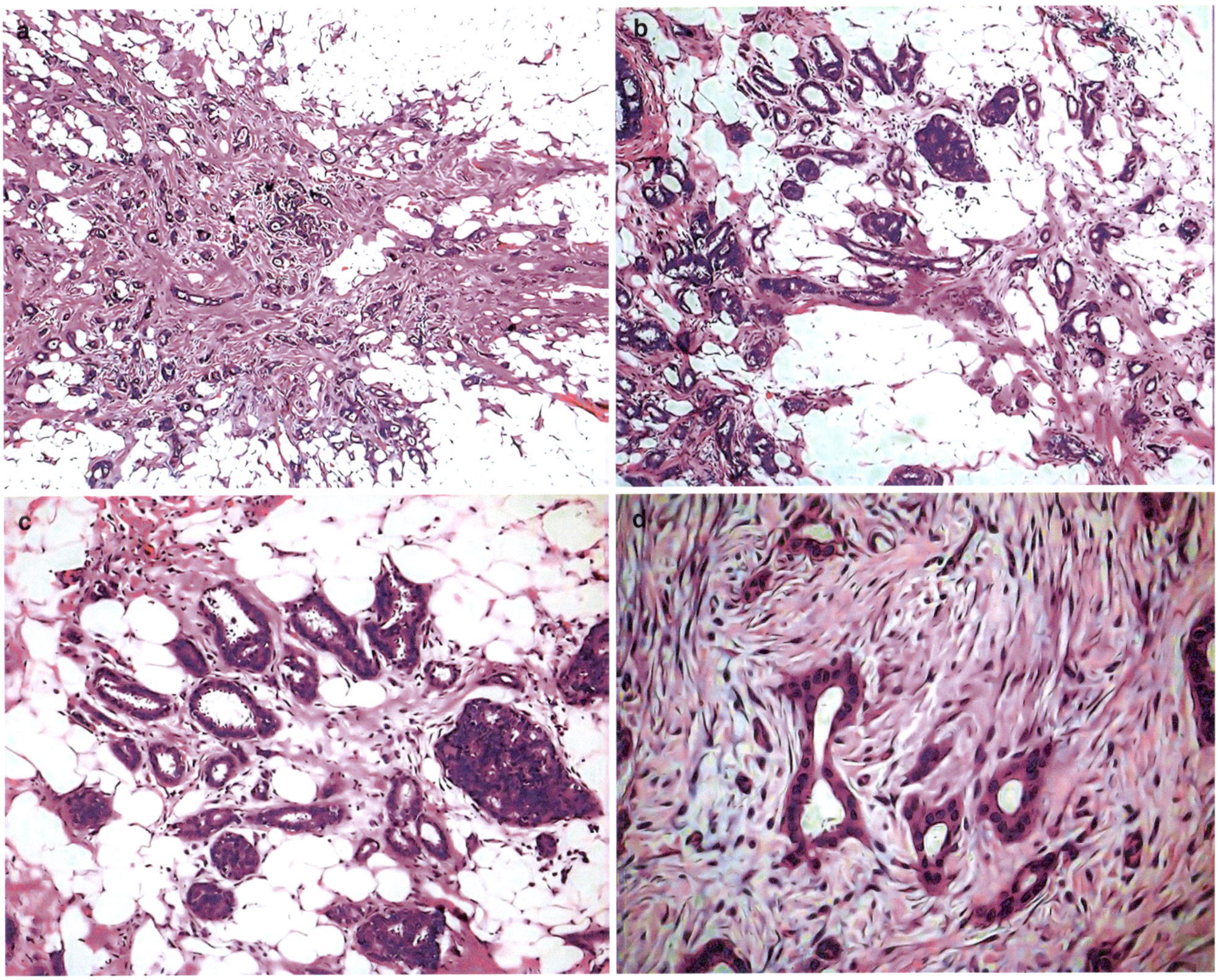

Sections show an infiltrative growth pattern, often with invasion into adipose tissue and with an associated fibrous or desmoplastic stromal response. >90% of the tumor is composed of small, ovoid, or angulated tubules with open lumina. Tubules are lined by a single layer of epithelial cells with low-grade nuclei and sparse mitoses (grade 1). Tumor cells often have apical cytoplasmic tufting or snouts. Cells lining the neoplastic tubules are cuboidal to columnar with uniform, small to intermediate-sized nuclei. No significant cytologic atypia, multilayering, or high mitotic activity (the presence of these would rule out tubular carcinoma). There may be luminal secretions or calcifications.

Pearls

A research study shows that the actual structure is not tubular; instead, it simulates a beaded necklace. 2-dimensional microscopy and 3-dimensional modeling studies revealed that the structure resembled a necklace formed by a string of beads, with the tubules visualized as blebs bridged together by solid cords of cells; continuous or branching tubules were not seen [8].

Micropapillary Carcinoma (a, b)

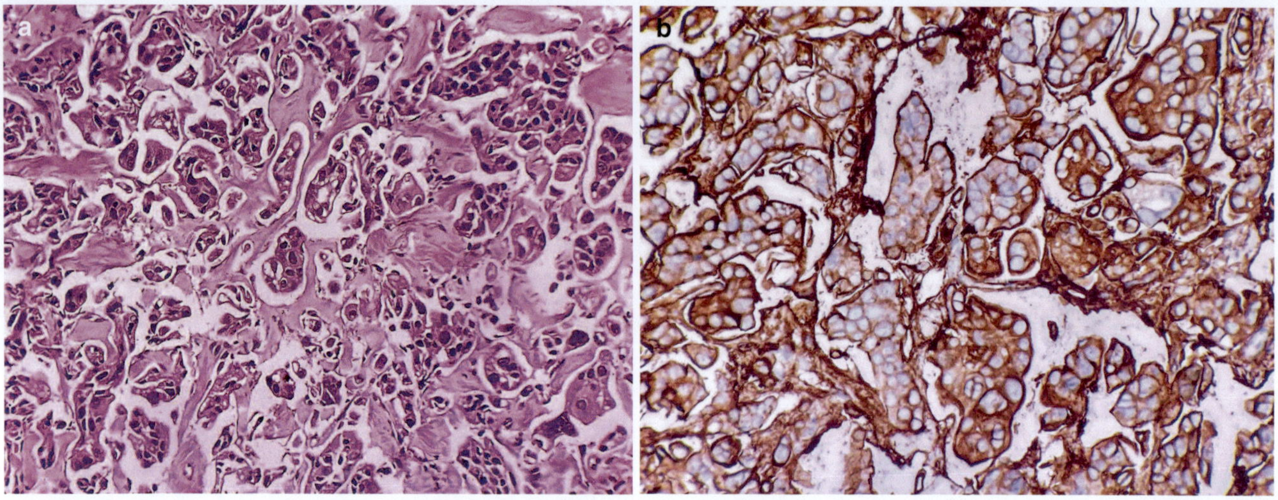

The section shows tufts of cells arranged in pseudopapillae, hollow tubules, and morula that are surrounded by empty, clear spaces formed by fibrocollagenous stroma. Cells show characteristic reverse polarity, also called inside-out pattern, with the apical surface abutting the epithelial stromal interface. Tumor cells have abundant eosinophilic cytoplasm. May have intracytoplasmic mucin. Nuclei around the periphery bulge with a knobby/serrated appearance. IHC for EMA (b) stains the apical membrane abutting the stroma, confirming inside out epithelial polarity.

Infiltrating Duct Carcinoma and Paget's Disease of the Breast with Metastases into Axillary Lymph Nodes (a, b)

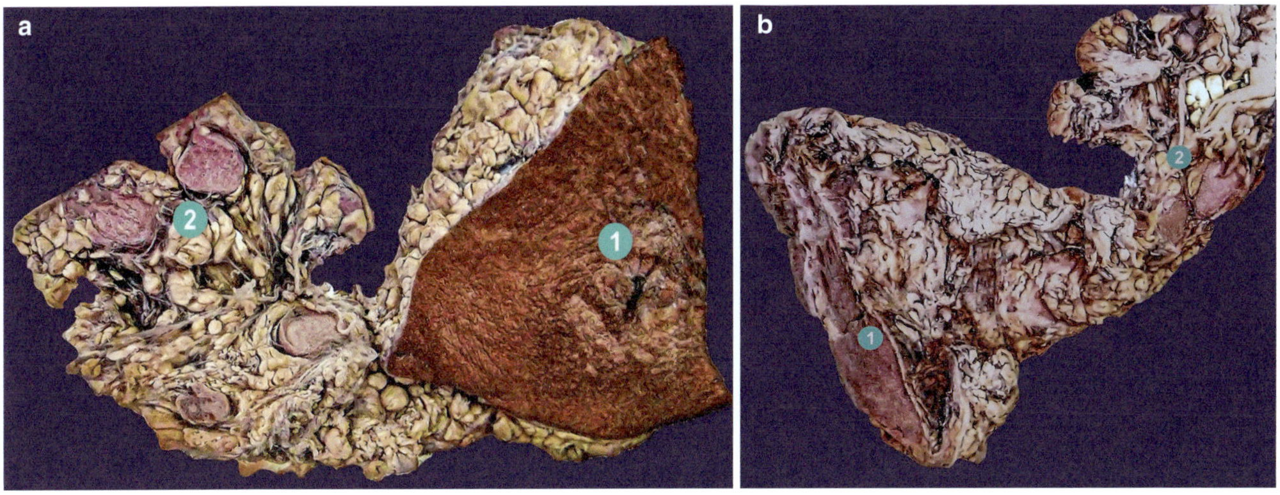

A specimen of breast tissue is mounted.

1. The cut section of the breast shows a gray-white, firm, irregular mass. The tumor mass is seen under the areola infiltrating the overlying skin with retraction and ulceration of the nipple.
2. The axillary lymph nodes are enlarged with a gray-white cut section denoting infiltration by tumor cells.

Microscopic Picture of Paget's Disease of Breast (c, d)

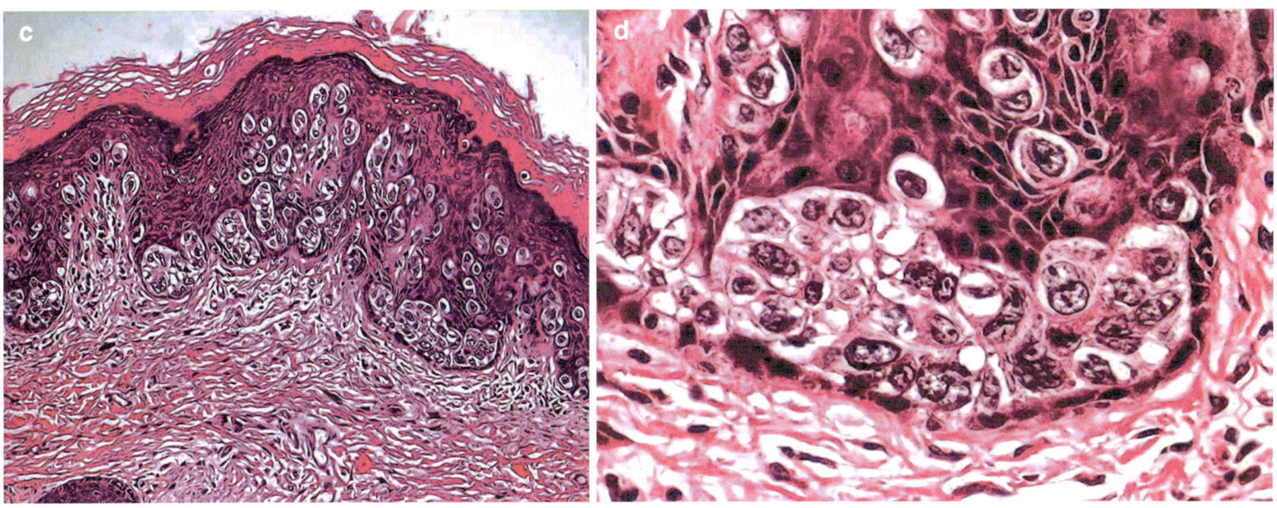

Sections show the epidermis is permeated by malignant cells arranged singly and in groups, often more numerous in the basal region. There is associated chronic inflammation in the superficial dermis. Cells have abundant pale cytoplasm and large irregular nuclei with prominent nucleoli.

Ancillary Tools

IHC [9]:

- CK7 (>90%)
- HER2 (80–100%)
- CAM5.2 (70–100%)
- ER (10–40%)
- PR (0–30%)

Microscopic Picture of Metastatic Lobular Carcinoma of Breast in Lymph Node (e–g)

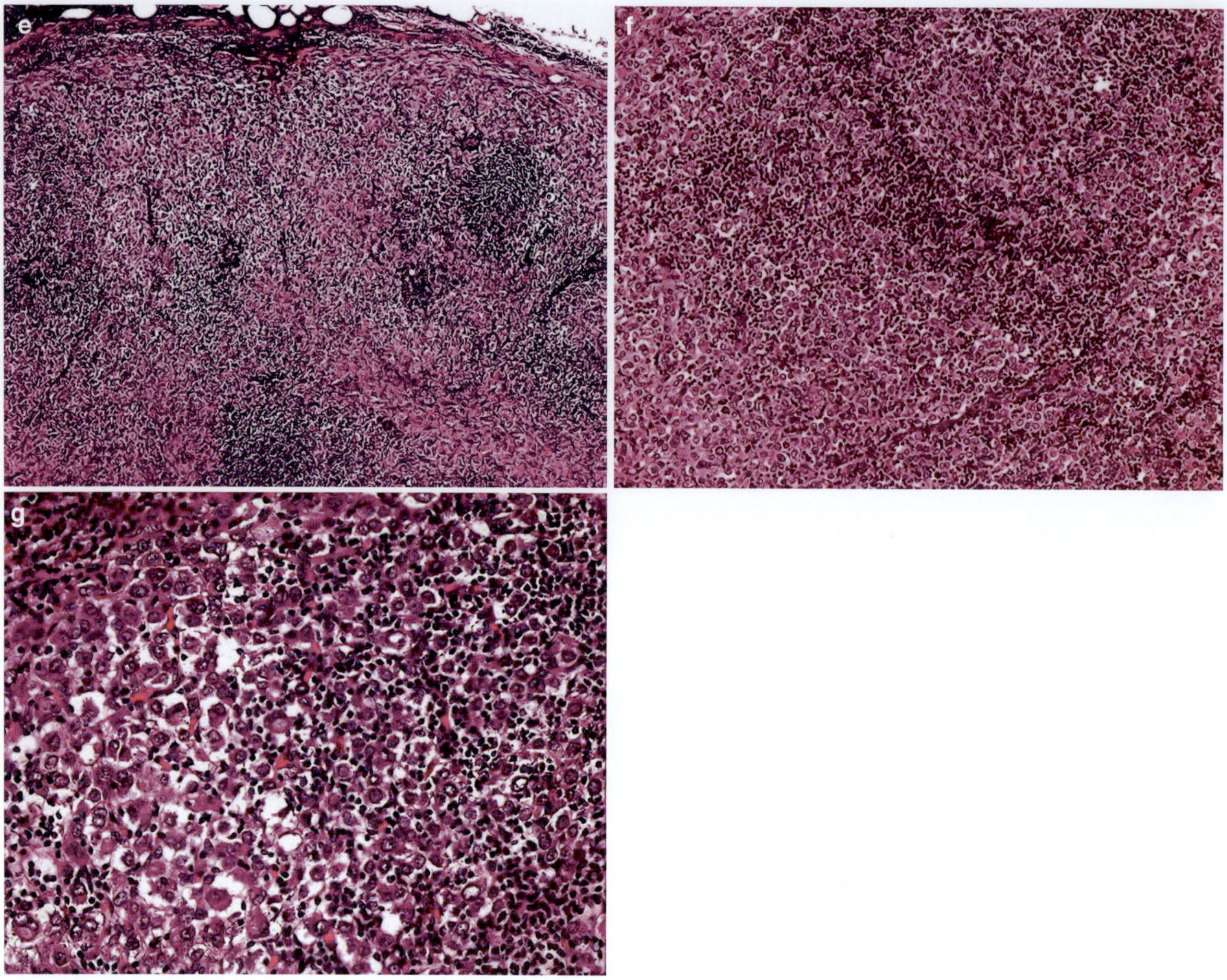

Sections of lymph nodes show diffuse infiltration by clusters of malignant epithelial cells of lobular breast carcinoma.

Mucinous (Colloid) Carcinoma

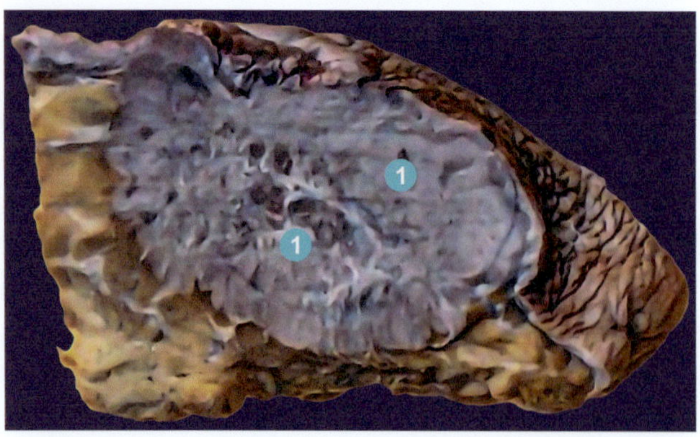

A specimen of breast tissue is mounted.

1. There is a large infiltrative, bluish-white gelatinous mass with central areas of degeneration and necrosis.

Microscopic Picture of Mucinous (Colloid) Carcinoma (a–c)

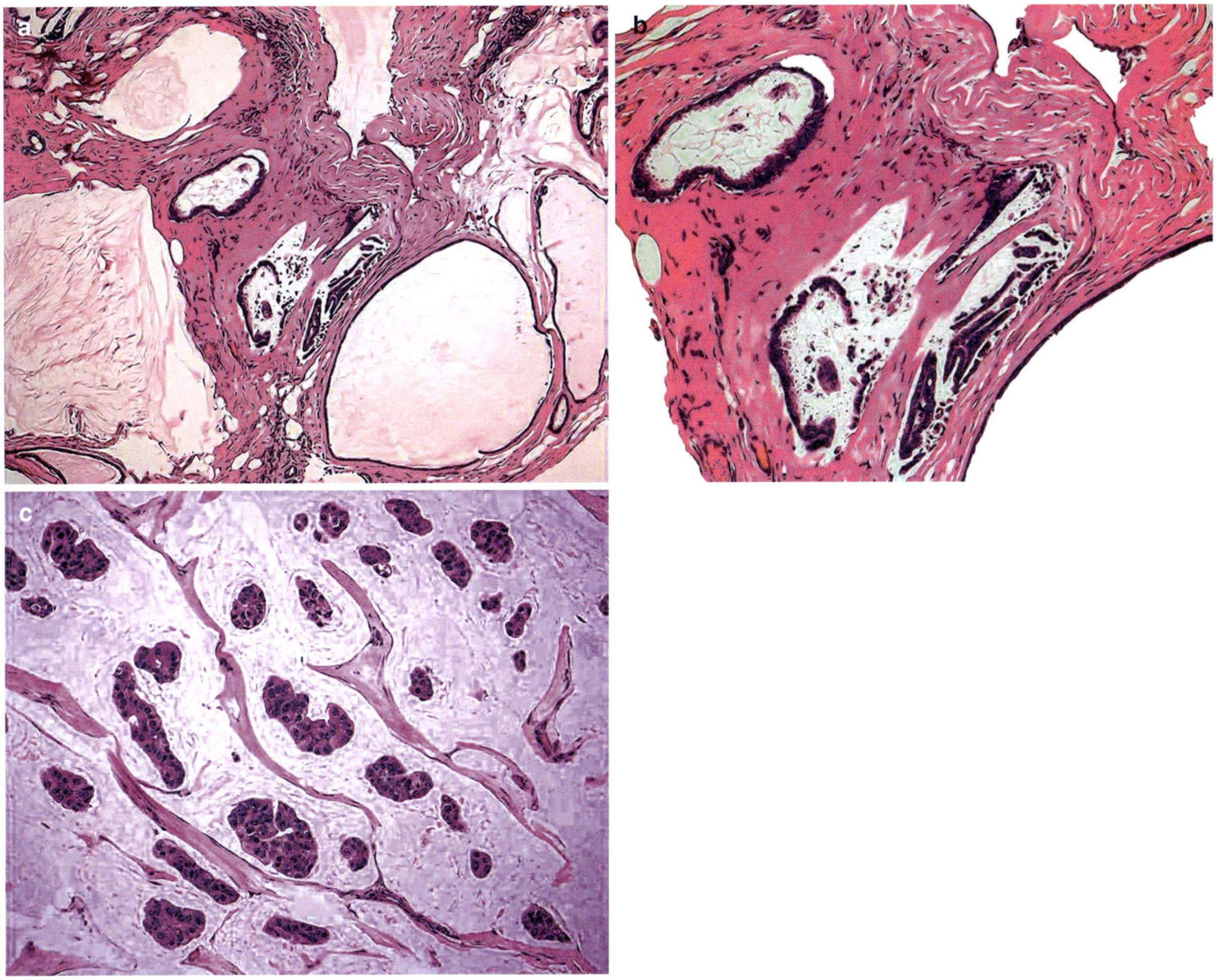

Sections show scattered small epithelial clusters/nests of tumor cells with low or intermediate nuclear grade floating in pools of extracellular mucin separated by fibrous septa with capillaries. The mucinous component comprises >90% of the tumor (Capella type A tumor).

Ancillary Tools

IHC [10]:

ER (94%), PR (80%)

MUC2

Type B: chromogranin, synaptophysin, neuron-specific enolase (NSE)

WT1

GATA3

Molecular/cytogenetics description [11]:

Categorized as luminal A with a favorable prognosis

Lacks 1p gains and 16q losses and somatic mutations of PIK3CA and AKT1, which are common in other ER+, HER2-invasive breast carcinomas. More often, diploid

Fungating Carcinoma of the Breast

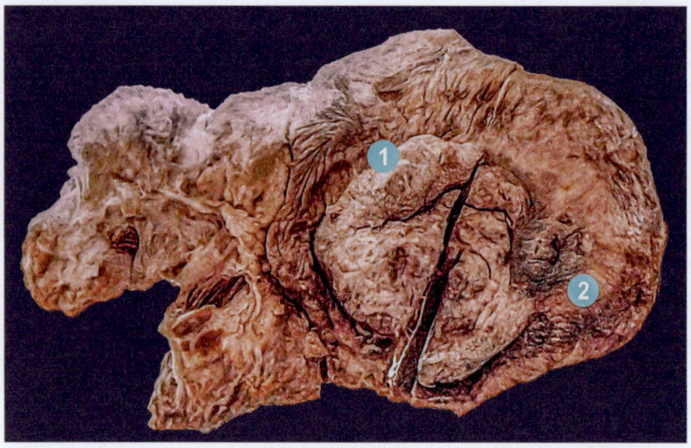

A specimen of breast tissue is mounted.

1. It shows a fungating malignant tumor tissue destroying the skin to form a raised malignant ulcer.
2. The retracted and ulcerated nipple is seen at the lower border of the mass.

Fungating Carcinoma of the Breast

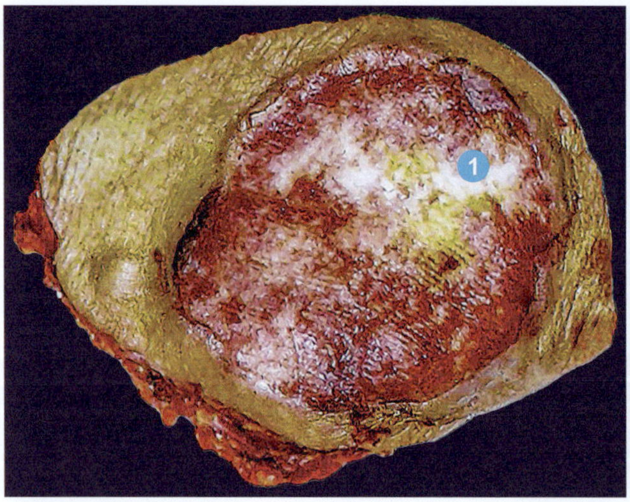

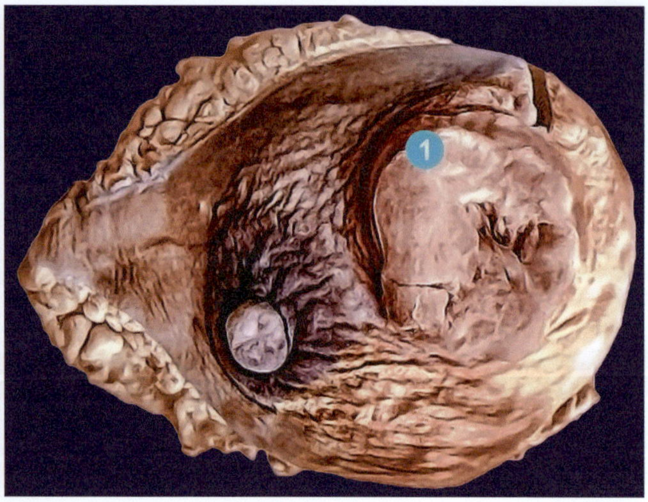

A specimen of breast tissue is mounted.

1. It shows a large, red, and necrotic mass protruding through the skin.

Carcinoma of Male Breast

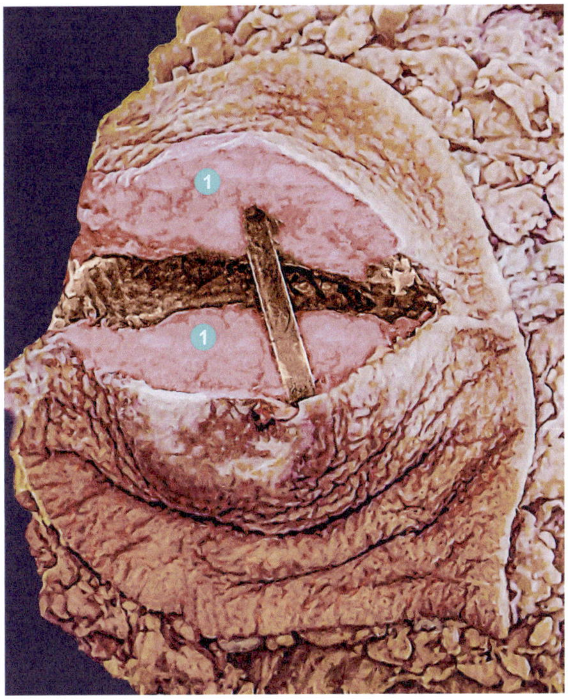

The male breast is mounted.

1. The cut section shows a gray-white malignant tumor mass eroding and destroying the nipple.

Microscopic Picture of Carcinoma of Male Breast (a–c)

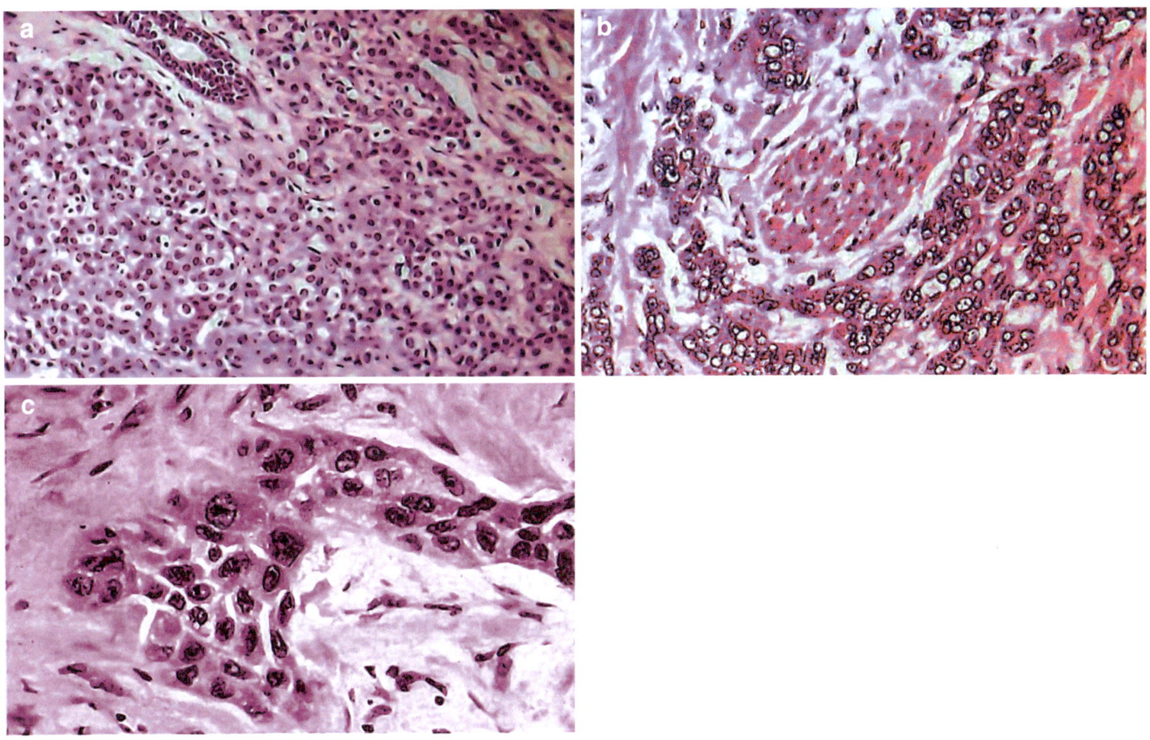

Sections show features of invasive duct carcinoma similar to those of the female counterpart. The cells are highly pleomorphic with an area of perineural invasion.

Ancillary Tools

IHC [12]:

ER (85–90%), PR (85%), AR (90–95%), BCL2 (94%) (most luminal A or luminal B type)

Younger patients (under 45 years) tend to have HER2+

Molecular/cytogenetics description [13]:

p53 mutations in exon 6 found in over 90% of male cases

Gene expression performed in 66 male breast cancer tumors revealed 2 unique subgroups (luminal M1 and M2) that were different in biological features and outcome when compared to female breast cancers

EGFR and CCND1 genes are amplified more in male than female breast cancers

High methylation status of MSH6, WT1, PAX5, PAX6, GATA5, and CDH13 correlates with more aggressive phenotypes and poor survival

Male and female breast cancers share many of these methylated genes, but many genes are less frequently methylated in males

Methylation of RASSF1A (downregulation of ER alpha and microRNAs) is more common in male than female breast carcinomas

References

1. Maiorano E, Albrizio M. (1995). Tubular adenoma of the breast: an immunohistochemical study of ten cases. Pathol Res Pract. 191(12):1222-30. doi: https://doi.org/10.1016/S0344-0338(11)81130-1. PMID: 8927570.
2. Darooei M. et al. (2019). MED12 somatic mutations encompassing exon 2 associated with benign breast fibroadenomas and not breast carcinoma in Indian women. J Cell Biochem. 120(1):182-191. doi: https://doi.org/10.1002/jcb.27293. PMID: 30230586.
3. Shubham S, Ahuja A, Bhardwaj M. (2019). Immunohistochemical expression of Ki-67, p53, and CD10 in phyllodes tumor and their correlation with its histological grade. J Lab Physicians. 11(4):330-334. doi: https://doi.org/10.4103/JLP.JLP_106_19. PMID: 31929699; PMCID: PMC6943865.
4. Sawyer EJ. et al. (2000). Molecular analysis of phyllodes tumors reveals distinct changes in the epithelial and stromal components. Am J Pathol. 156(3):1093-8. doi: https://doi.org/10.1016/S0002-9440(10)64977-2. PMID: 10702425; PMCID: PMC1876863.
5. Rakha E, Tozbikian G. Invasive breast cancer of no special type (NST). PathologyOutlines.com website. https://www.pathologyoutlines.com/topic/breastmalignantductalNOS.html.
6. Simpson, P.T. et al. (2005), Molecular evolution of breast cancer. J. Pathol., 205: 248-254. https://doi.org/10.1002/path.1691.
7. Christgen M. et al. (2021).Lobular Breast Cancer: Histomorphology and Different Concepts of a Special Spectrum of Tumors. Cancers (Basel). 13(15):3695. doi: https://doi.org/10.3390/cancers13153695. PMID: 34359596; PMCID: PMC8345067.
8. Marchiò C, Sapino A, Arisio R, Bussolati G. (2006). A new vision of tubular and tubulo-lobular carcinomas of the breast, as revealed by 3-D modeling. Histopathology. 48(5):556-62. doi: https://doi.org/10.1111/j.1365-2559.2006.02373.x. PMID: 16623781.
9. Sandoval-Leon AC. et al. (2013). Paget's disease of the nipple. Breast Cancer Res Treat. 141(1):1-12. doi: https://doi.org/10.1007/s10549-013-2661-4. PMID: 23929251.
10. Dumitru A. et al. (2015). Mucinous Breast Cancer: a Review Study of 5 Year Experience from a Hospital-Based Series of Cases. Maedica (Bucur). 10(1):14-8. PMID: 26225144; PMCID: PMC4496759.
11. Pareja F. et al. (2019). The Genomic Landscape of Mucinous Breast Cancer. J Natl Cancer Inst. 111(7):737-741. doi: https://doi.org/10.1093/jnci/djy216. PMID: 30649385; PMCID: PMC6624163.
12. Chavez-Macgregor M. et al. (2013). Male breast cancer according to tumor subtype and race: a population-based study. Cancer. 119(9):1611-7. doi: https://doi.org/10.1002/cncr.27905. PMID: 23341341; PMCID: PMC3971835.
13. Johansson I. et al. (2012). Gene expression profiling of primary male breast cancers reveals two unique subgroups and identifies N-acetyltransferase-1 (NAT1) as a novel prognostic biomarker. Breast Cancer Res. 14(1):R31. doi: https://doi.org/10.1186/bcr3116. PMID: 22333393; PMCID: PMC3496149.

Diseases of the Lymphoreticular System

10

The lymphoreticular system is an intricate network composed of the lymphoid tissues and the reticuloendothelial system, playing pivotal roles in the human body's defenses against a variety of pathogenic agents. As the staging ground for both the adaptive and innate immune responses, any pathological alterations in this system can significantly influence overall health.

This chapter delves into the gross and microscopic pathology of the lymphoreticular system, elucidating the diverse spectrum of diseases and conditions that can afflict it, from benign lymphadenopathy to malignant lymphomas. Each disorder will be examined in terms of its gross and microscopic changes.

We aim to provide a comprehensive, yet accessible, guide to the gross and microscopic pathology of the lymphoreticular system, serving as a valuable resource for medical students, pathology residents, and practicing pathologists, as well as clinicians in related fields.

The studied cases will be arranged according to the following scheme:

1. **Circulatory Disturbances**
   (a) Congestive splenomegaly
   (b) Infarction
2. **Inflammatory Lesions**
   (a) Tuberculosis
3. **Neoplastic Lesions**
   (a) Lymphoma
4. **Amyloidosis**

10.1 Circulatory Disturbances

Congestive Splenomegaly

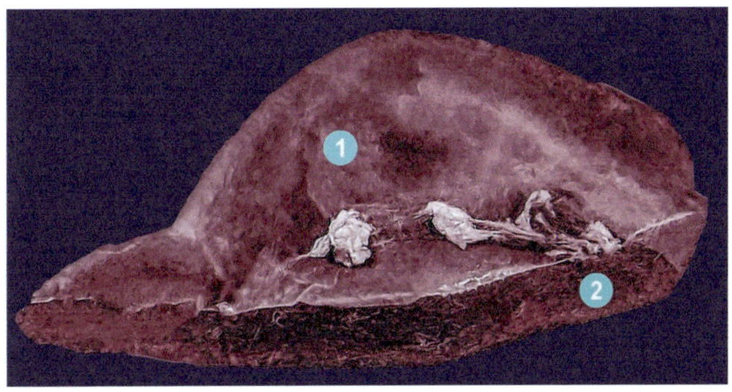

Half of a bisected spleen is mounted.

1. The spleen is enlarged and has a smooth, dark red surface and sharp edges indicative of firm consistency.
2. The cut section is dark brown due to chronic venous congestion (due to portal hypertension and bilharzial pigments).

G. Dawood, *Color Atlas of Human Gross and Microscopic Pathology*, https://doi.org/10.1007/978-3-031-76007-5_10

Congestive Splenomegaly

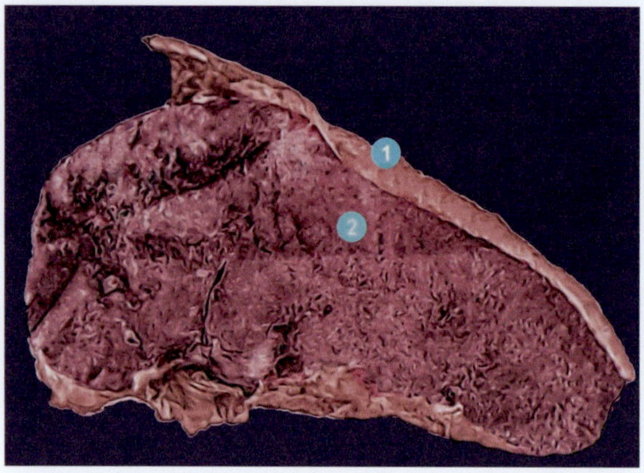

The cut section of the spleen is mounted.

1) The capsule is thickened and fibrous.
2) The cut section is congested with a muddy look.

Microscopic Picture of Congestive Splenomegaly (a, b)

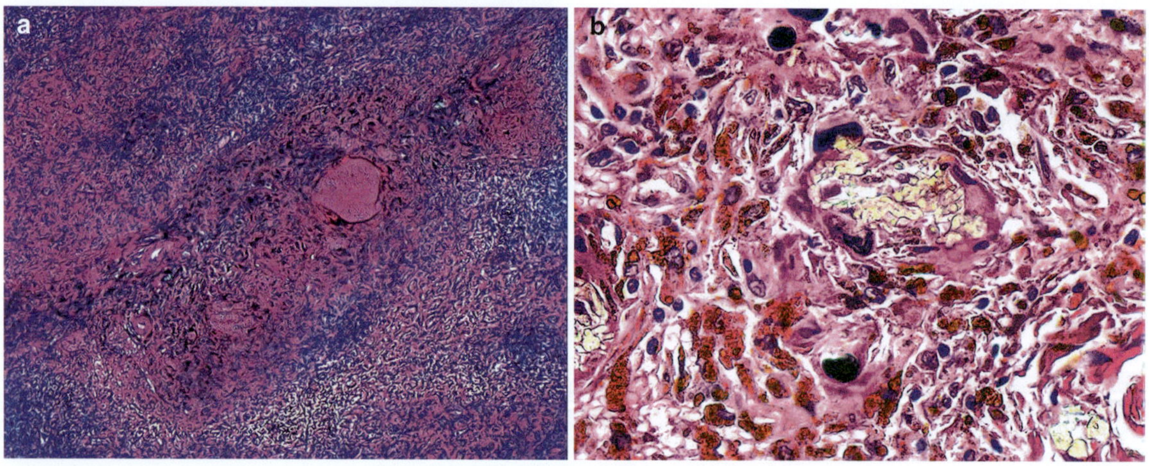

Sections show dilated veins and sinuses, fibrosis of red pulp, and hemosiderin-laden macrophages. Iron and calcium-containing fibrotic nodules (Gamna-Gandy bodies) secondary to hemorrhage are seen in areas.

Pearls

The muddy appearance of congested splenomegaly may be due to [1]:

1. Hemostasis and Blood Pooling: The spleen, being a highly vascular organ, holds a significant portion of the body's blood supply. In conditions leading to splenomegaly, this capacity is often increased, resulting in increased blood pooling. This causes a mottled or "muddy" appearance due to stagnant, coagulated blood mixed with the spleen's normal tissue.
2. Histopathological changes in the underlying disease process causing splenomegaly. These changes may include infiltration by inflammatory cells, fibrosis, or necrosis, all of which can contribute to a "muddy" appearance.
3. Hyperplasia of Splenic Tissue: Conditions causing splenomegaly often involve an increased production of splenic tissues, including white and red pulp. The red pulp, being rich in blood vessels, may contribute to a congested, muddy appearance.

Infarction of Spleen (a, b)

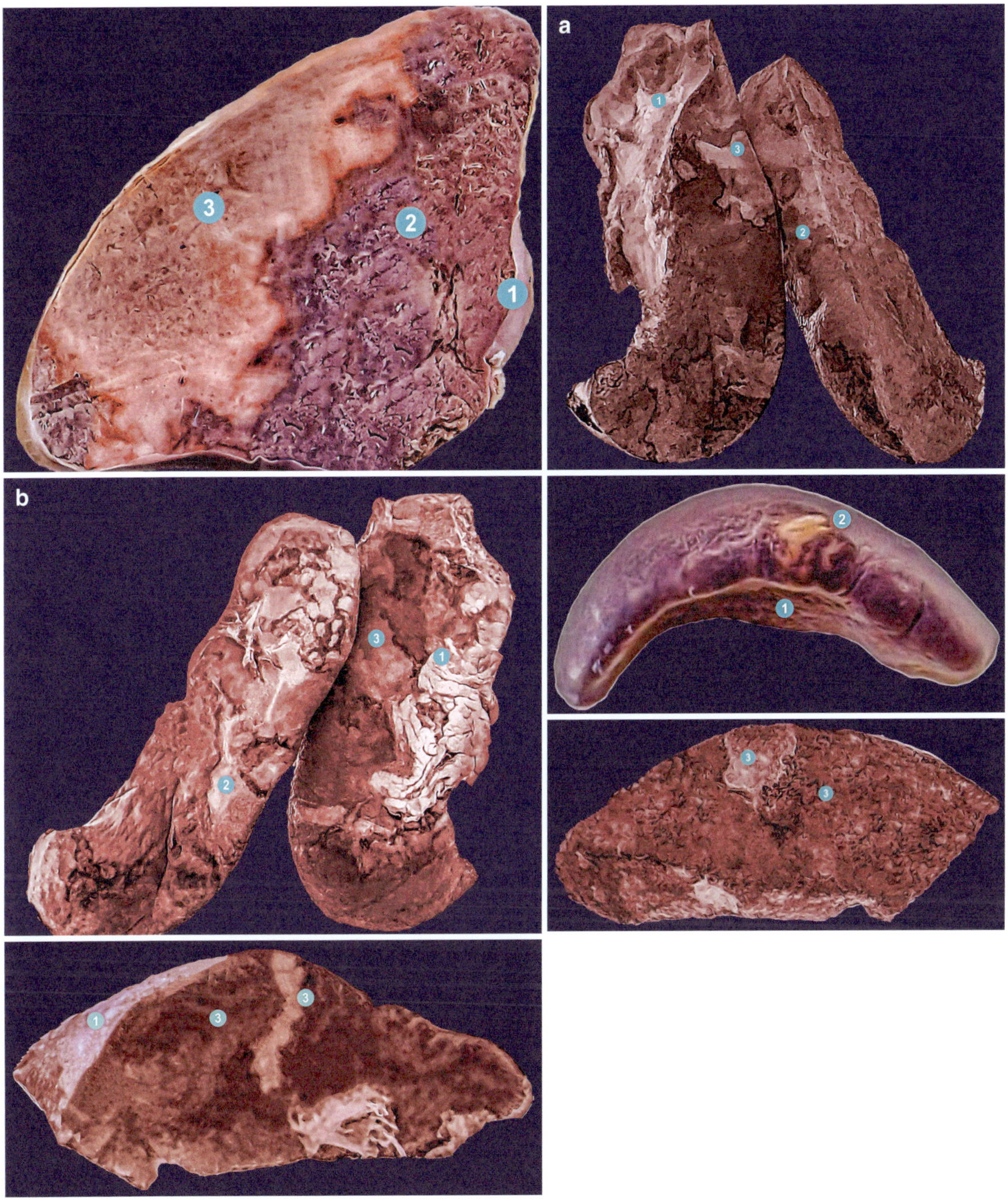

Half of a bisected enlarged spleen is mounted.

1. The capsule is white and thickened by fibrosis.
2. The surface shows a pale brown area surrounded by hemorrhagic zones.
3. The cut section is dark red with a pale area of infarction with dark congested borders. The broad base of the infarct is directed towards the surface.

Microscopic Picture of Infarction of Spleen (a–c)

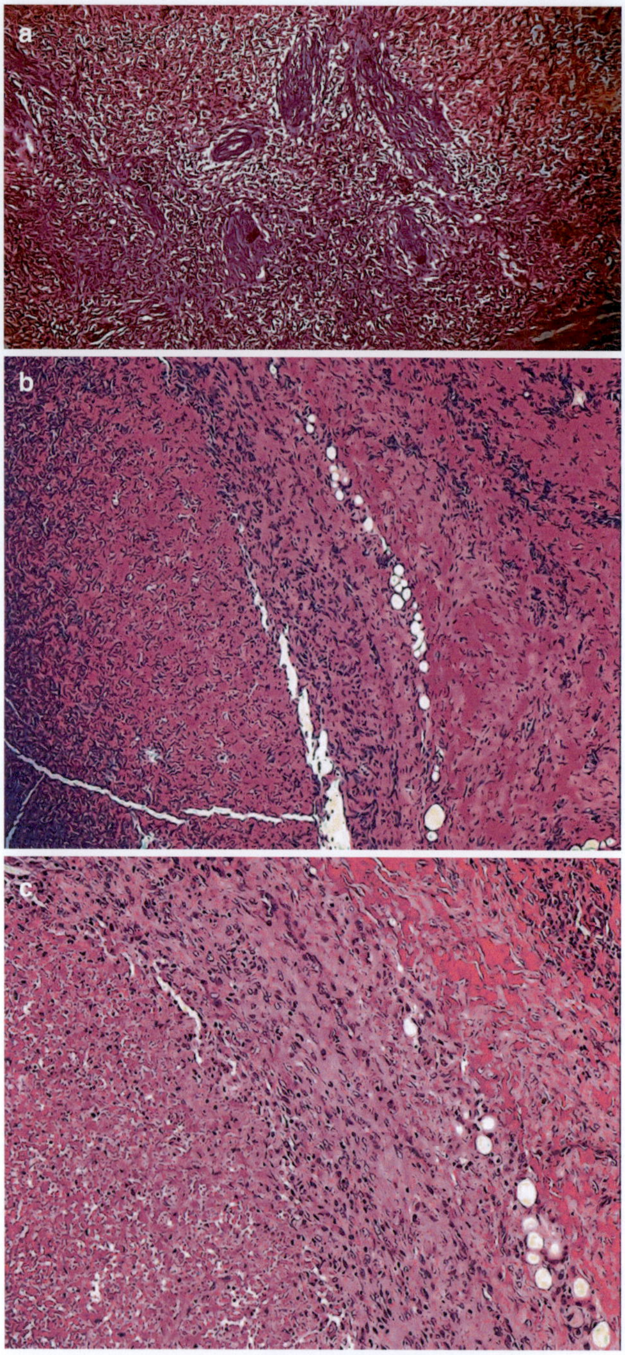

Sections show coagulative necrosis of the splenic parenchyma, with loss of nuclear detail and eosinophilic cytoplasm. The necrotic area is surrounded by a zone of congestion and hemorrhage, infiltrated with neutrophils.

10.2 Inflammatory Lesions

Miliary Tuberculosis of Spleen

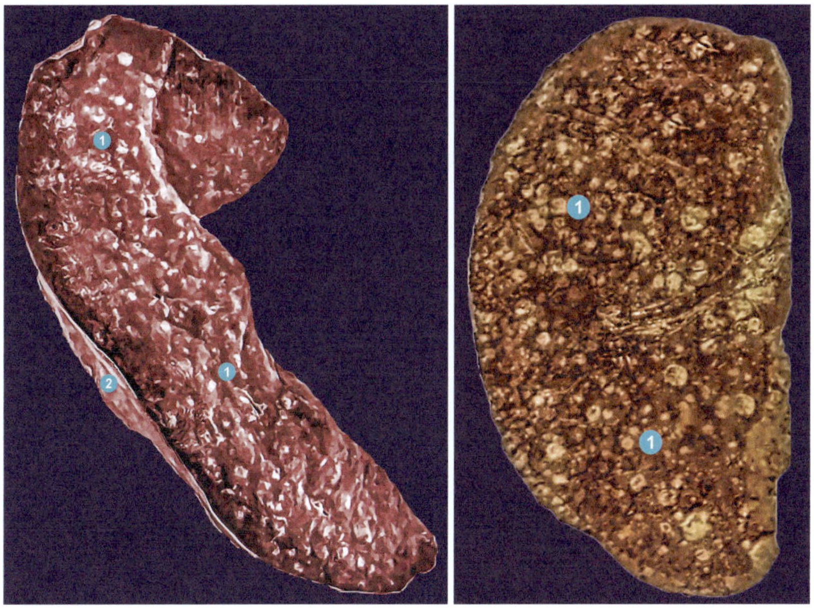

Half of a bisected spleen is mounted.

1. The cut section shows multiple, small, yellow caseous foci.
2. The capsule is thickened and fibrous.

Multiple Tuberculomata of Spleen (a, b)

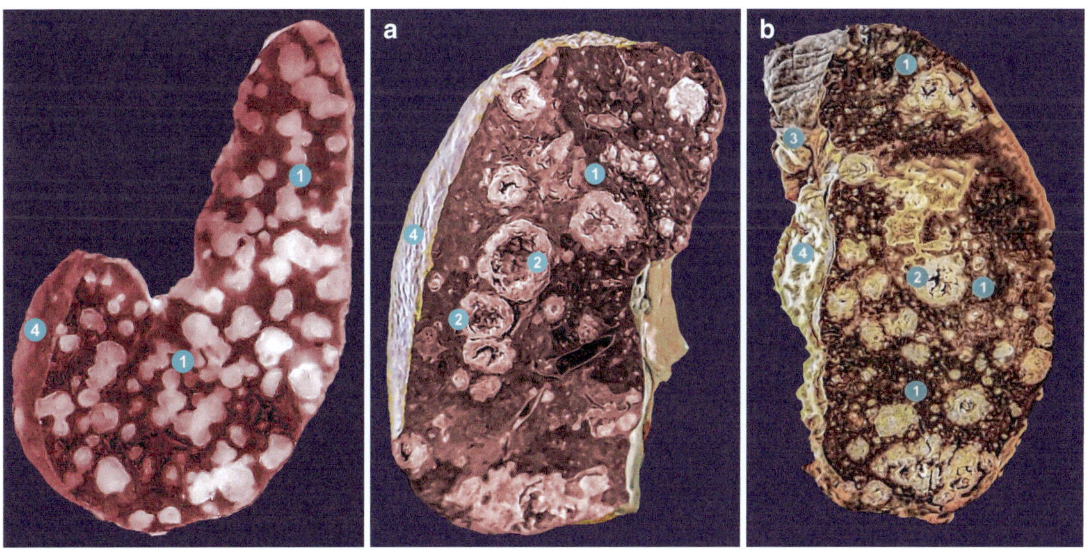

Half of a bisected spleen is mounted.

1. The cut section shows multiple, large, well-defined, yellow-white, caseous foci scattered all over.
2. The large one shows central cavitation due to the fall of caseous material.
3. An enlarged caseous lymph node is seen at the hilum.
4. The capsule is thickened and fibrous.

Microscopic Picture of Tuberculosis of Spleen (c, d)

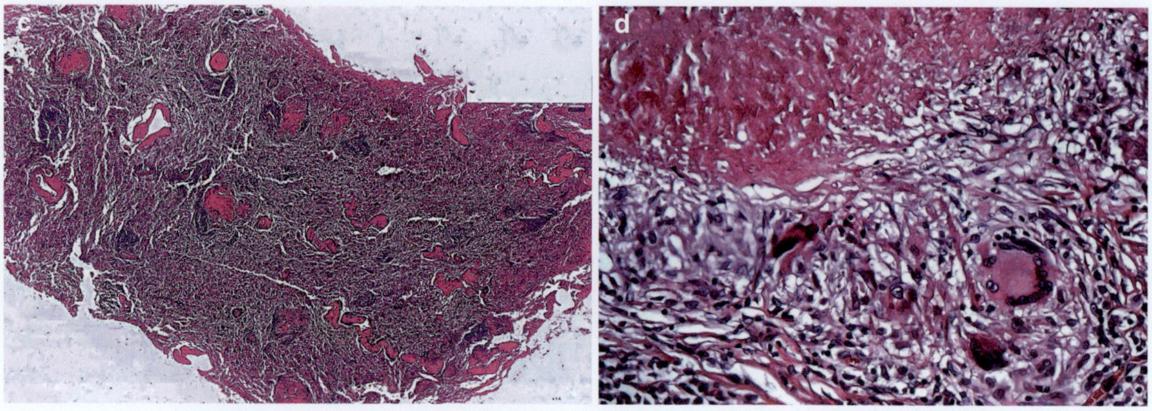

Sections show multiple tuberculoid granulomas formed of epithelioid cells, Langhans giant cells, and lymphocytes with the presence of areas of caseation necrosis.

Tabes Mesentrica

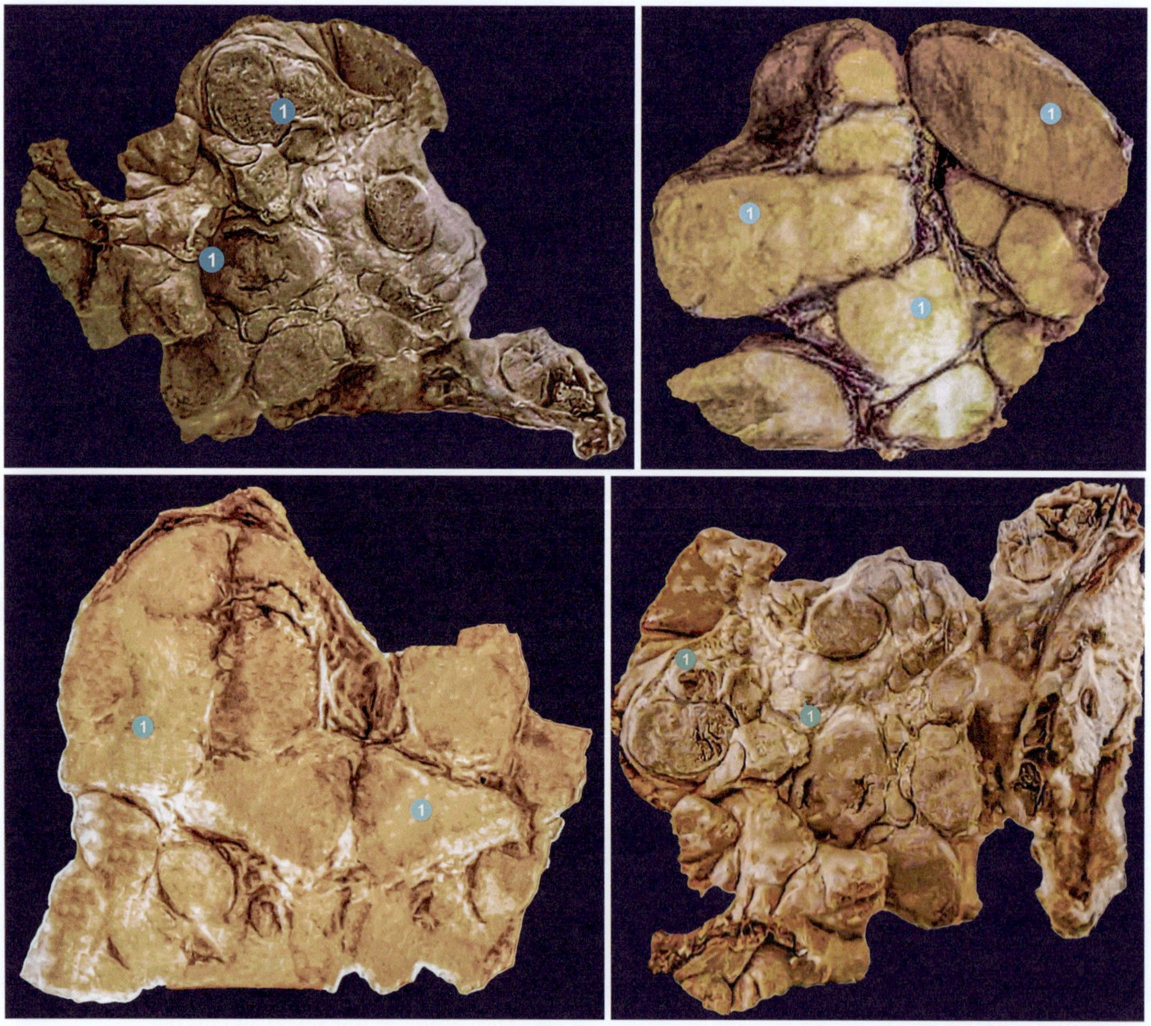

A part of the mesentery is mounted.

1. Multiple enlarged mesenteric lymph nodes, variable in size, matted, and with opaque yellow-cut sections are observed.

10.3 Neoplastic Lesions

Lymphoma of Lymph Nodes (Hodgkin's Lymphoma)

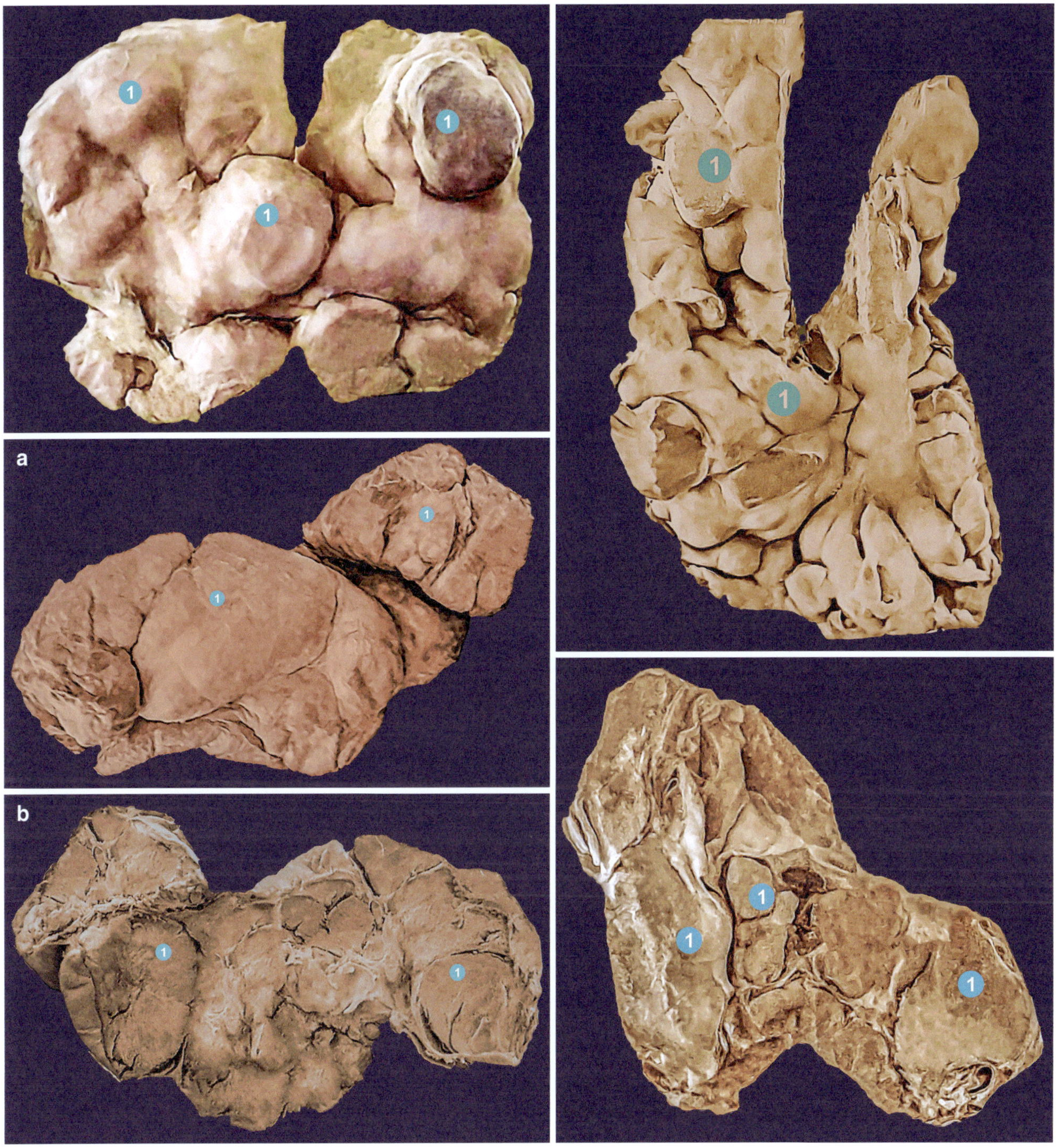

A group of enlarged lymph nodes is mounted.

1) They have a bossy nodular surface and a fleshy cut section (fish flesh appearance).

Microscopic Picture of Classic Hodgkin's Lymphoma—Nodular Sclerosis Type (a–o)

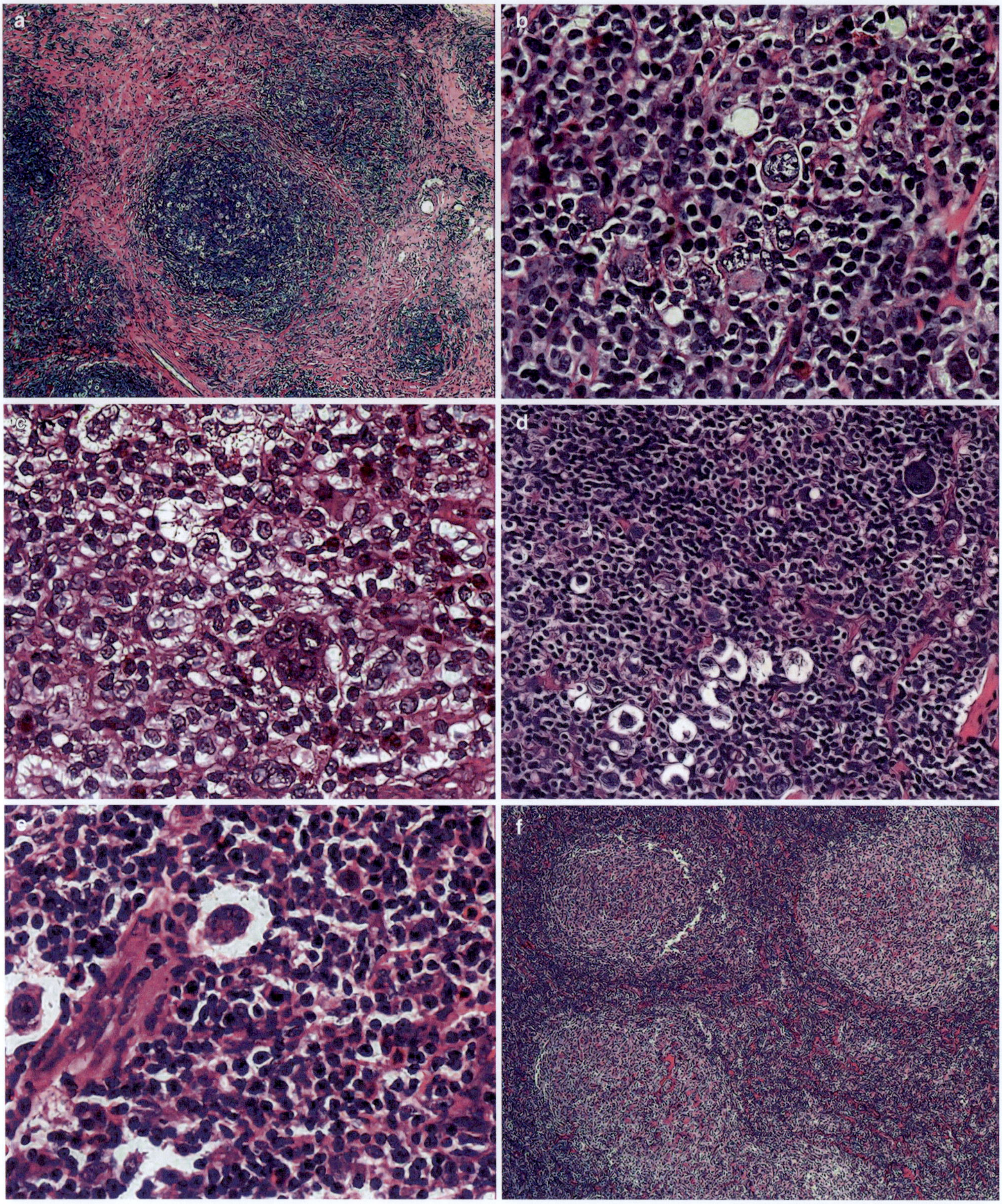

Sections show (a–e) effaced nodal architecture by nodular growth with a mottled or moth-eaten appearance due to clusters of lacunar cells, microabscesses, or areas of necrosis. The nodular growth is surrounded by broad fibrous, poor birefringent collagen bands. The nodular infiltrate has a highly variable number of HRS cells, small lymphocytes, and other inflammatory cells; often numerous eosinophils, histiocytes, and neutrophils; occasional foamy macrophages. Mitoses are uncommon.

HRS cells have more lobated nuclei, smaller lobes, less prominent nucleoli, and more cytoplasm than other types of classic Hodgkin's lymphoma. **Lacunar cells** have folded or multilobate nuclei surrounded by abundant pale cytoplasm

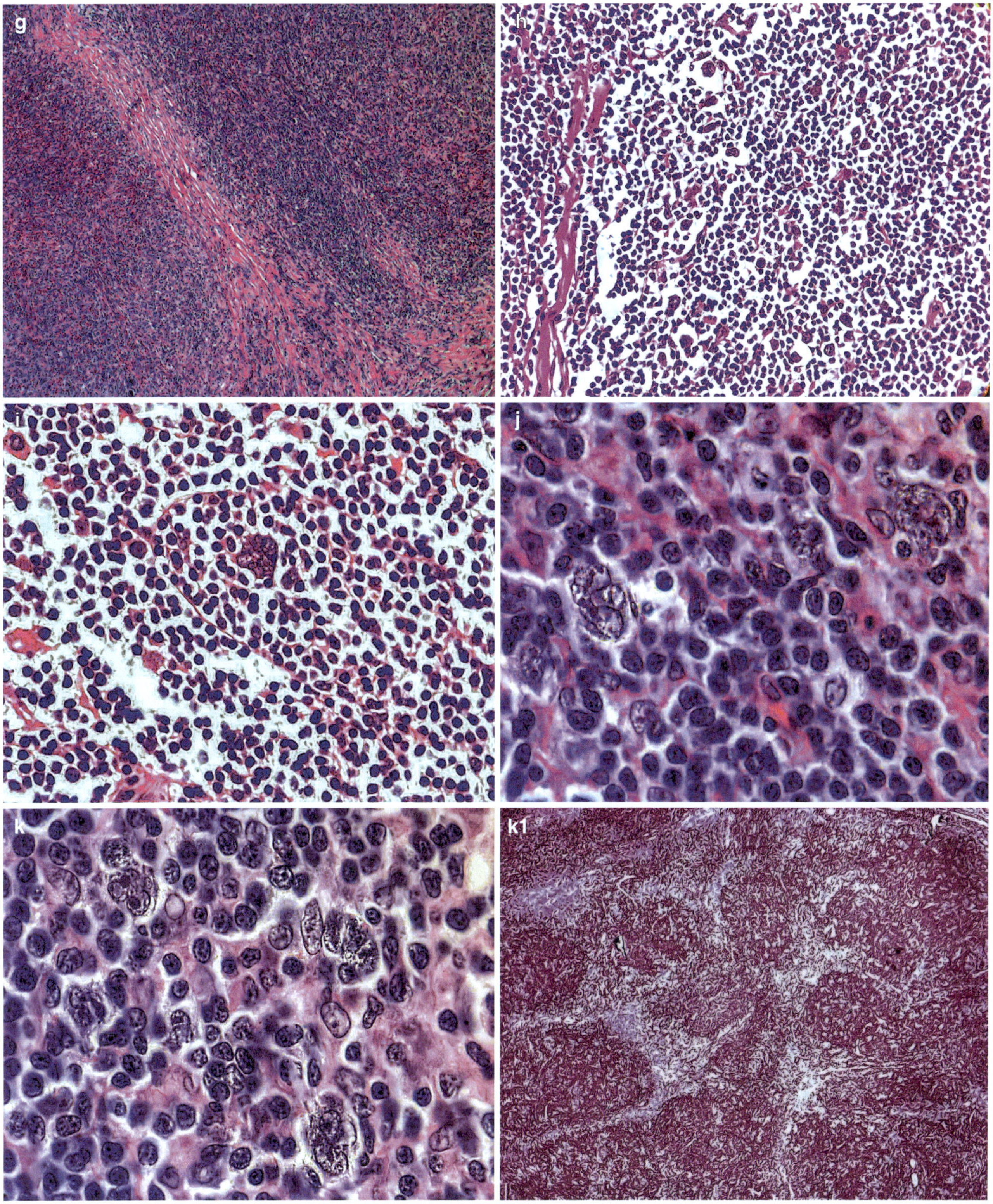

often disrupted or retracted during cutting of sections with formalin fixation (but not B5 or Zenkers), leaving a lacune (empty hole); associated with necrosis and histiocytes (necrotizing granuloma-like).

- **Nodular sclerosis lymphocytic predominant type (NLPHL)** (f–k) has similar features with few differences. It has vague nodules of small lymphocytes with sparse, relatively large tumor cells with multilobulated or round nuclei, a thin nuclear membrane, finely granular chromatin, and variable small nucleoli (popcorn cells). Large cells called LP cells, previously known as lymphocytic and histiocytic cells, are present and admixed with numerous small B lymphocytes, epithelioid histiocytes, and

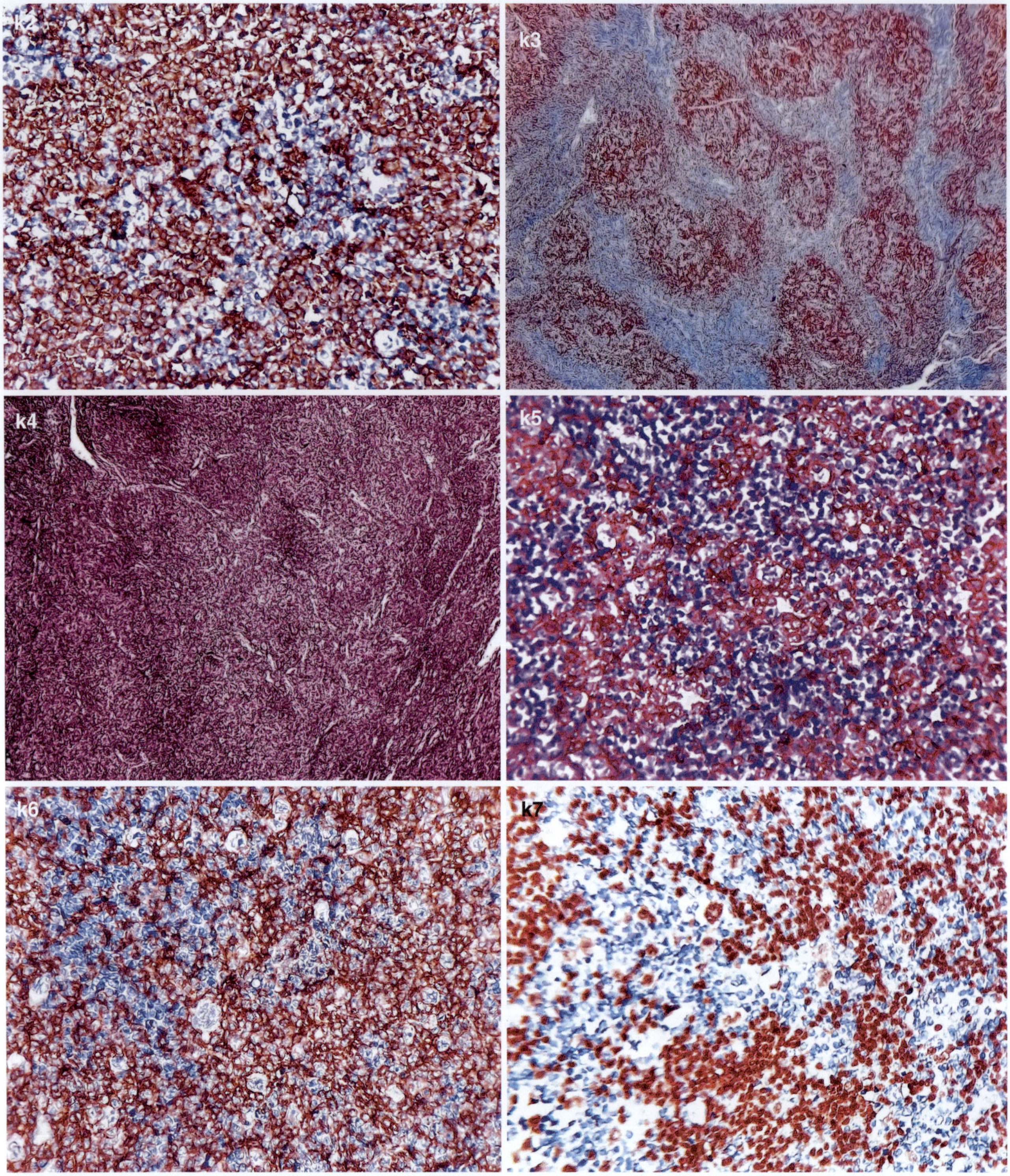

CD21+ follicular dendritic cells. Scant eosinophils, plasma cells, or fibrosis. Prominent sclerosis is unusual but may occur in older lesions. No/rare classic Reed-Sternberg (RS) cells, although LP cells may occasionally resemble Reed-Sternberg cells/variants.

Immunohistochemically, the tumor cells are stained positively for

CD20 (k1 & k2)
CD21 (k3)
CD3 (k4 & k5)
CD4 (k6)
PAX5 (k7)
OCT2 (k8)
Ki67 (k9)

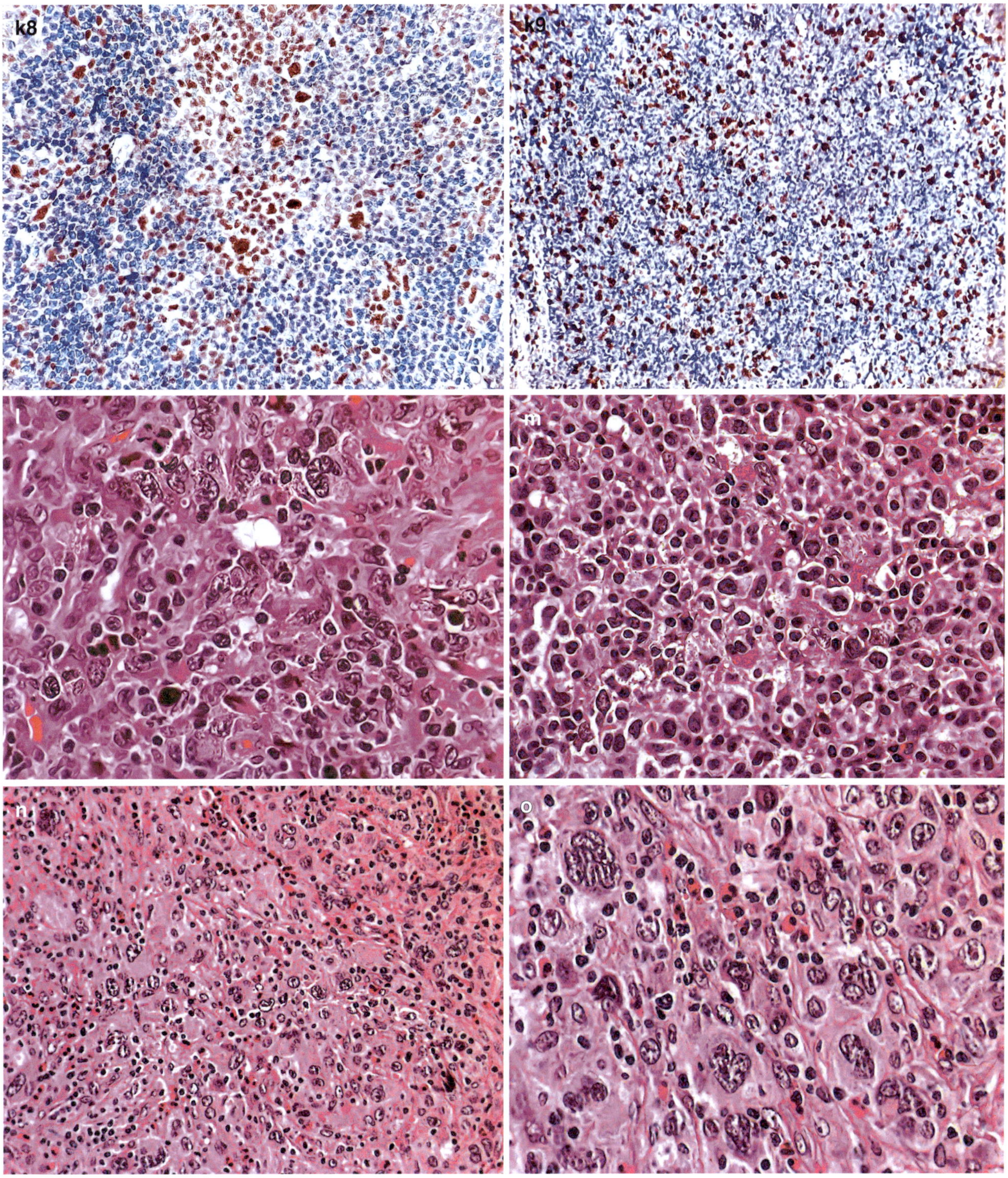

- **Syncytial variant** (l–o): characterized by numerous HRS cells that have a cohesive appearance and form confluent sheets in many of the tumor nodules and prominent aggregates of lacunar cells.

Microscopic Picture of Classic Hodgkin's Lymphoma—Mixed Cellularity Type (a–e)

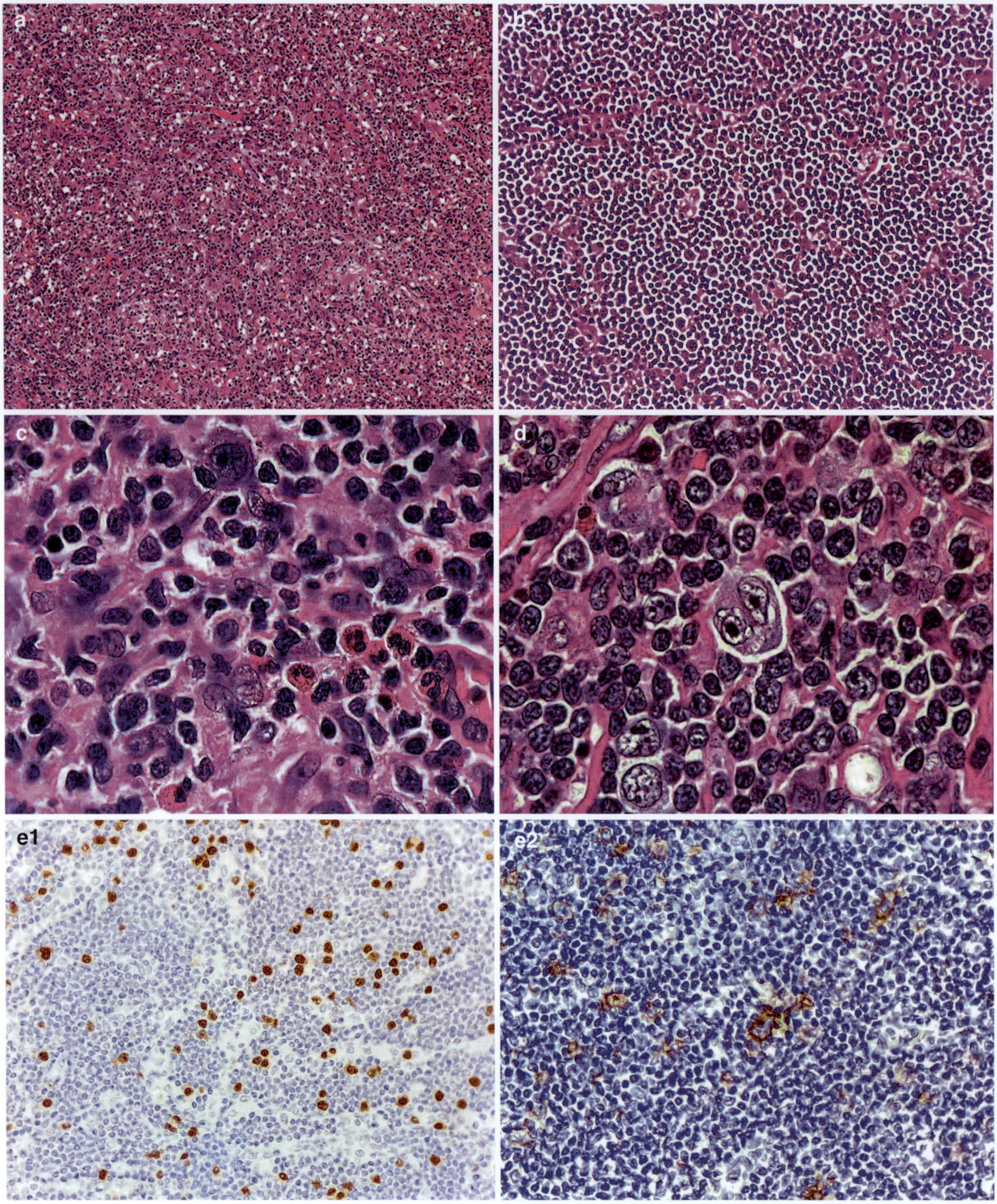

Sections show effaced nodal architecture by diffuse cellular infiltrate formed of lymphocytes, eosinophils, neutrophils, plasma cells, histiocytes, fibroblasts admixed with a proliferation of HRS cells (<10% of the cellularity), and Hodgkin cells. Tumor cells are positively stained with

MUM1 (e1) and
CD30 (e2)

Microscopic Picture of Classic Hodgkin's Lymphoma—Lymphocytic Rich Type (a, b)

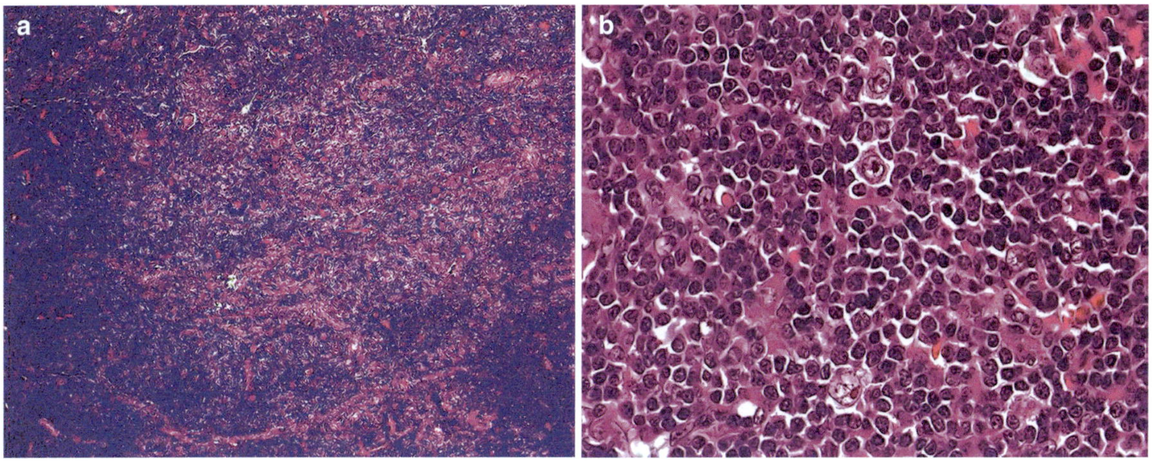

The section shows effaced nodal architecture by small lymphocytes forming either nodular or diffuse patterns. Nodules contain HRS cells within the nodules but outside of the germinal centers. In LRCHL diffuse cases, small lymphocytes of the background can be intermingled with histiocytes with or without epithelioid morphology.

Microscopic Picture of Classic Hodgkin's Lymphoma—Lymphocytic Depleted Type (a–d)

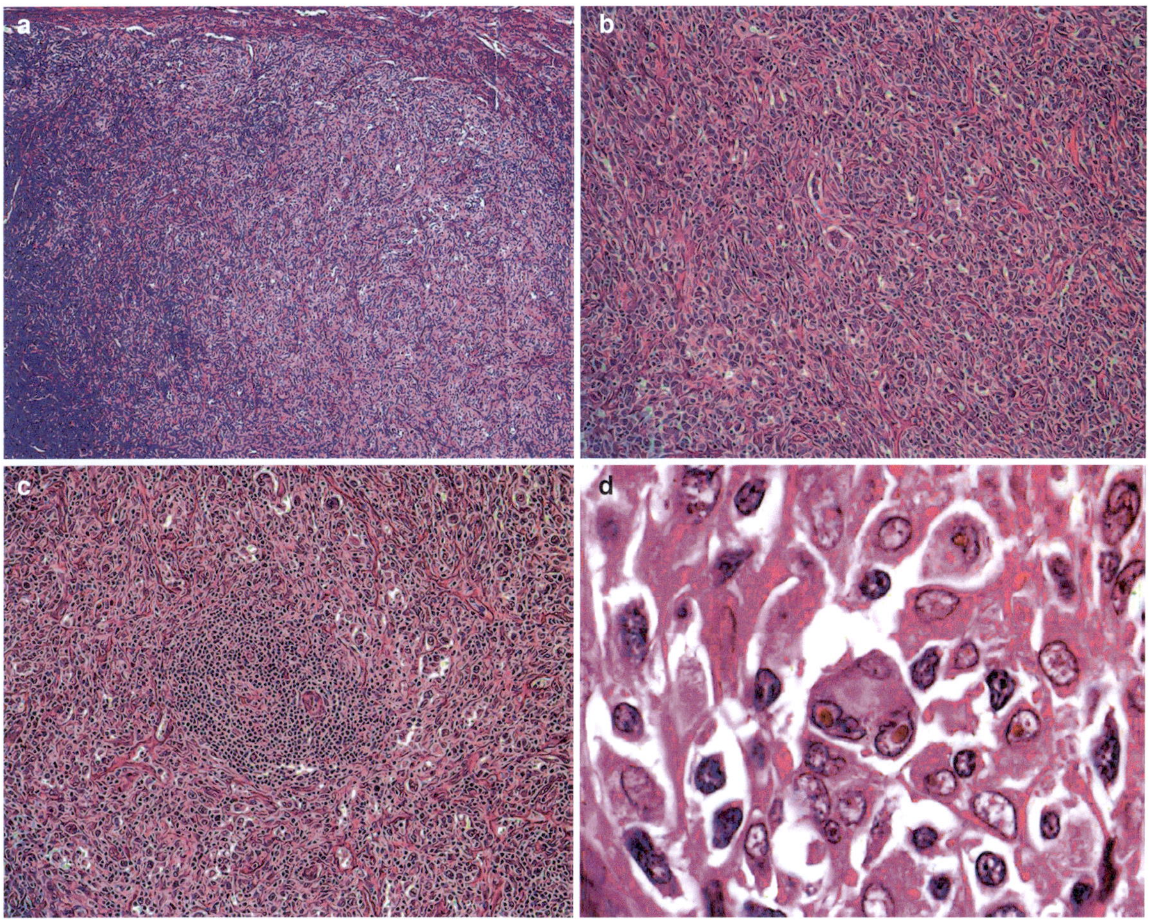

The section shows effaced nodal architecture by a diffuse cellular infiltrate formed of a predominance of Reed-Sternberg cells and scarce background lymphocytes with a lack of plasma cells or eosinophils. Reed-Sternberg cells have multilobated nuclei with prominent eosinophilic inclusion-like nucleoli.

Lymphoma of Lymph Nodes and Kidneys

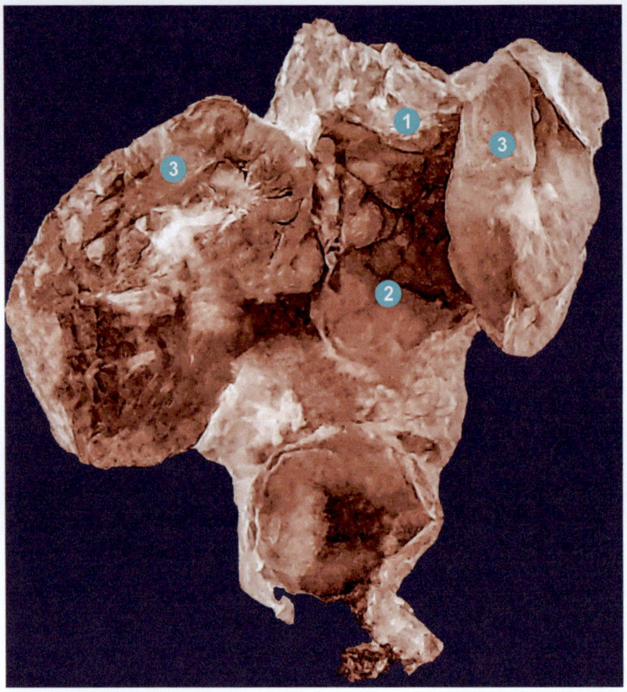

Para-aortic lymph nodes, both kidneys and the urinary bladder are mounted.

1. The lymph nodes are enlarged and fused.
2. Their cut section is fleshy and pale.
3. Both kidneys are enlarged due to infiltration by malignant lymphoid cells but retain their normal contour.

Microscopic Picture of Non-Hodgkin: Diffuse Large B Cell Lymphoma—Immunoblastic Variant (a–f)

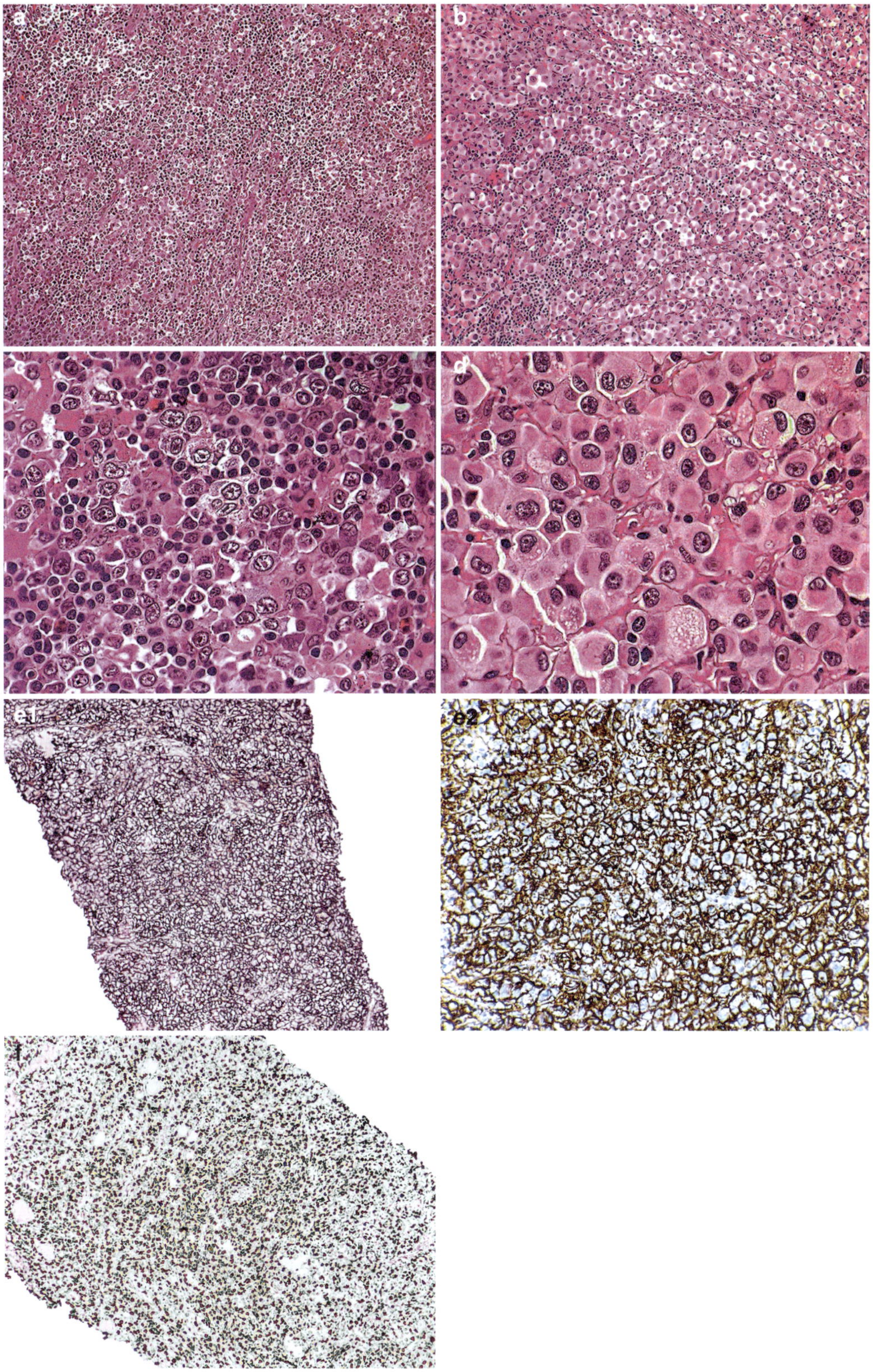

Sections show complete effacement of normal tissue architecture by a diffuse infiltrate of large (or occasionally medium size) atypical B lymphoid cells with vesicular chromatin and prominent nucleoli (large is defined as nucleus size $\geq$ histiocyte nucleus or >2 lymphocyte nuclei). Immunoblasts have ample eosinophilic cytoplasm and pleomorphic nuclei with vesicular chromatin and a single central nucleolus.

Ancillary Tools

IHC [2]:

B cell markers CD20 (**e1 & 2**)

Ki67 (**f**) (high)

CD30 (14%), associated with anaplastic morphology

PAX5, CD79a, CD19, CD22

Cell of origin subtyping: CD10 (30–50%), MUM1 (**e1**) (35–65%), BCL6 (60–90%)

Evaluation of double expresser/possible double hit status: BCL2 (47–84%), MYC

CD5 (12%)

Molecular/cytogenetics description [3]:

Gene expression profiling identifies activated B cell and germinal center B cell molecular subtypes of DLBCL, NOS.

FISH used to differentiate DLBCL and NOS from high-grade B cell lymphoma with MYC and BCL2 and/or BCL6 rearrangements:

- BCL2 rearrangement (20–30%; <5% activated B cell, 50% germinal center B cell)
- BCL6 rearrangement (30%; 30% activated B cell, 15% germinal center B cell)
- MYC rearrangement (8–14% for activated B cells and germinal center B cells; ~50% have co-occurring BCL2 or BCL6 rearrangements)

PCR B cell gene rearrangement studies show clonal immunoglobulin gene rearrangement.

The mutational landscape is very heterogeneous, with recurrent alterations identified in over 150 genes.

- Most frequently mutated genes include KMT2D (25%), MYD88 (17%), PIM1 (15%), CREBBP (12%), HIST1H1E (11%), BCL2 (10%), SPEN (10%), ARID1A (10%), and TP53 (9%) [3].

Multiple integrative genomic classification models have recently been proposed but none are currently incorporated into WHO classification guidelines

- Common DLBCL genomic subtypes that have emerged from multiple independent studies include those characterized by:
  - MYD88 L265P and CD79B mutations: mainly activated B cell subtype, 18q gain, genetically similar to primary extranodal lymphomas, poor survival
  - BCL6 translocations and NOTCH2 mutations: mainly activated B cell subtype, constitutive B cell receptor signaling, genetically similar to marginal zone lymphoma, more favorable survival
  - BCL2 translocations and mutations in EZH2/other chromatin modifiers: mostly germinal center B cell subtype with genetic features similar to other B cell lymphomas of germinal center origin

Lymphoma of Paratracheal Lymph Nodes

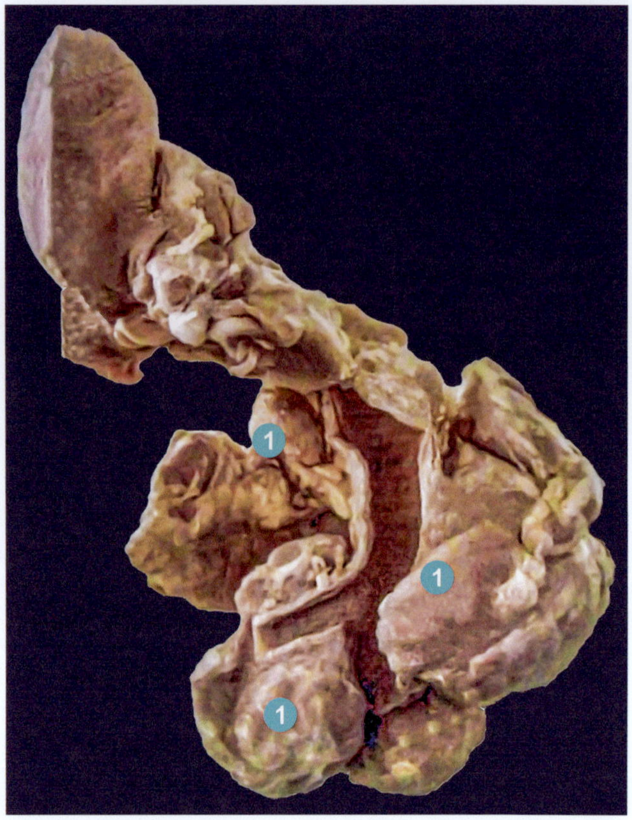

Tongue, tonsils, epiglottis, and trachea are mounted.

1. Paratracheal lymph nodes at the bifurcation of the trachea are enlarged and have a gray-white cut section. No evidence of caseation is observed.

Lymphoma of Spleen (Hodgkin's Lymphoma)

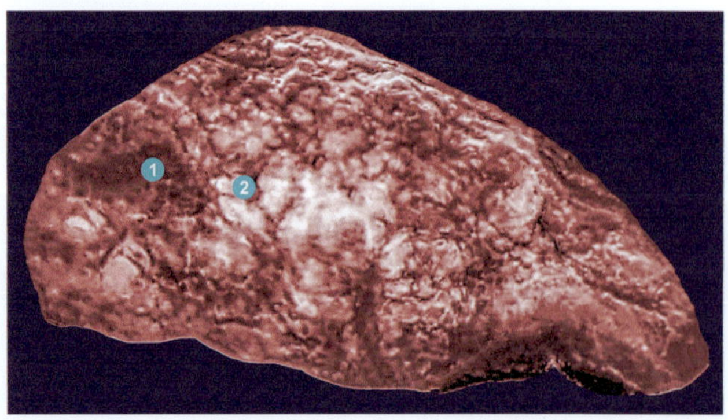

The spleen is mounted.

1. The spleen is enlarged and firm.
2. A pale area is present in the center. The specimen was taken from a boy suffering from Hodgkin's lymphoma.

Lymphoma of Spleen

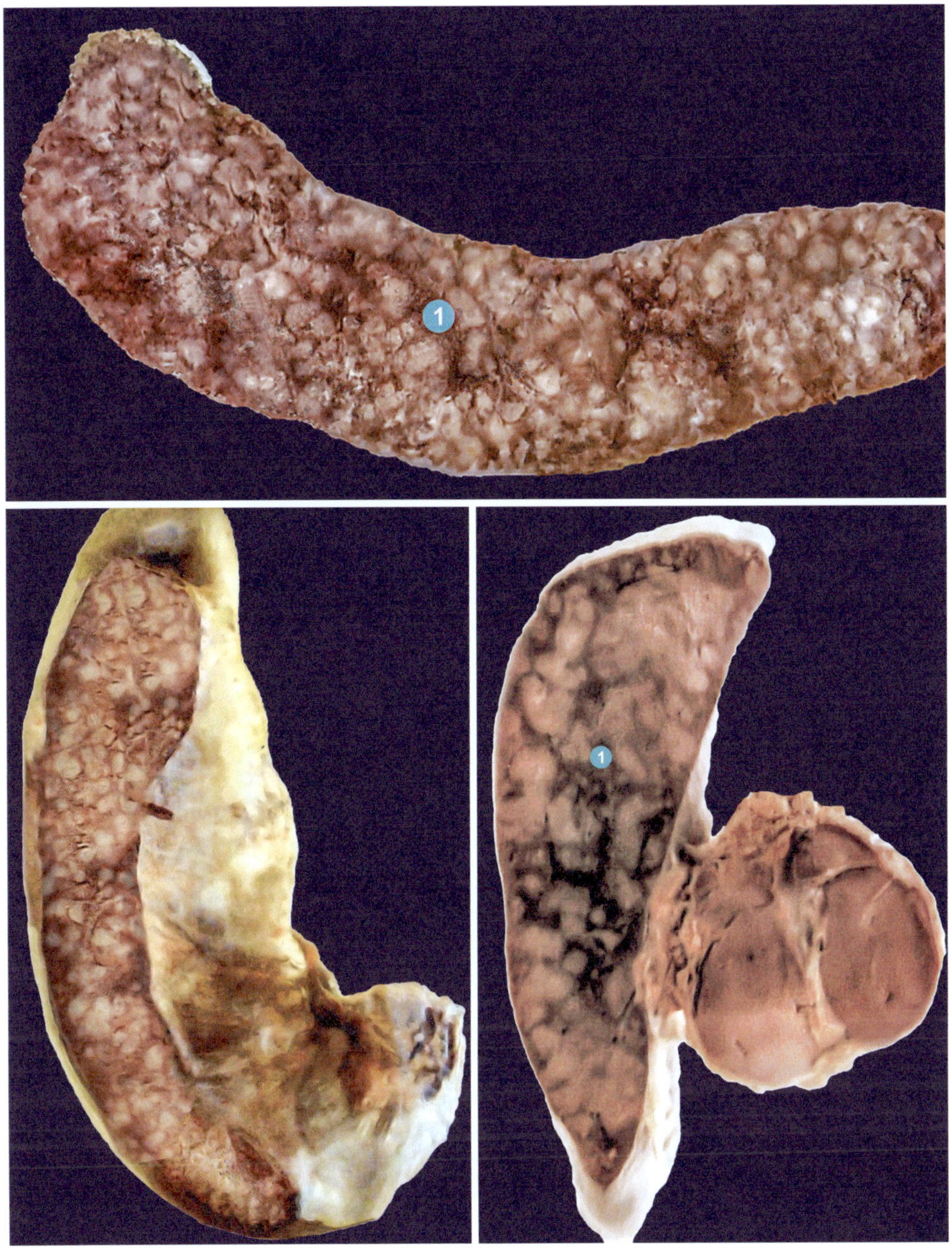

A slice of spleen is mounted.

1. The spleen is diffusely enlarged and firm. The cut surface shows a light brown appearance riddled with innumerable small pale foci.

Microscopic Picture of Non-Hodgkin: Follicular Lymphoma (a–j)

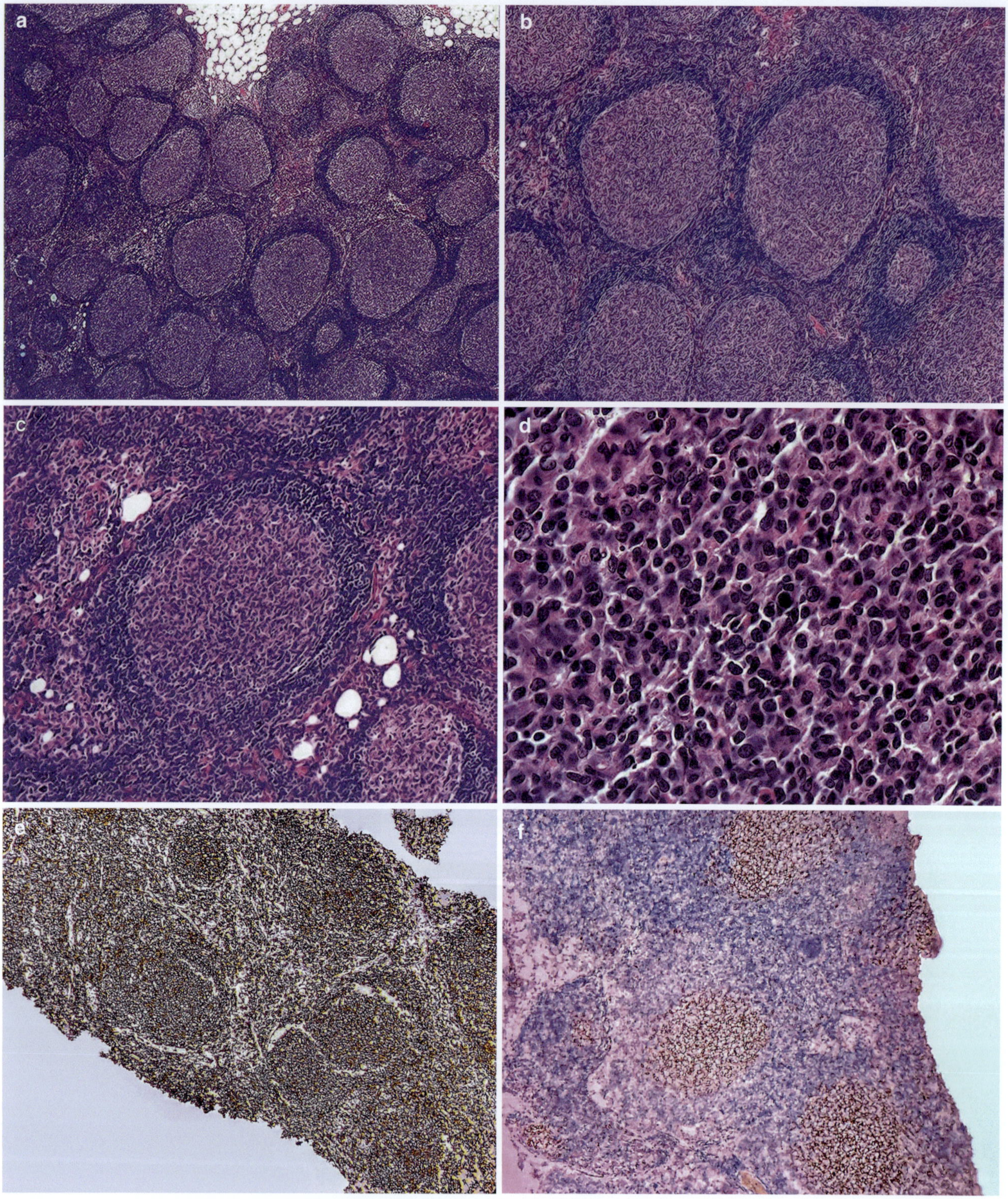

Sections show complete effacement of lymph node by multiple neoplastic nonpolarized follicles having similar size, attenuated or absent mantle zones, and lack of tingible body macrophages. The neoplastic follicles are formed of centrocytes or centroblasts with infrequent mitoses (except grade 3) with or without sclerosis. Follicular dendritic cell meshworks are absent in diffuse areas.

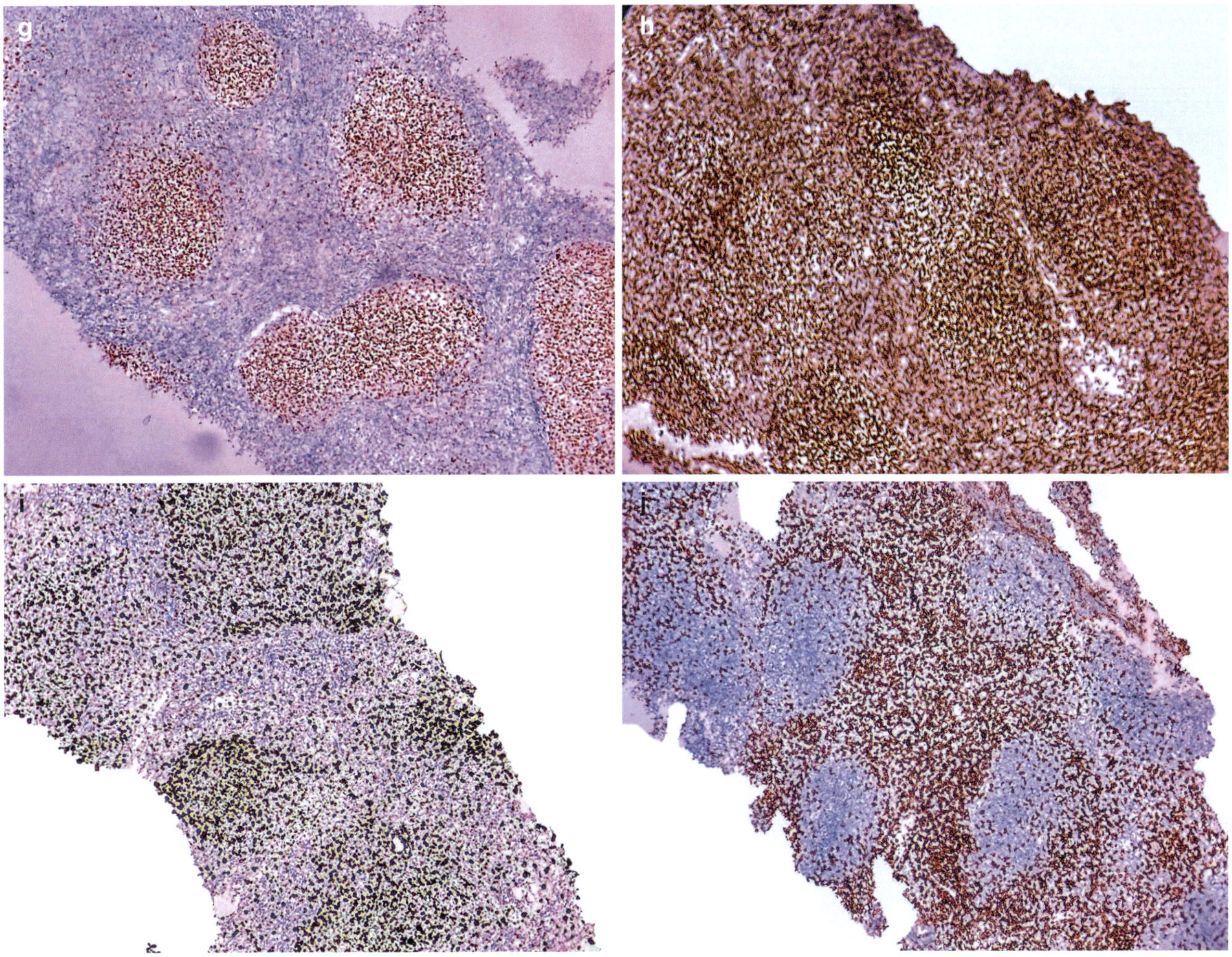

Ancillary Tools

IHC [4]:

Pan-B cell markers: CD20 (**e**), CD19, CD22 and CD79a

Germinal center markers: CD10 (**f**), BCL6 (**g**), HGAL, LMO2

BCL2 (**h**): + (85–90%)

Ki67 (**i**): The findings are consistent with involvement by a follicular lymphoma WHO grade 3-A of 3.

CD3 (**j**): The pattern of CD3, accumulating around neoplastic follicles, can be used to highlight the nodular distribution of lymphoma cells.

CD10: + (95–100%)

Molecular and Cytogenetic Description [4]:

Monoclonal immunoglobulin (Ig) heavy and light chain gene rearrangements

FISH can detect t(14;18)(q32;q21) IGH-BCL2 in up to 90% of follicular lymphoma cases.

FISH is more sensitive than PCR-based approaches.

- Variation in breakpoint regions

Juxtaposition of the Ig light chain promotors to BCL2: t(2;18) and t(18;22)

3q27 BCL6 rearrangement or amplification mostly in follicular lymphoma 3B

Loss of 1p36, which contains TNFRSF14, is common.

MYC rearrangement/activation of MYC is rare in follicular lymphoma (<5%).

- Associated with transformation to diffuse large B cell lymphoma
- Categorized as double-hit lymphoma if transformed and also has BCL2 or BCL6 translocation

Frequent genetic alterations

- BCL2 > KMT2D/MLL2 > EPHA7 > EZH2 > BCL6 > C REBBP > TNFRSF14

Lymphoma of Spleen

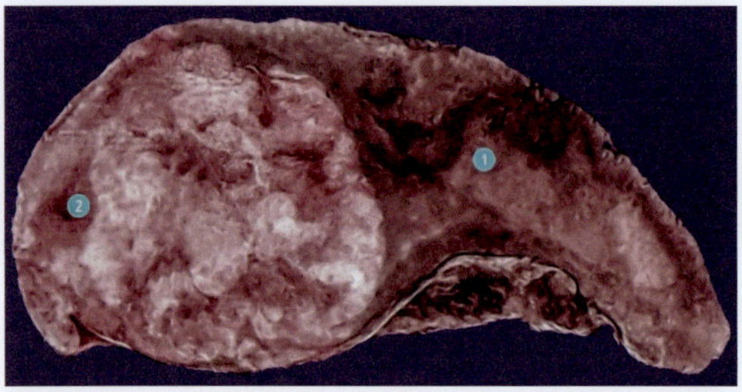

The spleen is mounted.

1. The spleen is enlarged and firm.
2. It shows a large round hemorrhagic area at the periphery with focal areas of necrosis.

Chronic Myeloid Leukemia of Spleen

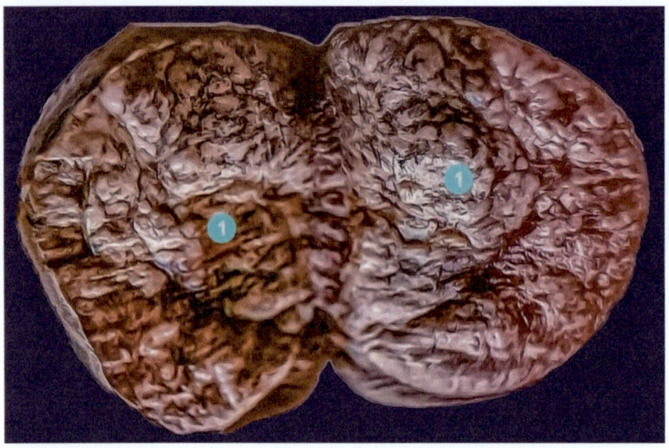

An enlarged spleen sectioned longitudinally is mounted.

1. It shows diffuse replacement of splenic tissue by extensive infiltration, forming a vague nodular pattern with areas of hemorrhage.

Ancillary Tools

IHC [5]:

Chronic phase:

Myeloperoxidase, specific esterase (naphthol AS-D chloroacetate esterase)

BB1 (basogranulin) stains basophils [5]

Blast phase/accelerated phase:

Myeloid differentiation: CD34, CD117, myeloperoxidase

B lymphoid differentiation: CD19, CD79a, PAX5, CD34, TdT

T lymphoid differentiation: CD3, CD2, CD4 or CD8, CD5, CD7, CD34, TdT, CD1a

Pearls

Chronic myeloid leukemia (CML) is a type of myeloproliferative neoplasm involving hematopoietic stem cells that results in overexpression of cells of myeloid lineage, especially granulocytes. It is caused by a reciprocal translocation between chromosomes 9 and 22, resulting in the formation of the Philadelphia chromosome, which contains the BCR-ABL1 fusion gene. The BCR-ABL1 fusion gene encodes a hybrid tyrosine kinase with increased enzymatic activity that leads to the unregulated proliferation of hematopoietic stem cells. These cells subsequently differentiate into mature myeloid cells, resulting in CML. CML has three distinct phases: the chronic phase (CP-CML), the accelerated phase (AP-CML), and the blast phase (BP-CML, also referred to as blast crisis). Patients with CP-CML may be asymptomatic or present with nonspecific symptoms (e.g., fever, weight loss, night sweats) and splenomegaly [6].

10.4 Amyloidosis

Sago Spleen

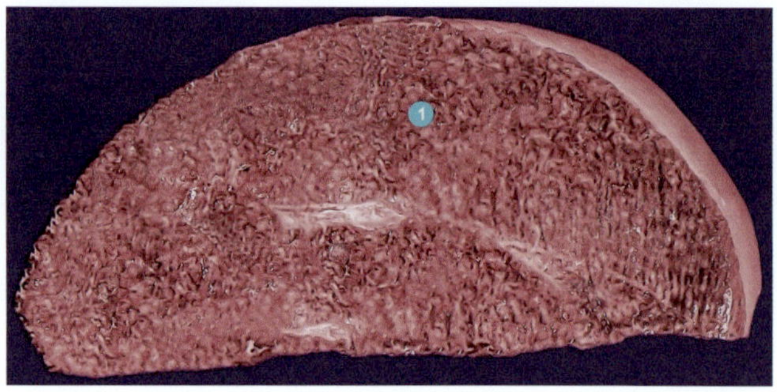

Half of a bisected spleen is mounted.

1. The cut section is studded with multiple tiny brownish spots representing amyloid in lymphoid follicles.

References

1. Chapman J, Goyal A, Azevedo AM. (2024). Splenomegaly. [Updated 2023 Jun 26]. In: StatPearls [Internet]. Treasure Island (FL): StatPearls Publishing. https://www.ncbi.nlm.nih.gov/books/NBK430907/.
2. Hu S. et al. (2013). CD30 expression defines a novel subgroup of diffuse large B-cell lymphoma with favorable prognosis and distinct gene expression signature: a report from the International DLBCL Rituximab-CHOP Consortium Program Study. Blood. 121(14):2715-24. doi: https://doi.org/10.1182/blood-2012-10-461848. PMID: 23343832; PMCID: PMC3700465.
3. Reddy A. et al. (2017). Genetic and Functional Drivers of Diffuse Large B Cell Lymphoma. Cell. 171(2):481-494.e15. doi: https://doi.org/10.1016/j.cell.2017.09.027. PMID: 28985567; PMCID: PMC5659841.

4. Khanlari M, Chapman J. Follicular-usual. PathologyOutlines.com website. https://www.pathologyoutlines.com/topic/lymphomafollicularnodalusual.html.
5. Agis H. et al. (2006). Identification of basogranulin (BB1) as a novel immunohistochemical marker of basophils in normal bone marrow and patients with myeloproliferative disorders. Am J Clin Pathol. 125(2):273-81. doi: https://doi.org/10.1309/M9FQ-MQGF-6616-7N2X. PMID: 16393678.
6. Mughal TI. et al. (2016). Chronic myeloid leukemia: reminiscences and dreams. Haematologica. 101(5):541-58. doi: https://doi.org/10.3324/haematol.2015.139337. PMID: 27132280; PMCID: PMC5004358.

11 Diseases of Bones

The osseous system, or skeleton, is a complex system of bones that provides support, movement, protection, and other essential functions.

Osseous system pathology encompasses a wide range of conditions that can affect bone health, including developmental abnormalities, injuries, cancers, metabolic conditions, and degenerative diseases.

Understanding the gross and microscopic features of osseous pathologies is crucial for accurate diagnosis and management.

This chapter provides a comprehensive overview of osseous pathologies, including their classification, gross presentations, and microscopic features.

By the end of this chapter, readers should be able to:

Define osseous system pathology and list its major categories.

Describe the gross and microscopic features of common osseous pathologies.

Apply their knowledge of osseous pathology to recognize and manage these conditions in clinical practice.

The chapter will be organized as follows:

1. **Inflammatory Lesions**
   (a) Chronic Osteomyelitis (Sequestrum)
   (b) Chronic Osteomyelitis (Involucrum)
   (c) Syphilitic Gumma of the Skull
2. **Benign Cystic Lesions**
   (a) Simple Bone Cyst
3. **Neoplastic Lesions**
   (a) **Primary Tumors**
   - Bone-Forming Tumors
     – Osteosarcoma
   - Cartilage-Forming Tumors
     – Osteochondroma (Exostosis)
     – Chondroma
     – Chondrosarcoma
   - Fibrous Tumors
     – Fibrosarcoma
   - Osteoclastic Giant Cell Rich Tumors
     – Benign Tumors
       Aneurysmal Bone Cyst
     – Intermediate (locally aggressive, rarely metastasizing)
       Giant cell tumor of bone, NOS

   (b) **Metastatic Tumors**

11.1 Inflammatory Lesions

Chronic Osteomyelitis (Sequestrum)

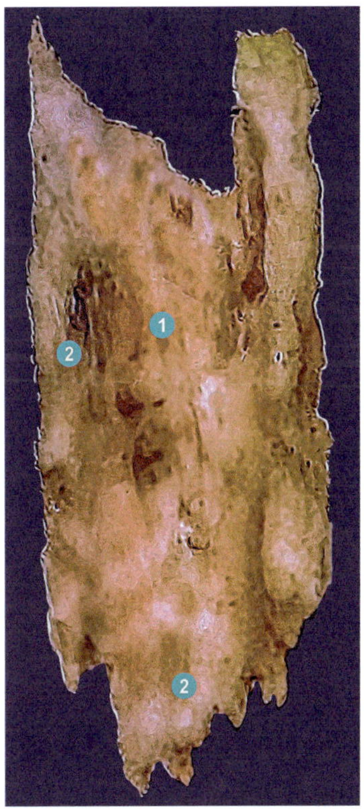

1. An irregular piece of necrotic long bone is mounted.
2. The surface and ends of the bone are irregular and appear eroded.

G. Dawood, *Color Atlas of Human Gross and Microscopic Pathology*, https://doi.org/10.1007/978-3-031-76007-5_11

Chronic Osteomyelitis (Involucrum)

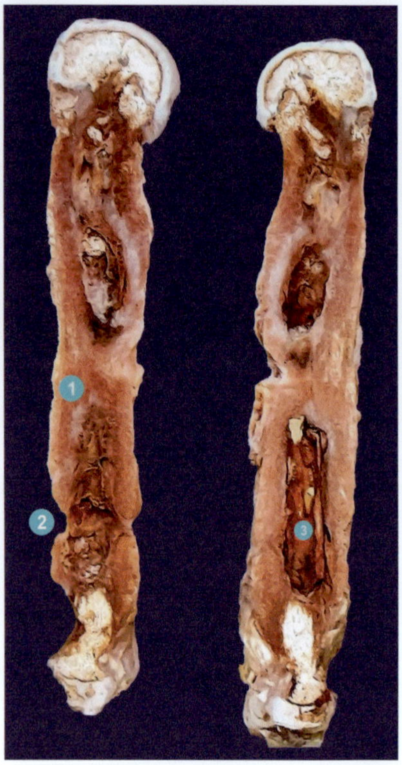

1. An irregular, sclerotic, thickened piece of bone.
2. Irregular holes representing cloacae.
3. Parts of sequestrum

Microscopic Picture of Chronic Osteomyelitis (a, b)

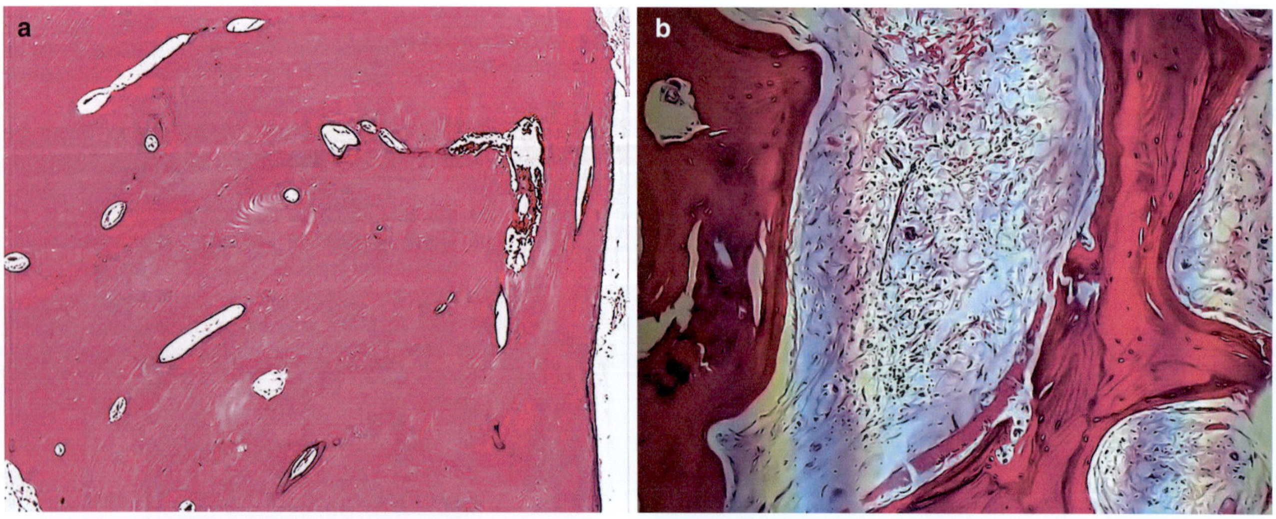

Sections show osteonecrosis bone trabeculae with visually empty osteocyte cavities are detectable as a criterion for necrotic bone tissue. The bone trabeculae have irregular contours and are fragmented. Lymphocytes, macrophages, and plasma cells infiltrate, and bacterial colonies are seen in fibrosed medullary spaces.

Syphilitic Gumma in the Vault of the Skull

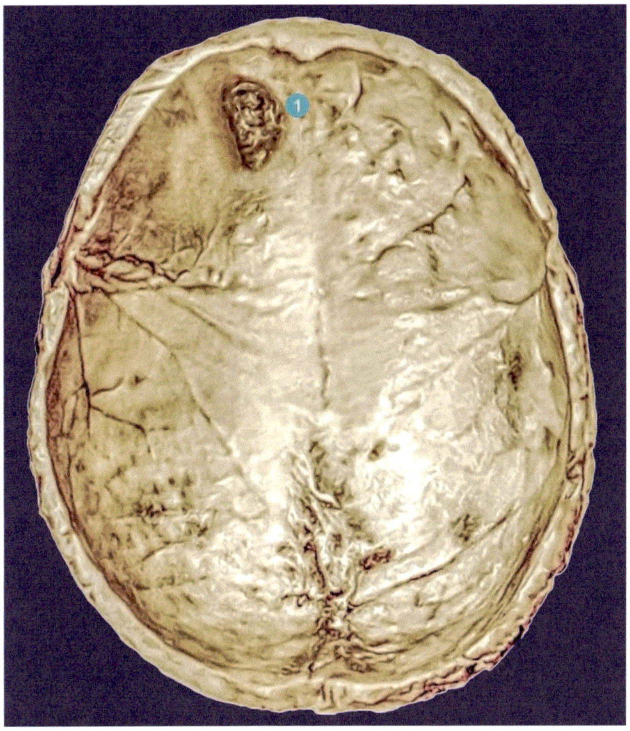

The vault of the skull is mounted.

1. A single irregular and necrotic lesion is seen in the parasagittal area to the left of the midline. The lesion is brown and measures up to 3–4 cm in maximum diameter. The lesion has eroded the inner table of the skull.

11.2 Benign Cystic Lesions

Simple Bone Cyst

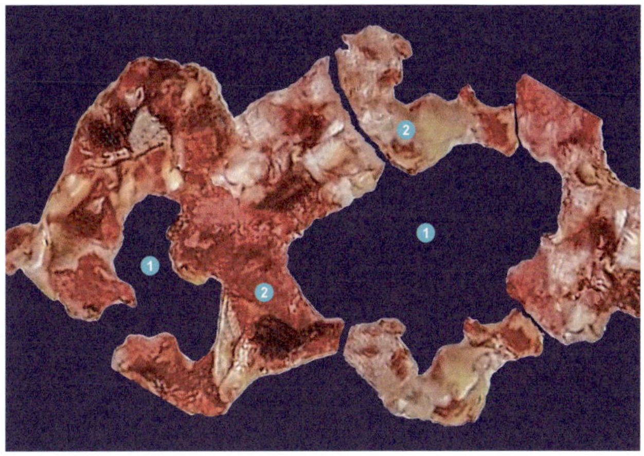

Fragments of the removed lining of a bone cyst present in the proximal femur were assembled to figure out the cyst shape.

1. The cyst is bilocular
2. The lining is thin, with areas of fibrosis and focal areas of hemorrhage.

Microscopic Picture of Simple Bone Cyst (a–c)

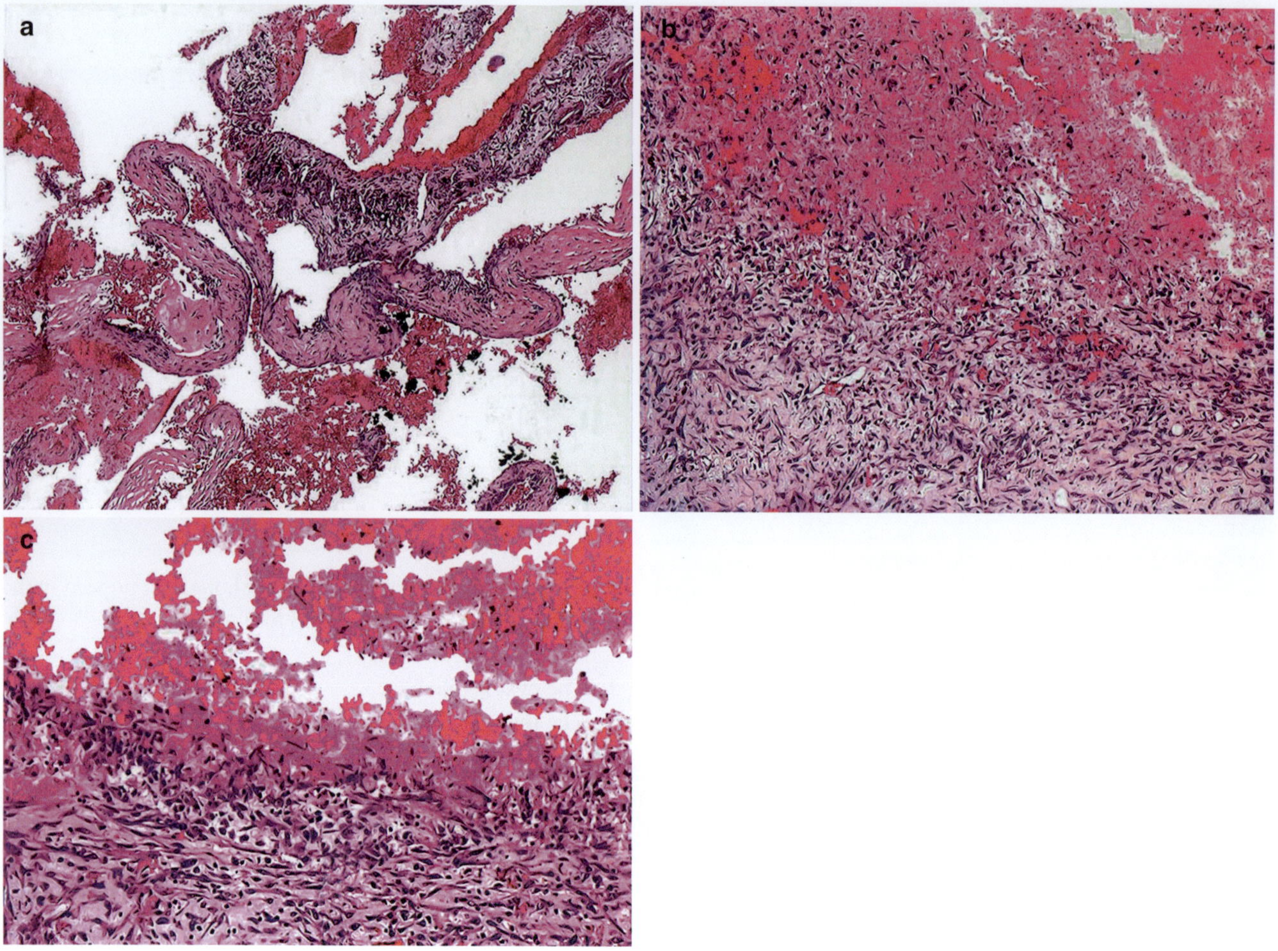

Sections show a thin fibrous cyst wall lacking an epithelial lining. It is composed of fibroblasts, irregular bands of fibrin-like material with focal areas of hemorrhage. The cyst wall is infiltrated with occasional osteoclast-type giant cells, foamy histiocytes, and hemosiderin pigment.

11.3 Neoplastic Lesions

11.3.1 Primary Tumors

11.3.1.1 Bone-Forming Tumors

Osteosarcoma of Femur

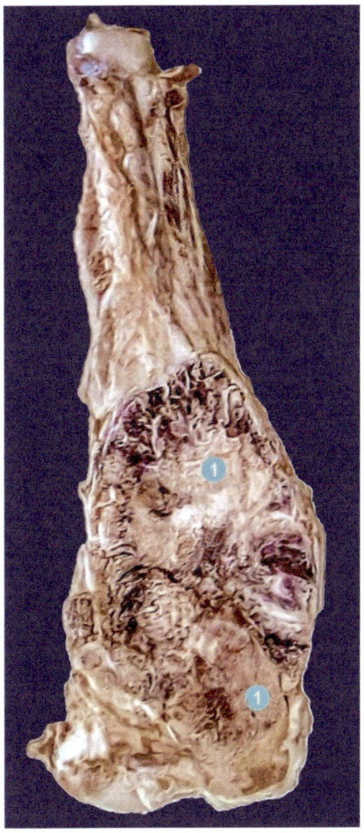

The lower end of the femur is mounted.

1. A large, gray-white, firm mass is seen filling the medullary cavity, destroying the cortical bone but sparing the articular cartilage.

Osteosarcoma of Femur

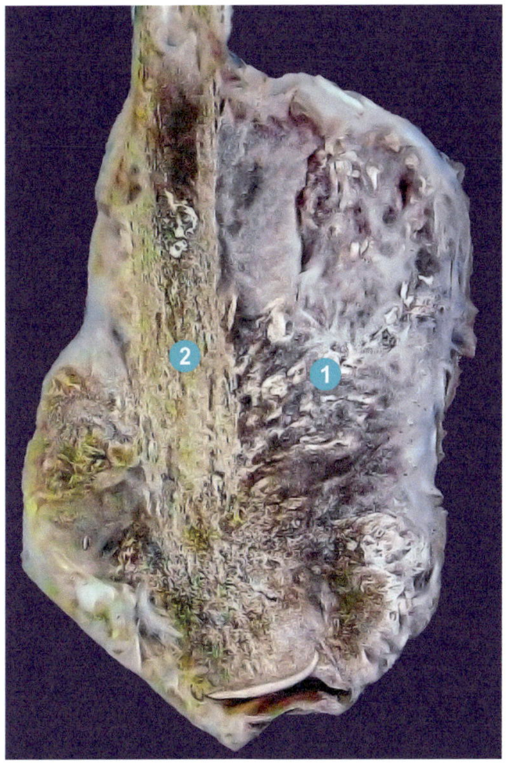

The lower end of the femur is mounted.

1. A large, gray-white, firm mass with focal semitranslucent areas of cartilaginous formation and other chalky white linear areas perpendicular to the shaft is observed.
2. The mass is filling the medullary cavity, destroying the cortical bone but sparing the articular cartilage.

Osteosarcoma of Radius

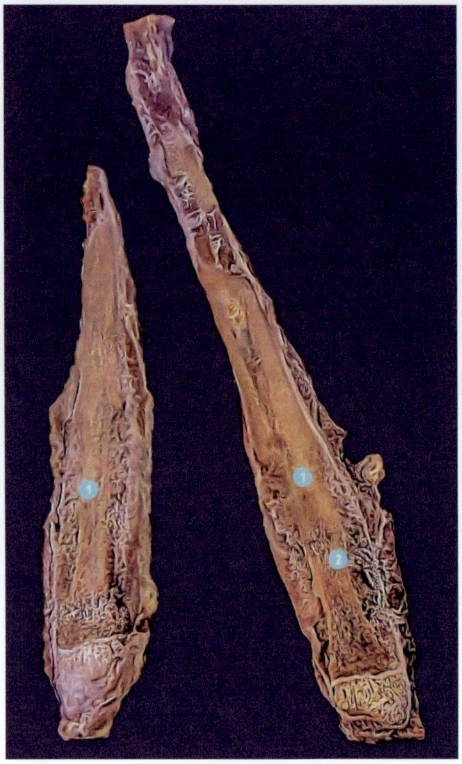

A radius with a well-formed epiphyseal line is mounted.

1. A gray-white and firm mass fills the medulla enveloping the bone around the metaphysis with partial infiltration of cortical bone.
2. The tumor shows white streaks perpendicular to the shaft.

Osteosarcoma with Pathological Fracture

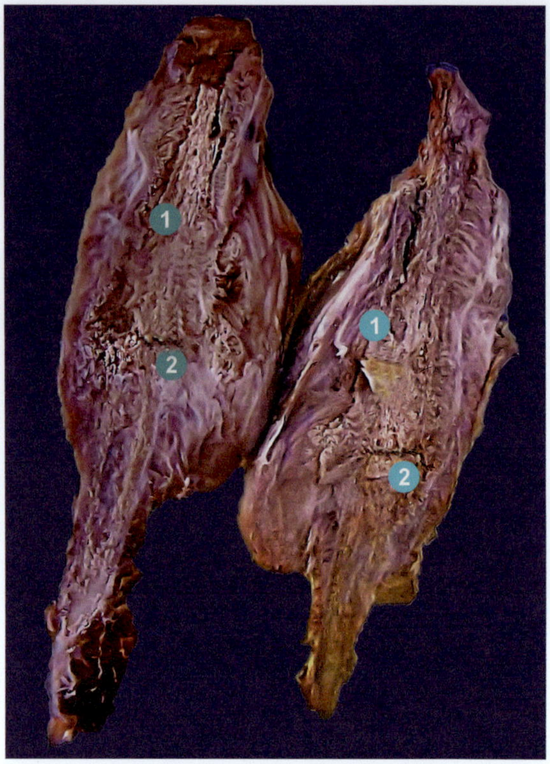

The shaft of a long bone is mounted.

1. A large, brown, firm mass enveloping the diaphysis with complete replacement of the medullary cavity and cortex.
2. The bone is fractured at the site of the tumor.

Microscopic Picture of Osteoblastic Osteosarcoma (a–d)

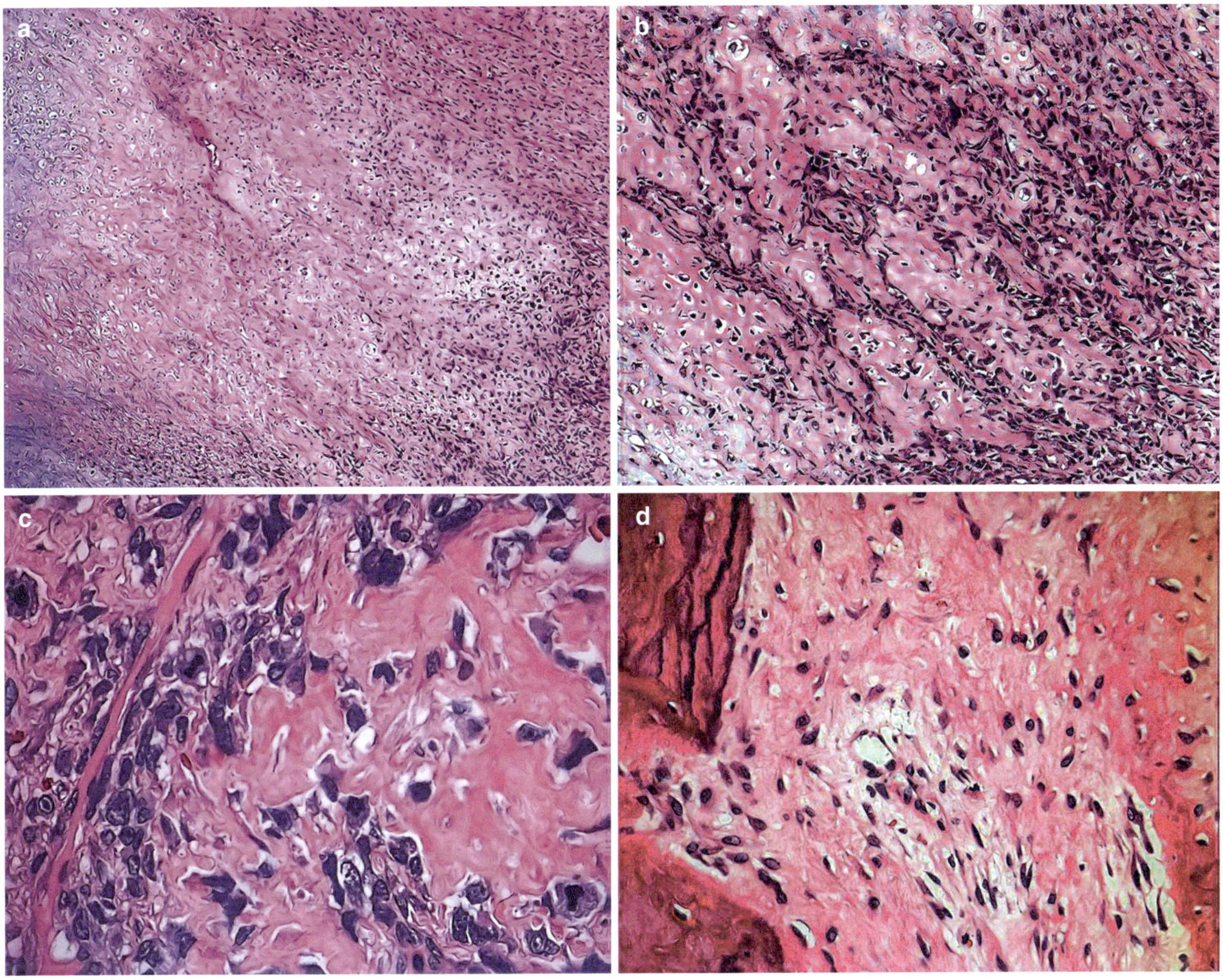

Sections show malignant spindle cells that produce osteoid arranged in sheets and trabeculae. The tumor cells are typically pleomorphic with hyperchromatic nuclei and eosinophilic cytoplasm. Mitotic figures are numerous and atypical. Focal areas of fibrosis and chondroid differentiation are observed.

The osteoid produced by osteoblastic osteosarcoma is typically immature and poorly mineralized. It may be arranged in a variety of patterns, including lace-like trabeculae, sheets, or globules.

Ancillary Tools

IHC [1]:

Often positive: SATB2, SMA, CD99, osteocalcin

SOX9 (not reliable distinguisher with chondrosarcoma)

Occasionally focally positive: cytokeratin, EMA

Molecular/cytogenetics description [2]:

Complex karyotype

TP53 inactivation: ~40% (Li-Fraumeni syndrome increases risk of osteosarcoma)

Rb inactivation: ~35% (germline RB1 mutation increases risk for post-radiation osteosarcoma)

Amplification/gain of 8q21-24 (contains c-Myc): 45–55%

MDM2 amplification: ~10%

11.3.1.2 Cartilage-Forming Tumors

Osteochondroma (Exostosis)

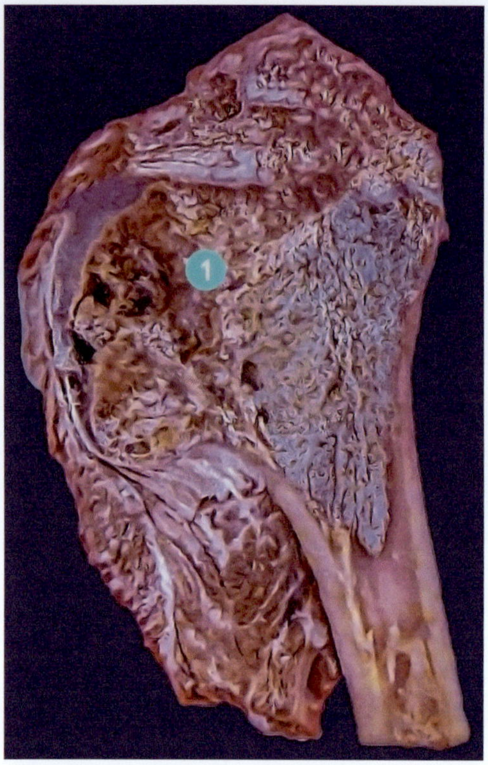

The upper part of the fibula is mounted.

1. The metaphyseal end shows a mass formed of cancellous bone and covered by a cartilaginous cap projecting at the metaphysis in relation to the metaphyseal cartilage.

Osteochondroma (Exostosis)

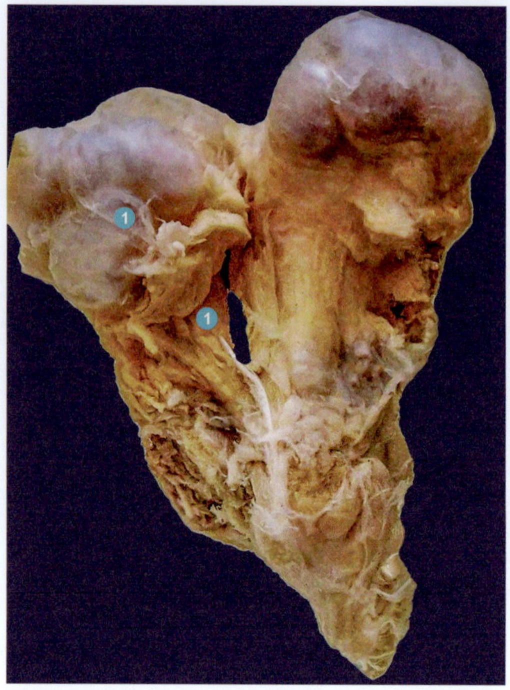

The metaphyseal end of a long bone is mounted.

1. A bony outgrowth or protuberance capped by a cartilaginous layer is observed. The outgrowth is pedunculated and protrudes from the surface of the bone covered with a hyaline cartilage cap.

Osteochondroma

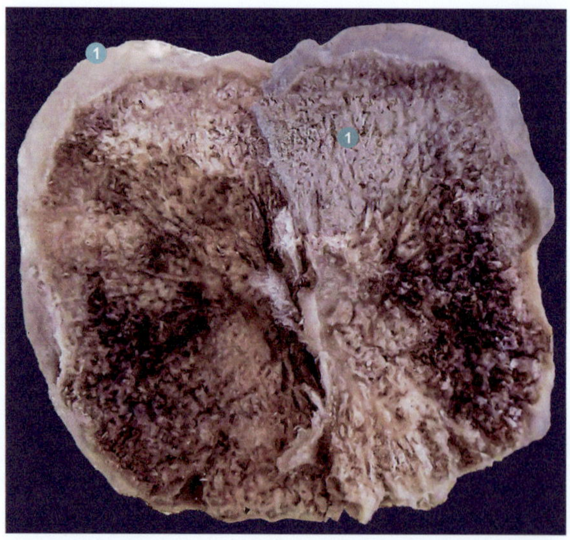

1. A mass formed of cancellous bone and covered by a cartilaginous cap.

Microscopic Picture of Osteochondroma (a–c)

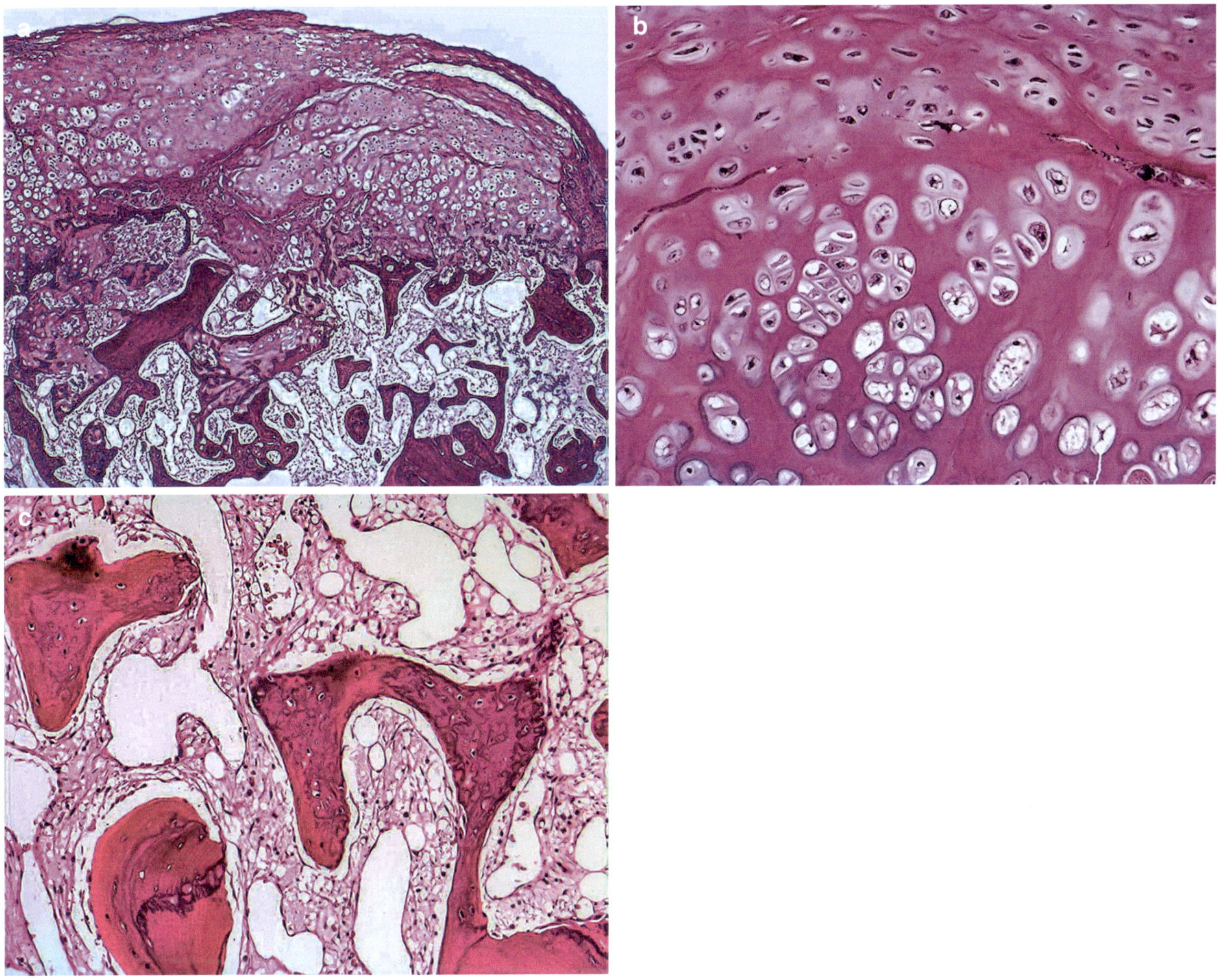

Sections show a cap of mature hyaline cartilage with overlying fibrous. perichondrium, covering mature bone that may contain bone marrow.

Enchondroma

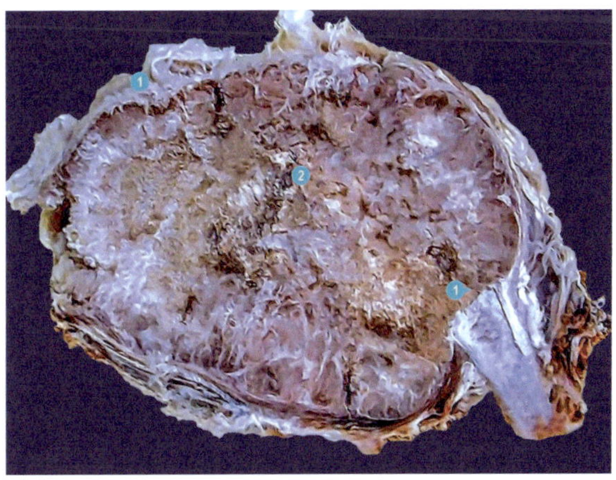

1. A well-encapsulated, lobulated mass arising from the center of the bone.
2. The cut section shows gray-white and glistening cartilage.

Microscopic Picture of Enchondroma (a–d)

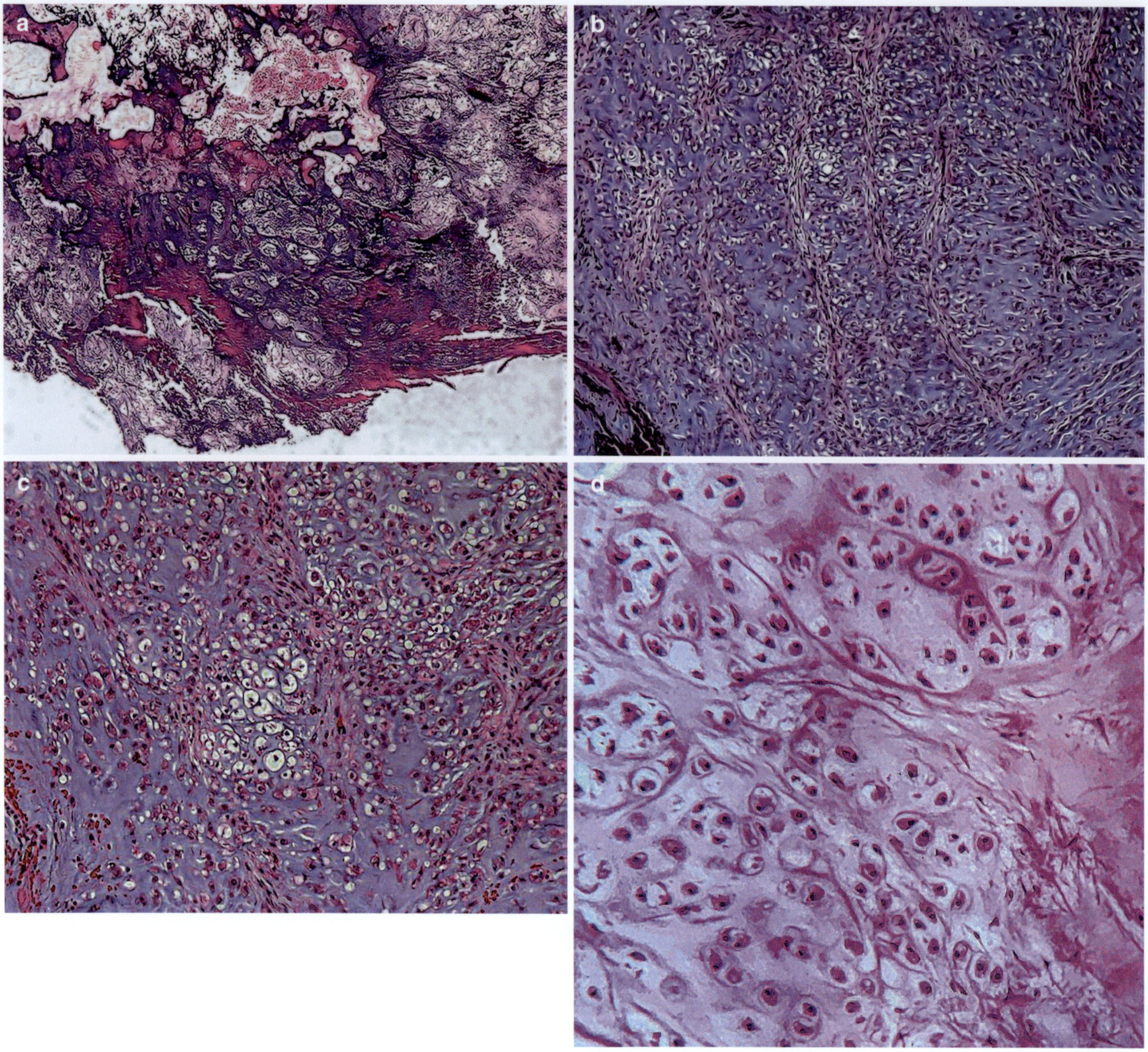

Sections show multiple nodules of mature cartilage cells embedded in an abundant hyaline cartilage matrix. The tumor cells are embedded within lacunar spaces and evenly dispersed. Tumor cells have small and round nuclei with condensed chromatin (lymphocyte-like) and eosinophilic cytoplasm. Cytologic atypia and mitoses are absent.

Ancillary Tools

IHC [3]:

S100

Estrogen receptor beta GADD45β

Chondrosarcoma of Iliac Bone (a, b)

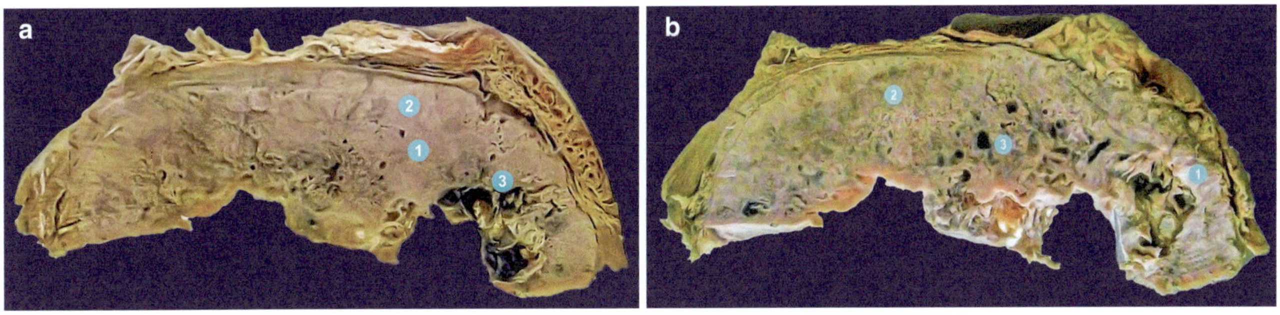

A large tumor mass covered by skin, subcutaneous fat, and muscle is mounted.

1. The tumor is gray-white with the presence of semitranslucent cartilaginous areas.
2. Blotchy chalky white calcification areas.
3. Areas of hemorrhage, necrosis, and cyst formation.

Chondrosarcoma (a, b)

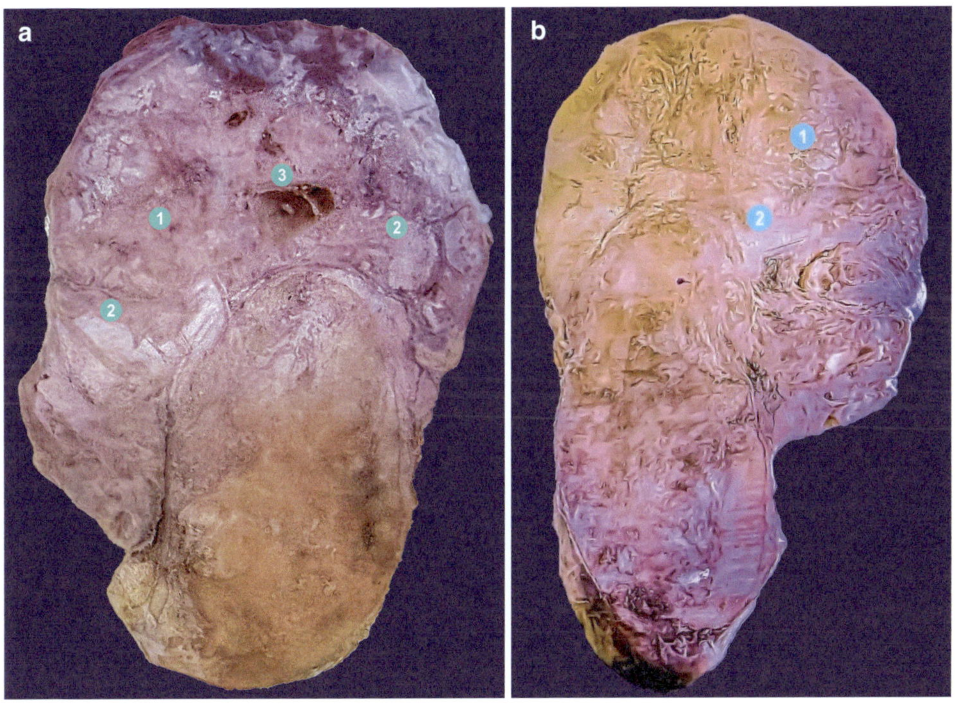

A large tumor mass is mounted.

1. The tumor is gray-white with the presence of semitranslucent cartilaginous areas.
2. Blotchy chalky white areas of calcification.
3. Areas of hemorrhage, necrosis, and cyst formation.

Chondrosarcoma of Femur (a, b)

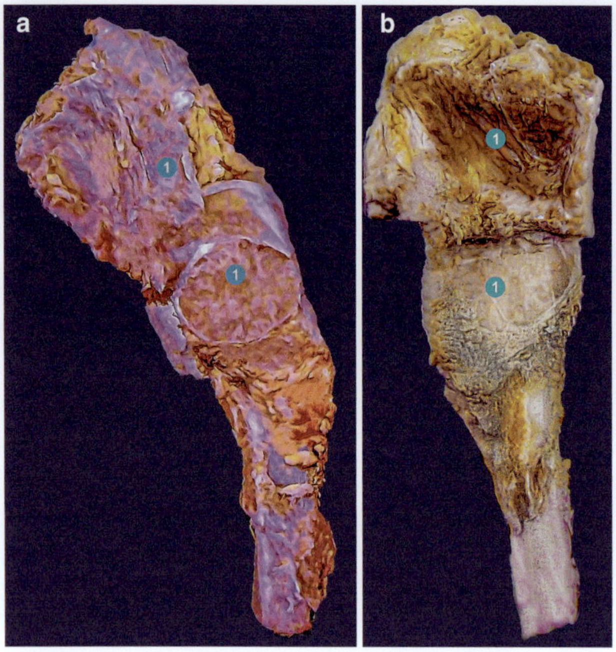

The lower end of the femur and upper end of the tibia are mounted.

1. The lower end of the femur and upper end of the tibia are destroyed by a lobular, semitranslucent, pale blue growth infiltrating the medullary cavity and cortex but sparing the articular cartilage.

Periosteal (Juxtacortical) Chondrosarcoma of Femur

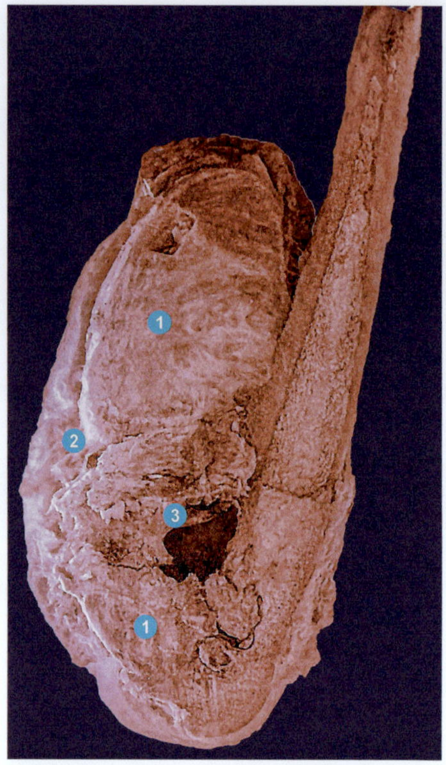

The lower end of the femur is mounted.

1. A mass is sharply defined, attached to the outer surface of the cortex, which is destroyed by a lobular, semitranslucent, pale blue growth infiltrating the medullary cavity and cortex but sparing the articular cartilage.
2. There is blotchy chalky white calcification.
3. Areas of hemorrhage, necrosis, and cyst formation are observed.

Pearls

Periosteal chondrosarcoma is a malignant cartilage-forming tumor that originates from the periosteum and grows on the surface of the bone. The tumor is extremely rare, accounting for less than 0.5% of all chondrosarcomas; it occurs in adults, primarily in the second to fourth decades of life, with a slight male predominance. Typically, it involves the metaphysis of long tubular bones, most commonly the distal femur and the humerus [4].

Microscopic Picture of Chondrosarcoma (a–c)

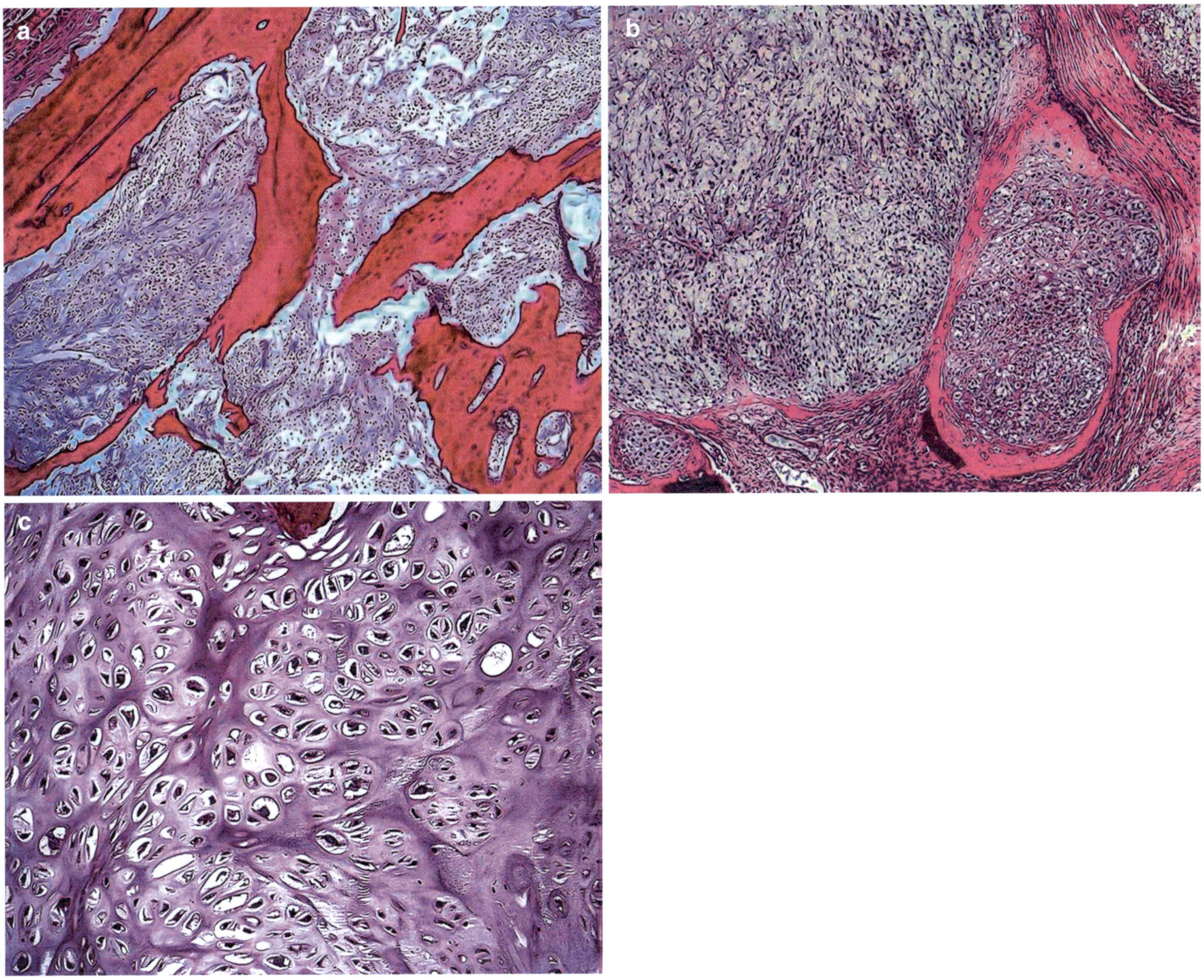

Sections show irregular nodules of an abundant cartilaginous matrix with high cellularity of chondrocytes embedded in lacunae, destroying lamellar bone spicules. The tumor cells show marked atypia with a pleomorphic appearance and easily identifiable mitotic figures.

Ancillary Tools

Molecular/cytogenetics description [5]:

IDH1 and IDH2 mutations in approximately 50% of cases.

Aneuploidy is seen with increasing histologic grade.

TP53 mutations and affected active signaling pathways (RB1, CDKN2A, CDK) are identified particularly in high grade chondrosarcomas.

11.3.1.3 Fibrous Tumors

Fibrosarcoma of Tibia

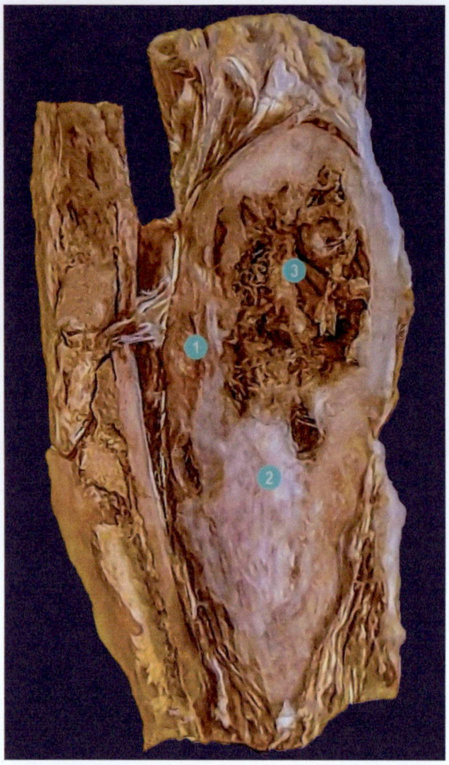

The tibia and fibula are mounted.

1. The metaphysis of the tibia shows a large, firm, gray-white, and fleshy mass.
2. The mass is seen infiltrating the medulla and cortical bone.
3. Areas of hemorrhage and necrosis are seen.

Fibrosarcoma of Femur (a, b)

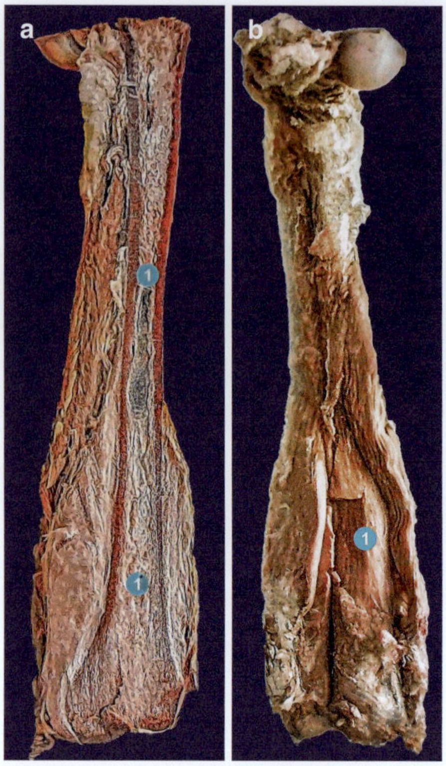

The femur is mounted.

1. It shows a large, firm, fleshy, hemorrhagic mass infiltrating the medulla and cortical bone.

Microscopic Picture of Fibrosarcoma of Femur (c–f)

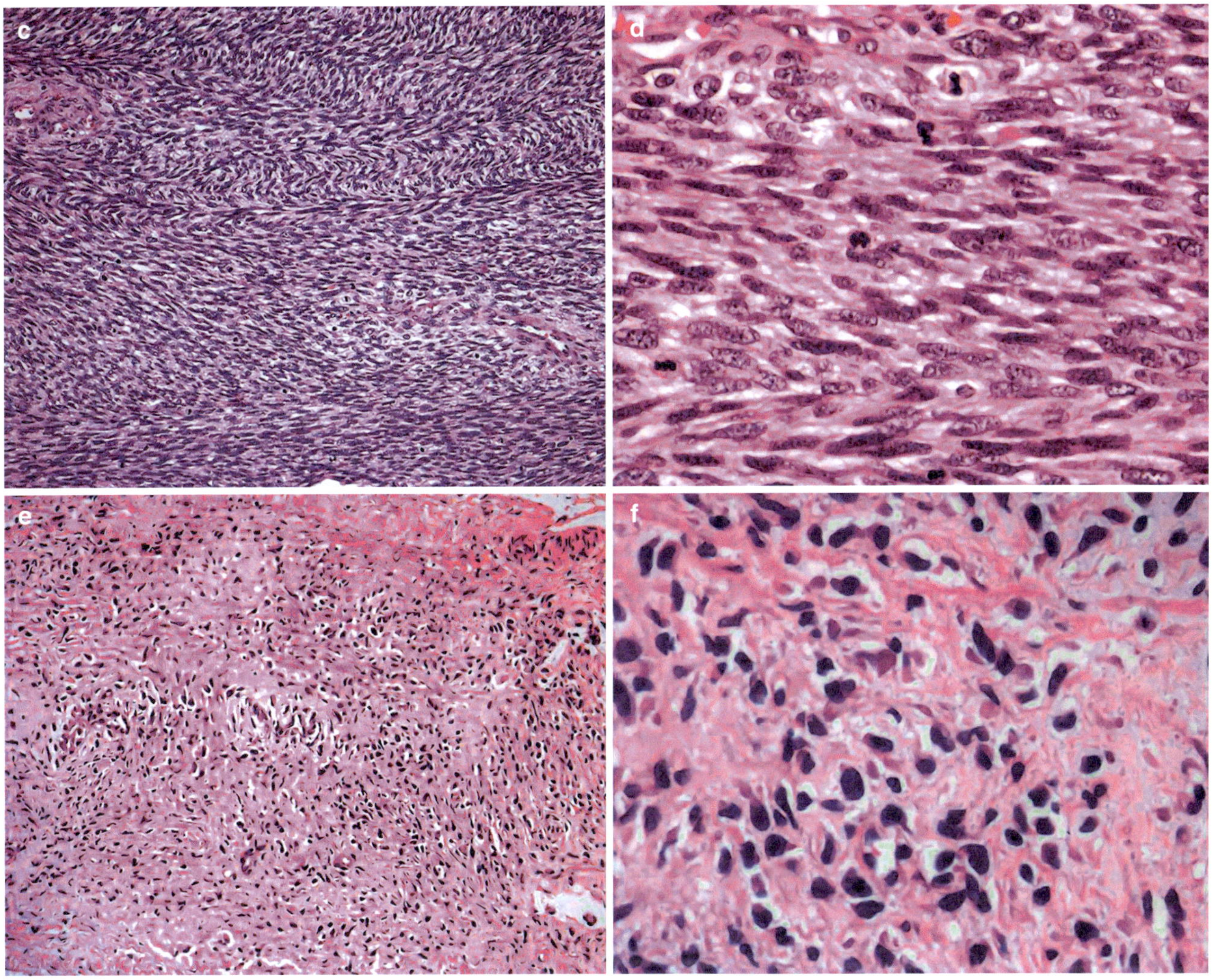

Sections show a highly cellular tumor formed of malignant spindle-shaped cells arranged in fascicles in a herringbone fashion. The nuclei of the tumor cells are enlarged and cigar-shaped, with prominent nucleoli and an increased number of mitoses.

11.3.1.4 Osteoclastic Giant Cell Rich Tumors

Benign Tumors

Aneurysmal Bone Cyst

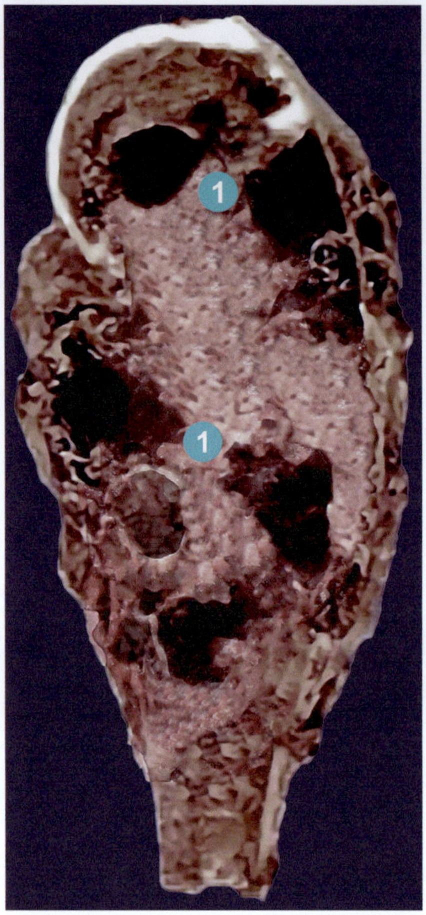

The metaphyseal end of a long bone is mounted.

1. A spongy, multiloculated, and hemorrhagic lesion with irregular, sharply demarcated borders with a thin shell of reactive bone and a variable amount of solid component.

Microscopic Picture of Aneurysmal Bone Cyst (a–d)

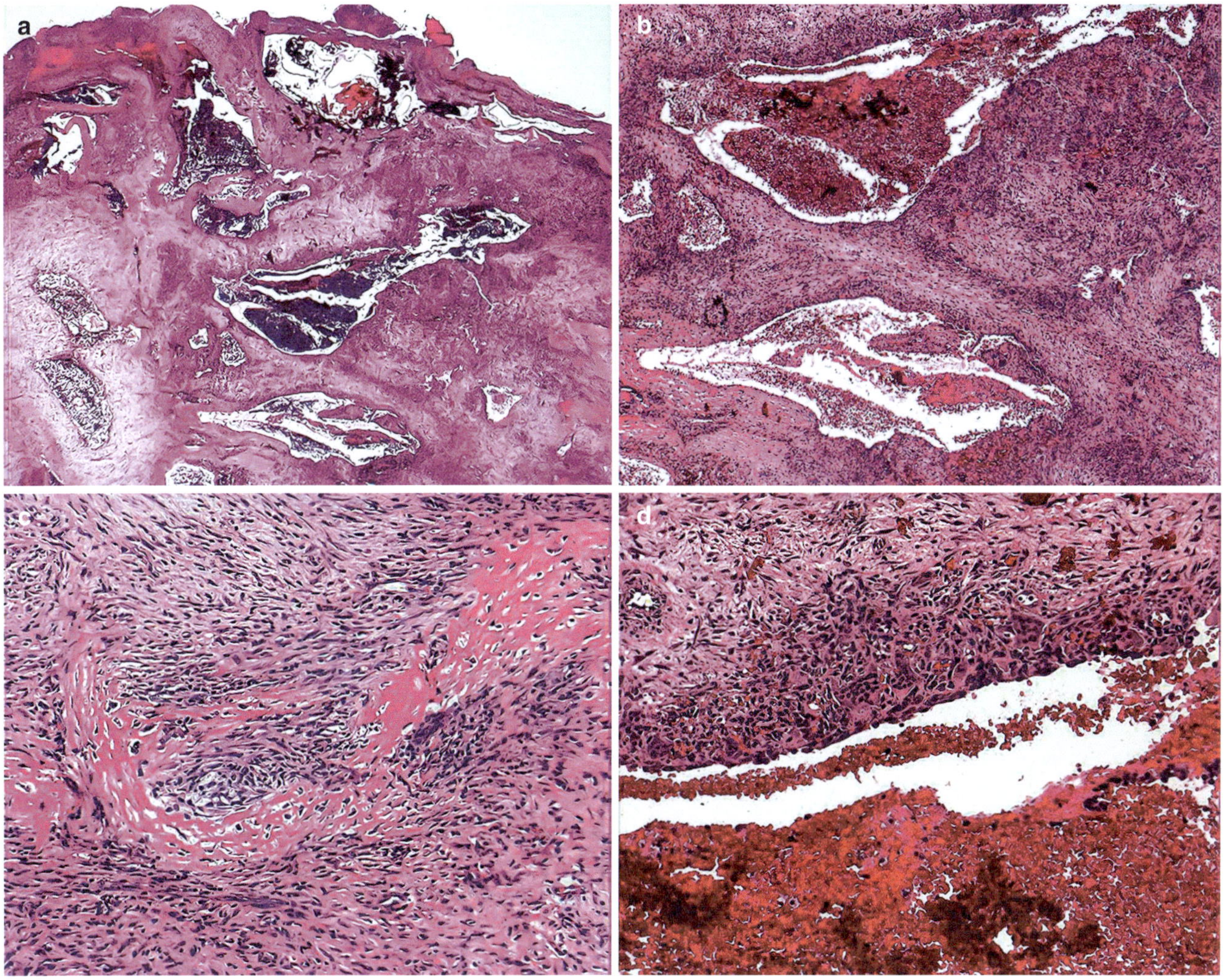

Sections show multiloculated blood-filled cystic spaces separated by cellular septa containing fibroblasts, giant cells, and woven bone. Mitotic activity is easily identified but no cytologic atypia. Numerous giant cells in connective tissue that line large sinusoidal spaces.

Ancillary Tools

Molecular/cytogenetics description [6]:

Abnormalities of the 17p13.2 locus in 63%

Fusion of USP6 with:

CDH11 (most frequent, approximately 30%), TRAP150 (THRAP3), ZNF9 (CNBP), OMD, COL1A1, RUNX2, PAFAH1B1, CTNNB1, SEC31A, E1F1, FOSL2, STAT3, USP9X, ASAP1, FAT1, SAR1A, TNC Rearrangement of the USP6 gene can be detected by FISH or fusion panel analysis by next-generation sequencing.

Intermediate (Locally Aggressive, Rarely Metastasizing) Tumors

Giant cell tumor of bone, NOS

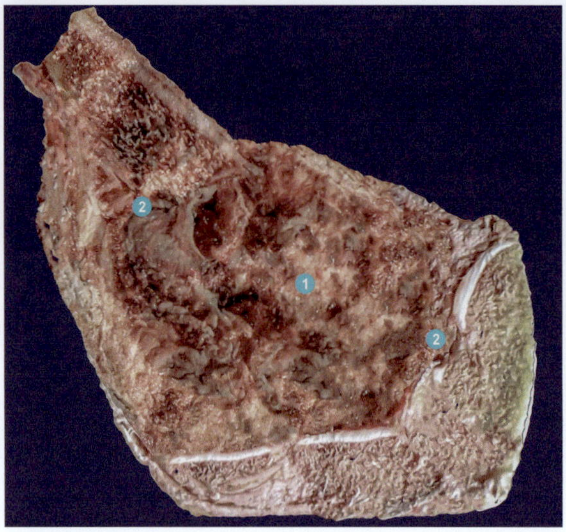

A piece of bone sectioned longitudinally is mounted.

1. Soft, friable, slightly brownish or red-tan, somewhat poorly defined neoplasm at the end of a long bone with yellow and firm white areas corresponding to xanthomatous change and fibrous tissue.
2. The surrounding cortex is thinned and may be destroyed in an area.

   The tumor involves epiphysis, metaphysis, and extends to articular cartilage.

Microscopic Picture of Giant Cell Tumor of Bone, NOS (a, b)

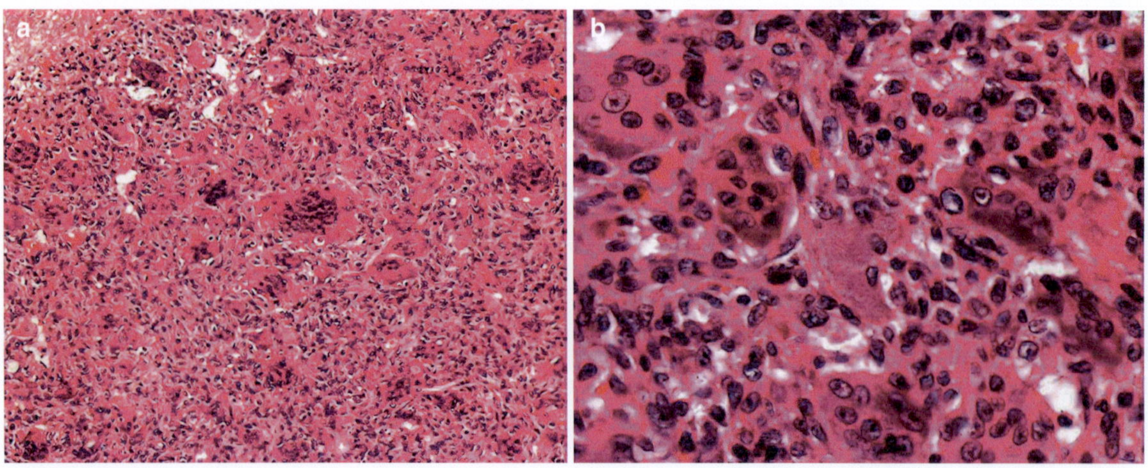

Sections show a highly cellular lesion composed of a large number of nonneoplastic osteoclast-like giant cells, between which mononuclear neoplastic cells are embedded. Mononuclear neoplastic cells exhibit a variety of morphological appearances, including round to oval cells and spindle cells with pale eosinophilic cytoplasm and nuclei with dispersed chromatin and small nucleoli. Mitoses are commonly present and can be numerous.

Ancillary Tools

IHC [7]:

- H3G34W
- p63
- SALL4 SATB2
- CD68

11.3.2 Metastatic Tumors

Metastatic Deposits in Vault of Skull

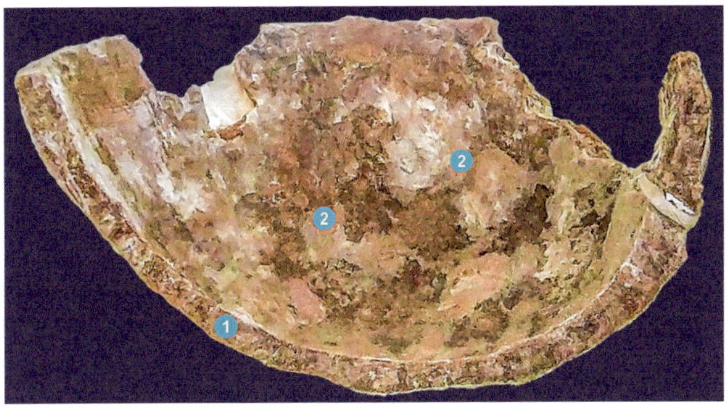

Half of the skull vault is mounted.

1. The bone is thickened.
2. Multiple, irregular, small, yellow deposits of tumor tissue are seen infiltrating bone and projecting inside the skull.

Microscopic Picture of Osteoblastic Metastatic Deposits of Adenocarcinoma in Bone (a)

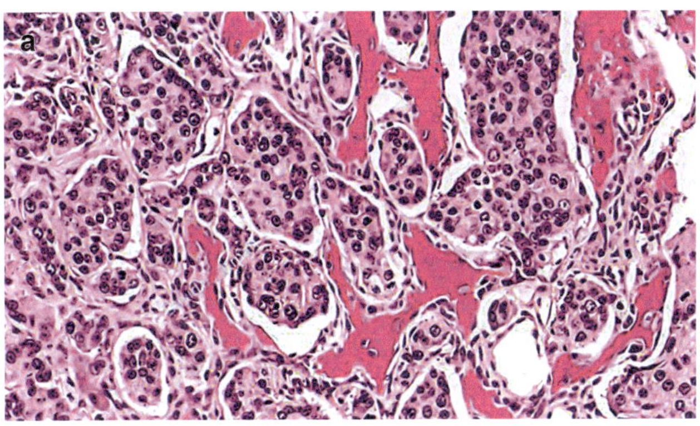

Sections show clusters of adenocarcinoma cells with an infiltrative growth pattern interspersed with thickened bony trabeculae rimmed by osteoblasts.

Metastatic Deposits in Vault of Skull

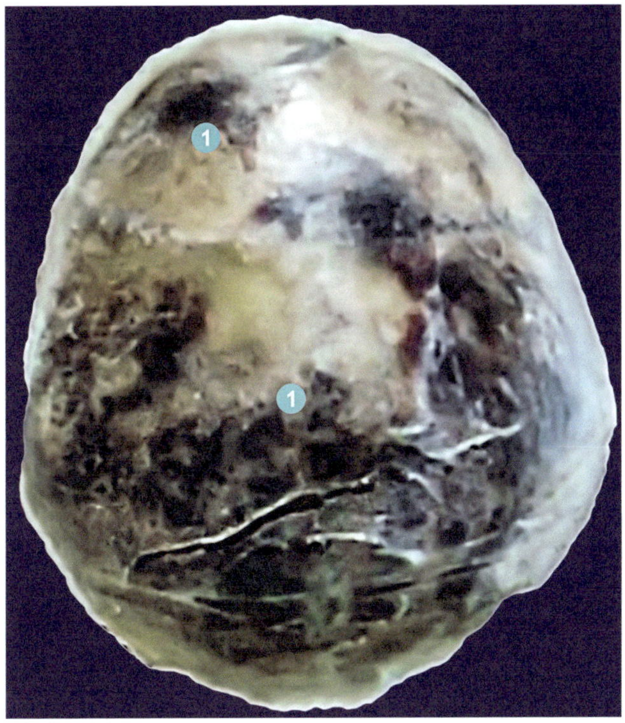

The vault of the skull is mounted.

1. Widespread osteolytic lesions with extensive hemorrhage are seen.

Microscopic Picture of Osteolytic Metastatic Deposits of Multiple Myeloma in Bone

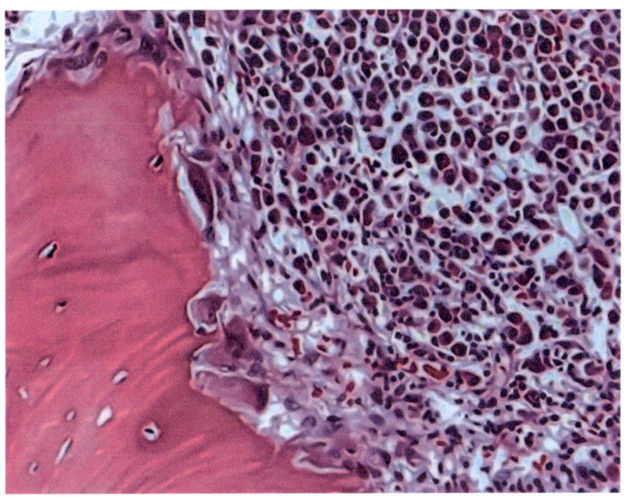

The section shows malignant plasmacytoid cells infiltrating bone marrow with the presence of osteoclasts actively resorbing bone adjacent to the tumor cells.

Metastatic Deposits in Skull

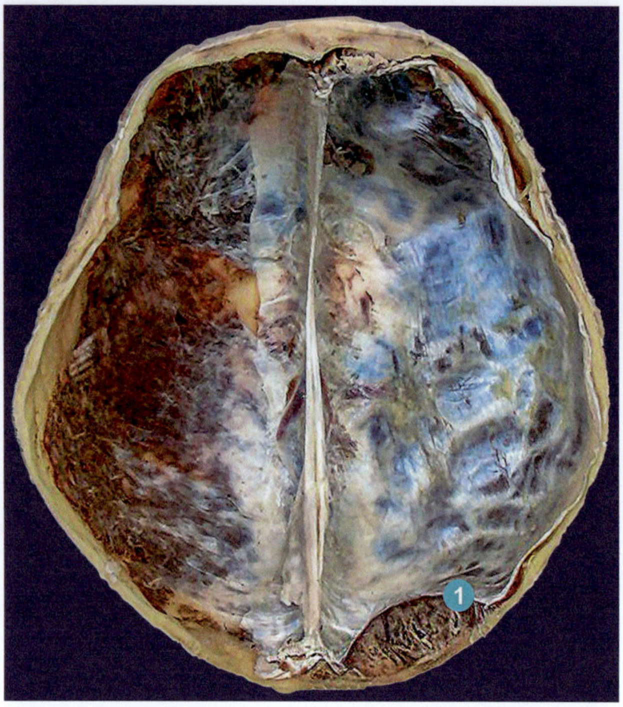

The vault of the skull covered with dura is mounted.

1. An epidural mass is seen projecting inside the skull.

Pearls

Bone metastasis is classified as osteolytic, osteoblastic, or mixed, according to the primary mechanism of interference with normal bone remodeling:

1. Osteolytic, characterized by destruction of normal bone, present in multiple myeloma (MM), renal cell carcinoma, melanoma, non-small cell lung cancer, non-Hodgkin lymphoma, thyroid cancer, or Langerhans-cell histiocytosis. The great majority of BC produces osteolytic metastases. This bone destruction is primarily mediated by osteoclasts and is not a direct effect of tumor cells.
2. Osteoblastic (or sclerotic), characterized by deposition of new bone, present in prostate cancer, carcinoid, small cell lung cancer, Hodgkin lymphoma, or medulloblastoma. The mechanisms of osteoblastic metastases are still poorly understood. In some instances, the new bone formation is not necessarily preceded by bone resorption [3]. Transforming growth factor, bone morphogenic proteins (BMP), and endothelin-1 are associated with osteoblast generation [8].

References

1. Lam S. et al. (2020). Utility of FOS as a diagnostic marker for osteoid osteoma and osteoblastoma. Virchows Arch. 476(3):455-463. doi: https://doi.org/10.1007/s00428-019-02684-9. PMID: 31768625; PMCID: PMC7085481.
2. Mejia-Guerrero S. et al. (2010). Characterization of the 12q15 MDM2 and 12q13-14 CDK4 amplicons and clinical correlations in osteosarcoma. Genes Chromosomes Cancer. 49(6):518-25. doi: https://doi.org/10.1002/gcc.20761. PMID: 20196171.
3. Grifone TJ, Haupt HM, Podolski V, Brooks JJ. (2008). Immunohistochemical expression of estrogen receptors in chondrosarcomas and enchondromas. Int J Surg Pathol. 16(1):31-7. doi: https://doi.org/10.1177/1066896907306774. PMID: 18203781.
4. Nakagawa M. et al. (2022). Clinical, Radiological, and Histopathological Characteristics of Periosteal Chondrosarcoma with a Focus on the Frequency of Medullary Invasion. Journal of Clinical Medicine 11, (7): 2062. doi:https://doi.org/10.3390/jcm11072062.
5. Schrage YM. et al. (2009). Central chondrosarcoma progression is associated with pRb pathway alterations: CDK4 down-regulation and p16 overexpression inhibit cell growth in vitro. J Cell Mol Med. 13(9A):2843-52. doi: https://doi.org/10.1111/j.1582--4934.2008.00406.x. PMID: 18624751; PMCID: PMC4498940.
6. Šekoranja D. et al. (2020). Novel ASAP1-USP6, FAT1-USP6, SAR1A-USP6, and TNC-USP6 fusions in primary aneurysmal bone cyst. Genes Chromosomes Cancer. 59(6):357-365. doi: https://doi.org/10.1002/gcc.22836. PMID: 32011035.
7. Liu TC, Ji ZM, Wang LT. (1989). Giant cell tumors of bone. An immunohistochemical study. Pathol Res Pract. 185(4):448-53. PMID: 2602217.
8. Macedo F et al. (2017). Bone Metastases: An Overview. Oncol Rev. 11(1):321. doi: https://doi.org/10.4081/oncol.2017.321. PMID: 28584570; PMCID: PMC5444408.

12 Diseases of Cutaneous and Soft Tissues

Skin is the largest organ of the body and provides a barrier against the external environment. It is made up of three main layers: the epidermis, dermis, and hypodermis. Pathologies of the skin can affect one or more of these layers, causing rashes, lesions, *ulcers*, discoloration, or abnormal growths.

Soft tissues include muscles, tendons, ligaments, fibrous tissues, fat, blood vessels, and other connective tissues. They surround and support organs and bones. Pathologies of soft tissues can cause swellings, deformities, or changes in texture or color. They can be caused by trauma, inflammation, infections, or tumors.

The study of gross and microscopic pathology of the skin and soft tissues can provide valuable information for diagnosing and managing patients.

This chapter will be organized as follows:

1. **Skin Pathology**
   (a) **Inflammatory Lesions**
   - Bacterial Infection
     - Leprosy
     - Mycetoma
     - Gangrene
   - Parasitic Infection
     - Leishmaniasis

   (b) **Neoplastic Lesions**
   - Squamous Cell Carcinoma
   - Basal Cell Carcinoma
   - Apocrine Carcinoma
2. **Soft Tissue Pathology**
   (a) **Benign Fibrohistiocytic Tumors**
   - Dermatofibroma

   (b) **Fibrohistiocytic Tumors of Intermediate Malignancy**
   - Dermatofibrosarcoma Protuberans (DFSP)

   (c) **Lipomatous Tumors**
   - Lipoma
   - Liposarcoma

   (d) **Malignant Vascular Tumor**
   - Angiosarcoma

   (e) **Malignant Tumors of Striated Muscle**
   - Rhabdomyosarcoma

   (f) **Primary Cutaneous Lymphoma**
   - Mycosis Fungoides (MF)

G. Dawood, *Color Atlas of Human Gross and Microscopic Pathology*, https://doi.org/10.1007/978-3-031-76007-5_12

12.1 Skin Pathology

12.1.1 Inflammatory Lesions

12.1.1.1 Bacterial and Fungal Infections

Hands of a Case of Lepromatous Leprosy (a, b)

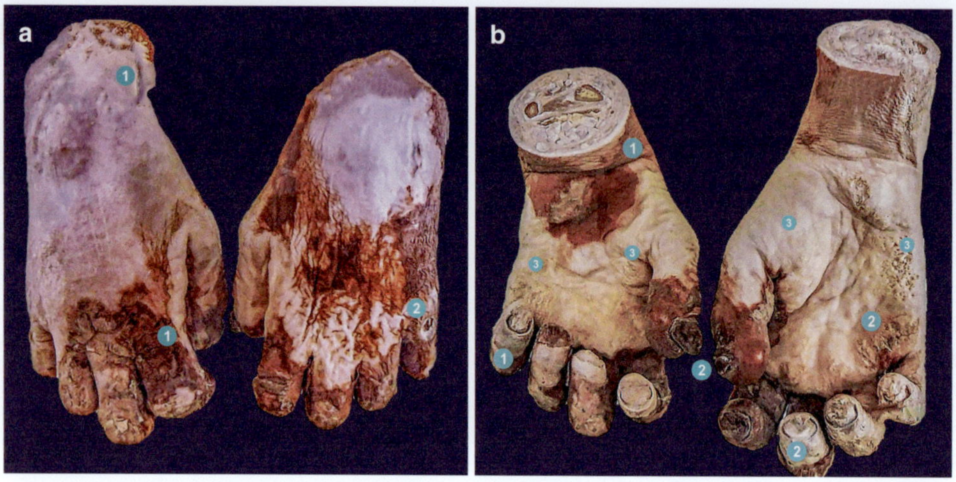

Both amputated hands of a patient having lepromatous leprosy (LL) are mounted.

1. Wrist drop and claw fingers.
2. The fingers show onycholysis and atrophy of distal phalanges. Trophic ulcers are seen.
3. Flattened thenar and hypothenar eminences.

The Hand of a Case of Lepromatous Leprosy

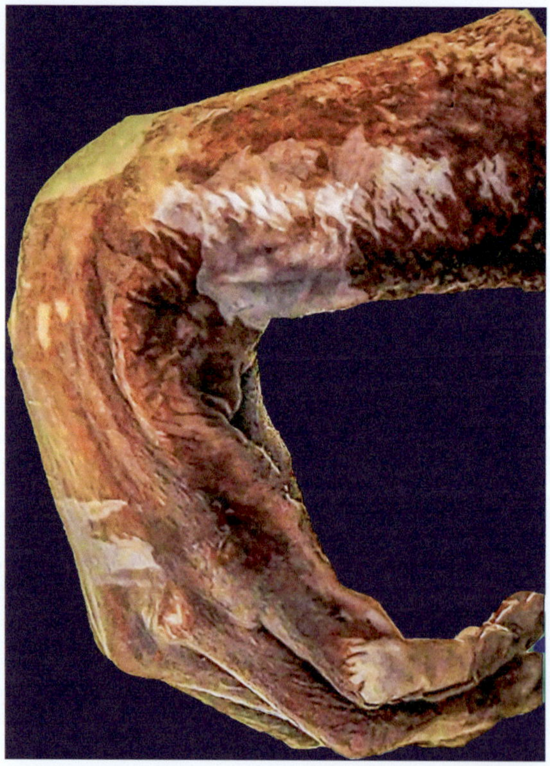

An amputated hand of a patient having lepromatous leprosy (LL) is mounted.

It shows wrist drops and claw fingers.

Microscopic Picture of Lepromatous Leprosy (a, b)

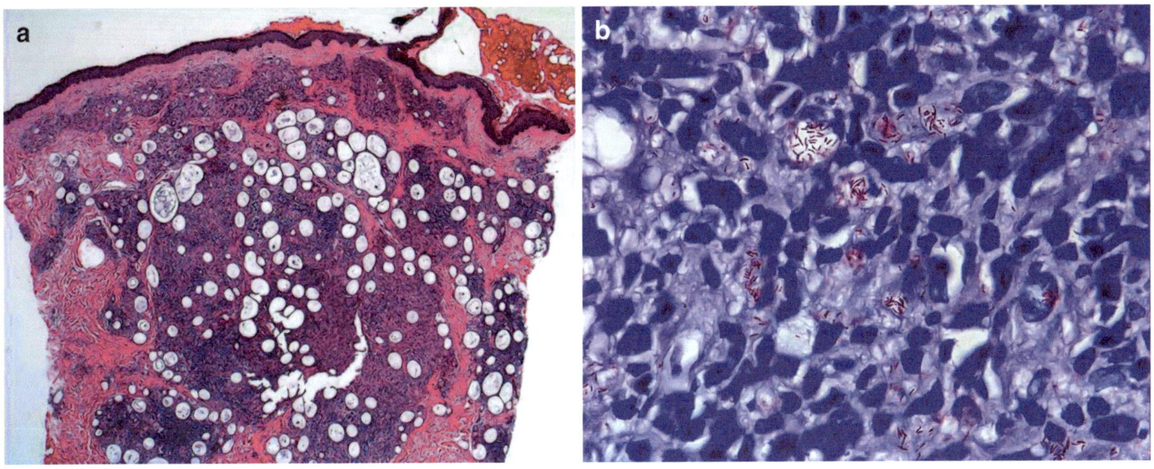

Sections show superficial and deep inflammatory-cell infiltrate, separated from the epidermis by a narrow zone of collagen (Grenz zone). The infiltrate is formed of lymphocytes, histiocytes, and foam cells, which form large nodules throughout the dermis. The lipid-containing acid-fast organisms that fill the cytoplasm of histiocytes and are responsible for their foamy appearance are well demonstrated by the Fite stain (d). The masses of densely packed acid-fast bacilli within histiocytes are called "globi."

Eumycetoma (Madura Foot) (a, b) (with a mirror in front of toes in b)

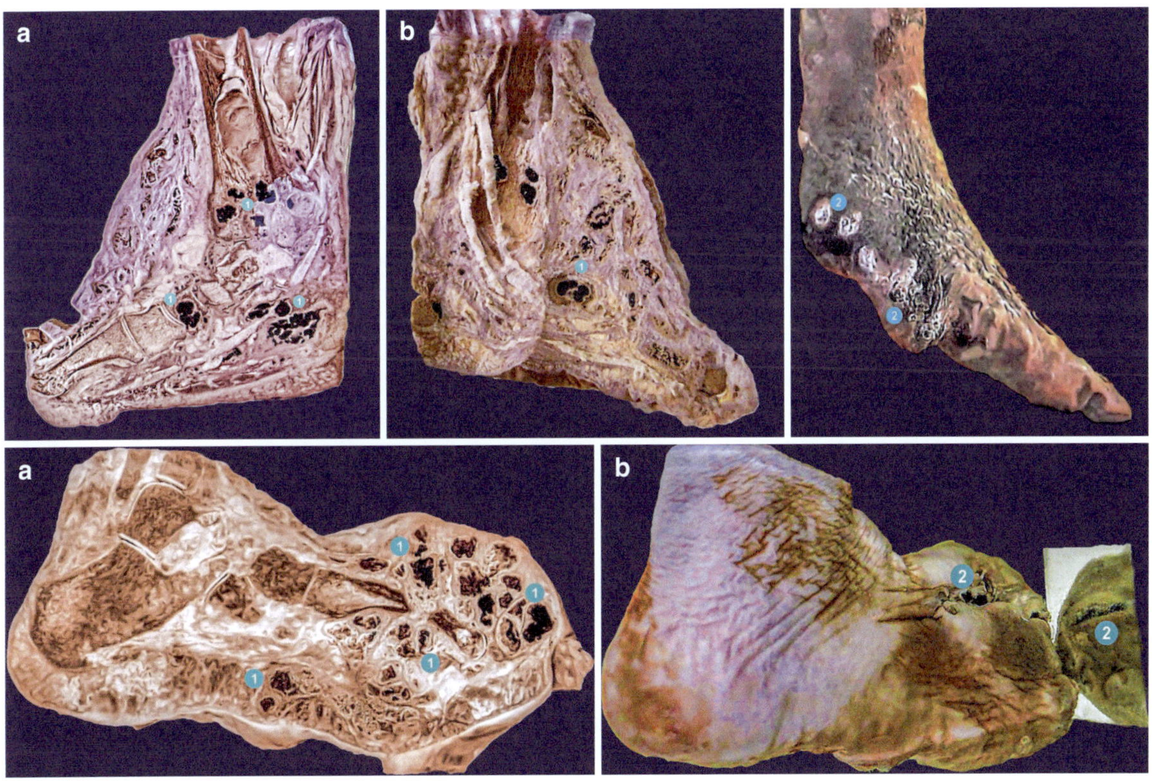

An amputated foot is sectioned longitudinally and mounted.

1. The cut section shows multiple black colonies destroying the bones and infiltrating soft tissue with the presence of areas of fibrosis.
2. Some colonies are seen in the sinuses opening on the skin surface.

Microscopic Picture of Eumycetoma (c–h)

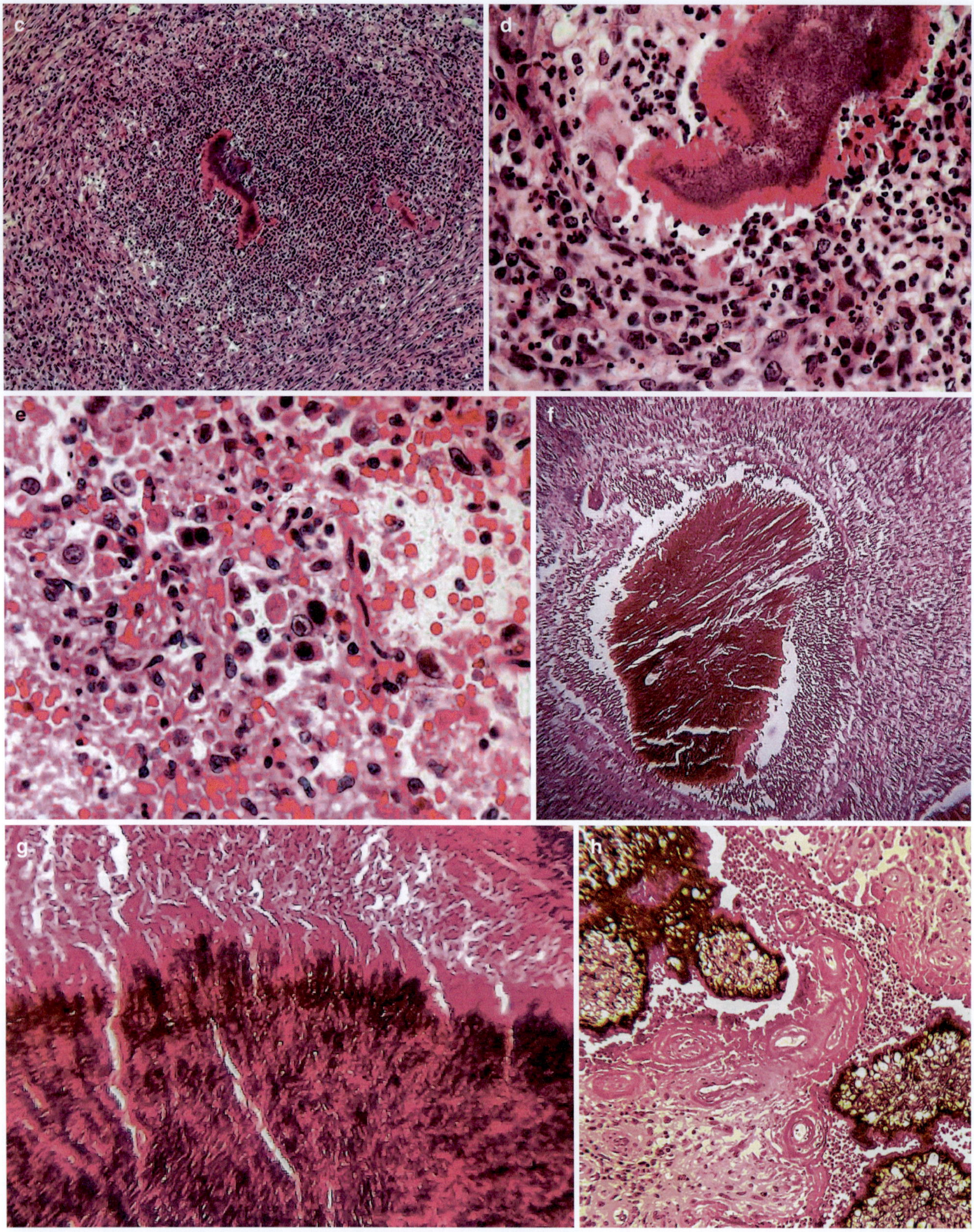

Sections show suppurative granulomatous inflammation around fungal colonies embedded in a fibrous stroma. The granuloma is formed of epithelioid cells, macrophages, giant cells, and lymphocytes admixed with a dense infiltrate of neutrophils. The fungal hyphae and spores are evident, while white grains are seen in (h).

Gangrene of Toes (a, b)

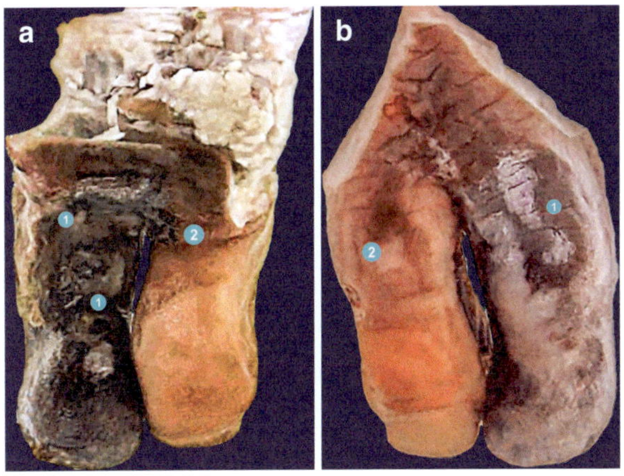

Two amputated toes are mounted.

1. The left toe is black, swollen, and with areas of skin ulceration.
2. The neighboring toes show skin mottling and extension of the gangrenous changes and ulceration to the ventral aspect at its base.

Gas Gangrene of Left Leg

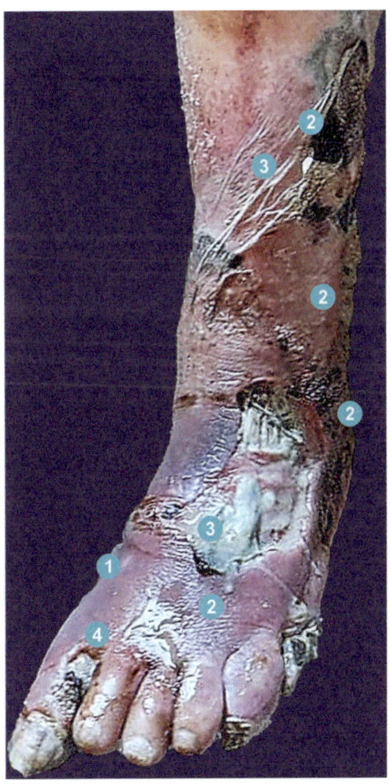

An amputated left leg is mounted.

1. The limb is swollen.
2. The dorsum of the foot is pale and turns red above the malleolus, with the presence of black areas in the foot and lateral side of the leg.
3. Thin-walled large bulla filled with pus is seen on the dorsum of the foot with the presence of remains of the thin roof of a ruptured bulla in the lower leg.
4. Interdigital infection and gangrene are seen between the first and second toes.

Microscopic Picture of Gas Gangrene (a)

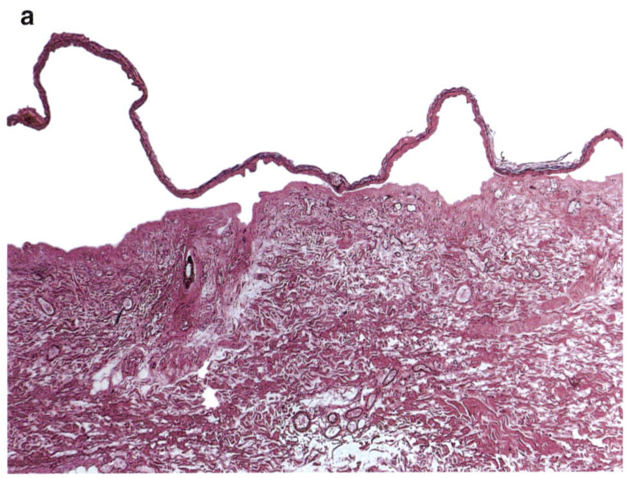

The section shows a subepidermal bulla, sweat gland necrosis, and no inflammatory cell infiltrate. Holes, representing gas bubbles, are seen in the dermis.

12.1.1.2 Parasitic Infection

Chronic Cutaneous Nodular Leishmaniasis

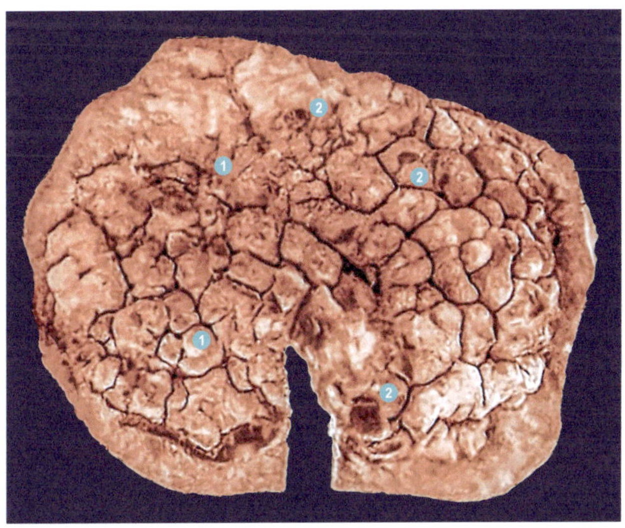

A piece of skin is mounted.

1. The skin has a rough nodular verrucous plaque with irregular borders.
2. Areas of superficial ulceration are observed.

Microscopic Picture of Cutaneous Leishmaniasis (a–c)

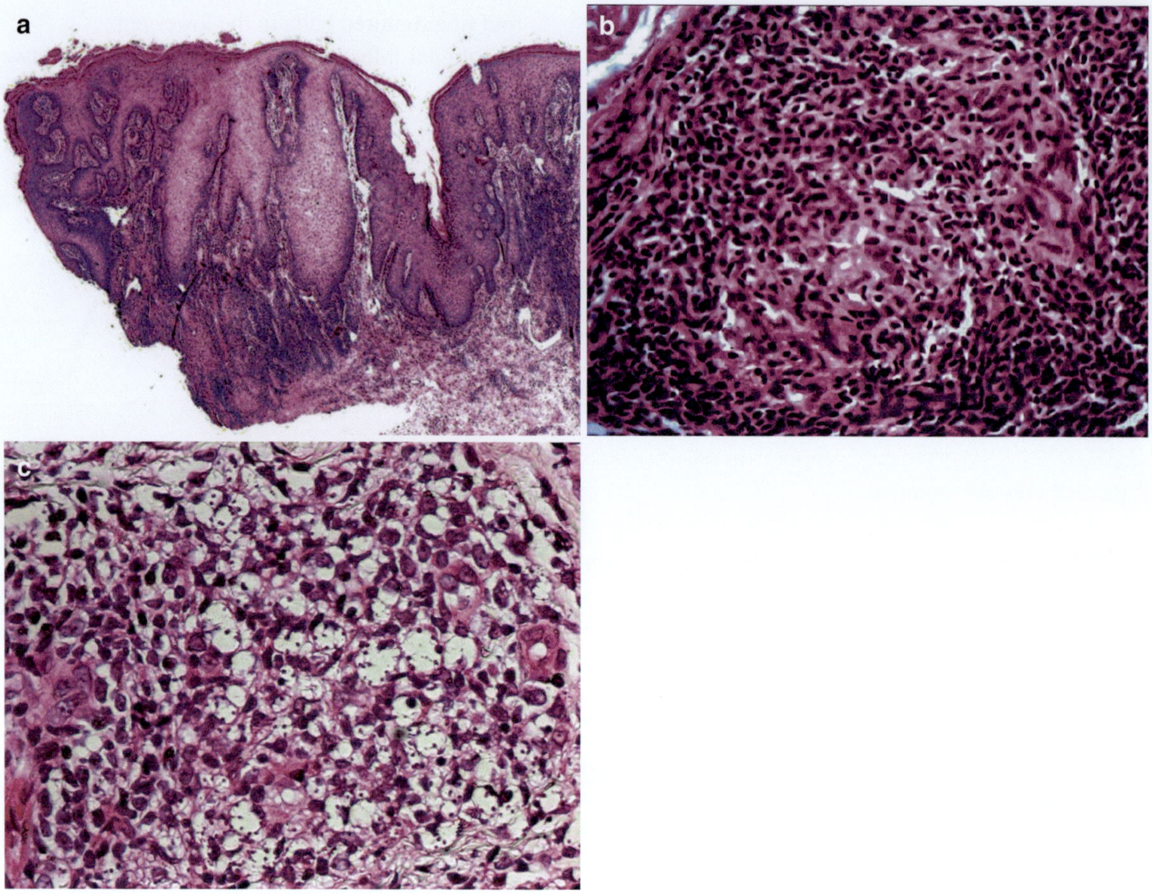

Sections show hyperkeratosis, irregular acanthosis, and superficial dermal infiltrate containing non-caseating granulomas, formed of epithelioid cells, macrophages, lymphocytes, and plasma cells, with the presence of sparse intracytoplasmic Leishman–Donovan bodies (LD bodies) in macrophages.

Pearls

The typical lesion of localized cutaneous leishmaniasis is initially a papule that progresses to an ulcer with a raised, infiltrated border and a granular background, which may be accompanied by regional lymphadenopathy and/or nodular lymphangitis. However, the clinical forms of pleomorphic and atypical aspects can hinder and delay the diagnosis and, consequently, adequate treatment. Among the atypical forms of ATL, the verrucous, lupoid, eczematous, zosteriform, tumor, acneiform, and sporotrichoid forms have been reported. The diagnosis should be based on epidemiology, lesion characteristics, direct examination, and culture. In atypical cases, histopathological examination and PCR are fundamental tools [1].

12.1.2 Neoplastic Lesions

Malignant Ulcer of Skin (a, b)

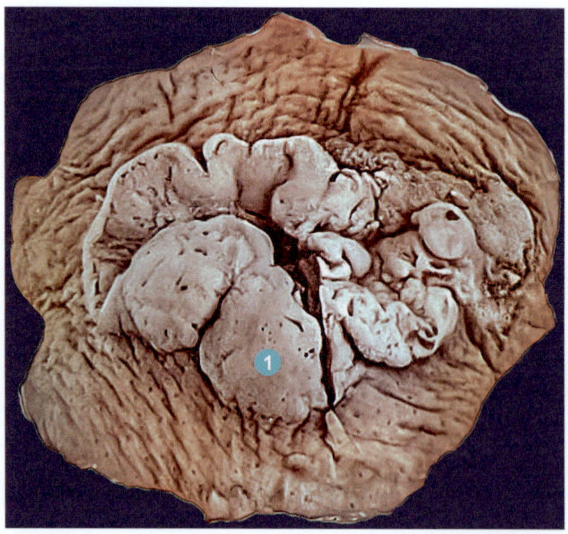

A piece of skin with the subcutaneous tissue is mounted.

1. A large ulcer with irregular borders, raised everted edges, and a necrotic floor.

Verrucous Carcinoma of the Skin (Carcinoma Cuniculatum)

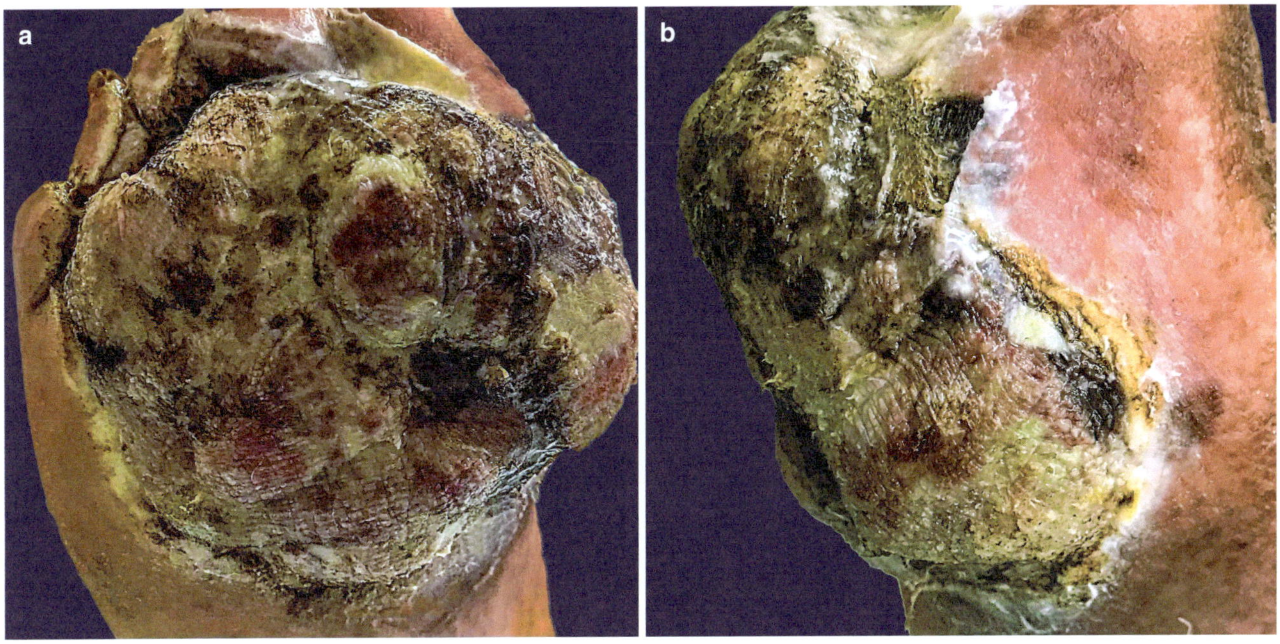

An amputated right foot with the heel facing up is mounted.

1. An exophytic, fungating, brownish-yellowish, and polypoid mass with a bossy hyperkeratotic surface and focal hemorrhage.
2. The lesion is traversed by deep keratin-filled sinuses.

Microscopic Picture of Verrucous Carcinoma of the Skin (a–e)

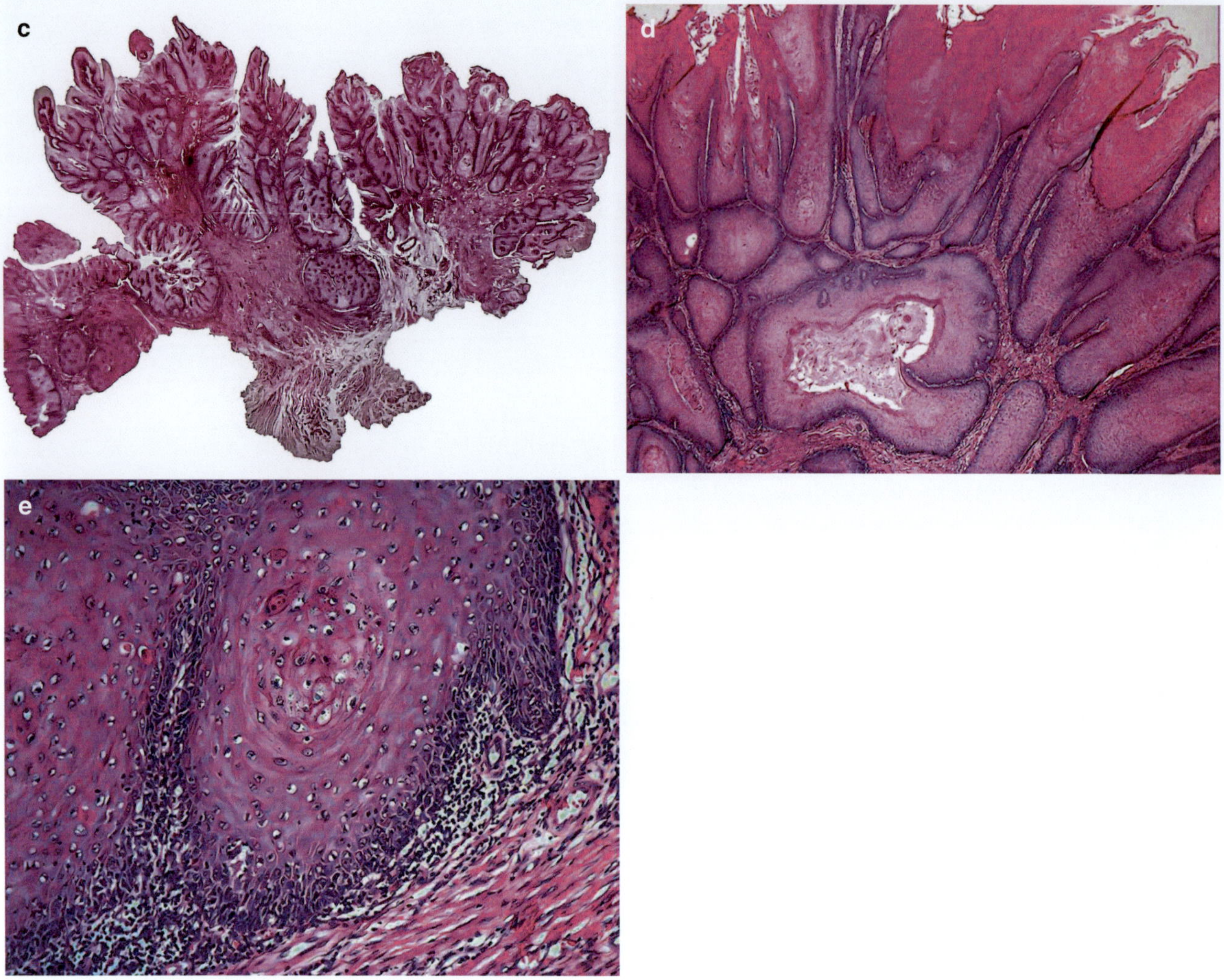

Sections show well-differentiated squamous proliferation with exophytic and endophytic components. The exophytic component is formed of papillomatosis and massive hyperkeratosis, often with an expanded granular layer with focal parakeratosis. Endophytic component with blunt projections of well-differentiated squamous epithelium with deep bulbous processes and a pushing margin. Tumor cells are large, polygonal squamous cells with abundant pink cytoplasm and enlarged nuclei with minimal nuclear atypia (apart from several layers at the interface of bulbous tips). The stroma is inflamed, edematous, and infiltrated with lymphoid cells.

Ancillary Tools

Molecular/cytogenetics description:

Association with somatic HRAS, PIK3CA, and BRAF mutations and less commonly PTEN, EGFR, and GNAS mutations has been described in the vulva in a spectrum of lesions from verrucous carcinoma to differentiated vulvar intraepithelial dysplasia [2].

Pearls

VC usually tends to show a less invasive and more indolent course than other skin cancers that originate from other parts of the body. The clinical features of VC are non-specific and similar to those of benign lesions such as verruca vulgaris. These indolent courses and non-specific presentations often lead to a delayed diagnosis [3].

Malignant Ulcer of the Skin (Marjolin Ulcer-Squamous Cell Carcinoma)

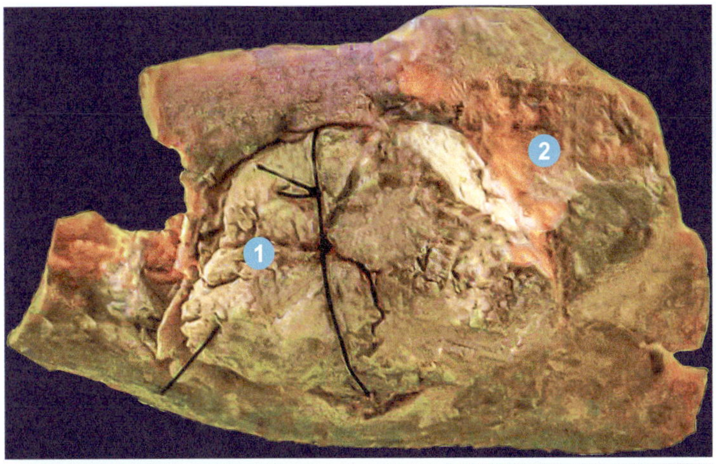

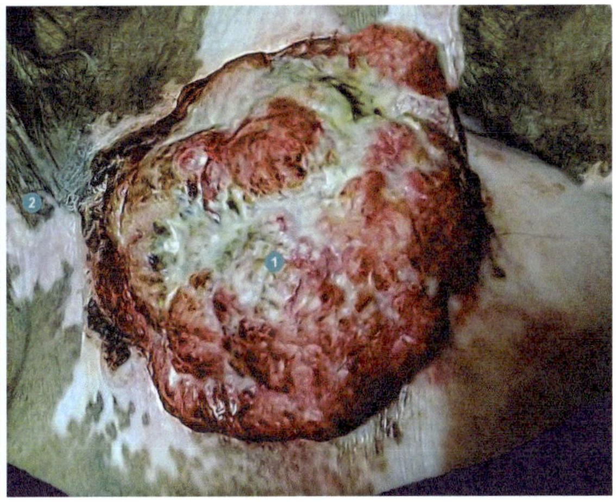

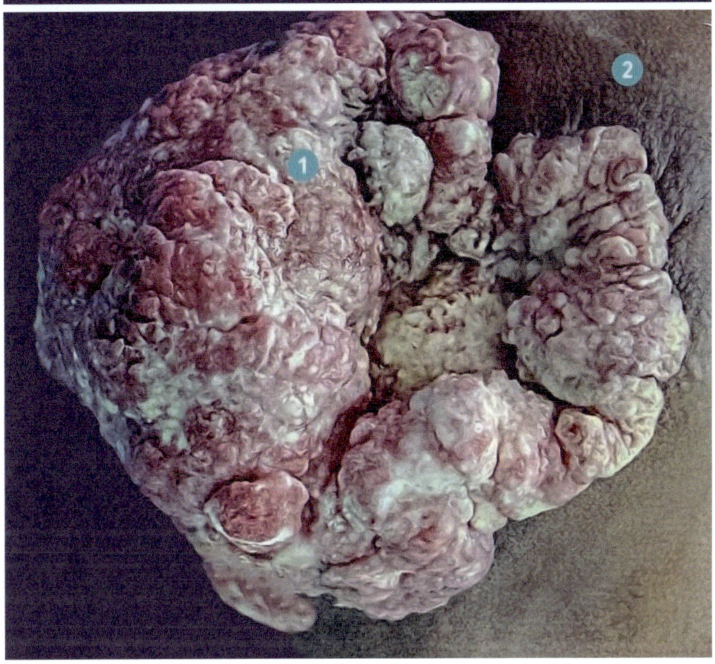

A piece of skin with the subcutaneous tissue is mounted.

1. A large, exophytic, and friable mass with irregular borders extending deep into the skin.
2. The skin around the ulcer is blotchy with the presence of hyper- and hypopigmented areas due to an old burn scar.

Microscopic Picture of Well-Differentiated Squamous Cell Carcinoma (a)

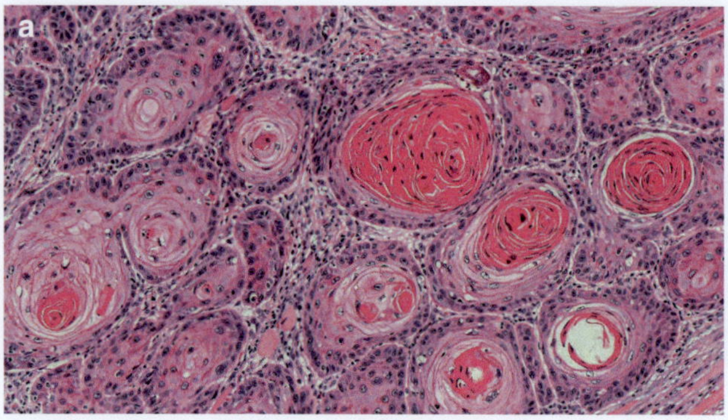

The section shows multiple cell nests of malignant squamous cells with central parakeratin infiltrating the stroma.

Ancillary Tools

IHC [4]:

Keratins: AE1/AE3, MNF 116, 34 beta E12, CK5/6, CK5
EMA
p63, p40

Rodent Ulcer (Basal Cell Carcinoma)

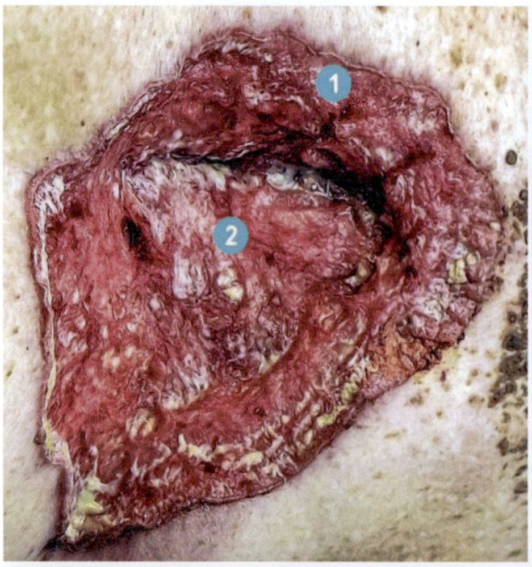

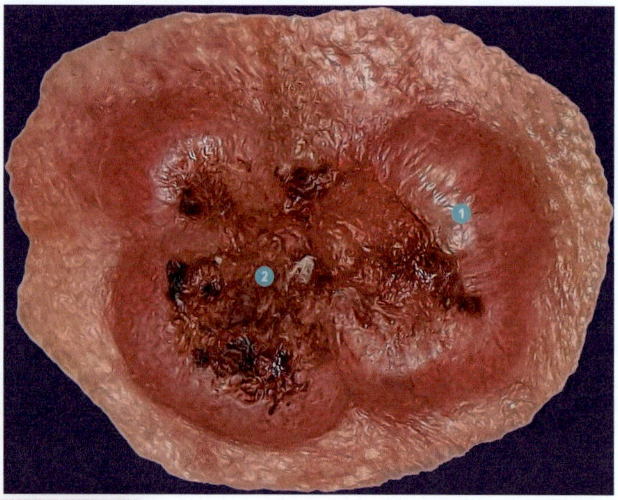

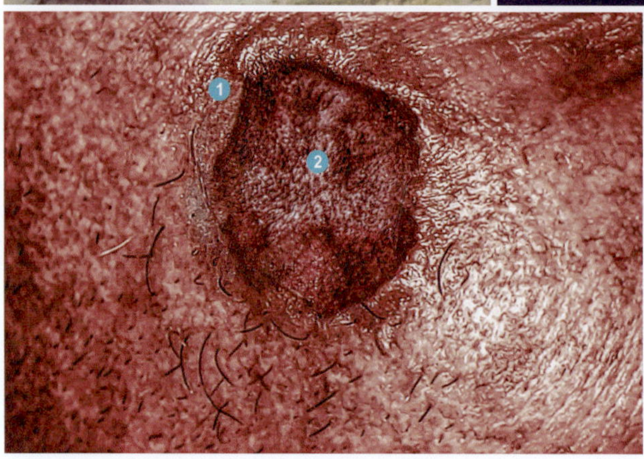

A piece of skin is mounted. It shows a large ulcer with

1. A rolled-in edge
2. necrotic floor.

Microscopic Picture of Nodulocystic Basal Cell Carcinoma (a–e)

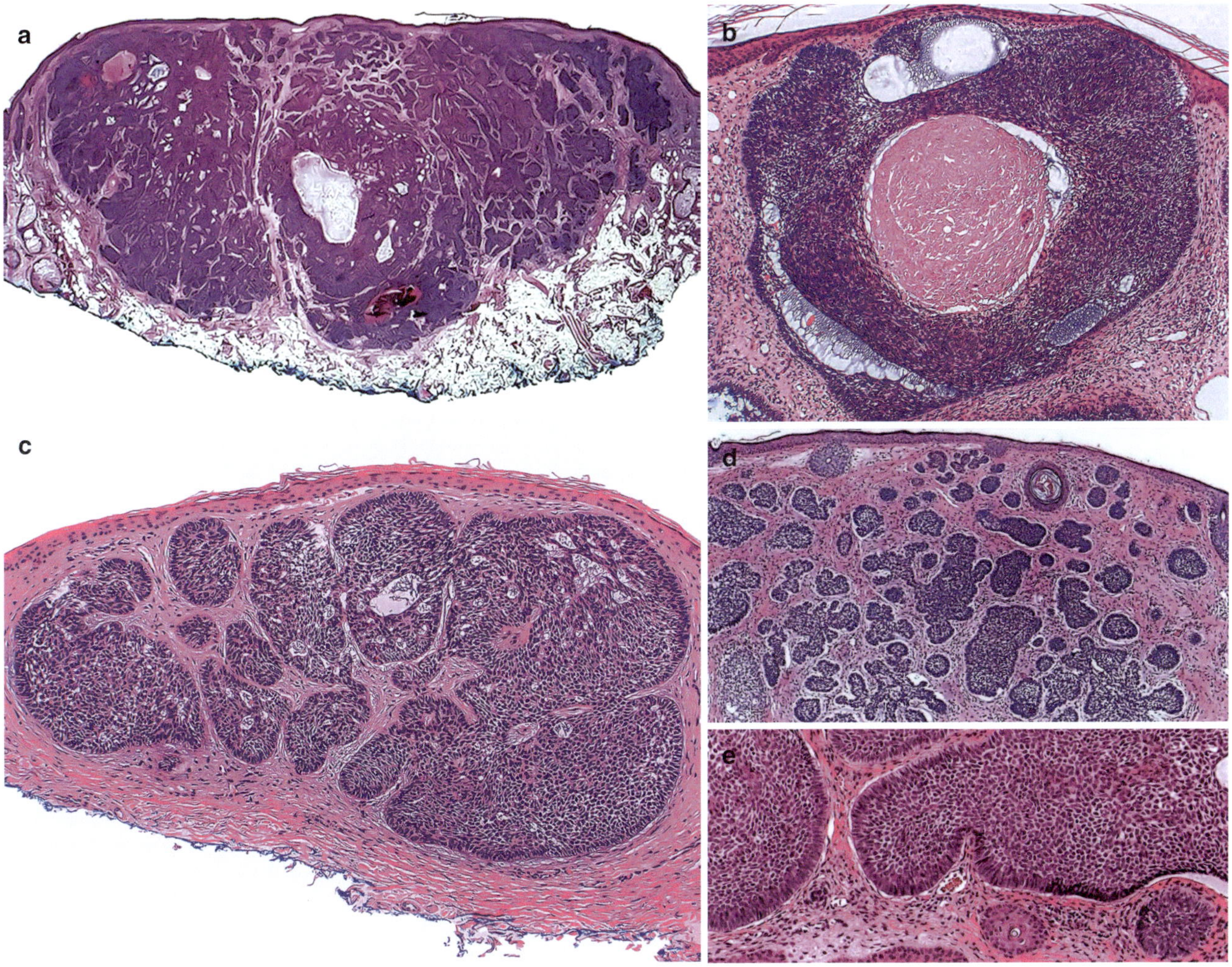

Sections show a large nodular tumor with cystic spaces. The tumor is formed of malignant basaloid cells infiltrating the dermis, reaching up to the subcutaneous fat. The tumor mass shows peripheral palisading of tumor cells. The surrounding stroma is immature and shows myxoid change and artifactual clefts.

Microscopic Picture of Adenoid Basal Cell Carcinoma (f, g)

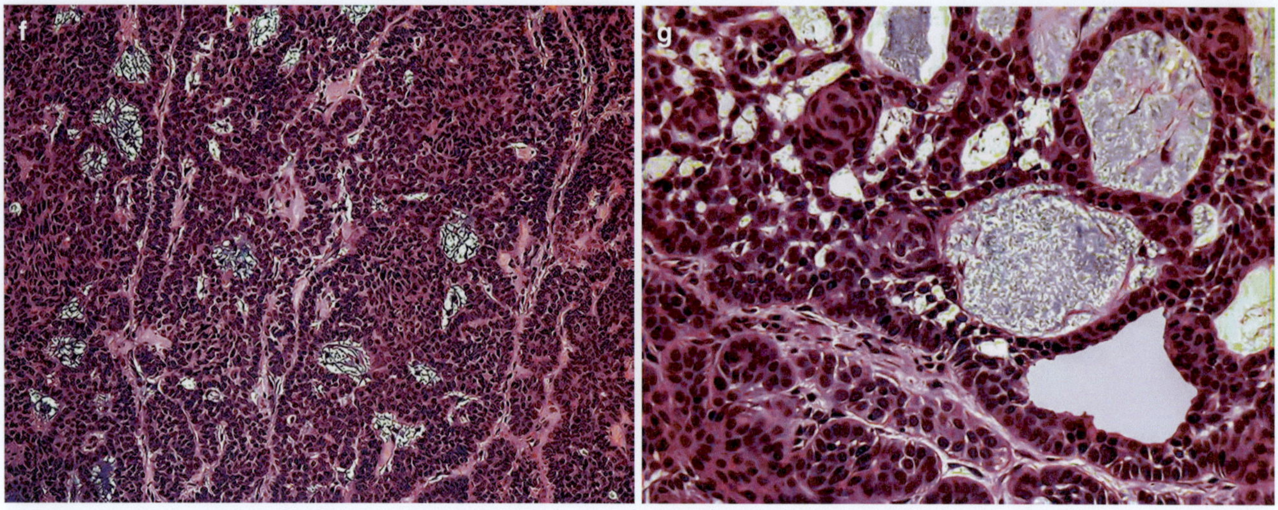

Sections show a reticulate pseudoglandular pattern of basaloid cells with peripheral palisading and mucinous stroma.

Microscopic Picture of Morpheaform (Sclerosing, Morphoeic) Basal Cell Carcinoma (h, i)

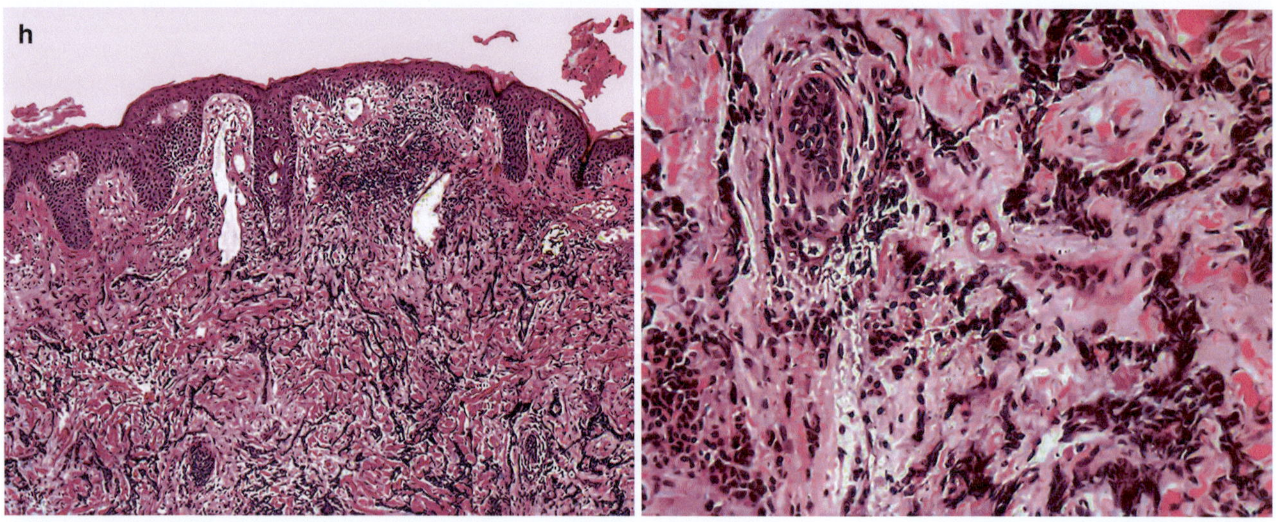

Sections show extensive dermal spread of thin strands and nests of basaloid cells enmeshed within collagen bundles with limited peripheral palisading. The stroma is dense and sclerotic.

Microscopic Picture of Fibroepitheliomatous Basal Cell Carcinoma (Fibroepithelioma of Pinkus) (j, k)

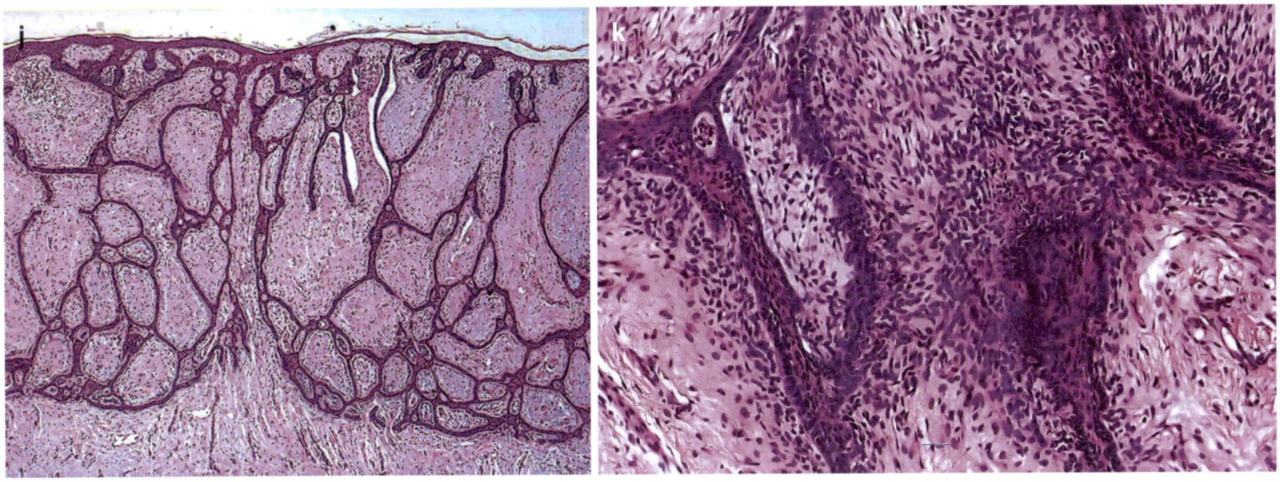

Sections show anastomosing strands and cords of basaloid cells connected to the epidermis. The tumor shows peripheral nuclear palisading with a formation of follicular germ-like structures.

Ancillary Tools [5]

IHC:

CK AE1 / AE3 (100%), BerEP4 (80–100%), p63 (100%), CAM 5.2 (20–95%), androgen receptor (33–66%), p53 (74.5–83%), 34 beta E12 (high molecular weight CK), BCL2 (diffuse pattern), CD10 (positive in tumor cells, negative in stroma).

Molecular/cytogenetics description:

chromosomal gains at 6p (47%), 6q (20%), 9p (20%), 7 (13%), and X (13%)

Regional loss on 9q in 33% of tested tumors encompassing 9q22.3 to which the patched gene has been mapped.

Primary Cutaneous Apocrine Carcinoma of Axilla (PCAC) (a, b)

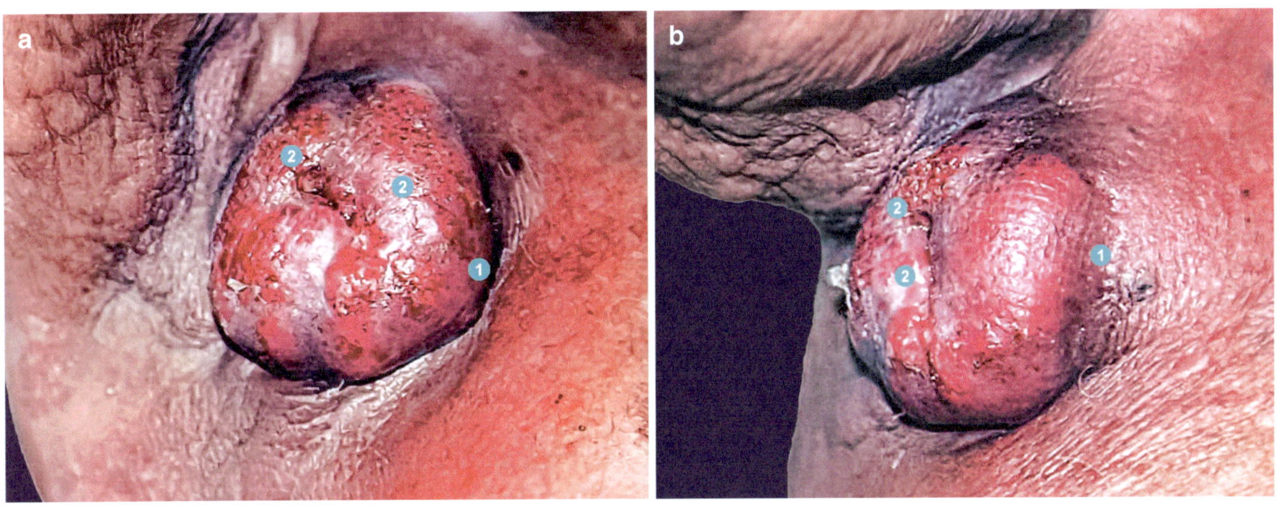

A mass is present in the axilla.

1. The mass is a large sessile nodule.
2. The overlying skin is blotchy with erythematous and white areas and shows a central ulcer.

Microscopic Picture of Primary Cutaneous Apocrine Carcinoma (c, d)

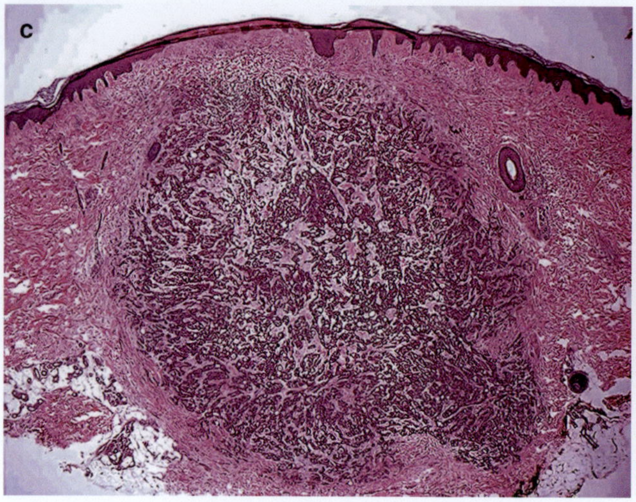

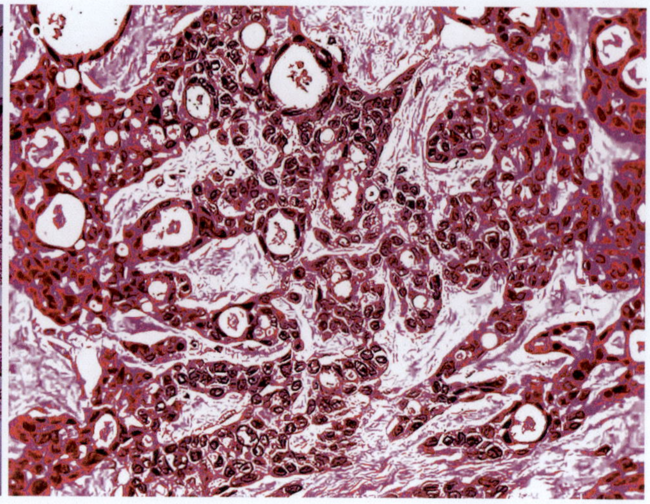

Sections show a nonencapsulated dermal neoplasm formed of solid nests and sheets of tubular structures and microcystic spaces. The tumor cells are large and polygonal with abundant eosinophilic cytoplasm and hyperchromatic nuclei. Lymphoid aggregates are present at the periphery of the neoplasm. The stroma shows mucinous change.

Ancillary Tools

IHC [6]:

Androgen receptors, p63, GCDFP-15, calretinin (variable in PCAC) D2–40, focal positive CK5/6, and GATA-3

Pearls

Apocrine carcinoma is a rare malignant sweat gland tumor that has only been reported in approximately 200 cases. Apocrine carcinoma primarily develops between the ages of 60 and 70 years among Caucasians, and its cause remains unknown. It mainly occurs in the axilla, which has a high concentration of apocrine glands. However, in rare cases, it has been reported to develop on the scalp, anogenital region, ear canal, chest, wrist, finger, and eyelid. Apocrine carcinoma is an indolent, asymptomatic, cutaneous, or subcutaneous mass, and its color varies from red to purple. PCAC is characterized by the presence of cells with abundant eosinophilic cytoplasm, eccrine basally located nuclei, and decapitation secretions that are generally observed in luminal cells [7].

Congenital Melanocytic Hairy Nevus (a, b)

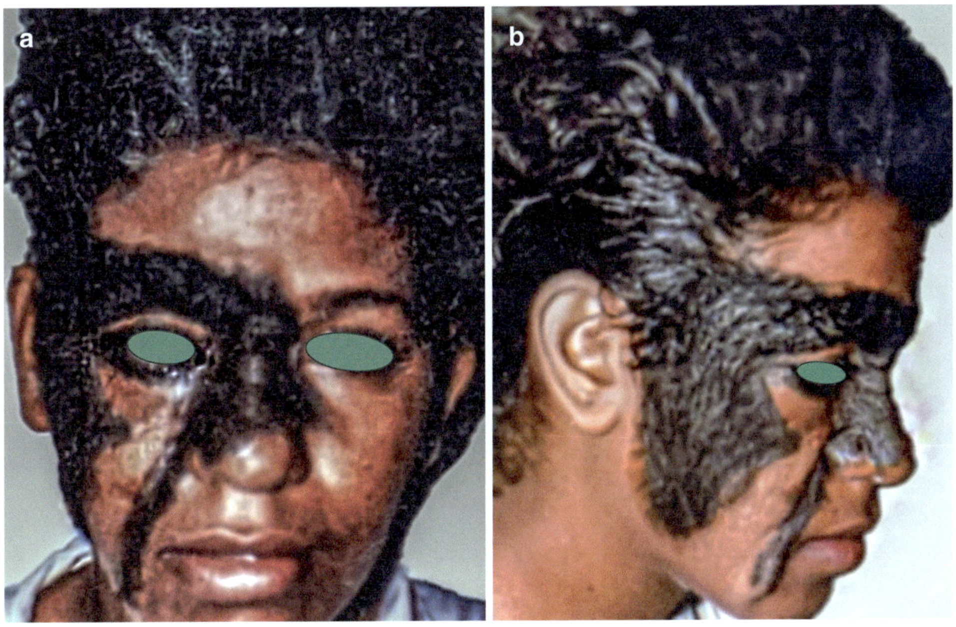

Clinically, the lesion is a black-colored, medium-sized patch covered with coarse black hairs with sharp borders blending with the surrounding skin present on the face and extending to the scalp.

Microscopic Picture of Congenital Melanocytic Hairy Nevus (c–f)

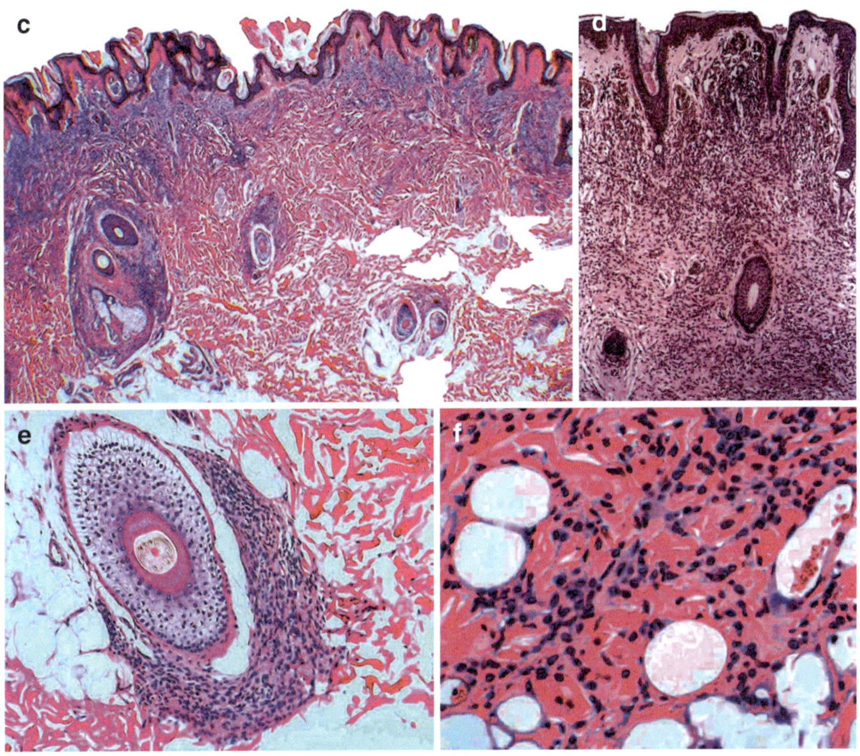

Sections show diffuse melanocytic proliferation in the dermis with extension into subcutaneous fat. The Grenz zone is identified between the epidermis and melanocytes. Nevus cells encircle and extend to walls of dermal appendages, perineural space, and blood vessels and can dissect through collagen bundles. Variable pigmentation and focal neurotization may be present. Sparse mitotic activity.

Ancillary Tools

IHC [8]:

S100

SOX10

MelanA/MART1

HMB45 (positive only in superficial part)

Molecular/cytogenetics description [9]:

NRAS mutation

BRAF mutations are also reported in CMN; however, they are uncommon.

Nodular Malignant Melanoma

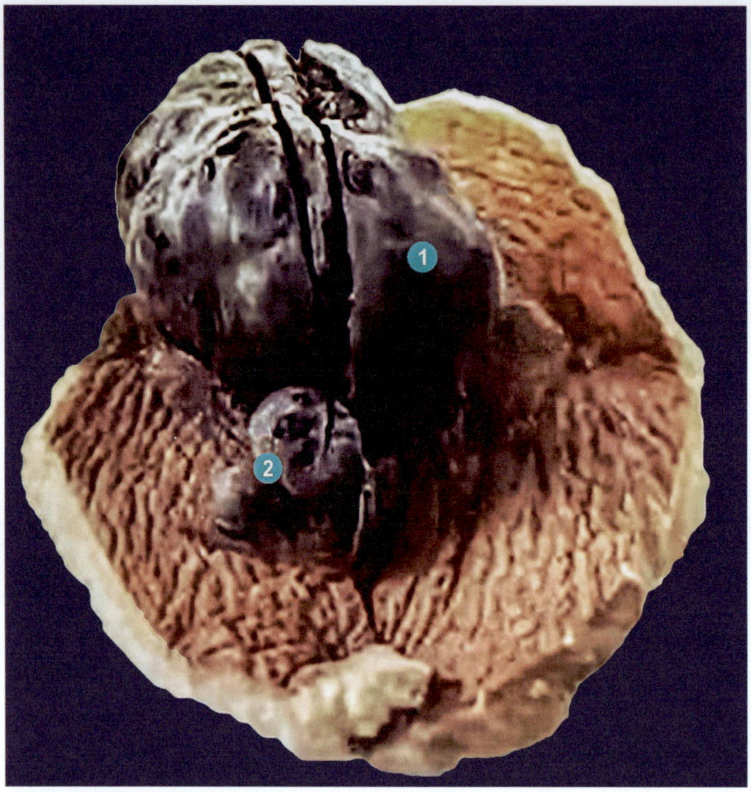

A piece of skin is mounted. It shows:

1. A large black nodule with a bossy ulcerated surface
2. Two adjacent tumor satellites are seen close to the main mass.

Microscopic Picture of Nodular Malignant Melanoma (a–g)

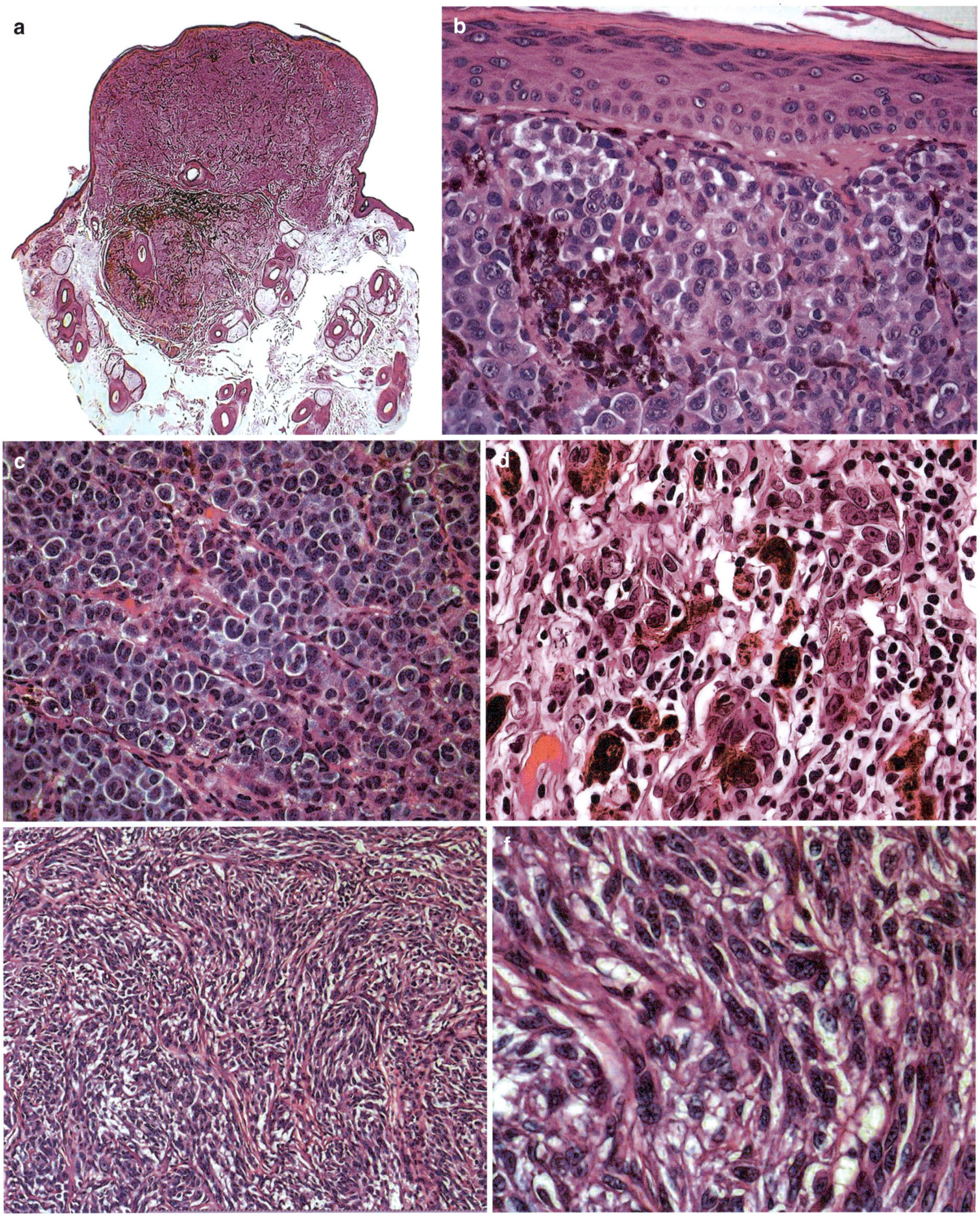

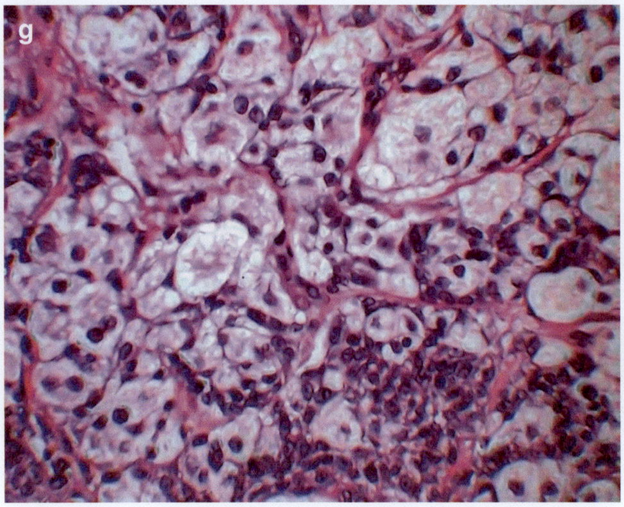

Sections show a large, raised, dome-shaped tumor mass of the skin. There is a proliferation of malignant melanocytes growing throughout the dermis with upward epidermal invasion but minimal adjacent epidermal spread or horizontal growth. Tumor cells are predominantly round and epithelioid, arranged focally in nests with the presence of melanin pigment, mixed with a lesser component of spindle-shaped cells. Both types of cells have hyperchromatic nuclei with an increased number of mitoses. In some areas, the malignant cells acquire balloon cell change.

Ancillary Tools

IHC1 [10]:

S100 (nuclear and cytoplasmic)
SOX10 (nuclear)
MelanA/MART1 (cytoplasmic)
HMB45 (cytoplasmic)
Tyrosinase (cytoplasmic)
MiTF (nuclear)
PRAME (nuclear)
PNL2 (cytoplasmic)
KBA62 (cytoplasmic)
Ki67/MIB1

Molecular/cytogenetics description [11]:

Molecular alterations do not constitute proof of malignancy per se and have to be interpreted in light of the clinical and histological findings.

In contrast with benign nevi, melanomas harbor multiple chromosomal copy number aberrations.

- Main chromosomal copy number aberrations (detected by FISH, comparative genomic hybridization [CGH], array CGH, and single nucleotide polymorphism array)
  - Gain: 6p, 7q, 17q, 20q, 4q, 8q, 1q, 11q
  - Loss: 9p21, 10, 21q
- Main genetic driver alterations (detected by PCR, Sanger, and next-generation sequencing)
  - BRAF, NRAS, NF1, KIT (Cell 2015;161:1681)
  - Telomerase reverse transcriptase promoter (TERT-p) (Sci Rep 2015;5:11200)
  - CDKN2A, PTEN, TP53
- Generally high tumor mutational burden (TMB > 10 mut/Mb)
- Gene expression profile (GEP), mRNA expression level of uveal and cutaneous melanoma-related genes

12.2 Soft Tissue Pathology

12.2.1 Benign Fibrohistiocytic Tumors

Dermatofibroma

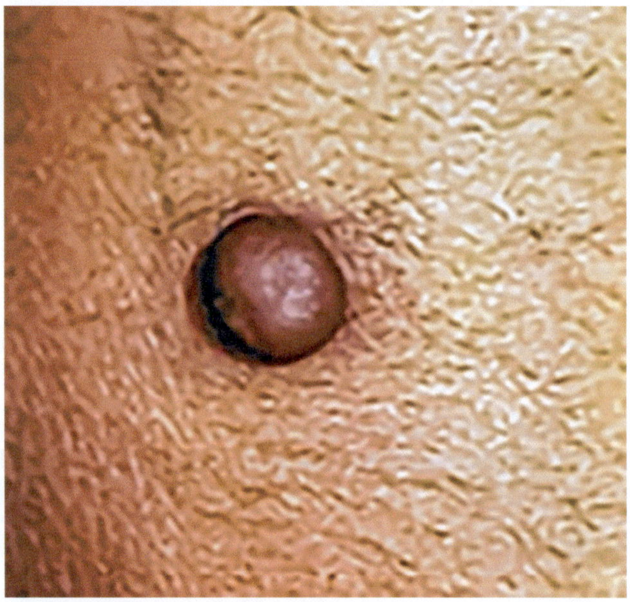

A piece of skin is mounted.

1. A round, red-brownish skin nodule is seen.

Microscopic Picture of Dermatofibroma (a–h)

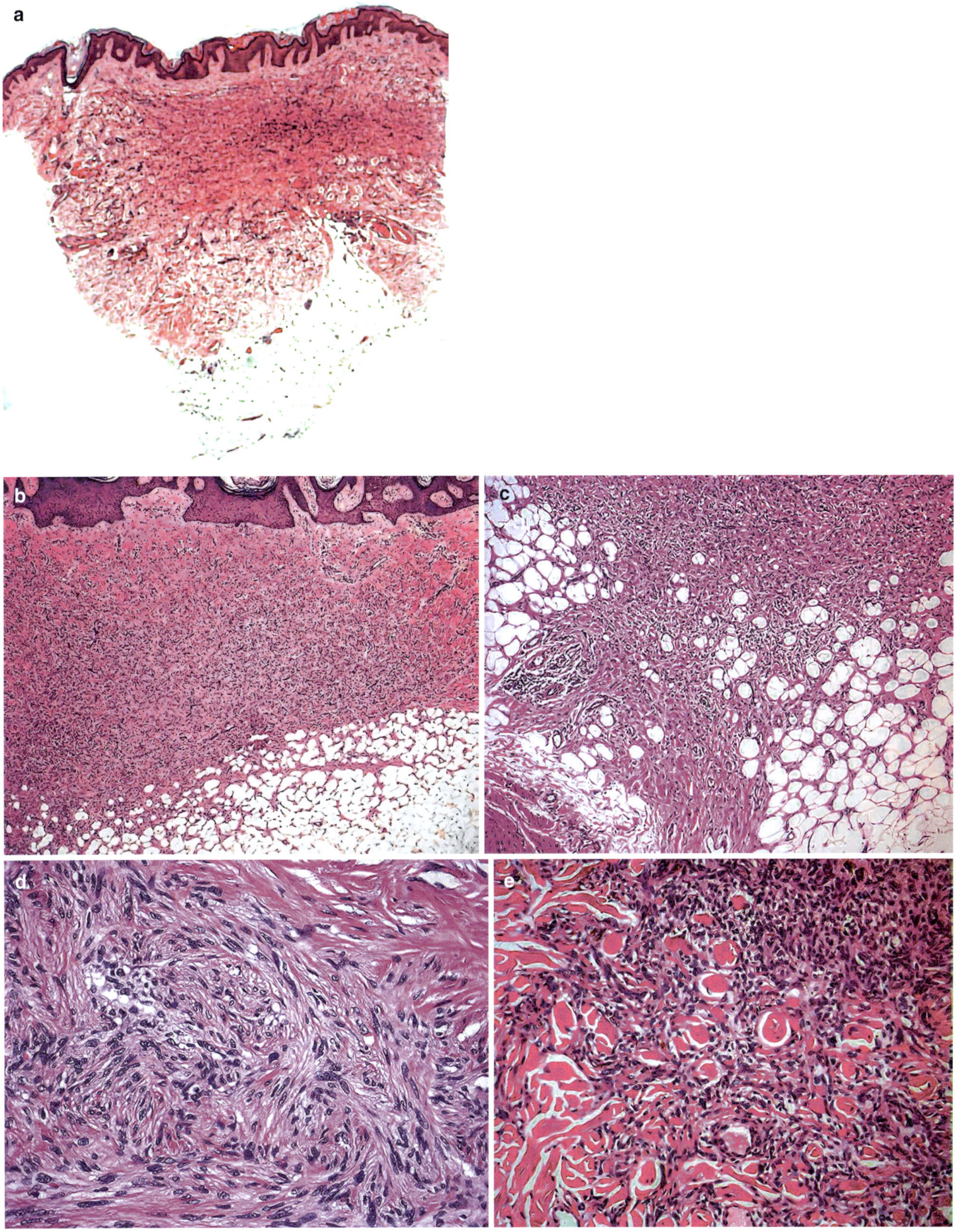

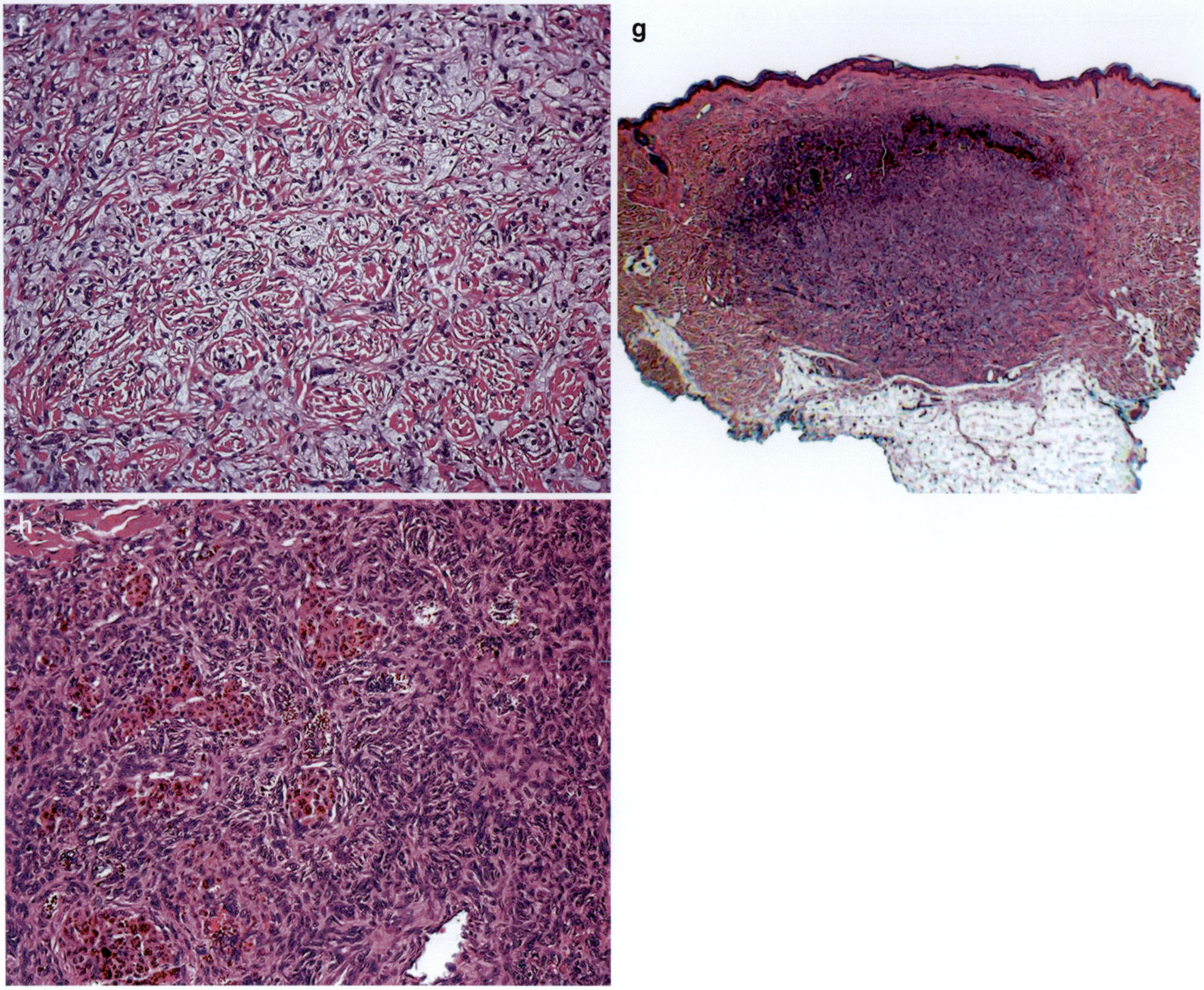

Sections show a well-circumscribed dermal lesion, separated from the epidermis by the Grenz zone (sparing of the superficial papillary dermis), with a central zone of fibroblastic proliferation and collagen deposition. The fibroblasts are arranged in a storiform pattern, forming whorls or fascicles. Collagen trapping is present at the periphery, forming spheres of eosinophilic collagen (collagen balls) surrounded by fibroblast proliferation. There are scattered inflammatory cells, such as lymphocytes and histiocytes, within the lesion. Areas of ringed lipidized siderophages are present.

Aneurysmal and hemosiderotic variants (g, h) are both characterized by numerous multinucleate cells and prominent hemosiderin deposition due to red blood cell extravasation; the distinction between these two is the pseudovascular spaces with blood in aneurysmal type.

Ancillary Tools

IHC [12]:

The most useful stain based on evidence is CD163; factor XIIIa is variable, and CD68 and CD10 are less specific for fibrohistiocytic lineage.

Ki67 and PHH3 can also be used to show an increased proliferation index in dermatofibroma (compared to a low index in dermatofibrosarcoma protuberans).

ALK nuclear and cytoplasmic reactivity in epithelioid fibrous histiocytoma due to ALK rearrangement and overexpression.

12.2.2 Fibrohistiocytic Tumors of Intermediate Malignancy

Dermatofibrosarcoma Protuberans (DFSP) of Toes (a–c)

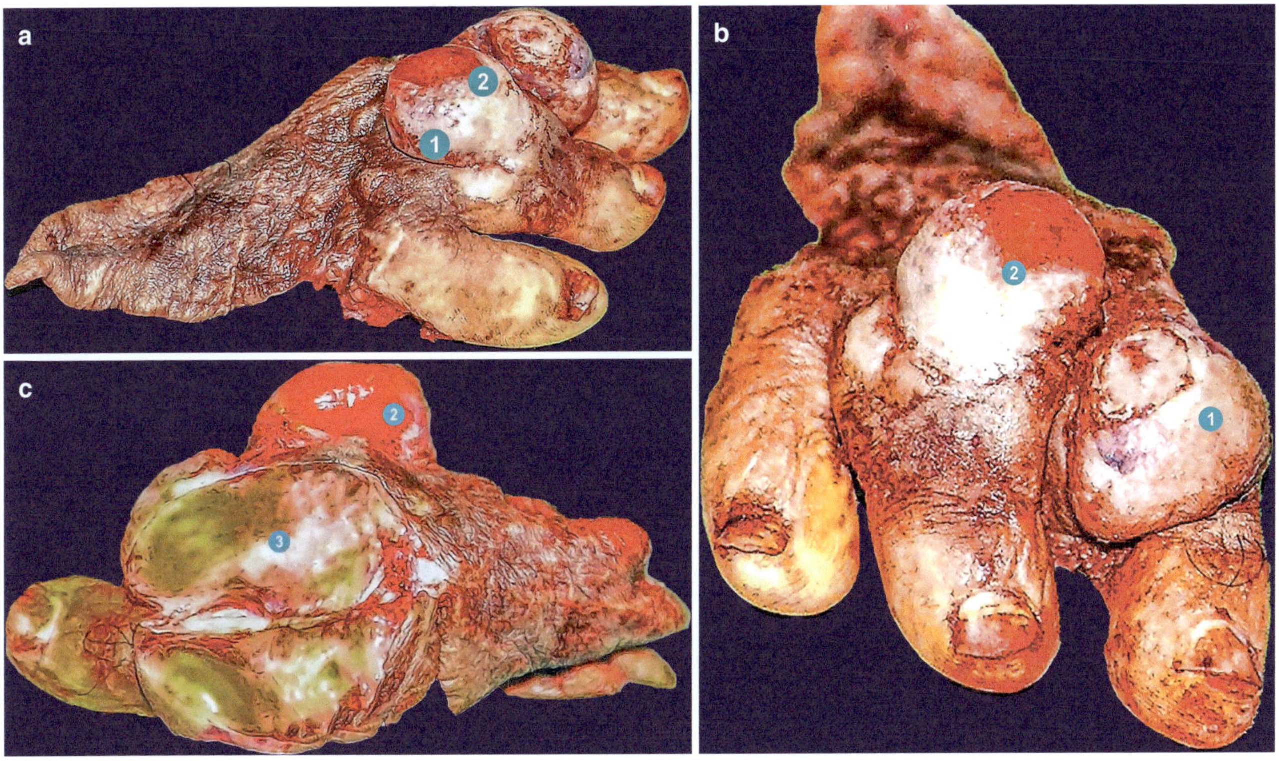

Digital amputation of 3 toes.

1. They show 2 large nodular masses projecting on the skin surface.
2. The overlying skin is white with an area of ulceration.
3. The cut section is gray-white showing a tumor involving the skin and subcutis.

Microscopic Picture of Dermatofibrosarcoma Protuberans (DFSP) (d–i)

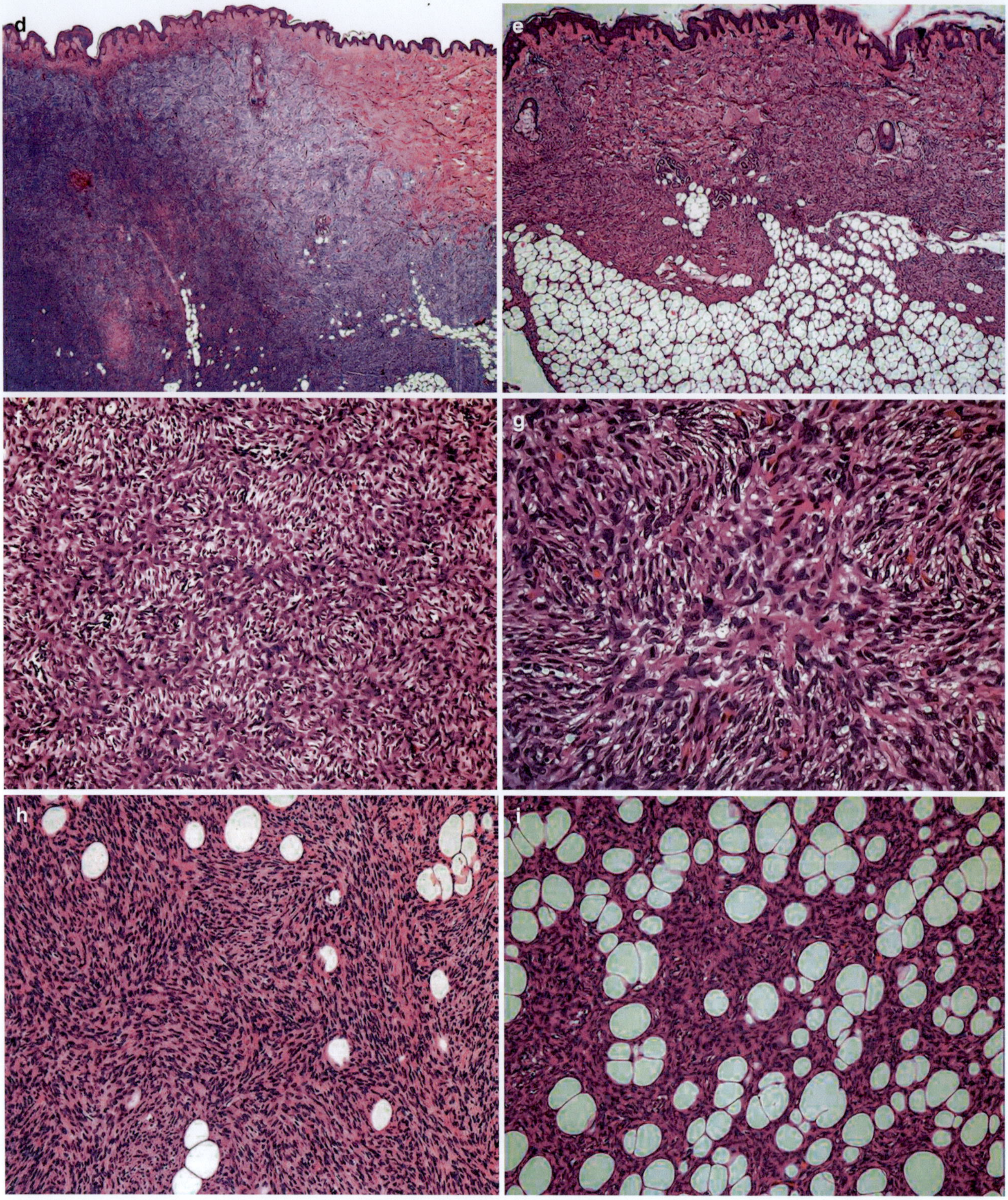

Sections show a dermal tumor sparing the adnexal structures. The tumor is formed of spindle cells with a storiform to whorled pattern. The tumor infiltrates and expands fibrous septa; interdigitation among lobules of fat yields a honeycomb pattern. The cytoplasm of tumor cells is generally abundant and eosinophilic; nuclei are monomorphic and ovoid to elongated with variable mitotic activity. The tumor cells are embedded in a collagenous stroma.

Ancillary Tools

IHC [13, 14]:

CD34: may be diminished/absent with fibrosarcomatous transformation

Vimentin, and p53.

Molecular/cytogenetics description [15, 16]:

Early cytogenetic studies identified a supernumerary ring chromosome in most cases; this led to the identification of t(17;22)(q22;q13)

The most common fusion is COL1A1::PDGFB

Less common fusions include

COL1A2::PDGFB

COL6A3::PDGFD

EMILIN2::PDGFD

TNC::PDGFD

Pearls

Dermatofibrosarcoma protuberans (DFSP) is an uncommon, low-grade dermal soft-tissue neoplasm with high recurrence but low metastatic potential. It mainly occurs on the trunk, proximal extremity, head, and neck, but rarely on the toes, with only a few cases reported. Histologically, DFSP on the toes typically presents uniformly monomorphous spindle cells with little atypia and mitotic activity arranged in storiform fascicles. The cellular nuclei are elongated with even chromatin and low to moderate quantities of cytoplasm. The neoplastic cells often infiltrate the surrounding adipose tissue in a honeycomb pattern. Variants, including fibrosarcomatous and myxoid types, were reported [17].

12.2.3 Primary Cutaneous Lymphoma

Mycosis Fungoides (a, b)

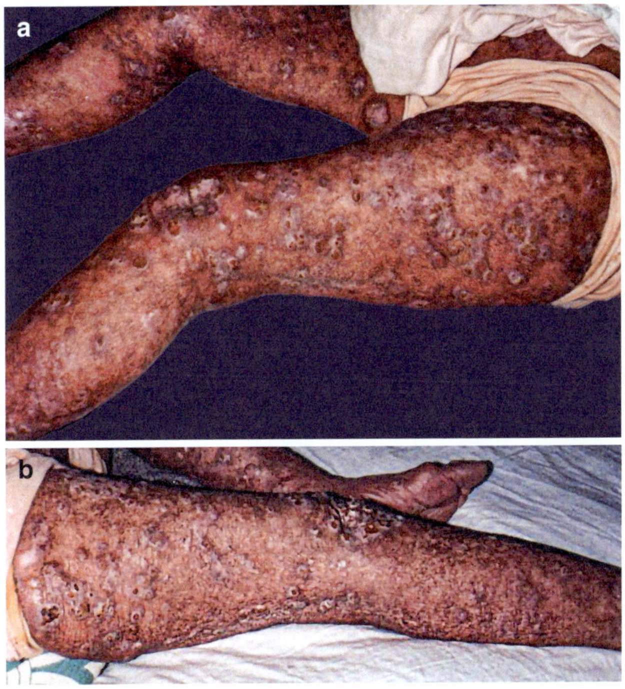

Wide-spread bilateral lower limb and lower abdominal lesions. They are well-demarcated annular or arciform, excoriated, and thickened plaques. Plaques are red, violaceous, or brown, sometimes scaly. Individual plaques can become quite large with central regression. The upper inner side of the right thigh shows a large round nodule with a shiny surface.

Microscopic Picture of Mycosis Fungoides (c–f)

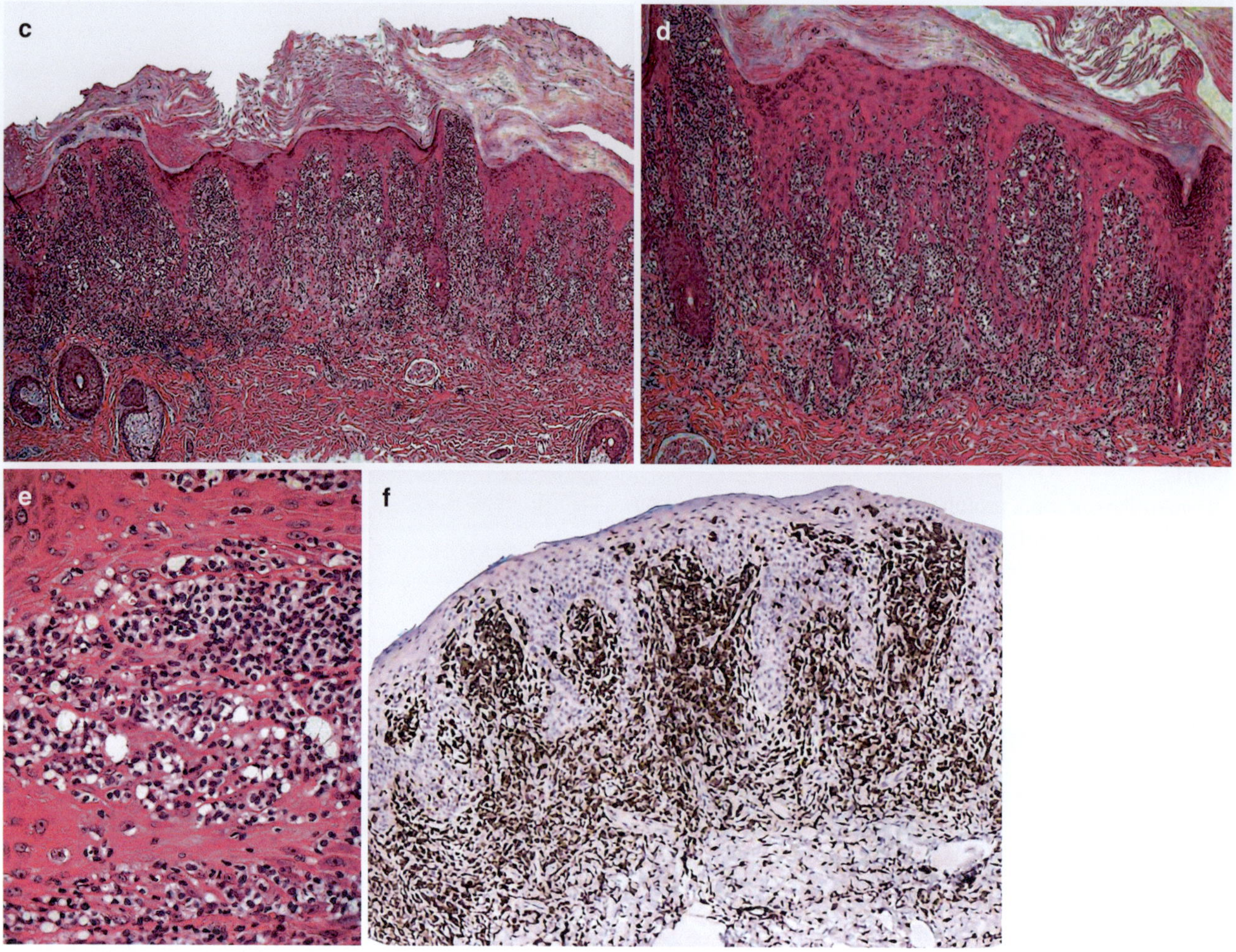

Sections show parakeratosis and irregular acanthosis of epidermis with focal areas of epidermal thinning. The dermis is infiltrated by dense cellular infiltrate, tagging the lower epidermis with areas of epidermal infiltration to form Pautrier's microabscesses. The infiltrate is formed mainly of lymphoid T-cells with hyperchromatic nuclei and perinuclear halos stained positively for CD4 (f).

12.2.4 Benign Lipomatous Tumors

Lipoma (a, b)

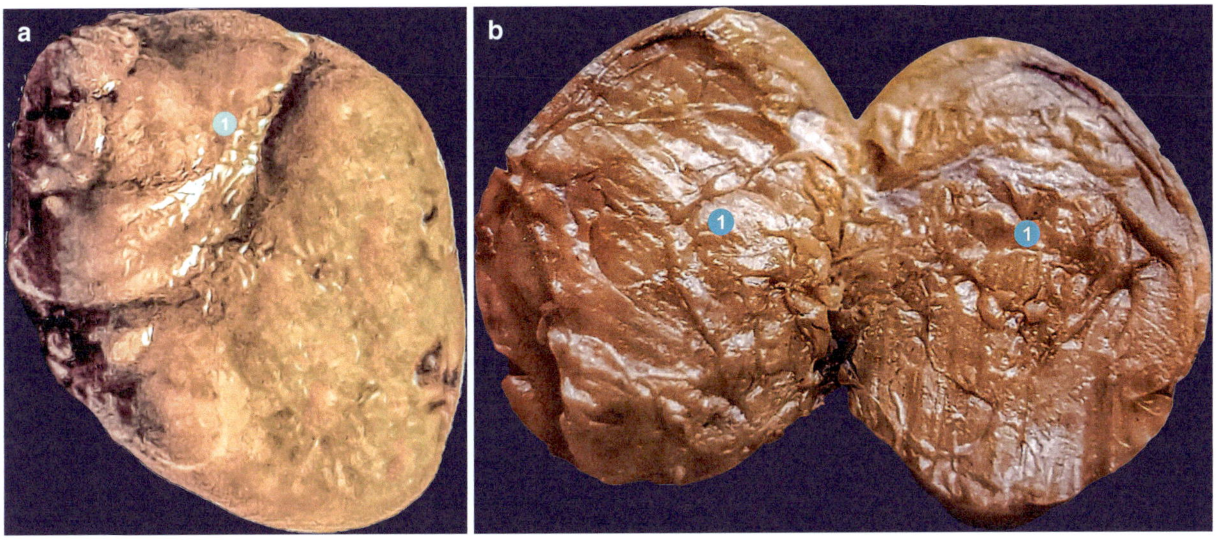

1. A well-defined, encapsulated mass with a smooth lobulated yellow surface and cut section.

Microscopic Picture of Lipoma (c)

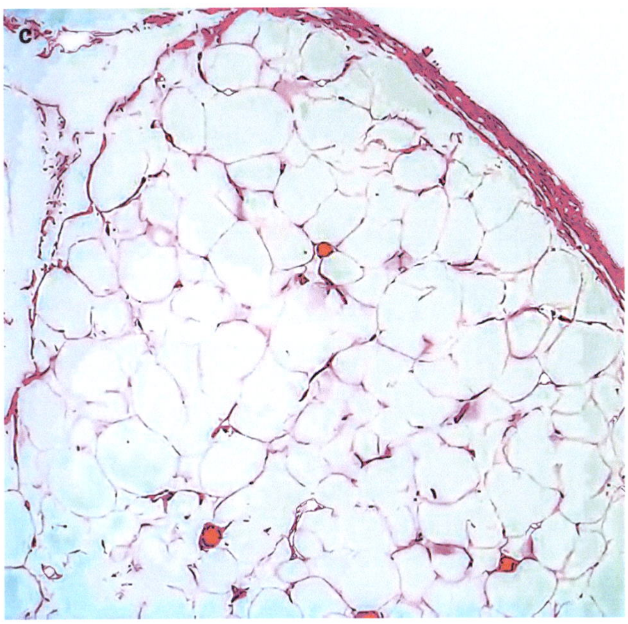

The section shows an encapsulated and lobulated tumor. The lobules are separated by thin fibrovascular septa. The tumor cells are mature adipocytes with small and bland nuclei often compressed at the periphery of the cells, giving a signet-ring appearance.

Lipoma with Fat Necrosis

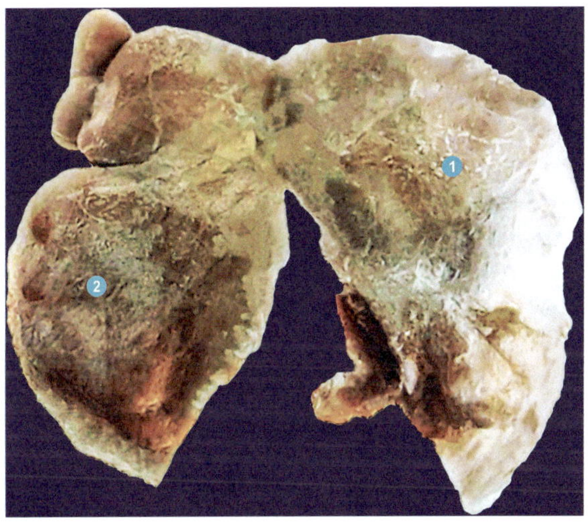

1. A large piece of fatty tissue covered with a thin capsule.
2. In the center of the mass, a gray-white area is seen representing fat necrosis.

Ancillary Tools

IHC [18]:

Rb (G3–245) preserved positivity (lost in spindle cell pleomorphic lipoma).

HMGA2 (negative in normal fat).

Molecular/cytogenetics description [19]:

Structural rearrangement of chromosome bands 12q13-q15 or HMGA2 gene

Structural rearrangement of chromosome bands 6p21 or HMGA1 gene

12.2.5 Liposarcoma

Retroperitoneal Liposarcoma (a, b)

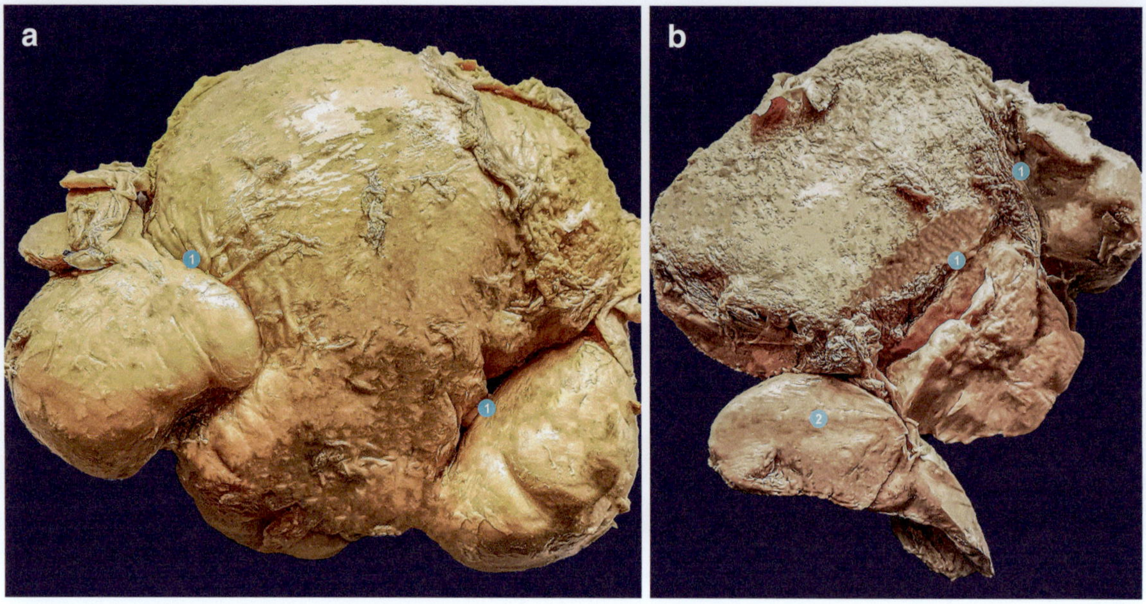

A part of a large tumor mass resected from the retroperitoneum is mounted.

1. The tumor is yellow, well-defined, and multinodular.
2. A yellow-cut section is devoid of necrosis or hemorrhage with the presence of yellow-tan areas.

Microscopic Picture of Myxoid Liposarcoma (c–h)

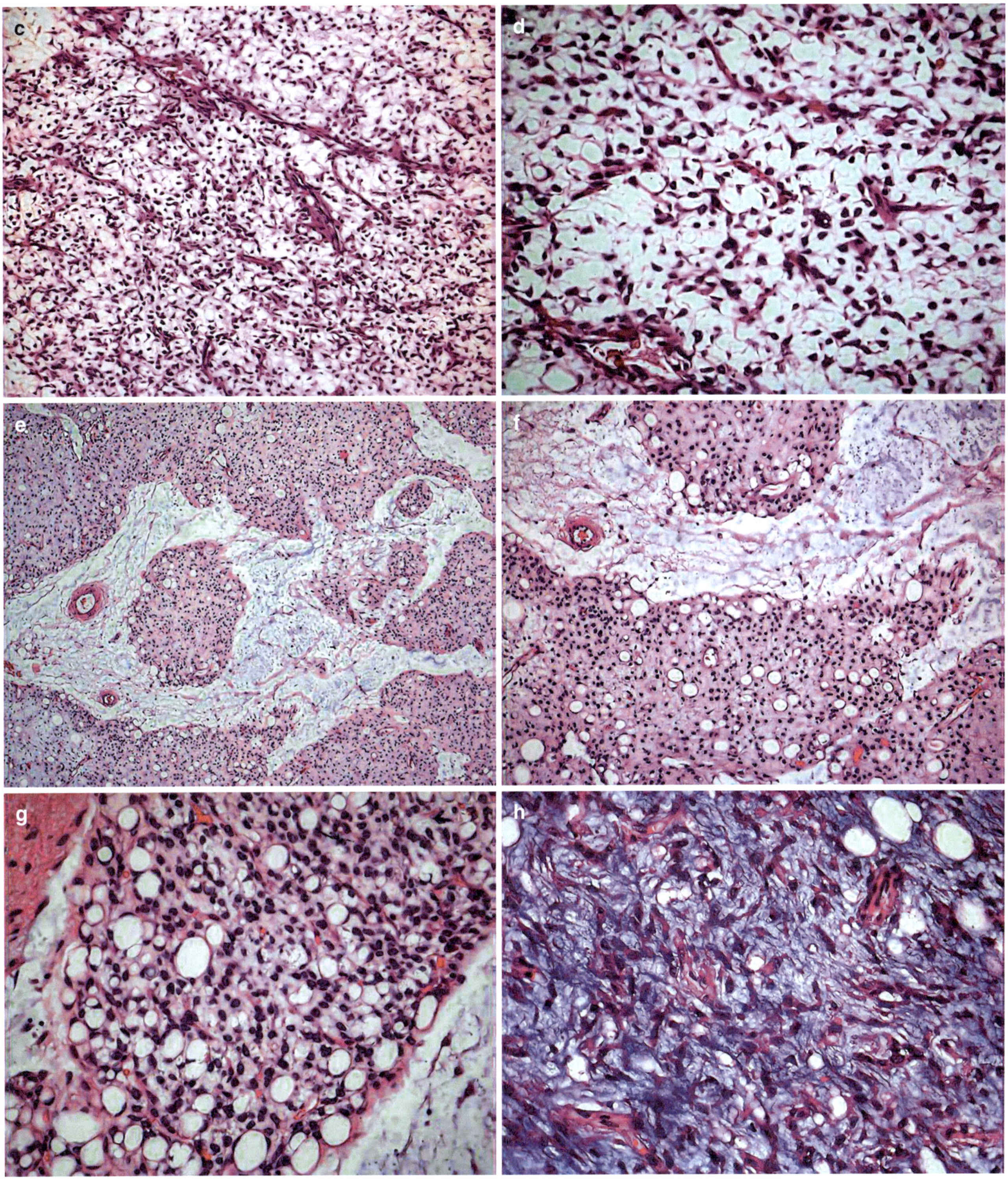

Sections show numerous signet ring lipoblasts, particularly at the periphery of lobules with the presence of prominent plexiform vasculature (delicate thin-walled arborizing and curving capillaries that form a network reminiscent of chicken wire fencing). These are still present in high-grade tumors but are much less obvious. A mucoid matrix rich in hyaluronic acid forming large mucoid pools is also observed.

Ancillary Tools

IHC [20]:

CD34, p16, p53

Molecular/cytogenetics description [20]:

Sarcoma with complex genomics characterized by structural chromosomal aberrations and monoallelic RB1 deletion.

Array comparative genomic hybridization (aCGH): frequently shows a distinctive genomic profile with whole chromosome gains (usually chromosomes 1, 6–8, 19–21, and X) and losses (2–5, 10–17, and 22).

Methylation profiling: myxoid pleomorphic liposarcoma and classic pleomorphic liposarcoma have overlapping profiles (suggesting that they are closely related).

Liposarcoma of Subcutaneous Tissue (a, b)

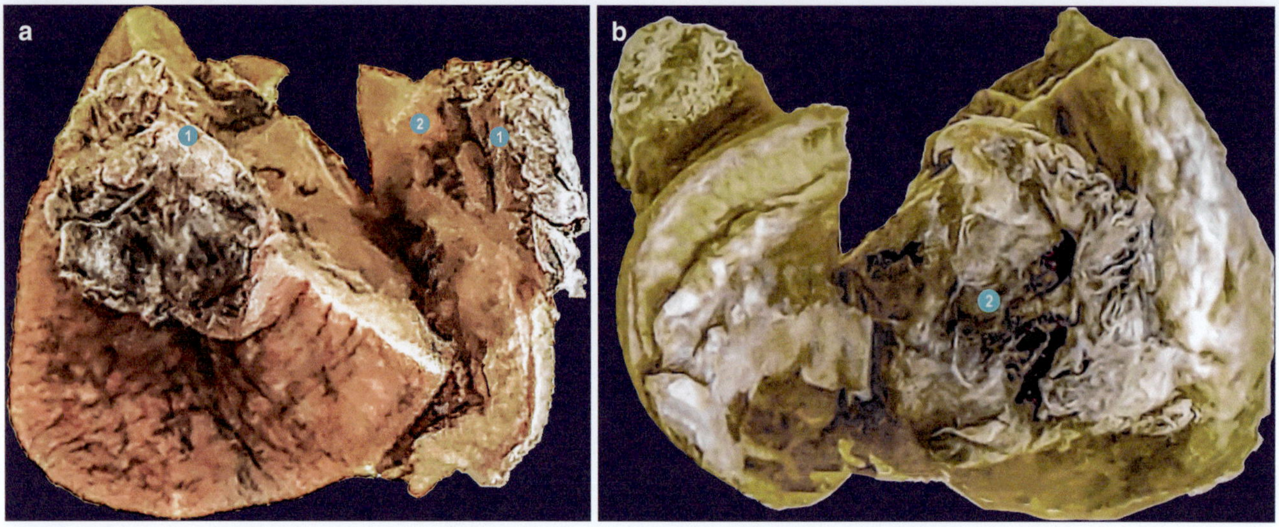

A piece of skin with a protruding mass is mounted.

The cut section shows:

1. An uncapsulated gray-white mass arising in the subcutaneous tissue and fungating through the skin.
2. Extensive areas of hemorrhage and necrosis.

12.2.6 Malignant Vascular Tumors

Primary Cutaneous Angiosarcoma

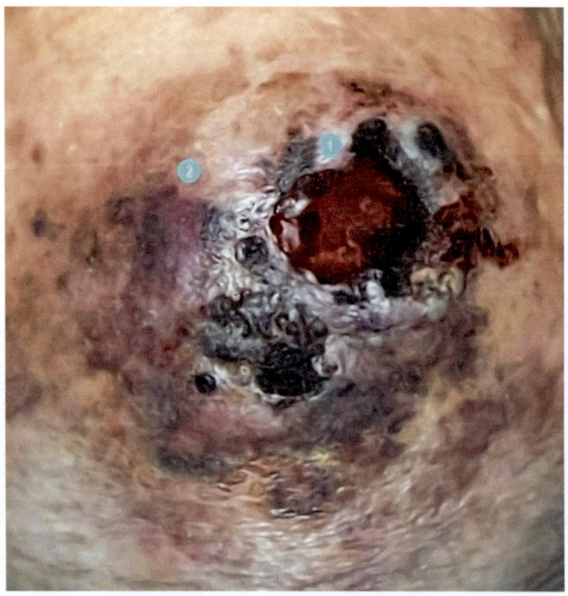

A piece of skin is mounted.

1. A large, ulcerated, infiltrative, and hemorrhagic nodule
2. Bruise-like discoloration of the skin around the nodule.

Microscopic Picture of Cutaneous Angiosarcoma (a–g)

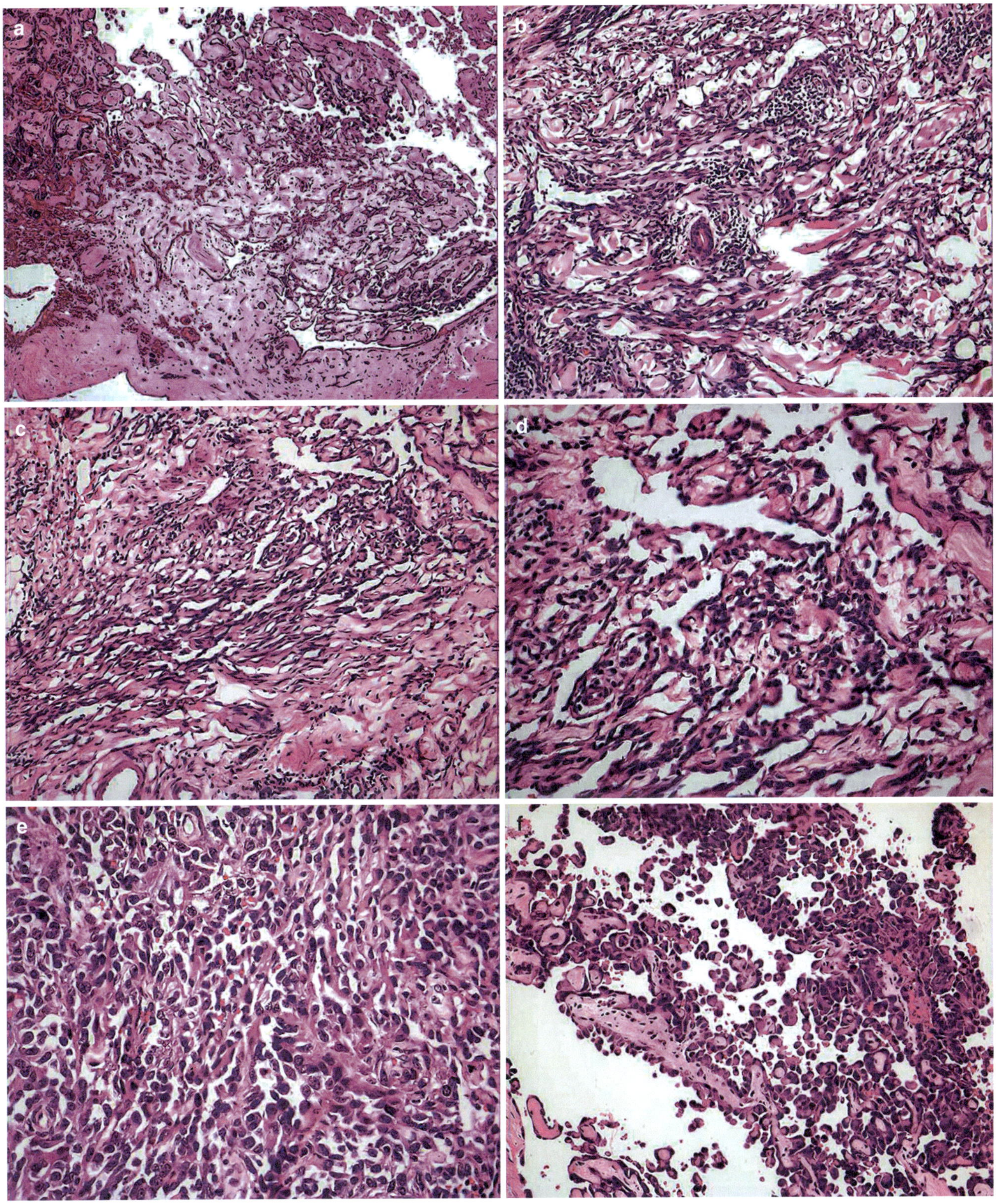

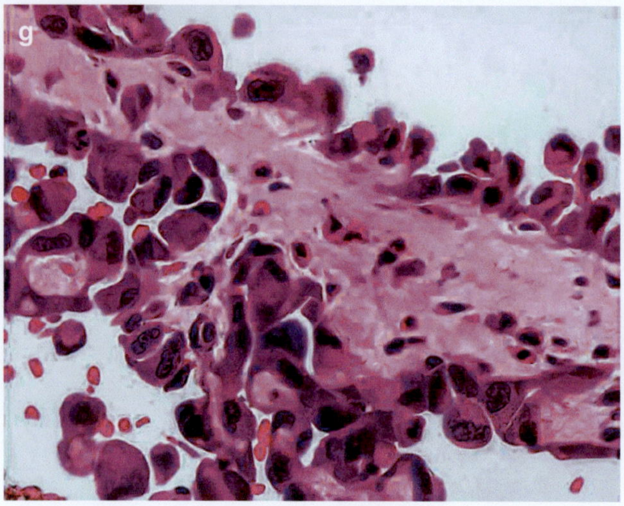

Sections show numerous irregularly shaped anastomosing vascular channels ramifying and dissecting through the dermis and intercalating through dermal collagen and subcutaneous soft tissues. The vascular channels are lined by atypical plump, pleomorphic, and mitotically active endothelial cells. They are polygonal, epithelioid, and primitive round cells, forming papillae or solid nests within vascular lumina. A solid growth pattern is seen in areas with other areas of intratumoral hemorrhage and lymphoid infiltration.

Ancillary Tools

IHC [21]:

Angiosarcoma expresses endothelial cell markers, including CD31, CD34, ERG, FLI1, VEGF, and factor VIII.

Cytokeratin, EMA, and CD30 may be expressed in a subset of epithelioid angiosarcoma.

Lymphatic marker Podoplanin, as determined by D2–40 immunostain, is variably expressed and suggests focal lymphatic differentiation in the tumor.

Molecular/cytogenetics description [22]

Angiosarcoma is characterized by upregulation of vascular-specific receptor tyrosine kinases, such as TIE1, KDR, TEK, and FLT.

Has overexpression of HIF1 alpha and HIF2 beta, which are upstream regulators of VEGF.

A high level of c-MYC gene amplification by FISH is seen in radiation-induced and chronic lymphedema-associated angiosarcoma.

Some tumors harbor recurrent PTPRB and PLCG1 mutations, which are involved in angiogenesis.

12.2.7 Malignant Tumors of Striated Muscles

Rhabdomyosarcoma (a, b)

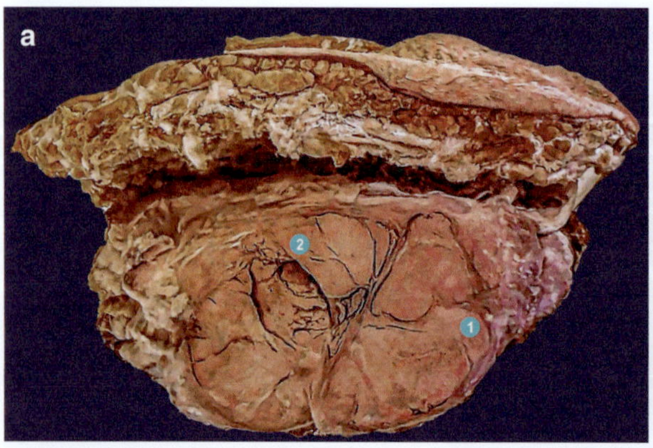

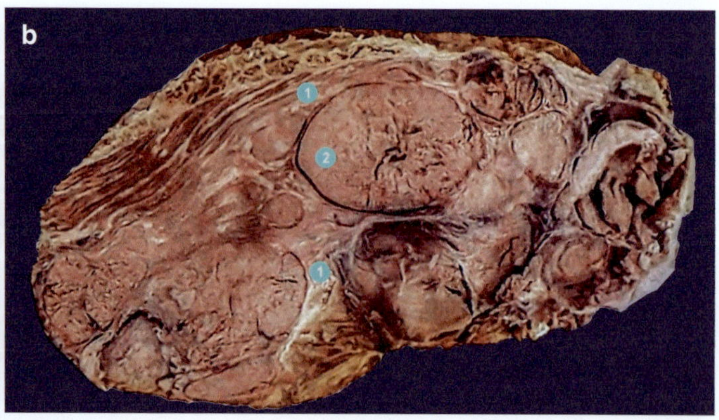

The gluteal muscles are mounted.

1. The muscles are infiltrated by a round tumor mass with a fleshy red-cut section.
2. The tumor is divided into several sections by bands of fibrous tissue septa with the presence of a focal area of hemorrhage.

Microscopic Picture of Alveolar Rhabdomyosarcoma (c–g)

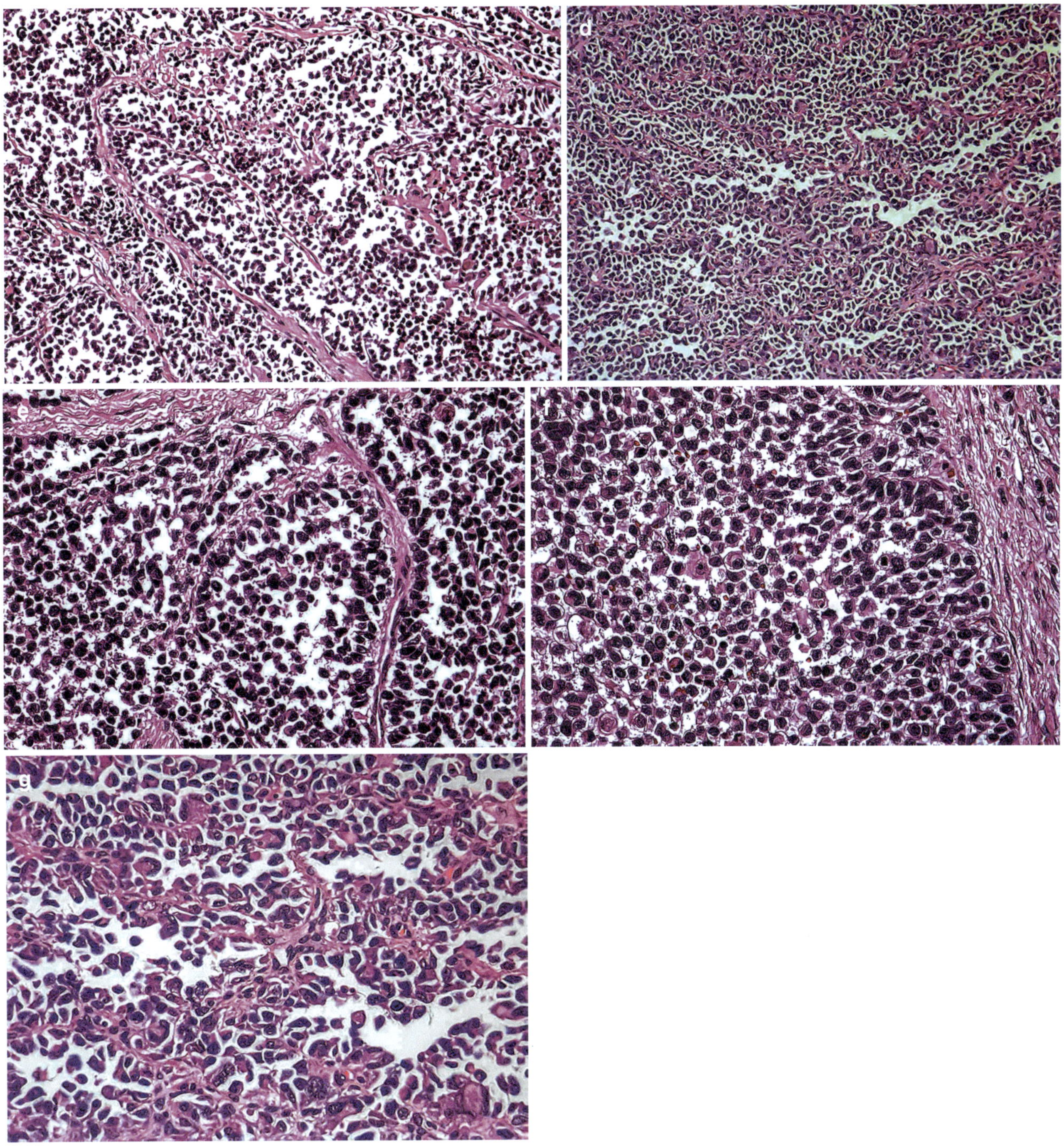

Sections show large clusters and trabeculae of primitive round cells with loss of cellular cohesion in the center, forming an alveolar-like, cystic, and vague papillary appearance, separated by variably thick fibrovascular septa. A layer of cells adheres to the periphery of the spaces and fibrous septa. The tumor cells are round, small to intermediate-sized, and monomorphic with scant cytoplasm and hyperchromatic nuclei with variable conspicuous small nucleoli and brisk mitoses. Round to oval rhabdomyoblasts with abundant acidophilic cytoplasm are present.

Ancillary Tools

IHC [23]:

Stains for myogenic differentiation:

Desmin

Myogenin (strong and diffuse)

MyoD1 (variable)

Muscle-specific actin (variable)

PAX3::FOXO1/PAX7::FOXO1 fusion-specific antibodies

Stains with variable expression:

PAX5

MUC4

ALK1 (cytoplasmic)

PAX7

AP2β

Cytokeratin

Synaptophysin

CD56

Chromogranin

CD99

P-cadherin

p80

Molecular/cytogenetics description [24, 25]

- PAX3::FOXO1/PAX7::FOXO1 fusion (85% of cases):
  t(2;13)(q36;q14): PAX3::FOXO1 in 70–90%
  Amplification of MYCN and CDK4 in PAX3::FOXO1 positive cases
  t(1;13)(p36;q14): PAX7::FOXO1 in 10–30%
  Amplification of PAX7 and MIR17HG in PAX7::FOXO1 positive cases
- Other fusions:
  PAX3::FOXO4 fusion
  PAX3::NCOA1 fusion
  PAX3::INO80D fusion
  FOXO1::FGFR1 fusion
  Inactivating mutation of TP53 and CDKN2
  Activating mutation of FGFR4
  Overexpression of ALK protein

References

1. Fabrício da Silva D. et al. (2023). Mutilating localized cutaneous leishmaniasis caused by Leishmania guyanensis. Letter—tropical/infectious and parasitic dermatology. Anais Brasileiros de Dermatologia (ABD).98(3).419-421. doi: https://doi.org/10.1016/j.abd.2022.04.014.
2. Akbari A. et al. (2020). Differentiated exophytic vulvar intraepithelial lesion: Clinicopathologic and molecular analysis documenting its relationship with verrucous carcinoma of the vulva. Mod Pathol. 33(10):2011-2018. doi: https://doi.org/10.1038/s41379-020-0573-5. PMID: 32427961.
3. Kim J.H. et al. (2022). Verrucous Carcinoma of the Toenail: A Case Report and Review of Literature. J Wound Manag Res.18(3):229-233. https://doi.org/10.22467/jwmr.2022.02194.
4. Yan S. Squamous cell carcinoma. PathologyOutlines.com website. https://www.pathologyoutlines.com/topic/skintumornonmelanocyticscc.html.
5. Kalmykova A, McKee PH. Basal cell carcinoma. Pathology Outlines.com website. https://www.pathologyoutlines.com/topic/skintumornonmelanocyticbcc.html.
6. Crabtree M. et al.(2021). Primary cutaneous apocrine carcinoma in a 50-year-old male. Human Pathology Reports. 26: 1-5. Doi: https://doi.org/10.1016/j.hpr.2021.300560.
7. Choi H.J. et al.(2022). Primary cutaneous apocrine carcinoma of the scalp. Two case reports and literature review. Medicine (Baltimore) 101(6): e28808. doi: https://doi.org/10.1097/MD.0000000000028808. PMCID: PMC8830877.
8. Gassenmaier M. et al.(2021). Histological and Immunohistochemical Changes of Congenital Melanocytic Nevi With Age. Am J Dermatopathol. 43(10):707-713. doi: https://doi.org/10.1097/DAD.0000000000001894. PMID: 33464753.
9. Roh MR. et al.(2015). Genetics of melanocytic nevi. Pigment Cell Melanoma Res. 28(6):661-72. doi: https://doi.org/10.1111/pcmr.12412. PMID: 26300491; PMCID: PMC4609613.
10. Pop AM. et al. (2023). The Importance of Immunohistochemistry in the Evaluation of Tumor Depth of Primary Cutaneous Melanoma. Diagnostics (Basel). 13(6):1020. doi: https://doi.org/10.3390/diagnostics13061020. PMID: 36980327; PMCID: PMC10046945.
11. Tímár J, Ladányi A. (2022). Molecular Pathology of Skin Melanoma: Epidemiology, Differential Diagnostics, Prognosis and Therapy Prediction. Int J Mol Sci. 23(10):5384. doi: https://doi.org/10.3390/ijms23105384. PMID: 35628196; PMCID: PMC9140388.
12. Hsi ED, Nickoloff BJ. (1996). Dermatofibroma and dermatofibrosarcoma protuberans: an immunohistochemical study reveals distinctive antigenic profiles. J Dermatol Sci. 11(1):1-9. doi: https://doi.org/10.1016/0923-1811(95)00409-2. PMID: 8867761.
13. Haycox CL.et al.(1997). Immunohistochemical characterization of dermatofibrosarcoma protuberans with practical applications for diagnosis and treatment. J Am Acad Dermatol. 37(3 Pt 1):438-44. doi: https://doi.org/10.1016/s0190-9622(97)70146-4. PMID: 9308560.
14. Abbott JJ, Oliveira AM, Nascimento AG. (2006). The prognostic significance of fibrosarcomatous transformation in dermatofibrosarcoma protuberans. Am J Surg Pathol. 30(4):436-43. doi: https://doi.org/10.1097/00000478-200604000-00002. PMID: 16625088.
15. Simon MP. et al. (1997). Deregulation of the platelet-derived growth factor B-chain gene via fusion with collagen gene COL1A1 in dermatofibrosarcoma protuberans and giant-cell fibroblastoma. Nat Genet. 15(1):95-8. doi: https://doi.org/10.1038/ng0197-95. PMID: 8988177.
16. Dadone-Montaudié B. et al.(2018). Alternative PDGFD rearrangements in dermatofibrosarcomas protuberans without PDGFB fusions. Mod Pathol. 31(11):1683-1693. doi: https://doi.org/10.1038/s41379-018-0089-4. PMID: 29955147.
17. Madden C. et al.(2019). Dermatofibrosarcoma Protuberans on Adult Toes: A Case Report and Review of the Literature. Anticancer Research. 39(4): 2105-2111. doi:https://doi.org/10.21873/anticanres.13323. PMID: 30952756.
18. Chen BJ. et al.(2012). Loss of retinoblastoma protein expression in spindle cell/pleomorphic lipomas and cytogenetically related tumors: an immunohistochemical study with diagnostic implications. Am J Surg Pathol. 36(8):1119-28. doi: https://doi.org/10.1097/PAS.0b013e31825d532d. PMID: 22790852.

19. Sirvent N. et al.(2007). Detection of MDM2-CDK4 amplification by fluorescence in situ hybridization in 200 paraffin-embedded tumor samples: utility in diagnosing adipocytic lesions and comparison with immunohistochemistry and real-time PCR. Am J Surg Pathol. 31(10):1476-89. doi: https://doi.org/10.1097/PAS.0b013e3180581fff. PMID: 17895748.
20. Creytens D. et al.(2021). Myxoid pleomorphic liposarcoma clinicopathologic, immunohistochemical, molecular genetic, and epigenetic study of 12 cases, suggesting a possible relationship with conventional pleomorphic liposarcoma. Mod Pathol. 34(11):2043-2049. doi: https://doi.org/10.1038/s41379-021-00862-2. PMID: 34168281.
21. Shustef E. et al.(2017). Cutaneous angiosarcoma: a current update. J Clin Pathol. 70(11):917-925. doi: https://doi.org/10.1136/jclinpath-2017-204601. PMID: 28916596.
22. Omiyale AO, Carton J. (2018). Clinical and Pathologic Features of Primary Angiosarcoma of the Kidney. Curr Urol Rep. 19(2):4. doi: https://doi.org/10.1007/s11934-018-0755-6. PMID: 29383452.
23. Machado I. et al. (2015). The Role of Immunohistochemistry in Rhabdomyosarcoma Diagnosis Using Tissue Microarray Technology and a Xenograft Model. Fetal Pediatr Pathol. 34(5):271-81. doi: https://doi.org/10.3109/15513815.2015.1042604. PMID: 26125949.
24. Mercado GE, Barr FG. (2007). Fusions involving PAX and FOX genes in the molecular pathogenesis of alveolar rhabdomyosarcoma: recent advances. Curr Mol Med. 7(1):47-61. doi: https://doi.org/10.2174/156652407779940440. PMID: 17311532.
25. Corao DA. et al.(2009). ALK expression in rhabdomyosarcomas: correlation with histologic subtype and fusion status. Pediatr Dev Pathol. 12(4):275-83. doi: https://doi.org/10.2350/08-03-0434.1. PMID: 18788887.

13 Diseases of the Central Nervous System

The central nervous system (CNS), comprised of the brain and spinal cord, is the primary control center for all bodily functions. It plays a critical role in how we move, think, and even feel. Given its central importance to life, understanding the pathological alterations or diseases that can affect it is crucial for medical professionals.

In this chapter, we delve into the pathologic study of some diseases as they affect the structure and function of the CNS, as revealed by macroscopic and microscopic examination.

This chapter's focus on the gross and microscopic pathology of the CNS offers an essential resource for students, researchers, and practitioners within the fields of medicine, particularly those in pathology, neurology, and neurosurgery.

The conditions in this chapter will be organized in the following order:

1. **Sellar Region Tumors**
   (a) Adamantinomatous Craniopharyngioma
   (b) Pituitary Neuroendocrine Tumor
2. **Cerebral Infection**
   (a) Hydatid Cyst
3. **Intracranial Hemorrhages**
   (a) Cerebral hemorrhage
   (b) Pontine hemorrhage
4. **Brain Tumors**
5. **Gliomas**
   (a) Astrocytoma
   (b) Pilocytic Astrocytoma
   (c) Glioblastoma
6. **Embryonal Tumors**
   (a) Medulloblastoma
7. **Vascular Malformation**
   (a) Arteriovenous Malformation

13.1 Sellar Region Tumors

Adamantinomatous Craniopharyngioma

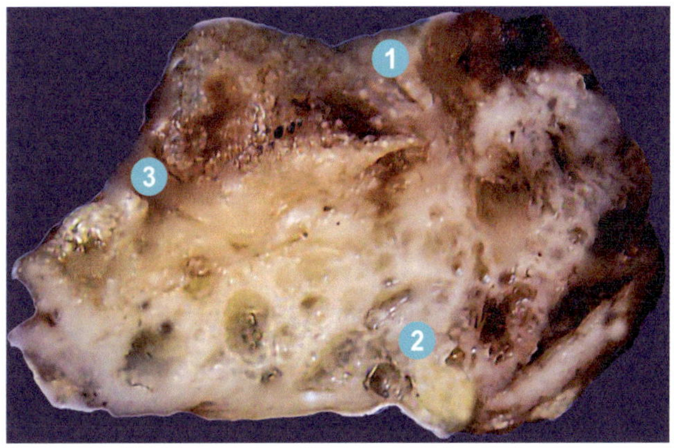

An irregular mass is mounted.

1. A lobular mass with solid and cystic areas with calcifications
2. Cysts with dark "motor oil" fluid composed of cholesterol and hemorrhage
3. The yellowish-white spots represent the nodules of so-called wet keratin, composed of clusters of anucleated squames.

G. Dawood, *Color Atlas of Human Gross and Microscopic Pathology*, https://doi.org/10.1007/978-3-031-76007-5_13

Microscopic Picture of Adamantinomatous Craniopharyngioma (a, b)

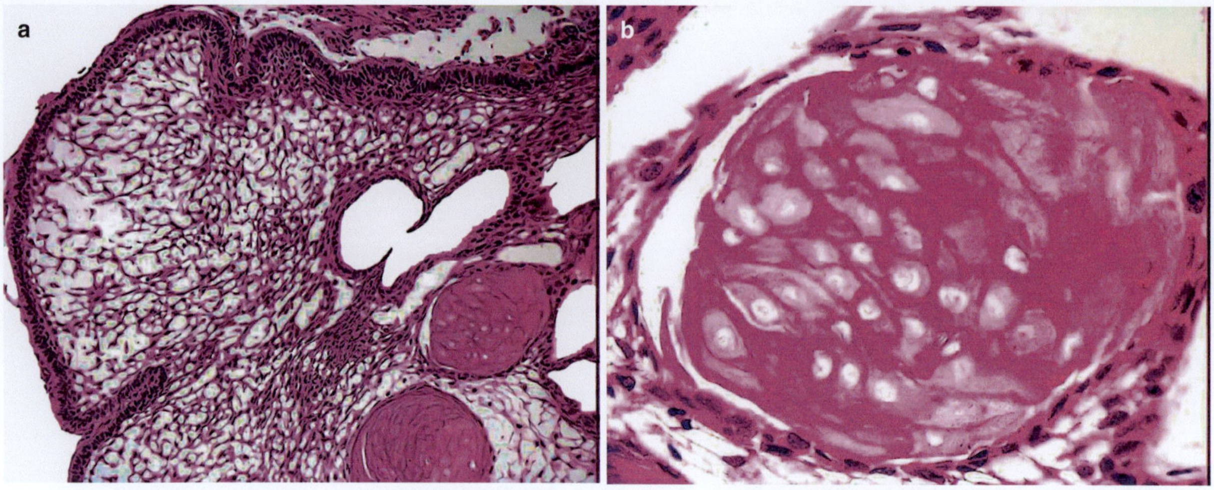

Sections show lobules of well differentiated squamous epithelium bordered by palisading columnar epithelium. Peripheral cells surround looser plumper cells called stellate reticulum.

Nodules of plump, anucleate squamous cells (ghost cells) and wet keratin are observed.

Ancillary Tools

IHC [1]:

CK7, CK8, CK19, pancytokeratin, CK5/6, EMA, and CK14

Beta-catenin: in whorls, both intranuclear (translocated) and cytoplasmic

Ki67 (low, usually concentrated along the peripheral palisading cells)

Pituitary Neuroendocrine Tumor

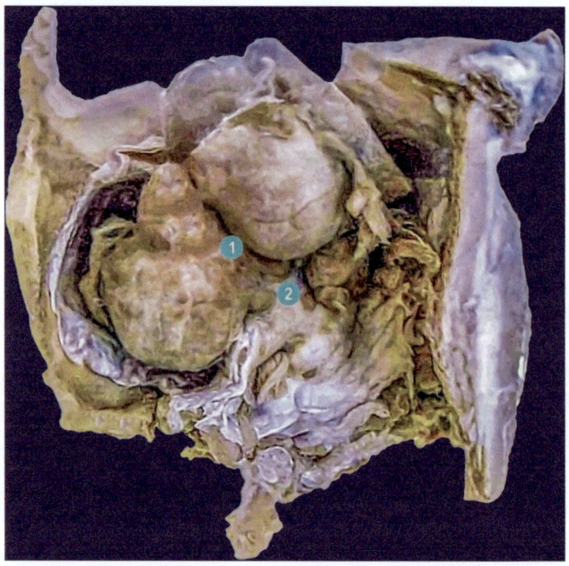

The specimen represents the anterior part of the base of the skull.

1. A large, nodular tumor projects in the region of the pituitary gland. The tumor is well-defined, encapsulated, multinodular, and gray-white.
2. The tumor destroyed the sella turcica to project upwards to destroy the optic chiasma.

The patient was blind and had manifestations of hypopituitarism: obesity, genital hypoplasia, mental retardation, hypoglycemia, low basal metabolic rate, and diabetes insipidus. He died in a coma.

Microscopic Picture of Pituitary Neuroendocrine Tumor (a, b)

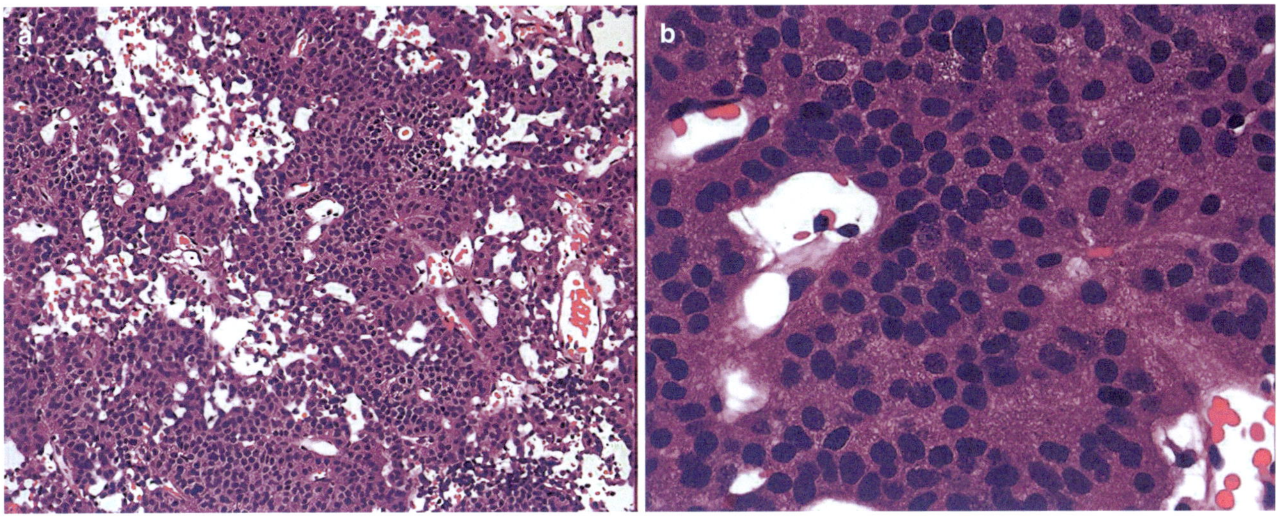

Sections show increased cellularity compared to normal pituitary tissue. The cells are arranged in sheets and clusters with focal formation of pseudorosettes around vascular channels. Tumor cells are epithelioid and show uniform nuclear morphology with stippled chromatin, inconspicuous nucleoli, and moderately abundant cytoplasm with focal mild atypia.

Ancillary Tools

IHC [2]:

All PitNETs must be classified based on lineage, cell type, and hormone production, as well as other ancillary features that allow the characterization of subtypes. In the ideal setting, all PitNETs should be stained for at least [1]:

1. The three main transcription factors, PIT1, TPIT, and SF1. Ideally, this panel should also include ERα and GATA3.
2. Staining for hormones should include ACTH, GH, PRL, βTSH, βFSH, and βLH, as well as the α-subunit of glycoprotein hormones (αSU).
3. Keratins: the most widely used antibody is the CAM5.2 clone, but others, including AE1/AE3 and CK18, are also satisfactory.
4. Ki67 is part of the assessment, but unlike other NETs, these tumors are not graded based on proliferation indices.

Molecular and Cytogenetics Description [3]:

- No specific molecular characteristics in routine clinical diagnostic workup.
- Most pituitary tumors are sporadic; the minority are part of hereditary or familial syndromes
- Somatic mutations in GNAS and USP8 genes have been found in ~40% of sporadic somatotroph tumors and 30–60% of sporadic corticotroph tumors, respectively

13.2 Cerebral Infection

Hydatid Cyst of Brain

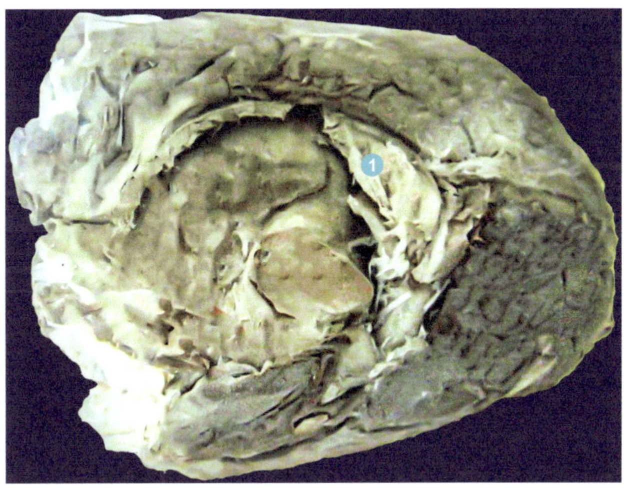

The right cerebral hemisphere is mounted.

1. It shows a solitary, spherical, and unilocular cyst with a pale yellow smooth lining.

13.3 Intracranial Hemorrhages

Cerebral Hemorrhage with Chronic "Cystic" Infarct

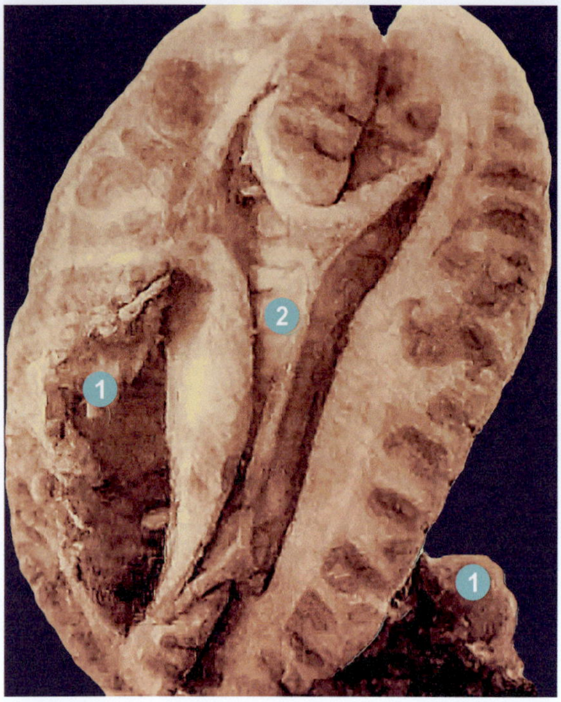

A transverse section of the cerebral hemisphere is mounted.

1. It shows a large cavity in white matter filled with clotted blood; a piece of which has fallen out of the cavity.
2. There is a shift in midline structures.

Microscopic Picture of Chronic Cystic Infarct (a)

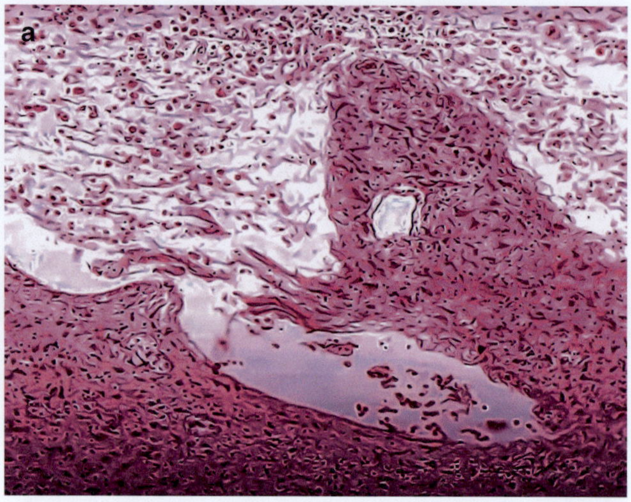

The section shows a cavitated lesion with vessels and macrophages surrounded by a glial scar while reactive astrocytes are seen at the edge of the cavitation.

Cerebral Hemorrhage with Chronic "Cystic" Infarct

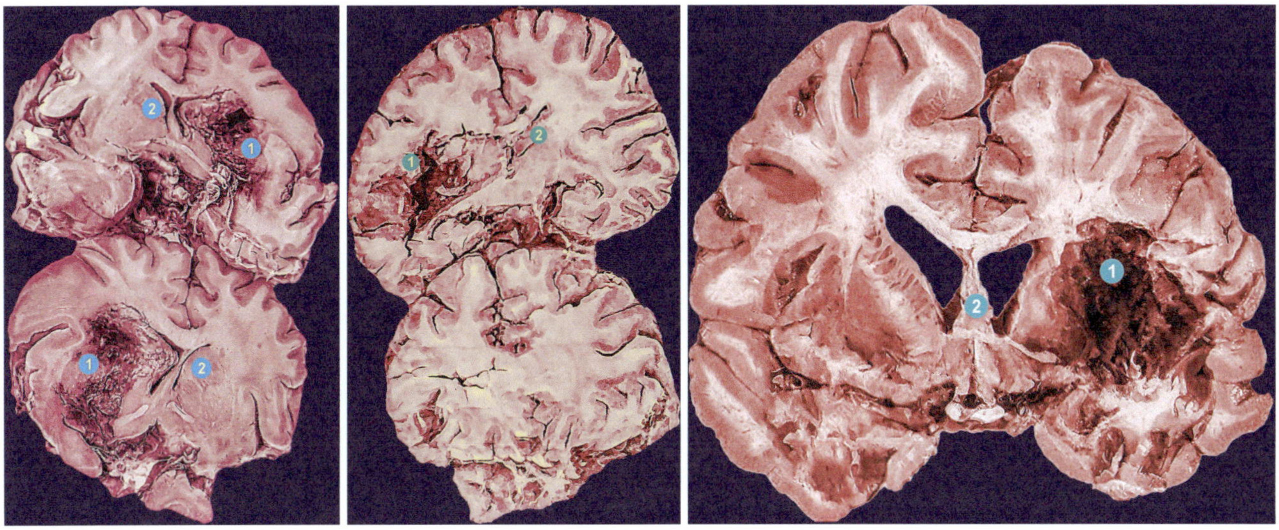

A coronal section of the cerebral hemisphere is mounted.

1. A large cavity in white matter filled with clotted blood and a thin cortical remnant overlying the cavitation.
2. There is a shift in midline structures.

Pontine Hemorrhage

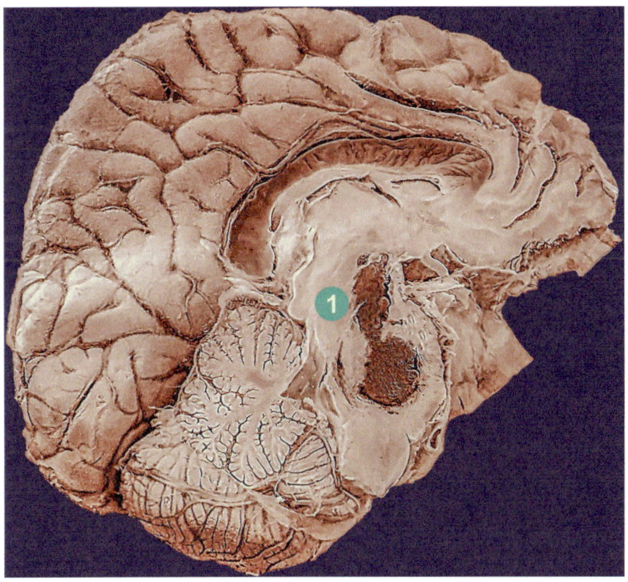

A sagittal section of the brain is mounted.

1. It shows a large, dark area of hemorrhage in the pons.

13.4 Brain Tumors

Astrocytoma Grade 3

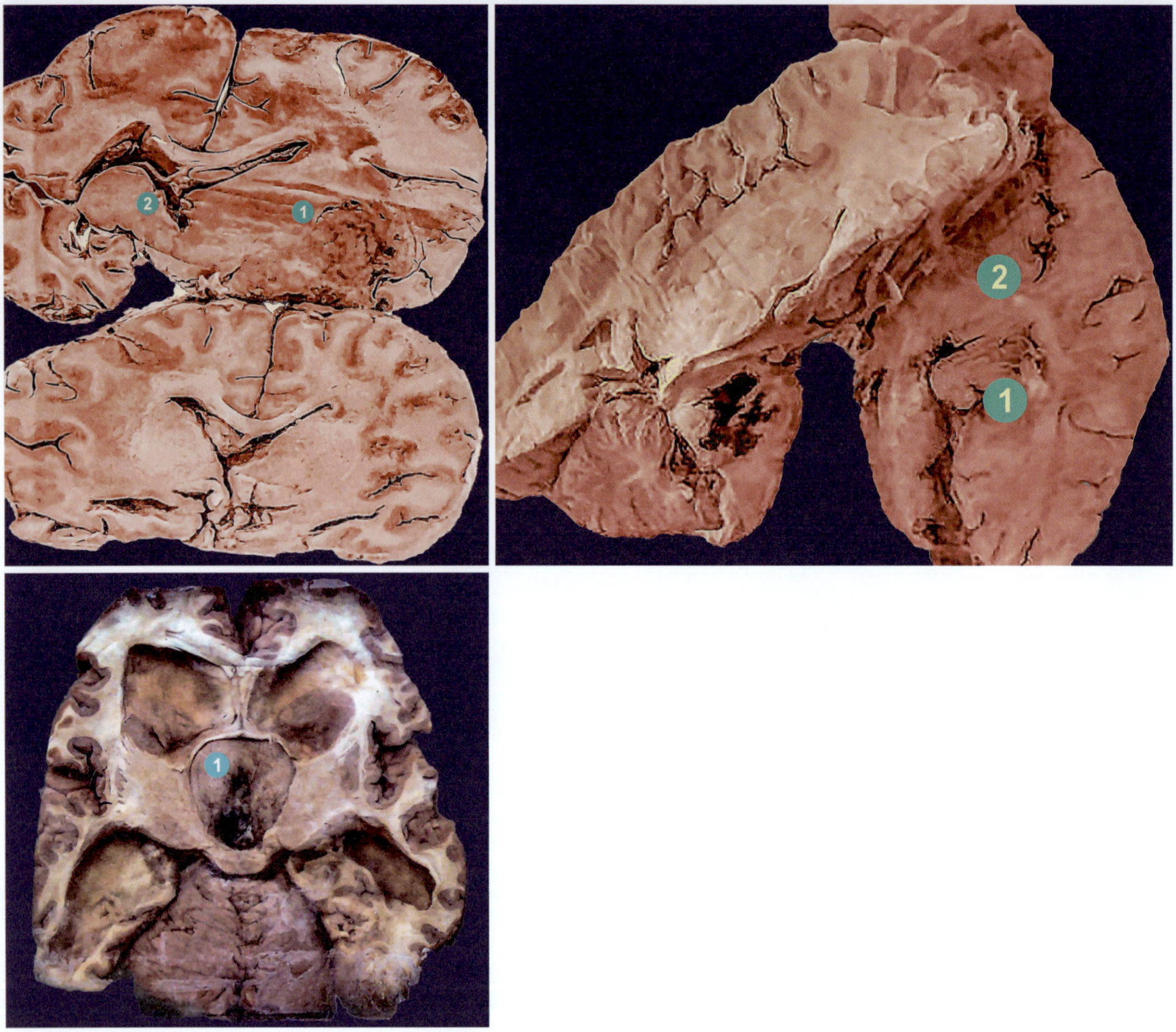

The left cerebral hemisphere is cut in a horizontal plane and mounted.

1. A pink, ill-defined tumor mass in the occipital lobe showing areas of hemorrhage.
2. Shifting of midline structures.

Microscopic Picture of Grade 2 Astrocytoma (a, b)

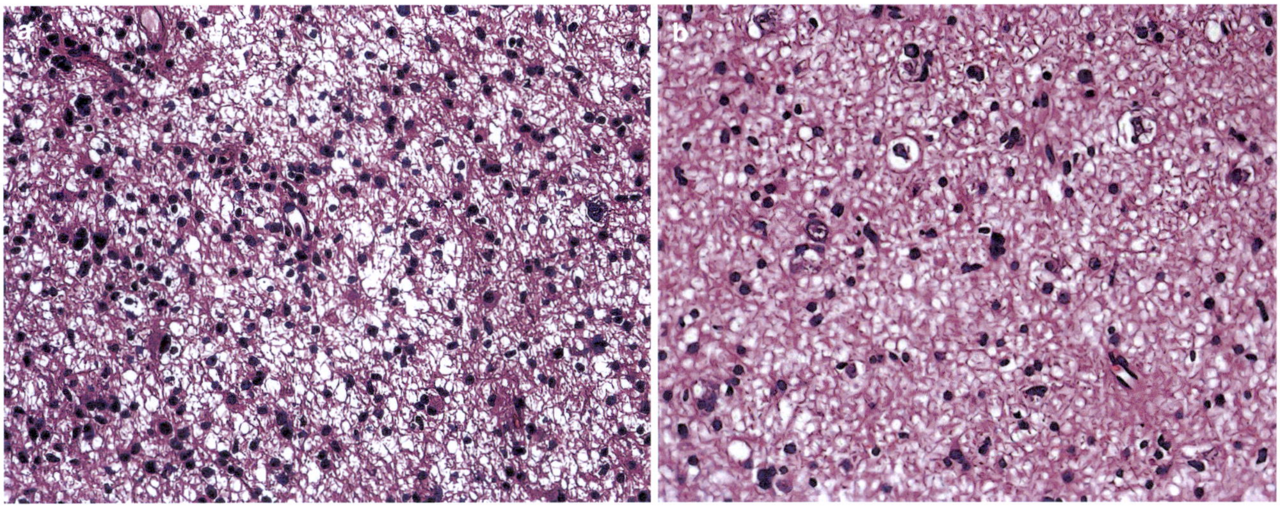

Sections show well-differentiated tumor cells with elongated hair-like processes (piloid appearance) present among Rosenthal fibers (eosinophilic, corkscrew-shaped structures). Microcysts containing mucinous fluid are seen among the tumor cells. The tumor has low mitotic activity and minimal invasion into surrounding tissue.

Microscopic Picture of Grade 3 Astrocytoma (c, d)

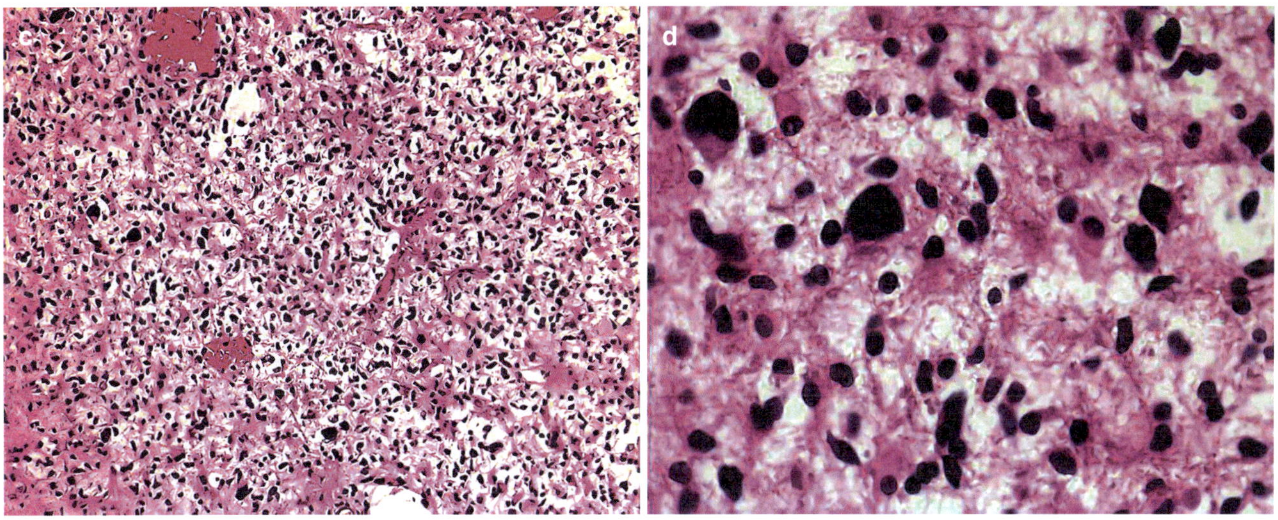

Sections show hypercellular astrocytic tumor cells, nuclear irregularities, and hyperchromasia with significant pleomorphism.

Ancillary Tools

IHC [4]:

- GFAP (variable)
- Olig2
- IDH1

- Marker of infiltrating gliomas, both astrocytic or oligodendroglial
- Recognizes only the most common mutation (IDH1 R132H, which accounts for about 90% of all glioma-associated IDH mutations).
- In the absence of immunohistochemical evidence for the IDH mutation, other IDH1/IDH2 mutations must be diagnosed by mutational analysis.
- Rare in children <14 years

p53

Ki67: increasing proliferation index with increasing grade

Neurofilament (highlights entrapped axons)

Molecular/cytogenetics description [5]:

IDH1 or IDH2 mutation necessary for the diagnosis, with the R132H IDH1 variant seen in >90% of cases

Tumors negative for R132H IDH1 immunohistochemistry require IDH1/IDH2 sequencing to determine IDH status.

p53 mutation and ATRX promoter mutation nearly always present (typically absent in oligodendroglioma, IDH mutant, and 1p19q codeleted).

Gain of chromosome 7

Usually lack TERT promoter mutations

The presence of CDKN2A/CDKN2B homozygous deletion portends a worse prognosis and is sufficient for a CNS WHO grade 4 designation regardless of histologic features present.

Microscopic Picture of Pilocytic Astrocytoma (e–j)

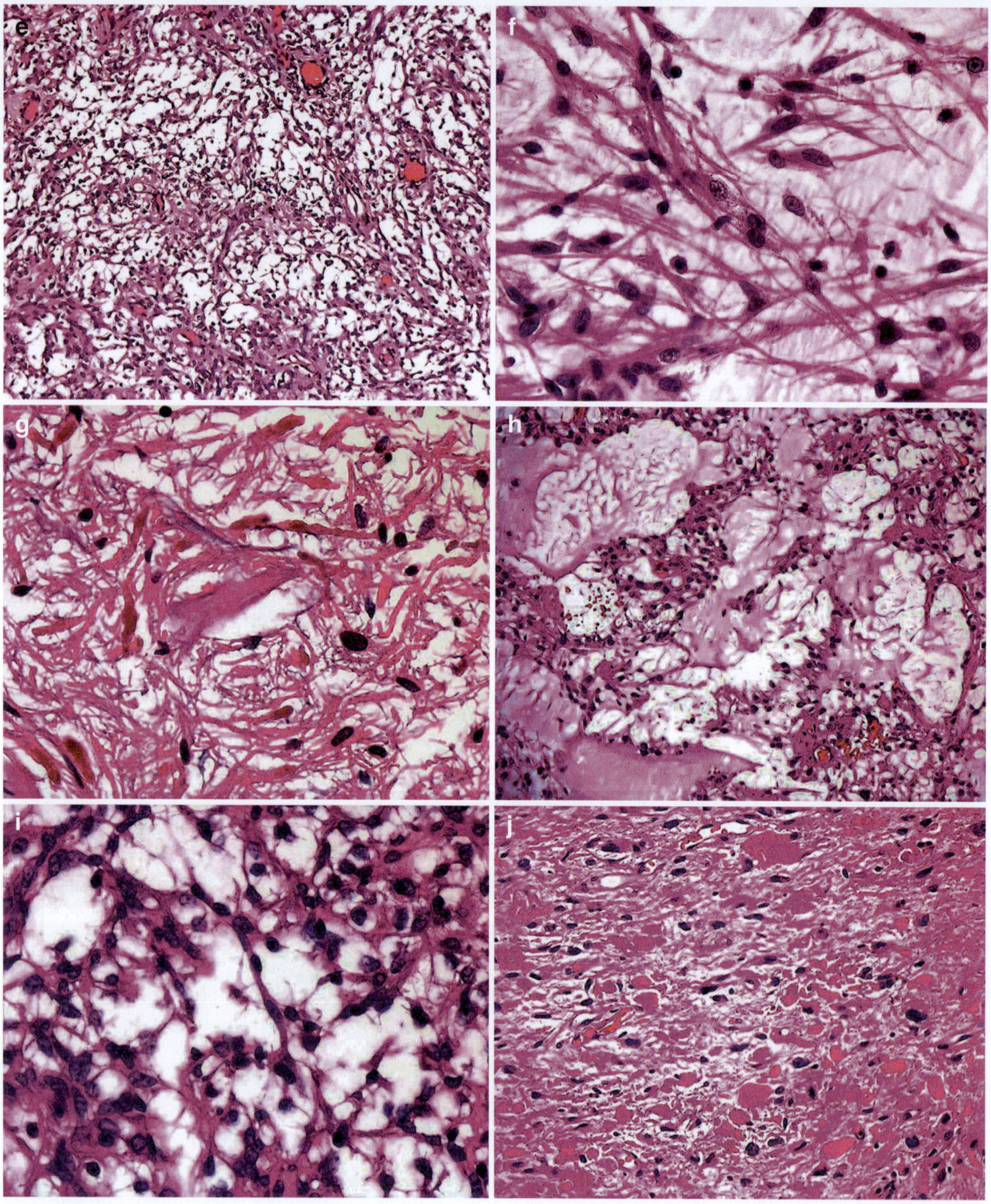

Sections show a tumor with a biphasic appearance formed of a compact fibrillar portion and a loose microcystic portion. The fibrillar portion has low to moderate cellularity and is formed of cells with elongated nuclei, bipolar piloid processes resembling hair, and Rosenthal fibers, which are elongated eosinophilic bundles. The loose microcystic portion has round to oval nuclei, cobweb-like processes, and eosinophilic granular bodies.

Ancillary Tools

IHC and Special Stains [6]:

Tumor cells are positive for:

- GFAP
- Olig2
- S100
- SOX10
- ATRX (retained nuclear staining)

Rosenthal fibers [7]:

- LFB (bright blue)
- Alpha B crystallin
- GFAP (limited to the periphery)

Eosinophilic granular bodies (EGBs):

- PAS/PASD
- Masson trichrome
- Alpha-1-antichymotrypsin
- Alpha-1 antitrypsin

Molecular/cytogenetics description [8]:

BRAF gene alterations (more common in pediatrics than in adult PCA)

MAPK signaling pathway alterations

KIAA1549-BRAF fusion mutation

Glioblastoma

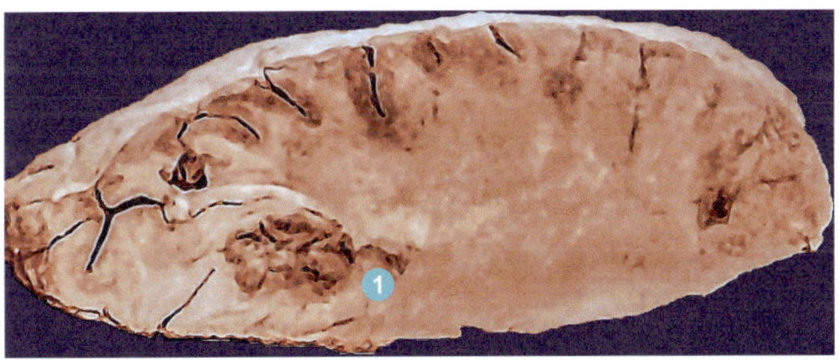

1. An ill-defined whitish-gray mass with areas of hemorrhage and necrosis.

Intrinsic Pontine Glioblastoma

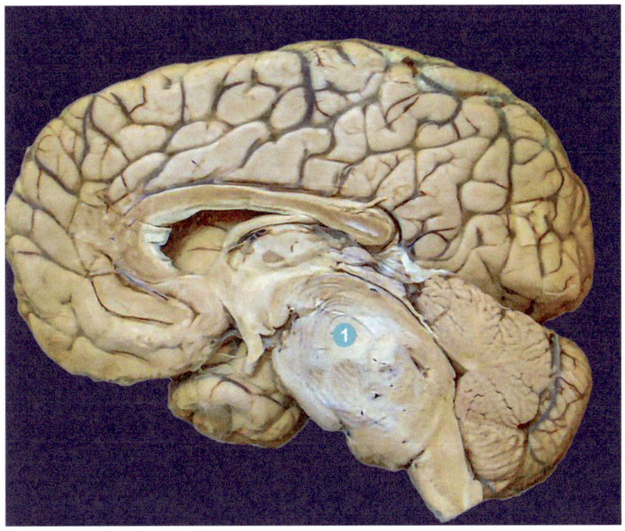

A sagittal section of brain stem and cerebellum is mounted.

1. Asymmetrical enlargement of the pons with focal areas of hemorrhage.

Microscopic Picture of Glioblastoma (a–g)

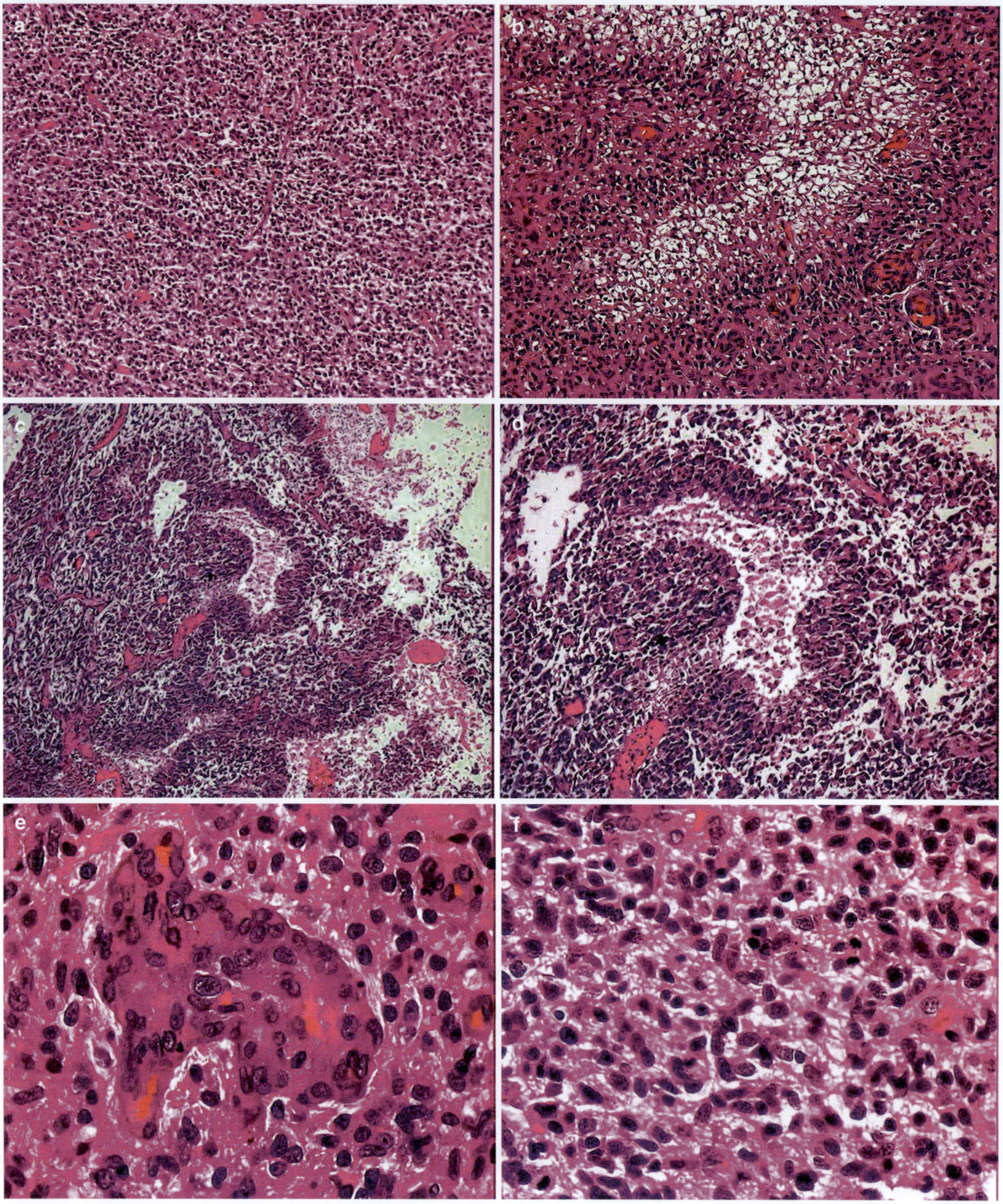

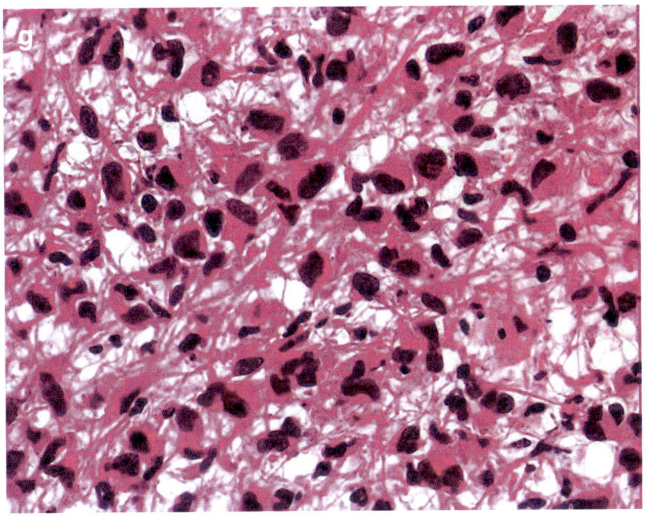

Sections show hypercellular and infiltrating astrocytic tumors. The tumor shows pseudopalisading necrosis, with neoplastic cells surrounding central necrosis, and microvascular proliferation in the form of multilayered, small caliber vessels with glomeruloid appearance. The tumor cells have hyperchromatic, elongated nuclei and irregular nuclear membranes with increased mitotic activity. The tumor has variable cell morphology, such as epithelioid cells, which are large eosinophilic cells with prominent nucleoli; rhabdoid cells with more eccentric nuclei; or small cells, which are monomorphic cells with small, round, or angulated, hyperchromatic nuclei and brisk mitotic activity.

Ancillary Tools

IHC [9]:

GFAP, Olig2, S100

GFAP may be lost in GBMs with sarcomatoid or primitive neuronal components.

Cytokeratin AE1/AE3 may cross-react with glial filaments

ATRX and H3K27 trimethylation are usually retained.

EGFR

Nuclear p53 in up to 30% of GBM; more common in giant cell GBM

BRAF V600E in epithelioid GBMs

Ki67 is usually high; it can be low in molecularly defined GBMs.

Molecular/cytogenetics description [10, 11]

Lacks mutations in IDH1/IDH2 and histone H3 genes

- Lack of IDH1 immunohistochemistry sufficient in patients ≥55 years of age meeting histologic criteria for glioblastoma with nonmidline tumors

Molecularly defined GBM: even in low-grade appearing tumors and tumors lacking necrosis or microvascular proliferation

- TERT promoter mutation
- EGFR gene amplification or combined whole chromosome 7 gain and whole chromosome 10 loss (+7/−10)

Alterations of RTK genes, PI3K pathway genes, and PTEN in up to 90% of GBM

CDKN2A/CDKN2B deletion can be present.

BRAF V600E in up to 50% of GBMs with epithelioid features

MYC or MYCN amplification associated with primitive neuronal component

Radiation-induced gliomas: PDGFRA, TP53, CDKN2A deletion

- Some radiation-associated gliomas with histologic features of glioblastoma may be molecularly more consistent with diffuse pediatric-type high-grade gliomas, H3 wild-type, and IDH wild-type.

If present, gene fusions most commonly involve the receptor tyrosine kinase (RTK) family.

- EGFR
- FGFR3
- MET
- NTRK1/NTRK2/NTRK3
- PDGFRA

Medulloblastoma

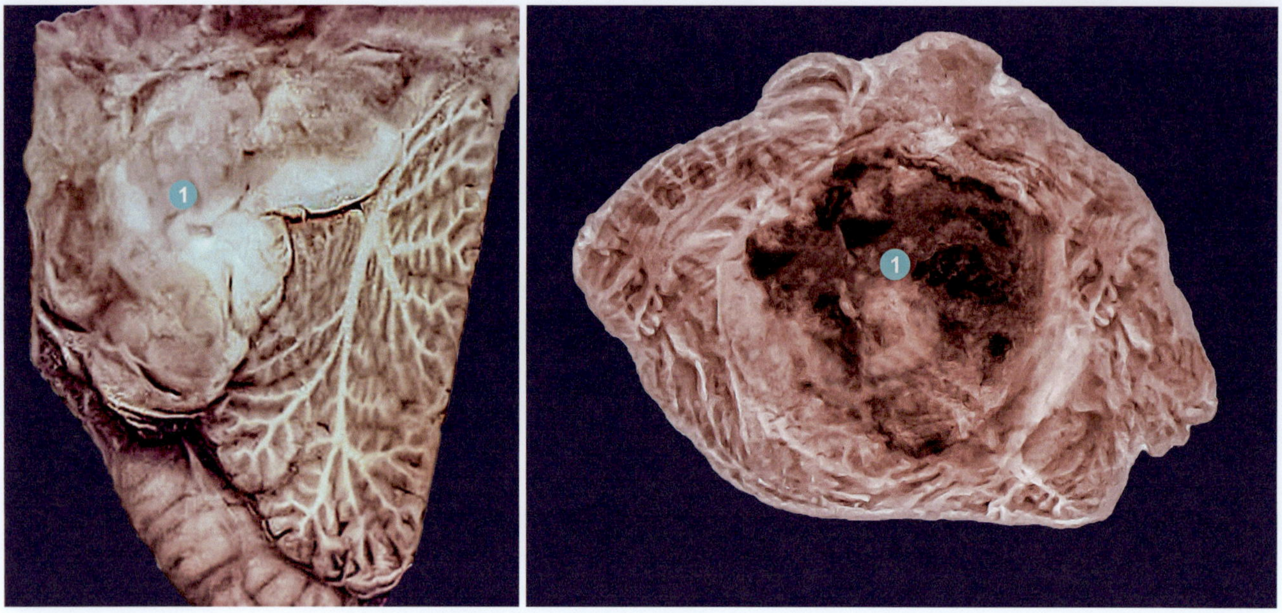

The cerebellum of a child is mounted.

1. It shows a tumor mass arising from the roof of the fourth ventricle in the middle of the cerebellum with areas of hemorrhage.

Microscopic Picture of Medulloblastoma (a–d)

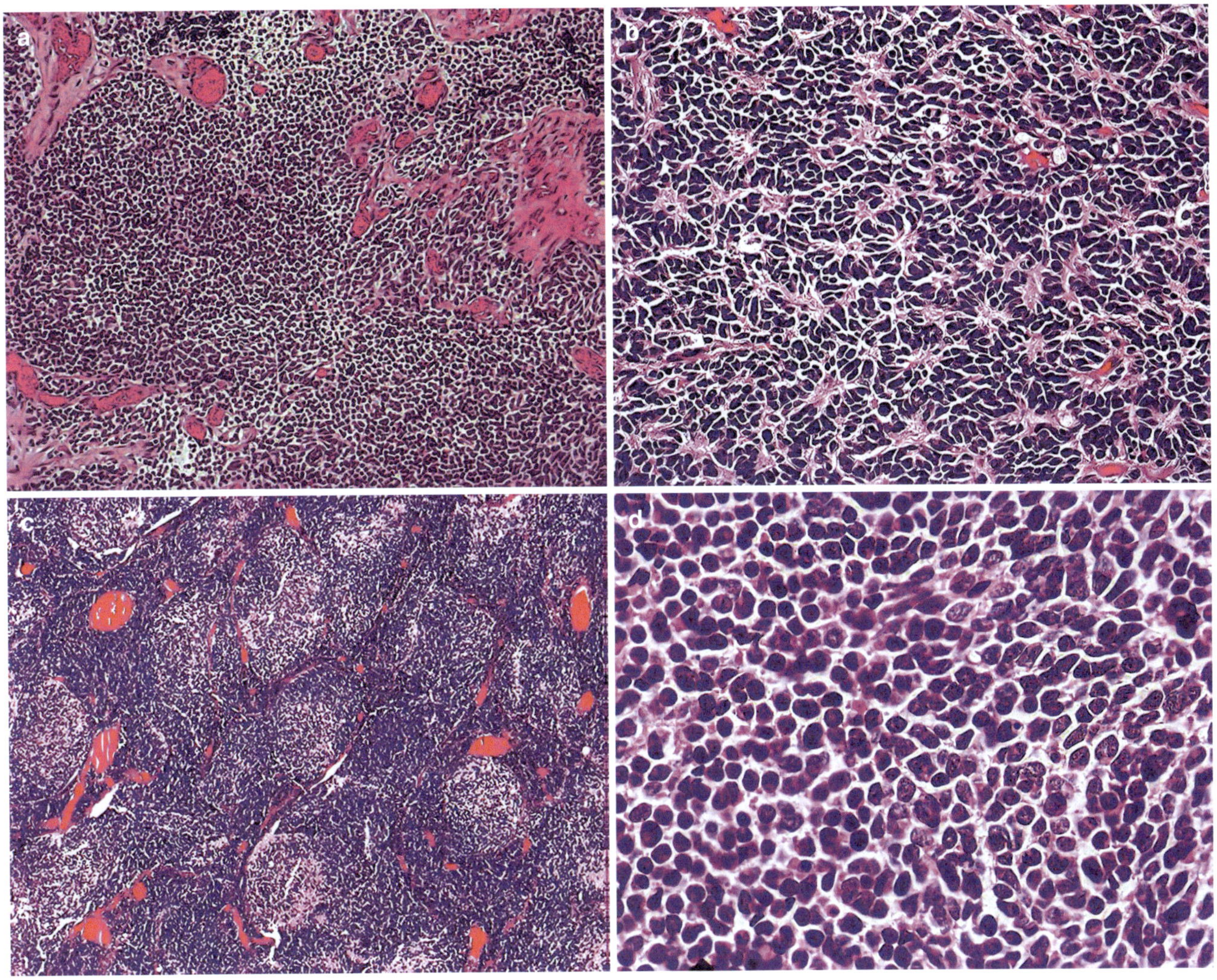

The tumor is composed of small, undifferentiated cells with round or oval nuclei. These cells are densely packed together and have a high nuclear-to-cytoplasmic ratio and increased mitotic figures. Tumor cells are arranged around a central lumen, resembling a rosette-like pattern forming Homer-Wright rosettes. The type of medulloblastoma with extensive nodularity shows expanded lobular architecture formed of pale nodules and densely packed, undifferentiated cells with hyperchromatic and pleomorphic nuclei.

Ancillary Tools

IHC [12]:

Synaptophysin, NeuN

Nuclear SMARCB1/INI1 and SMARCA4 are retained.

Medulloblastoma with melanocytic differentiation: HMB45, MelanA

Medulloblastoma with myogenic differentiation: desmin and myogenin

Molecular/cytogenetics description [13]

Molecular Subgroups of Medulloblastoma (MB)

1. WNT-activated MBs: these tumors are so named due to activation of the canonical Wingless (WNT) signal transduction pathway leading to cellular growth and proliferation of these tumors.
2. SHH-activated MBs: they exhibit a striking degree of biological, pathological, and clinical heterogeneity. Named for activation of the sonic hedgehog (SHH) signaling pathway. As such, the SHH MB with TP53 mutation is listed separately in the WHO classification and is considered very high risk clinically.
3. Group 3 MBs: Considered the most aggressive MB subgroup, Group 3 tumors confer a 5-year overall survival of <60%. Certain hallmark genomic features, such as MYC amplification, represent extremely high-risk disease. They are characterized by high-level MYC amplification.
4. Group 4 MBs: Group 4 tumors account for up to 40% of all cases and tend to occur in older children. Similar to their Group 3 counterparts, Group 4 MBs harbor gene-level amplifications of MYCN as well as somatic mutations in KBTBD4.

13.5 Vascular Malformation

Arteriovenous Malformation

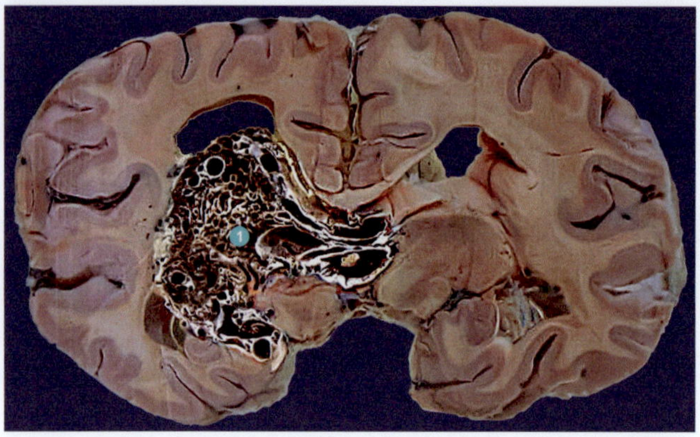

The coronal section of the brain is mounted.

1. A mass formed of tangles of abnormally developed arteries and veins without intervening capillaries. The mass occupies the medial temporal and hippocampus and extends to the lateral ventricle with areas of hemorrhage.

Microscopic Picture of Arteriovenous Malformation (a, b)

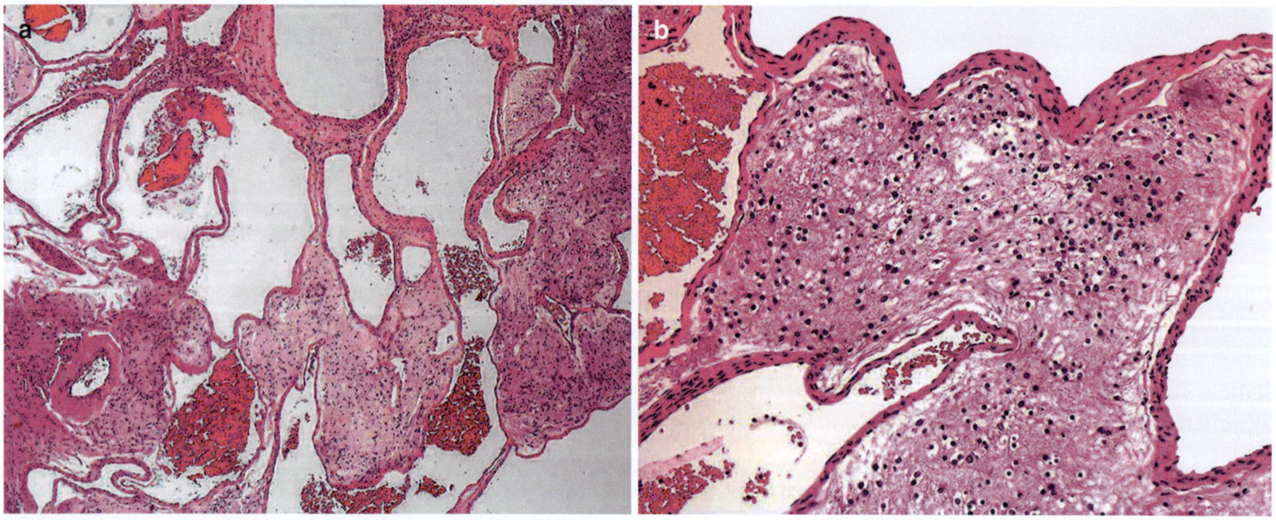

Sections show tortuous and disorganized vascular channels of varying diameter and wall thickness, some containing thrombus. Profound venous enlargement with intimal hyperplasia and microvessel accumulation is observed in some areas.

Ancillary Tools

IHC [14]:

- von Willebrand factor (FVIII)
- CD34 endothelial antigen
- Vimentin
- Alpha-smooth-muscle actin (SMA) cytoskeletal proteins

References

1. Jastania RA. et al. (2020). Adamantinomatous Craniopharyngioma in an Adult: A Case Report with NGS Analysis. Int Med Case Rep J. 13:123-137. doi: https://doi.org/10.2147/IMCRJ.S243405. PMID: 32368160; PMCID: PMC7183340.
2. Asa SL. et al. (2022). Overview of the 2022 WHO Classification of Pituitary Tumors. Endocrine Pathology. 33:6–26. https://doi.org/10.1007/s12022-022-09703-7.
3. Asa SL. et al. (2021). Genomics and Epigenomics of Pituitary Tumors: What Do Pathologists Need to Know? Endocr. Pathol.32(1):3-16. doi: https://doi.org/10.1007/s12022-021-09663-4. PMID: 33433883.
4. DeWitt JC. et al. (2017). Cost-effectiveness of IDH testing in diffuse gliomas according to the 2016 WHO classification of tumors of the central nervous system recommendations. Neuro Oncol. 19(12):1640-1650. doi: https://doi.org/10.1093/neuonc/nox120. PMID: 29016871; PMCID: PMC5716163.
5. Shirahata M. et al. (2018). Novel, improved grading system(s) for IDH-mutant astrocytic gliomas. Acta Neuropathol. 136(1):153-166. doi: https://doi.org/10.1007/s00401-018-1849-4. PMID: 29687258.
6. Tihan T. et al. (2012). Pathologic characteristics of pediatric intracranial pilocytic astrocytomas and their impact on outcome in 3 countries: a multi-institutional study. Am J Surg Pathol. 36(1):43-55. doi: https://doi.org/10.1097/PAS.0b013e3182329480. PMID: 21989351.
7. Machen SK, Prayson RA (1998). Cyclin D1 and MIB-1 immunohistochemistry in pilocytic astrocytomas: a study of 48 cases. Hum Pathol. 29(12):1511-6. doi: https://doi.org/10.1016/s0046-8177(98)90023-5. PMID: 9865840.
8. Collins VP, Jones DT, Giannini C.(2015) Pilocytic astrocytoma: pathology, molecular mechanisms and markers. Acta Neuropathol.129(6):775-88. doi: https://doi.org/10.1007/s00401-015-1410-7. PMID: 25792358; PMCID: PMC4436848.
9. Lee KS. et al. (2013). Immunohistochemical classification of primary and secondary glioblastomas. Korean J Pathol. 47(6):541-8. doi: https://doi.org/10.4132/KoreanJPathol.2013.47.6.541. PMID: 24421847; PMCID: PMC3887156.
10. Mao X, Hamoudi RA. (2000). Molecular and cytogenetic analysis of glioblastoma multiforme. Cancer Genet Cytogenet. 122(2):87-92. doi: https://doi.org/10.1016/s0165-4608(00)00278-8. PMID: 11106817.
11. Wang PF. et al. (2016). IDH-1R132H mutation status in diffuse glioma patients: implications for classification. Oncotarget. 7(21):31393-400. doi: https://doi.org/10.18632/oncotarget.8918. PMID: 27120786; PMCID: PMC5058765.
12. Ellison D. (2002). Classifying the medulloblastoma: insights from morphology and molecular genetics. Neuropathol Appl Neurobiol. 28(4):257-82. doi: https://doi.org/10.1046/j.1365--2990.2002.00419.x. PMID: 12175339.
13. Kumar R, Liu APY, Northcott PA.(2020). Medulloblastoma genomics in the modern molecular era. Brain Pathol. 30(3):679-690. doi: https://doi.org/10.1111/bpa.12804. PMID: 31799776; PMCID: PMC8018047.
14. Szeifert GT. et al. (2003). Immunohistochemical analysis of a cerebral arteriovenous malformation obliterated by radiosurgery and presenting with re-bleeding. Case report. Neurol Res. 25(7):718-21. doi: https://doi.org/10.1179/016164103101202228. PMID: 14579789.

14 Diseases of the Ocular System

The eye is a complex and unique part of the human organs that has been considered the window to the human soul. Broadly, the human eye is divided into two segments: anterior and posterior segments. The specific disease conditions of the eye are associated with each of these broad segments. The anterior segment involves the conjunctiva, ciliary body, iris, pupil, anterior chamber, cornea, and lens; the posterior segment consists of the sclera, choroid, retina, macula, and optic nerve.

Within its compact structure lies a complex interplay of light, tissue, and function that allows us to perceive the world around us. However, this intricate system is susceptible to a wide range of pathological processes. Understanding these processes, from inflammatory conditions to degenerative diseases and tumors, forms the foundation of ophthalmic pathology. This is crucial for ophthalmologists and other healthcare professionals to diagnose and manage eye disease effectively. By understanding the microscopic underpinnings of disease, we gain a powerful tool for accurate diagnosis and the development of targeted treatment strategies. Ultimately, this knowledge empowers us to preserve the precious gift of sight.

Please note: While pathology labs often receive small tissue samples or, in rare cases, orbital exenteration for examination, including clinical photos or gross images is not always feasible for this chapter. However, this chapter will still provide a comprehensive overview of the most common eye diseases, organized by the specific region of the eye or orbit affected.

14.1 Eye Lesions

1. Eyelid
   (a) Chalazion
   (b) Xanthelasma
   (c) Cutaneous Amyloid
   (d) Molluscum Contagiosum
   (e) Squamous Papilloma
   (f) Seborrheic Keratosis
   (g) Actinic Keratosis
   (h) Squamous Cell Carcinoma
   (i) Basal Cell Carcinoma
   (j) Apocrine Hidrocystoma
   (k) Syringoma
   (l) Trichoepithelioma
   (m) Sebaceous Hyperplasia
   (n) Sebaceous Carcinoma
   (o) Pyogenic Granuloma
2. Conjunctiva
   (a) Ligneous Conjunctivitis
   (b) Pinguecula
   (c) Epibulbar choristoma
   (d) Conjunctival Intraepithelial Neoplasia
   (e) Conjunctival Squamous Cell Carcinoma
   (f) Primary Acquired Melanosis (PAM)
3. Lacrimal duct/gland
   (a) Dacryocystitis/Canaliculitis
   (b) Adenoid Cystic Carcinoma
4. Uvea (iris, choroid, and ciliary body), Limbus, and Sclera
   (a) Lisch Nodule
   (b) Uveal Melanoma
5. Retina
   (a) Retinal Glioma
   (b) Retinoblastoma
6. Optic Nerve
   (a) Melanocytoma
   (b) Optic Nerve Meningioma
   (c) Optic Nerve Glioma
   (d) Optic Nerve Atrophy
7. Orbit
   (a) Orbital Dermoid Cyst
   (b) Embryonal Rhabdomyosarcoma

G. Dawood, *Color Atlas of Human Gross and Microscopic Pathology*, https://doi.org/10.1007/978-3-031-76007-5_14

14.2 Eyelid

Chalazion (a–c)

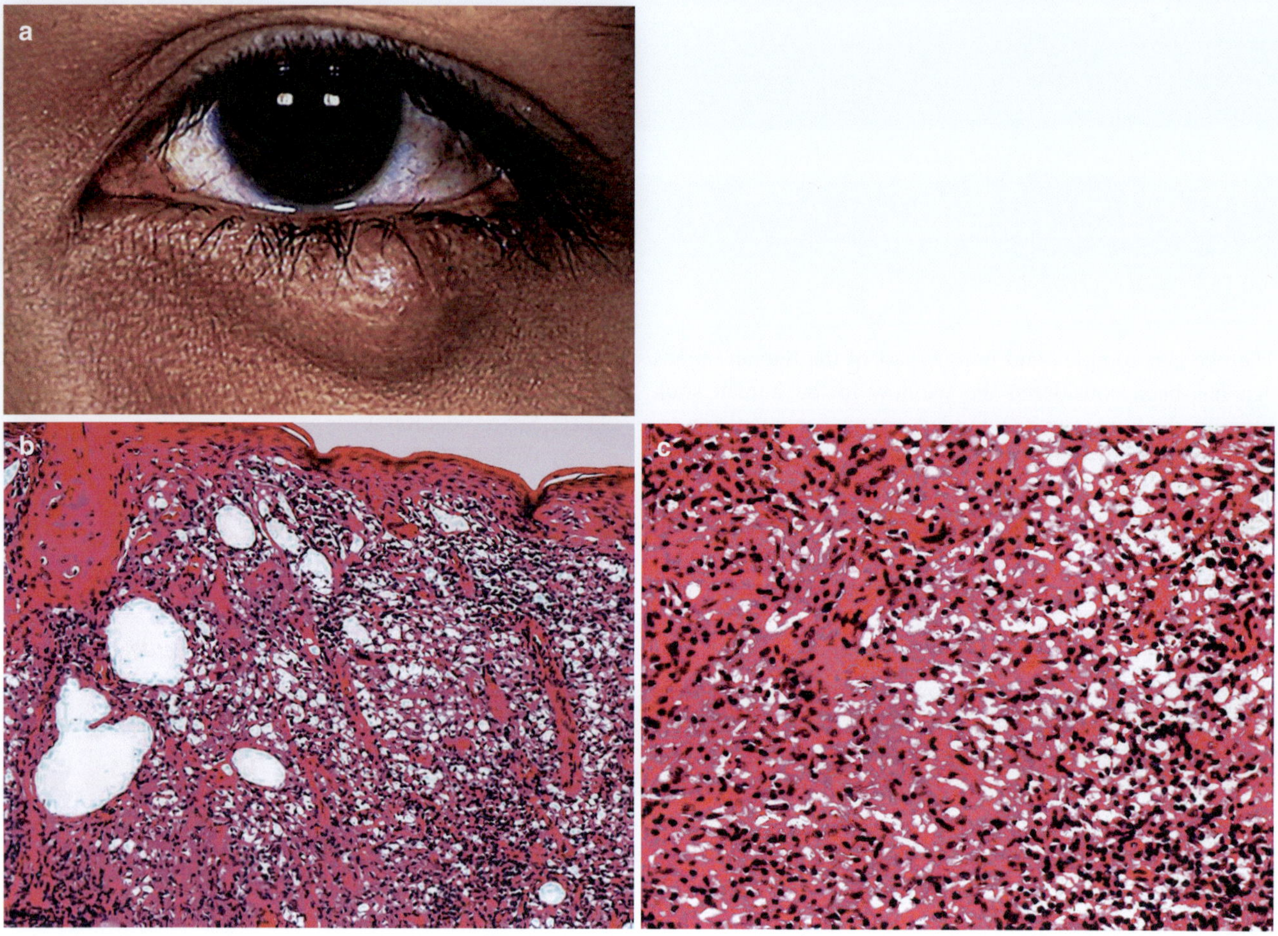

Clinically, the lesion is a solitary, non-tender nodule with a sloping edge and stretched skin over it. Lid eversion helps identify the lesion.

Sections show lipogranuloma formed of empty spaces surrounded by epithelioid and foamy histiocytes with multinucleated foreign body giant cells.

Xanthelasma (a–c)

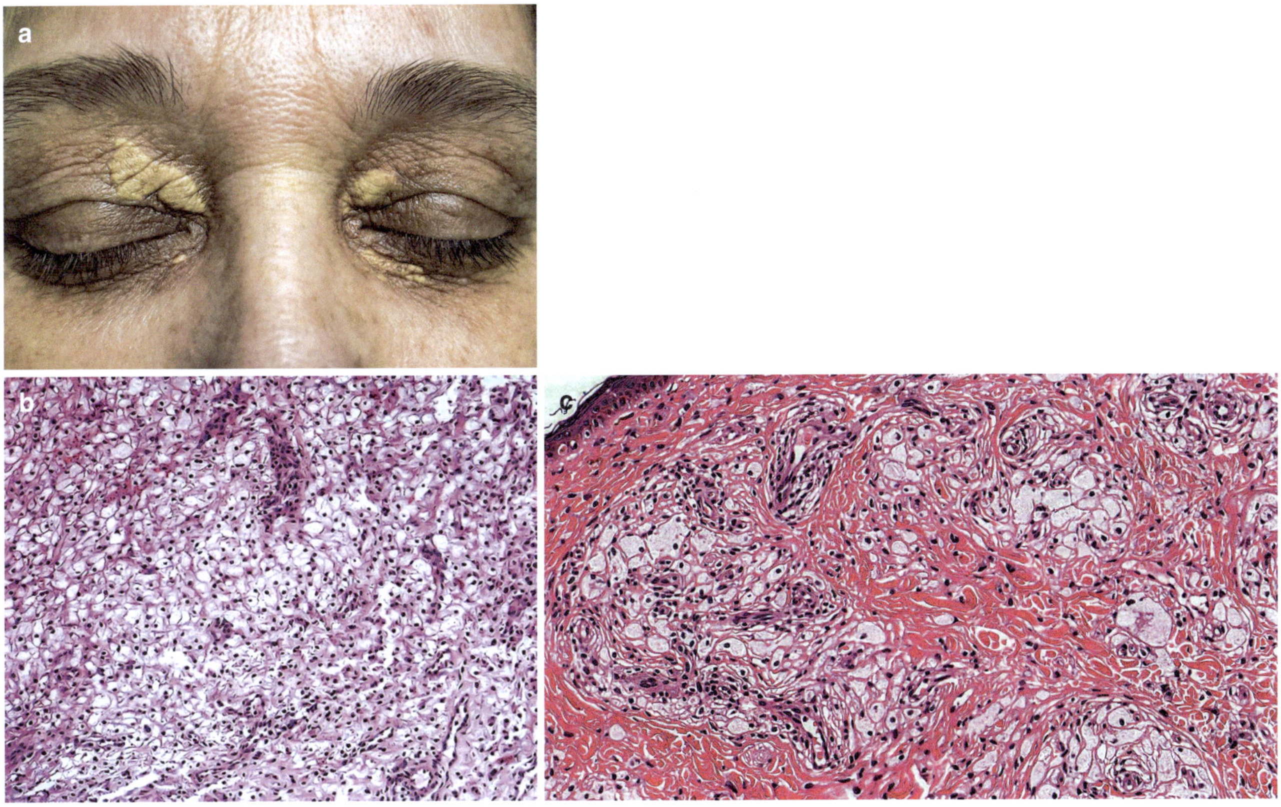

Clinically, the lesion is yellow elevated plaques in the upper and/or lower lid.

Sections show lipid-laden foamy histiocytes in the superficial dermis, clustering around blood vessels with the presence of multinucleated Touton giant cells. The lesion may also show thin, loose dermal collagen and skeletal muscle bundles.

Cutaneous Amyloidosis (a, b)

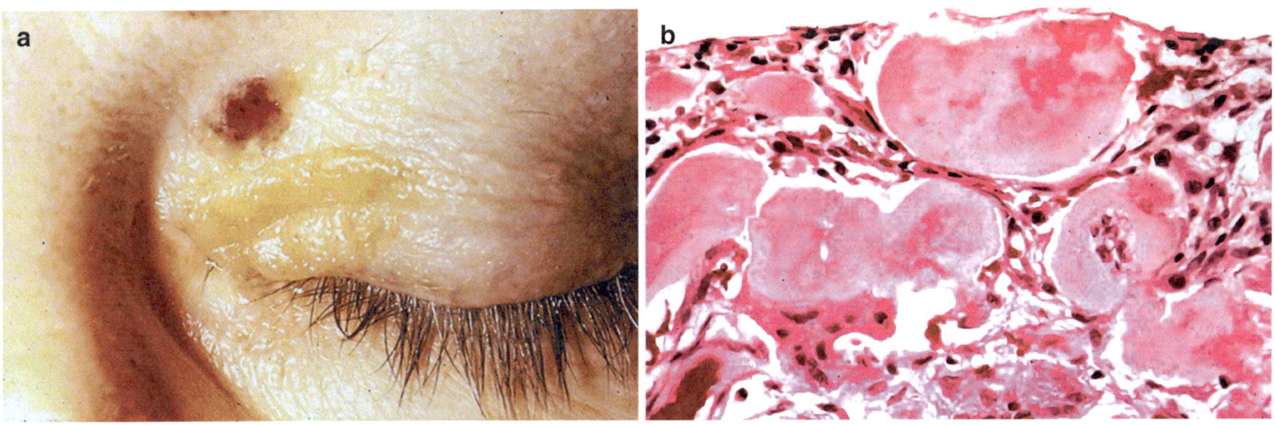

Clinically, the patient may present with a yellow-pink or hemorrhagic macule with obliteration of skin markings over the lesion.

The section shows homogeneous, amorphous eosinophilic material in the subepithelial stroma around and within blood vessel walls, causing its thickening.

Molluscum Contagiosum (a–c)

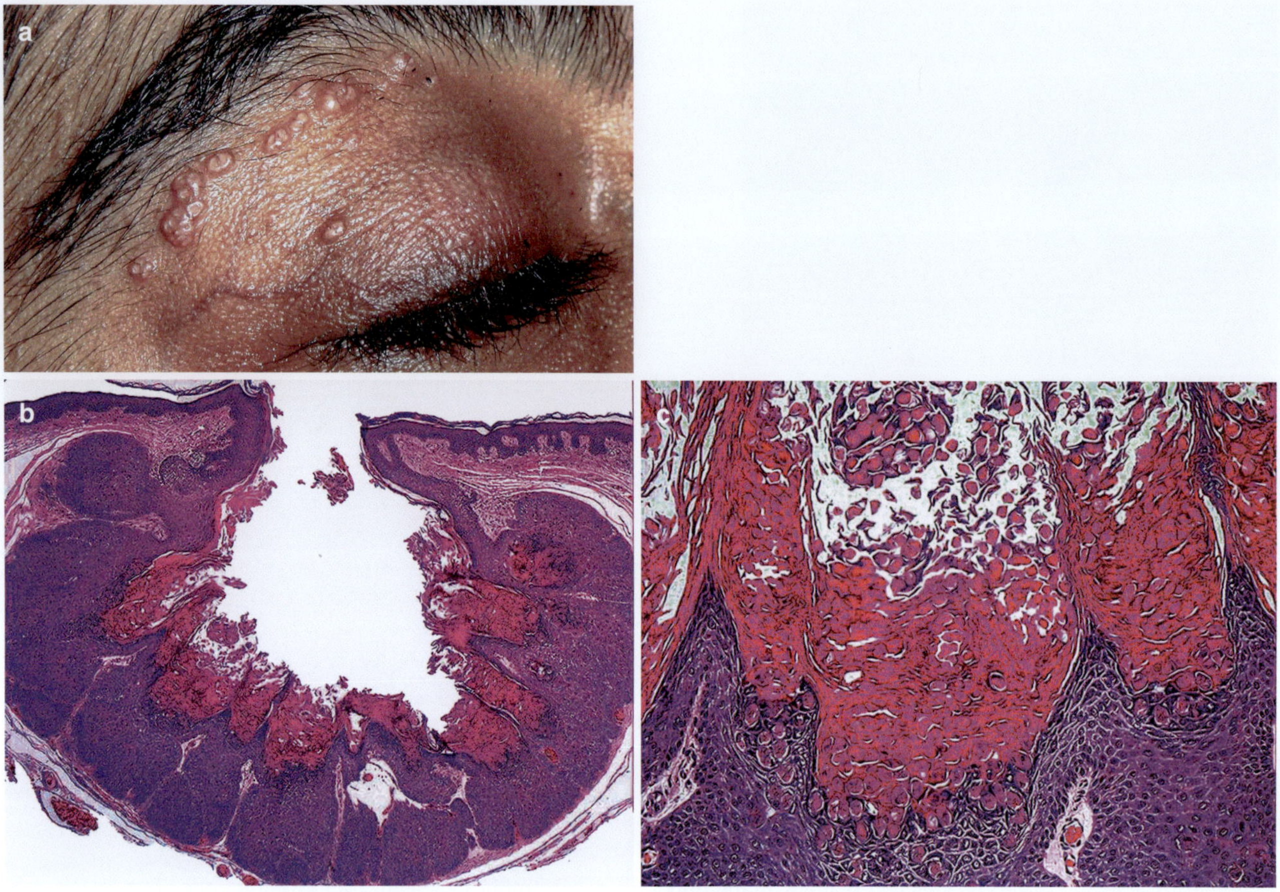

Clinically, the lesion is firm, white to flesh-colored, dome-shaped, pearly, and umbilicated papules.

Sections show a cup-shaped lesion with inverted lobules of acanthotic epidermis that expand into the underlying dermis. Henderson-Paterson (molluscum bodies) are large (up to 35 microns) intracytoplasmic eosinophilic inclusion bodies that start at the granular layer and become increasingly eosinophilic and occupy the entire cell.

Squamous Cell Papilloma (a, b)

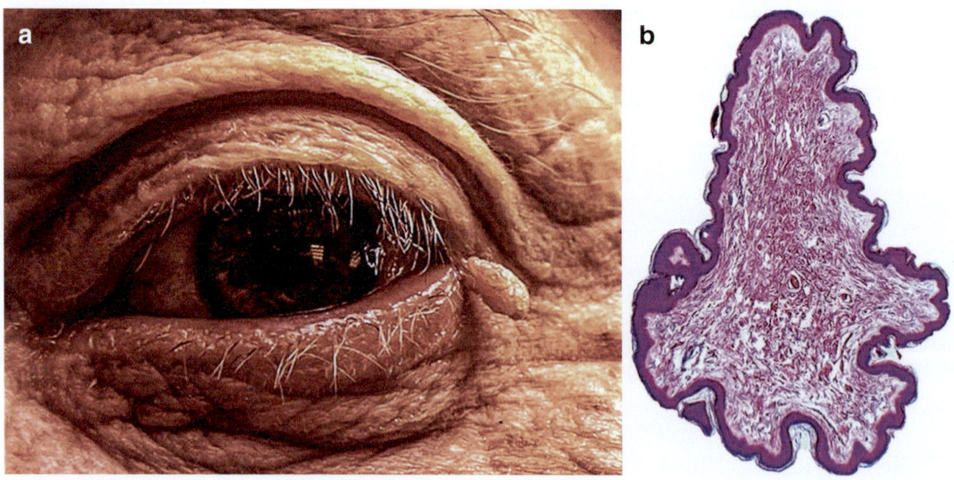

Clinically, the lesion is a pedunculated, soft, and flesh-colored polyp with a smooth, round surface.

The section shows a polyp formed of a fibrovascular core covered by epidermis.

Seborrheic Keratosis (a–d)

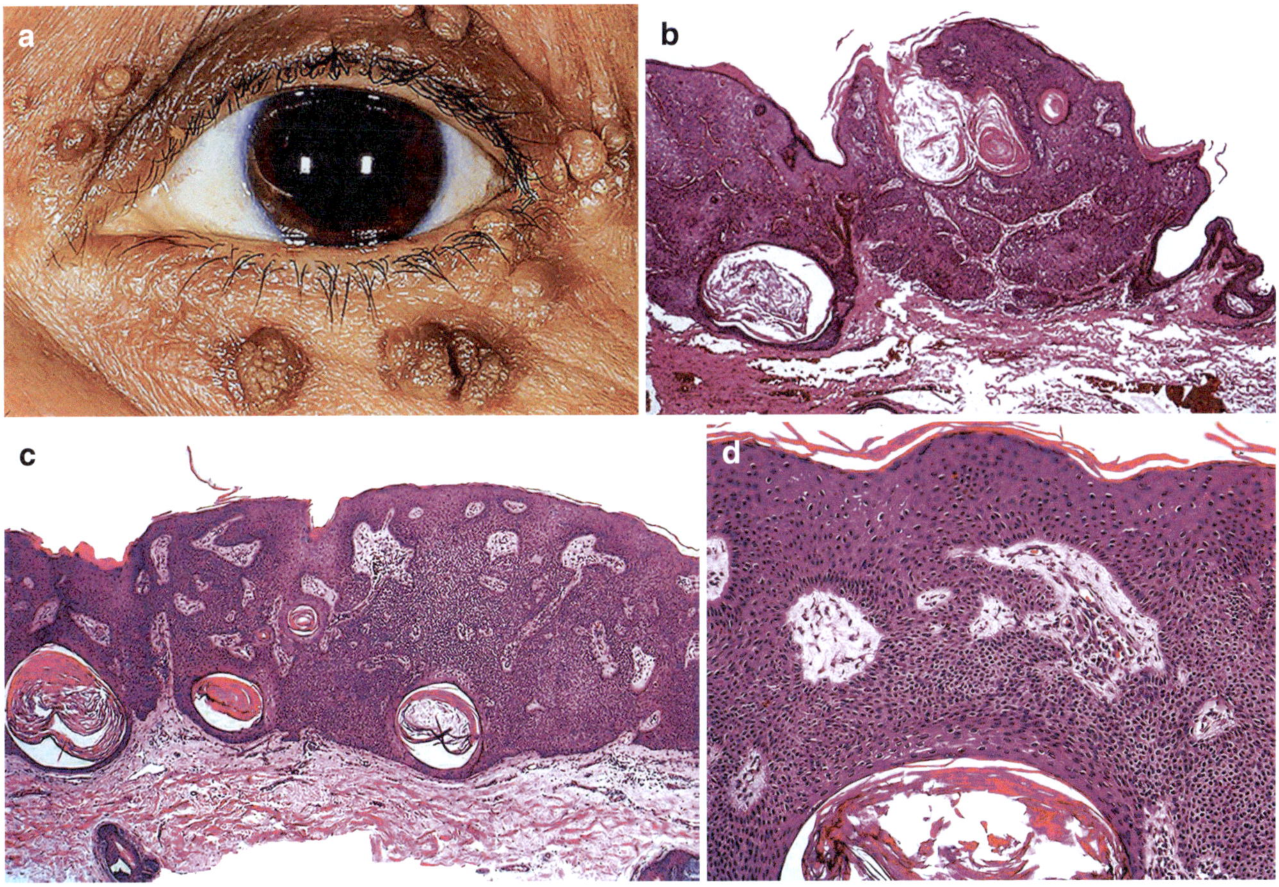

Clinically, the lesion is single or multiple, brown-black or gray, with papules or plaques with a stuck-on appearance (well-demarcated edges) and a waxy or greasy cerebriform surface.

Sections show acanthotic epidermis formed of the proliferation of basaloid and squamous cells with the formation of true and pseudo-horn cysts.

Actinic (Solar) Keratosis (a–c)

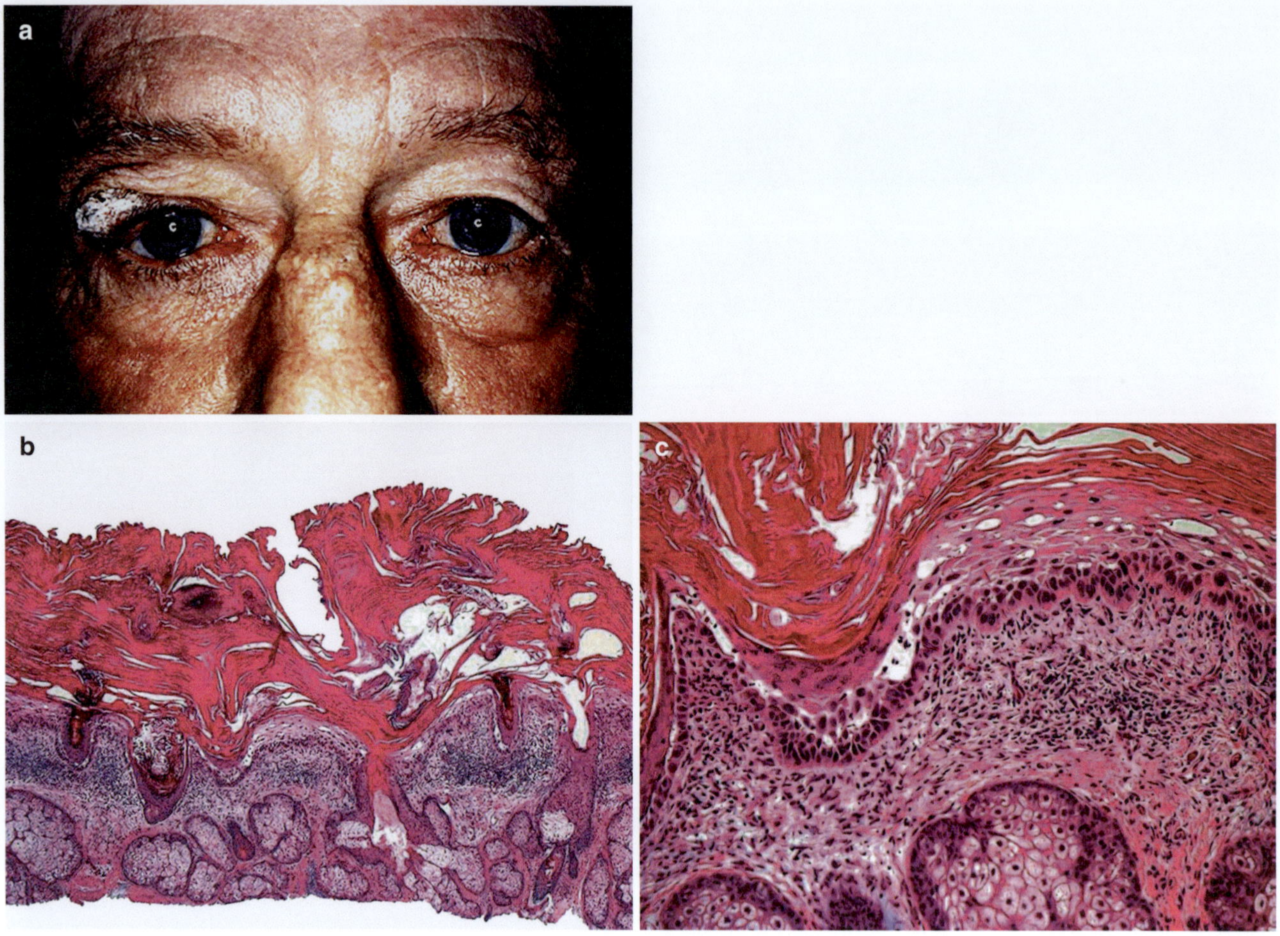

Clinically, the lesion is a thickened, white-yellow, and scaly plaque.

Sections show hyperkeratosis with focal parakeratosis and hypogranulosis with the presence of prominent irregular acanthosis. Basal keratinocytes are atypical with loss of polarization, crowding, and overlapping and with the presence of focal suprabasal acantholysis. The dermis shows superficial, mild-moderate inflammatory infiltrate.

Ancillary Tools

IHC [1]:

p53 (50%)

Cyclin D1 (50%)

Increased Ki67 expression

Molecular/cytogenetics description [2]:

Main driver mutations present in cutaneous invasive squamous cell carcinoma, such as TP53, NOTCH1, and NOTCH2, are already present in actinic keratosis.

MAPK pathway seems to play a leading role in invasion.

Squamous Cell Carcinoma of Eyelids (a, b)

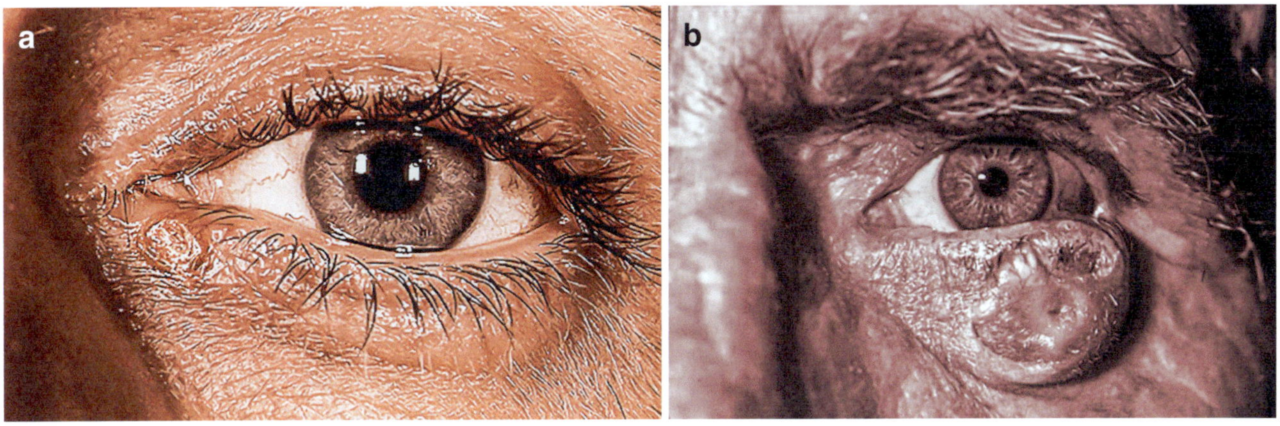

The lesion is a small ulcer with a raised, everted edge (a). The ulcer in (b) is larger with a raised everted edge and necrotic floor.

Basal Cell Carcinoma (a, b)

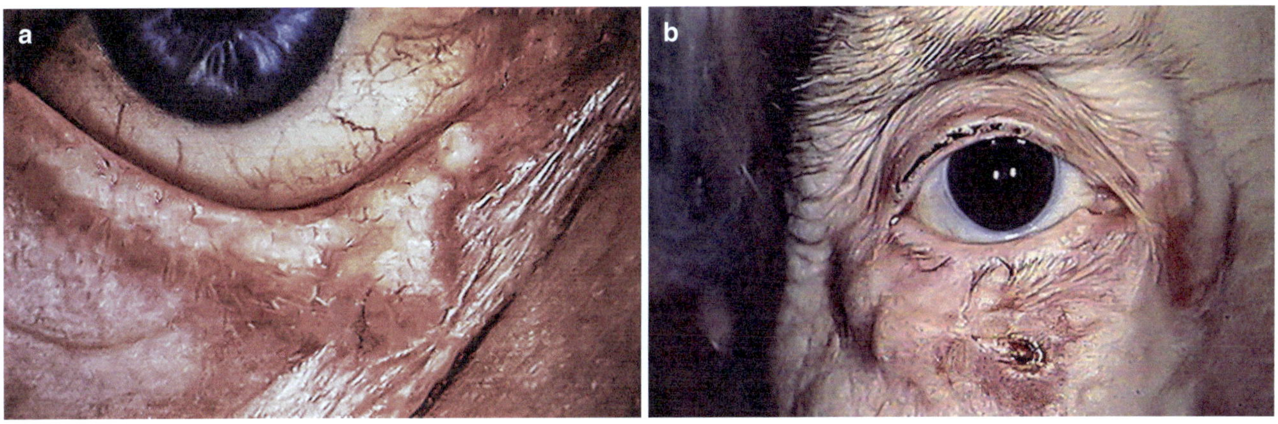

1. Infiltrative BCC: the white color results from the dense collagenous component. Note the dilated vessels coursing over the top of the lesion.
2. Nodular BCC: ulcerated lesion with a characteristic rolled border.

Apocrine Hidrocystoma (a–c)

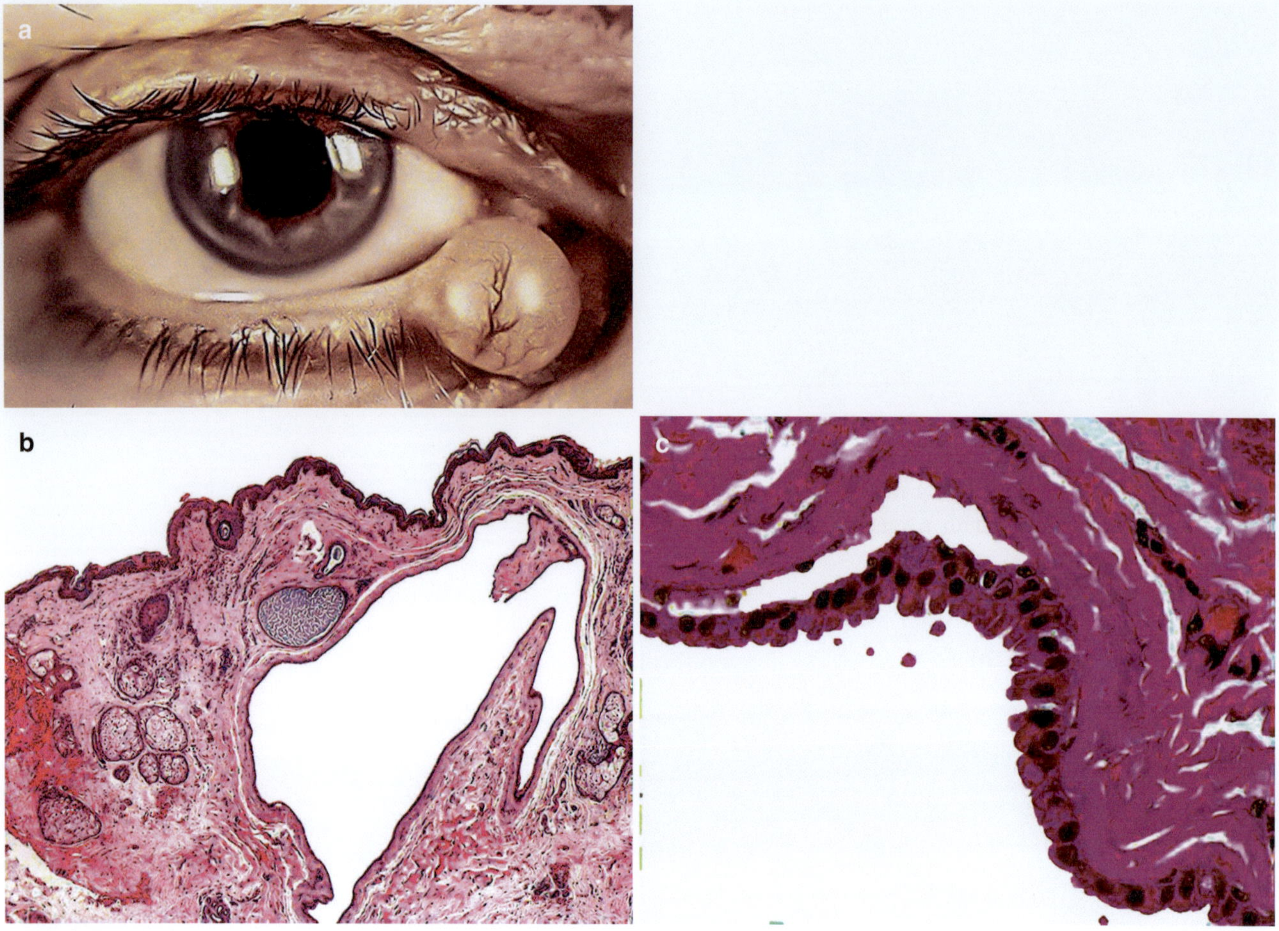

Clinically, the lesion is a thin-walled, translucent cyst with a smooth outer surface.

Sections show a unilocular subepithelial cyst with a clear/ empty cavity. The cyst is lined with an inner columnar, eosinophilic cell with apical snouts and decapitation and an outer myoepithelial cell layer.

Syringoma (a–c)

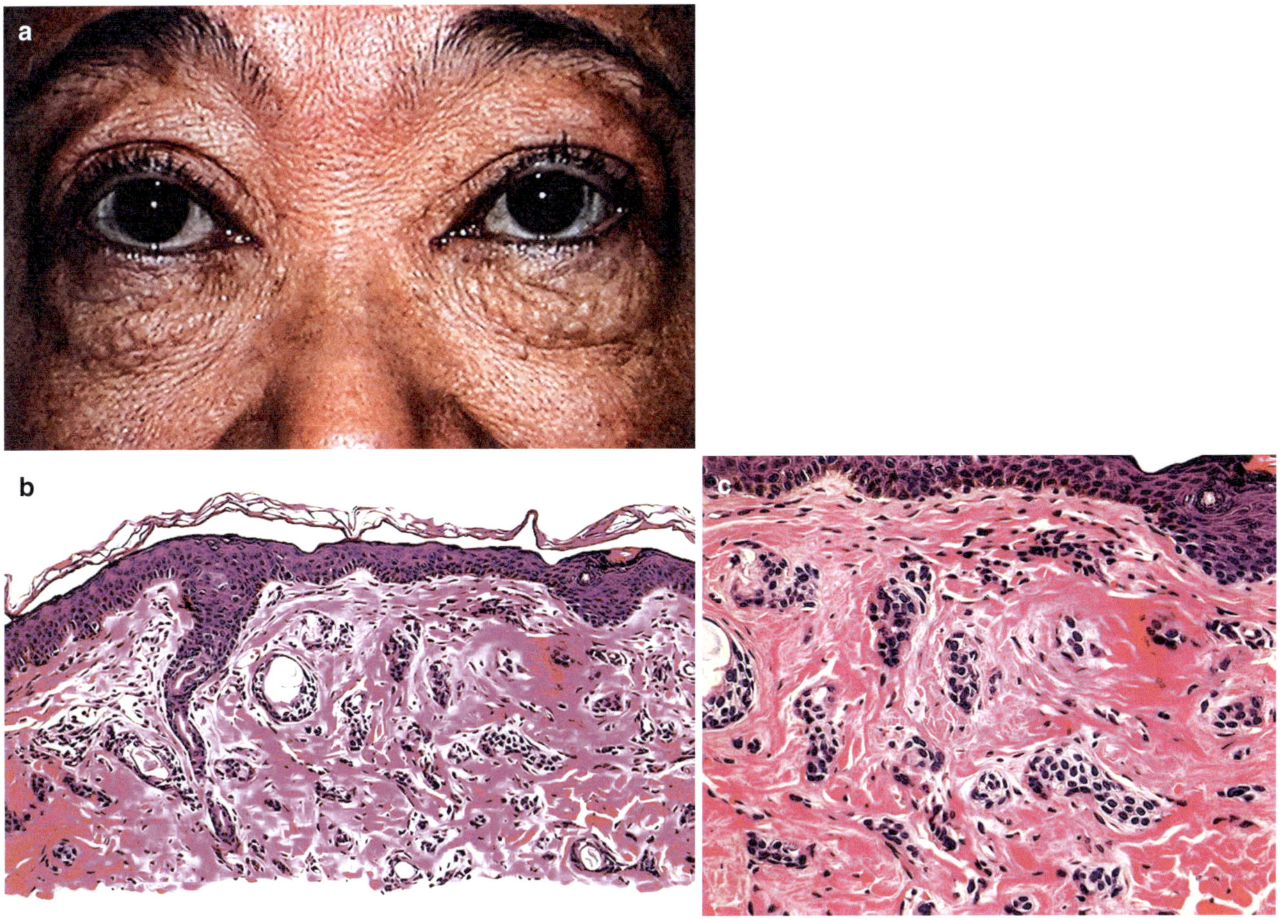

Clinically, the lesion is bilateral, multiple, skin-colored, small, and firm papules with a waxy surface.
Sections show a well-circumscribed proliferation of benign-appearing basaloid cells forming round and comma-shaped ductules, nests, and cysts in a fibrotic stromal background., usually in the superficial reticular dermis.

Ancillary Tools

IHC [3]:

CEA: the luminal surface of sweat ductal cells.

EMA: peripheral cells of dermal and intraepidermal ducts; solid strands.

CK5: outer cells of dermal ducts; solid strands.

Molecular/cytogenetics description [4].

Multiple syringomas may be inherited in an autosomal dominant fashion; linked to chromosome 16q22.

Trichoepithelioma (a–e)

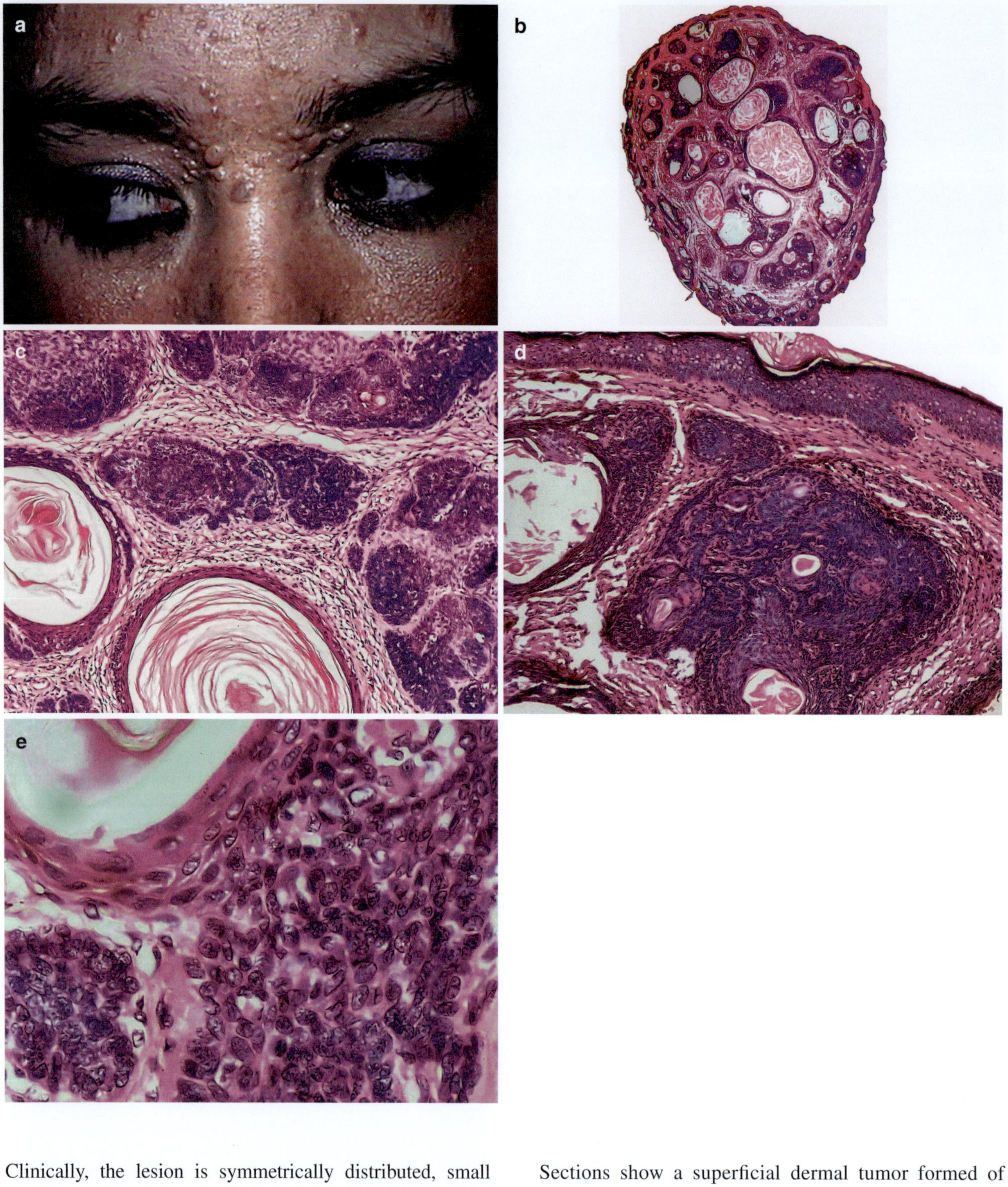

Clinically, the lesion is symmetrically distributed, small (usually <1 cm in diameter), firm, round, and flesh-colored papules, typically seen on the face, particularly the nose, eyelids, and forehead.

Sections show a superficial dermal tumor formed of nests of basaloid cells with keratin horn cysts. The fibrous cellular stroma is closely associated with the epithelial components.

Pilomatricoma (a–e)

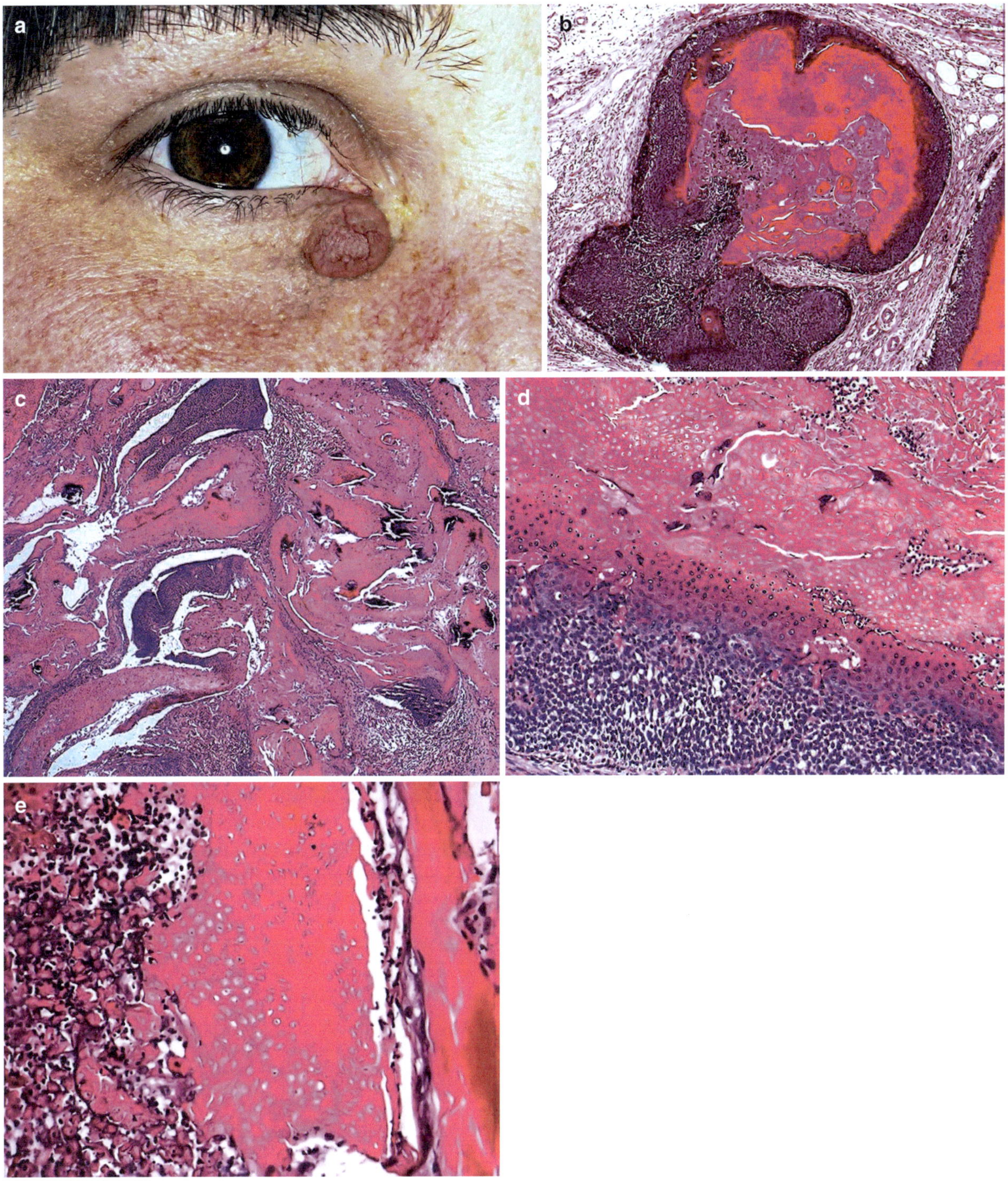

Clinically, the lesion is a circumscribed round, smooth, hard dermal tumor nodule and freely mobile from the underlying bone.

Sections show lobulated and circumscribed dermal-based neoplasm formed of islands of basaloid cells exhibiting abrupt keratinization without intervening granular layer (trichilemmal keratinization). Ghost/shadow cells may predominate. Intermediary cells have progressively more eosinophilic cytoplasm with a pyknotic nucleus. Tumor keratin may elicit an inflammatory response with foreign body giant cells, granuloma, cholesterol clefts, and calcification.

Sebaceous Hyperplasia (a–c)

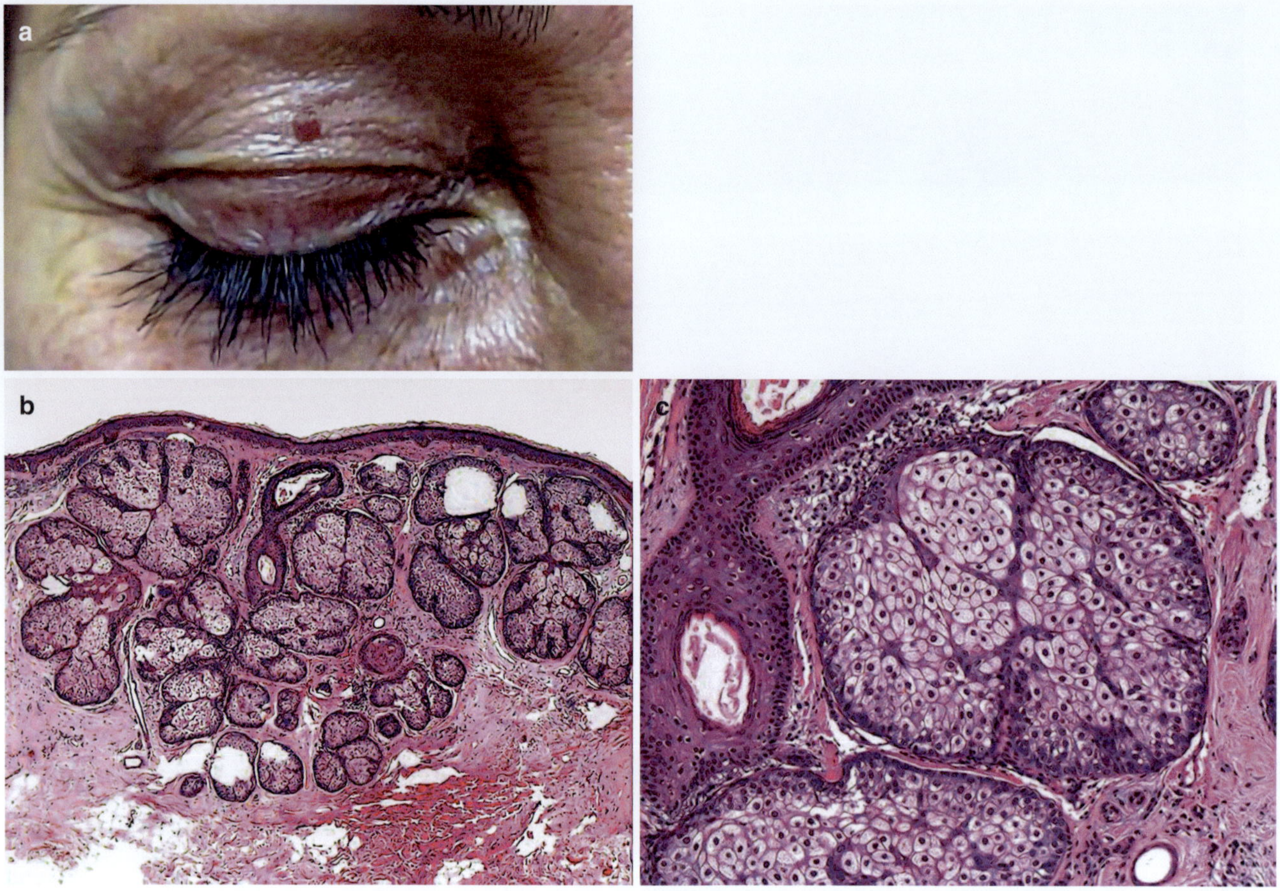

Clinically, the lesion is a brown, small, soft, dome-shaped papule, usually 2–5 mm in diameter, often with a central umbilication.

Sections show a large, mature sebaceous gland without thickening of the peripheral germinative layer of seboblasts with lateral lobules protruding the surface epithelium upward and a central dilated infundibulum.

Sebaceous Carcinoma (a–f)

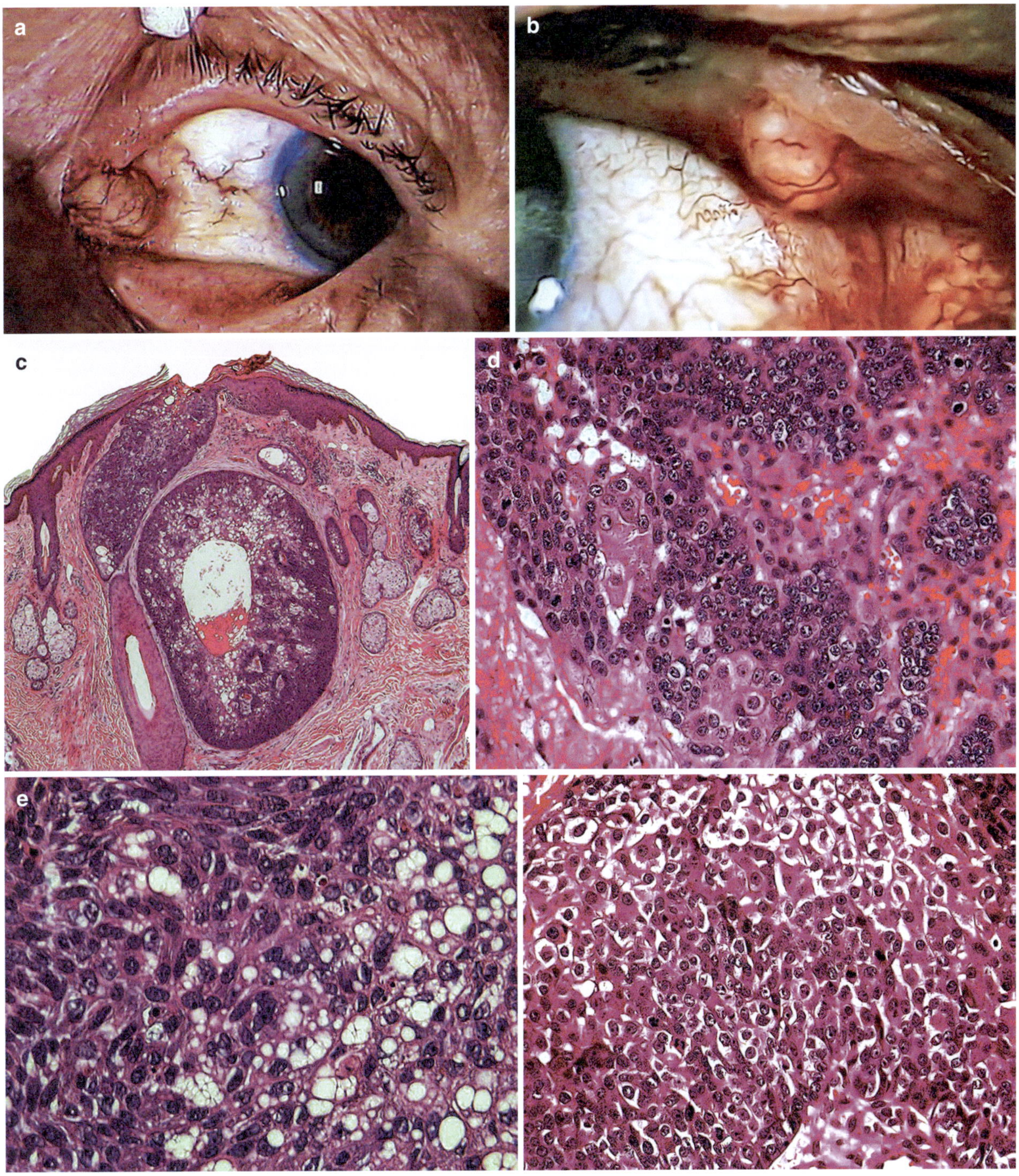

Clinically, the lesion is a yellow, small, circumscribed nodule with a smooth surface at the outer canthus with thin capillaries running over its surface. Another lesion is observed on lid eversion showing similar criteria and covered with conjunctiva.

Sections show a dermal-based tumor with a focal connection to the epidermis or follicular epithelium. The tumor is formed of lobular aggregates of cells separated by fibrovascular stroma and shows central comedo-type necrosis. The tumor lobules are formed of a higher proportion of atypical basaloid (undifferentiated) cells with minimal differentiation toward multivacuolated cells with prominent pleomorphism and atypia, frequent mitoses, and necrosis. Focal areas of squamous metaplasia are observed.

Ancillary Tools

IHC [5]

Androgen receptor

Adipophilin: membranous vesicular pattern (a granular pattern is considered negative)

Keratin

EMA

LeUM1

Ki67: increased relative to sebaceous adenoma and sebaceoma

p53: increased relative to sebaceous adenoma and sebaceoma

BerEP4

Pyogenic Granuloma (a, b)

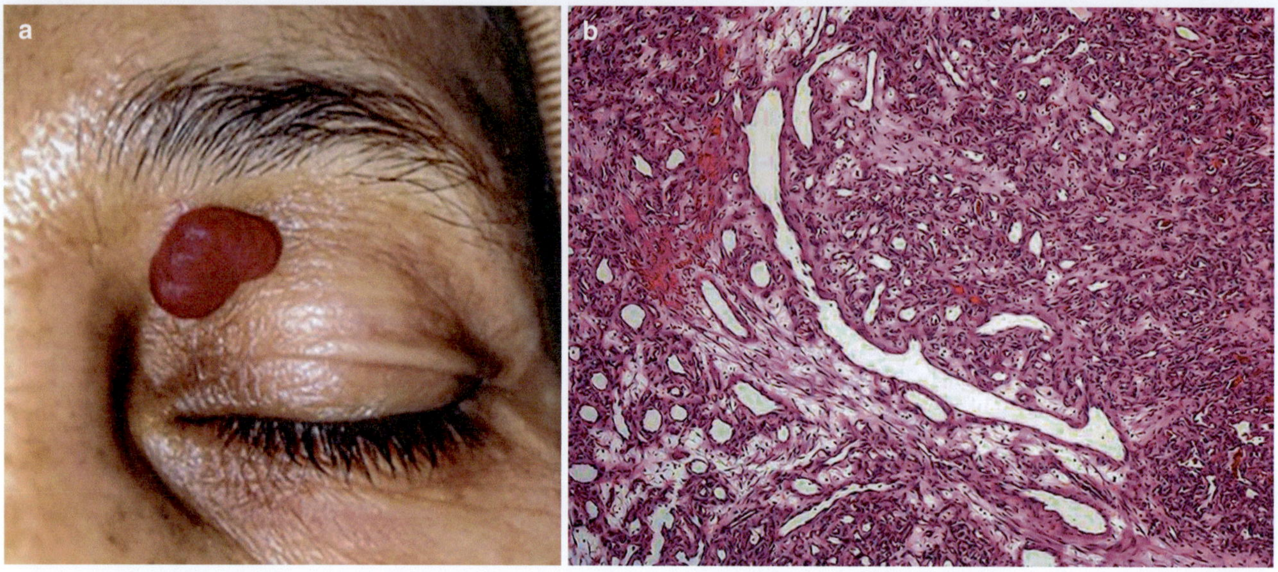

Clinically, the lesion is a smooth, red-purple, sessile nodule.

The section shows a lobular pattern of vascular proliferation with inflammation and edema resembling granulation tissue with a central branching vessel called a capillary or vascular lobule, with no / rare red blood cells, surrounded by endothelial cells. Deep lesions often lack edema and inflammation.

14.3 Conjunctiva

Ligneous Conjunctivitis (a, b)

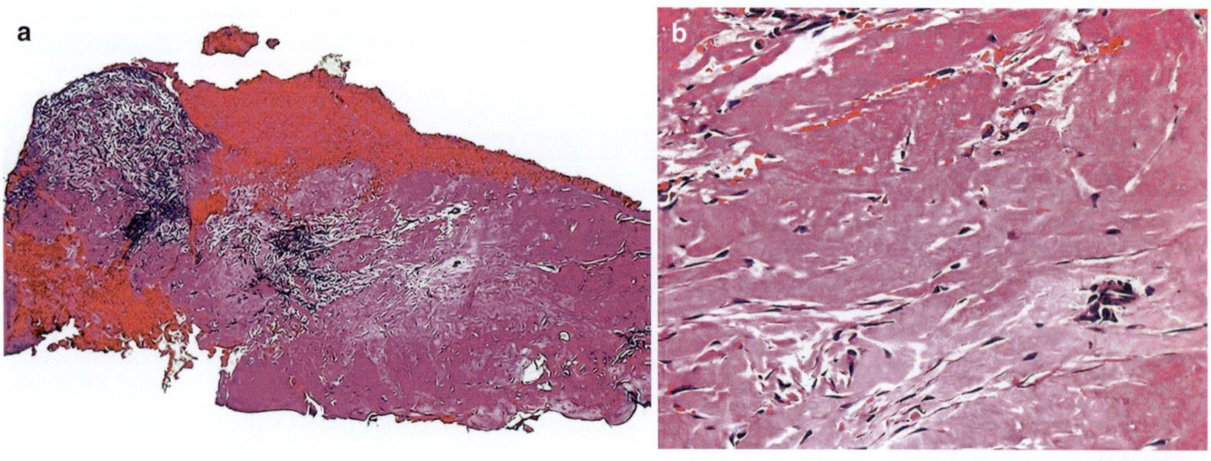

Sections show two components: granulation tissue and sheets of intensely eosinophilic acellular amorphous material, which is composed predominantly of fibrin. The conjunctival epithelium is thin and replaced focally with necrotic tissue.

Pinguecula (a–c)

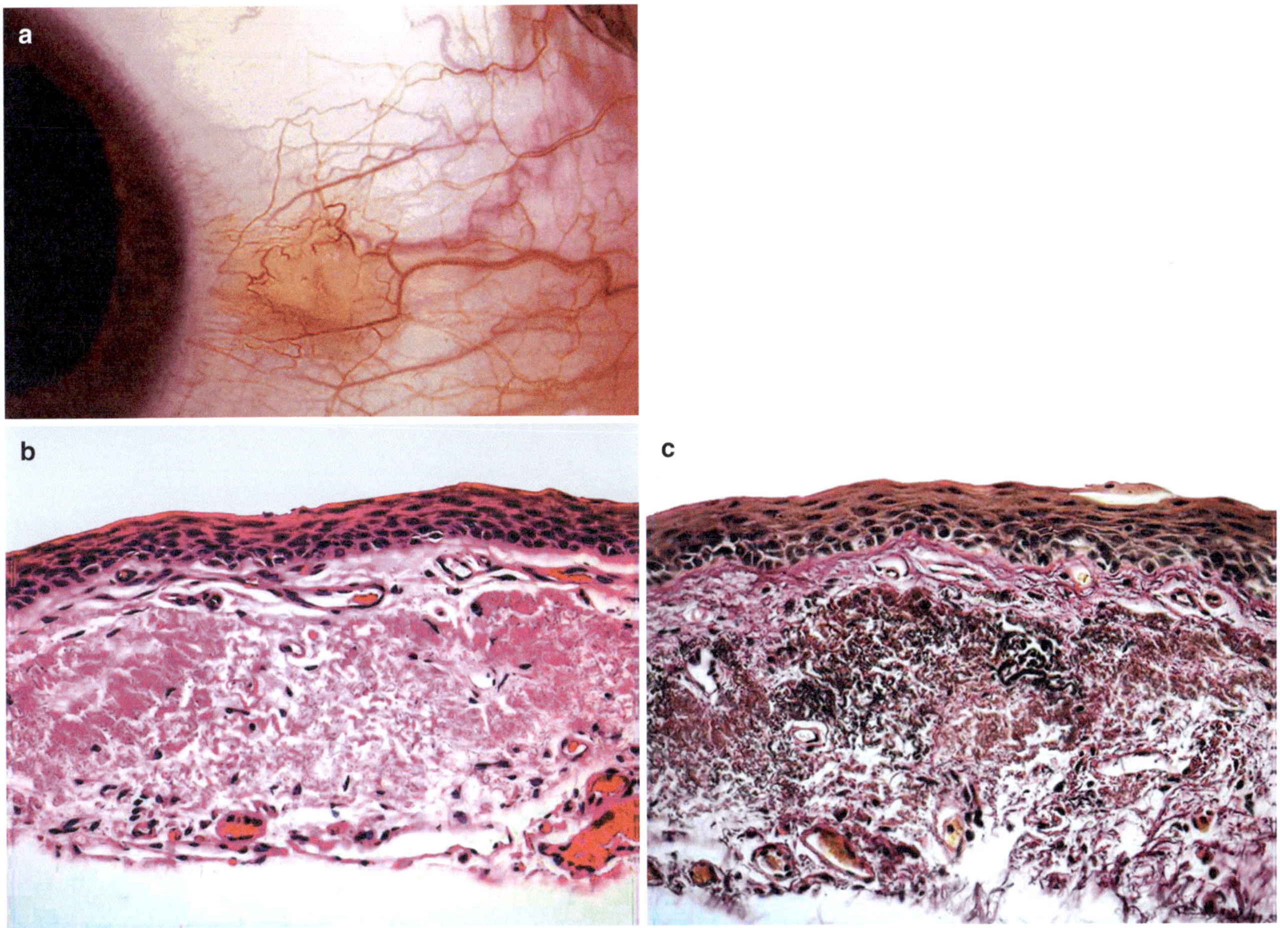

Clinically, the lesion is an elevated yellow mound near the limbus.

Sections show a cellular grayish granular deposit of extracellular matrix material beneath the limbal epithelium, which usually is elevated and thinned. The damaged matrix material stains positively (black) with the Verhoeff-van Gieson stain for elastic tissue.

Epibulbar Complex Choristoma (a–c)

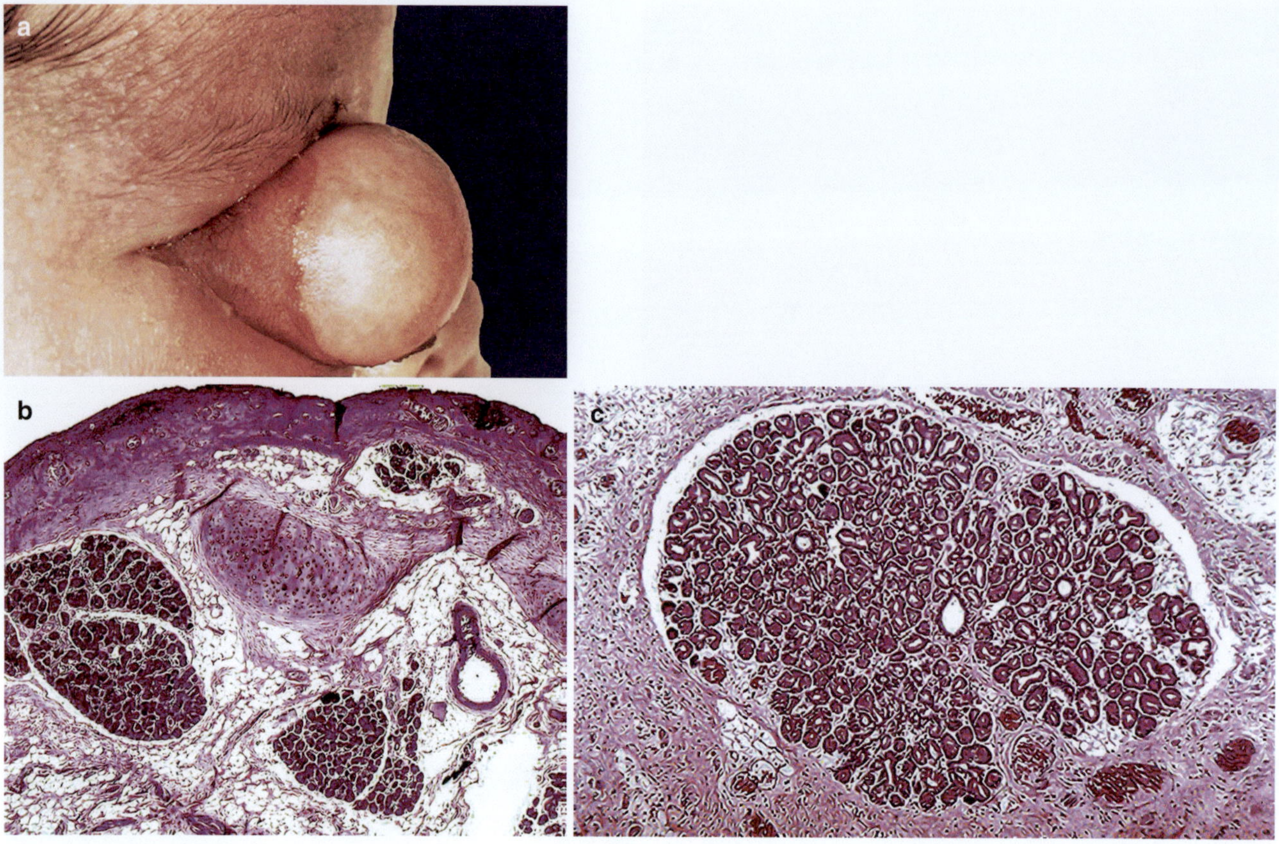

Clinically, the lesion is a firm, localized, elevated, opaque, yellow-white mass.

Sections show mature cartilage, lacrimal tissue, and adipose tissue.

Osseous Choristoma (a)

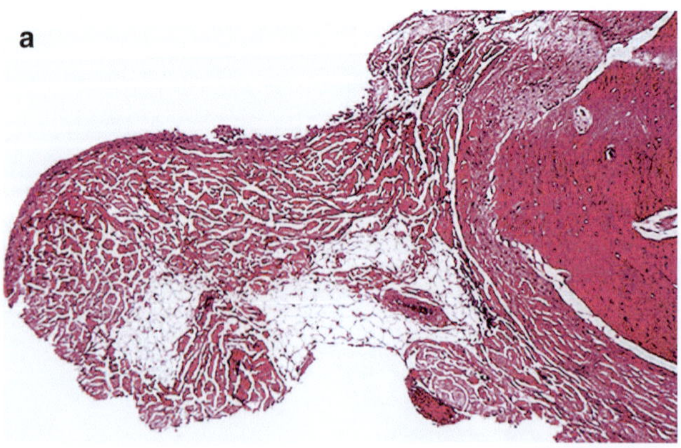

The section shows compact lamellar bone surrounded by dense, collagenous stroma.

Conjunctival Intraepithelial Neoplasia/CIS (a–h)

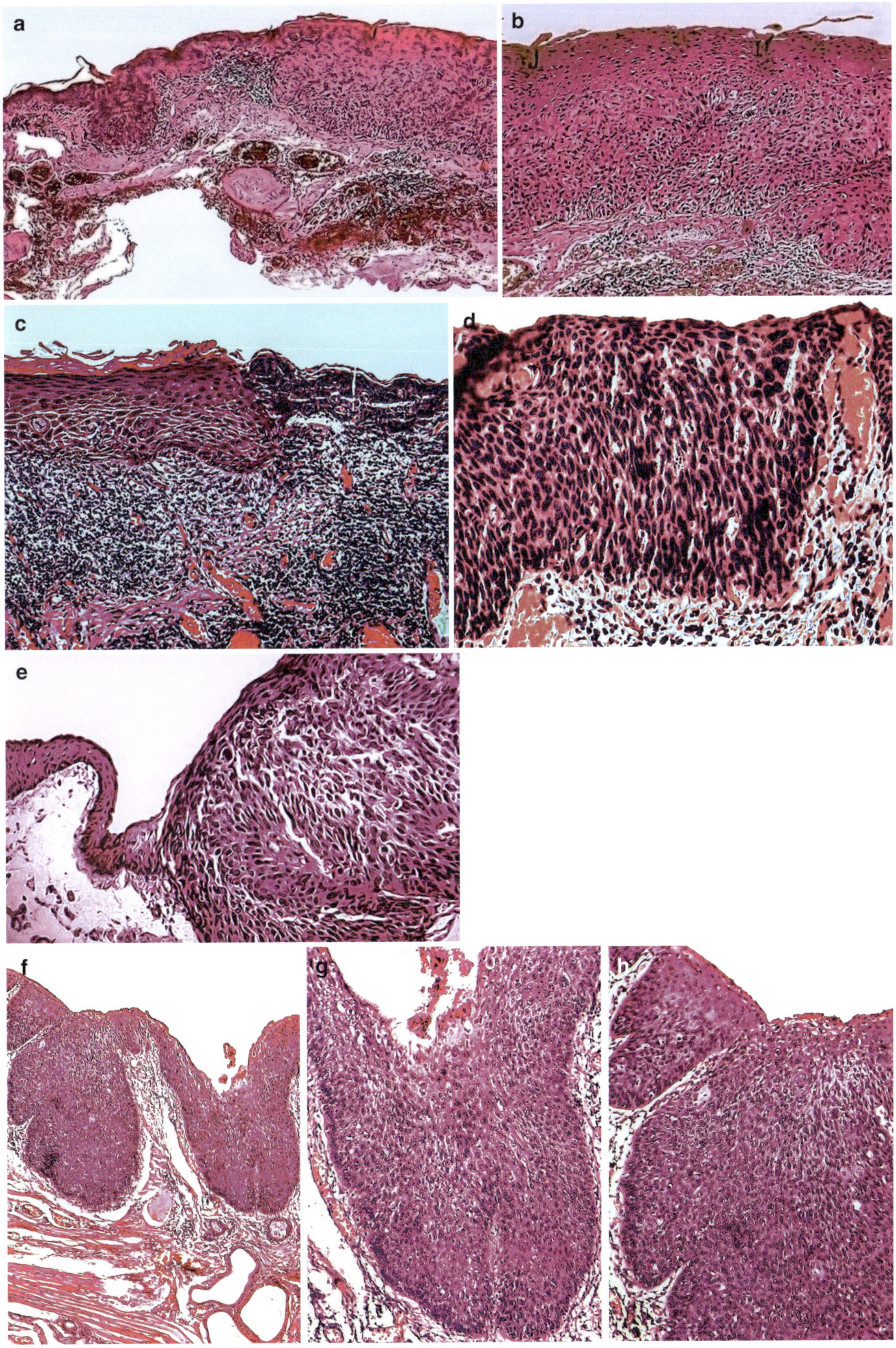

Sections show acanthosis, loss of normal maturation sequence with disorganization, and dysplasia with intact basement membrane. Dysplasia may be:

- **Grade 2 (moderate dysplasia)** (a–c), which involves lower two-thirds of thickness
- **Grade 3 (severe dysplasia) (d),** which involves > lower two-thirds of thickness surface maturation still present.

Carcinoma in situ (CIS) (e–h), which involves the entire epithelium (full thickness); no more surface maturation (surface epithelium replaced by dysplastic cells). The subepithelial connective tissue is fibrous and infiltrated by chronic inflammatory cells.

Conjunctival Well Differentiated Squamous Cell Carcinoma (a–h)

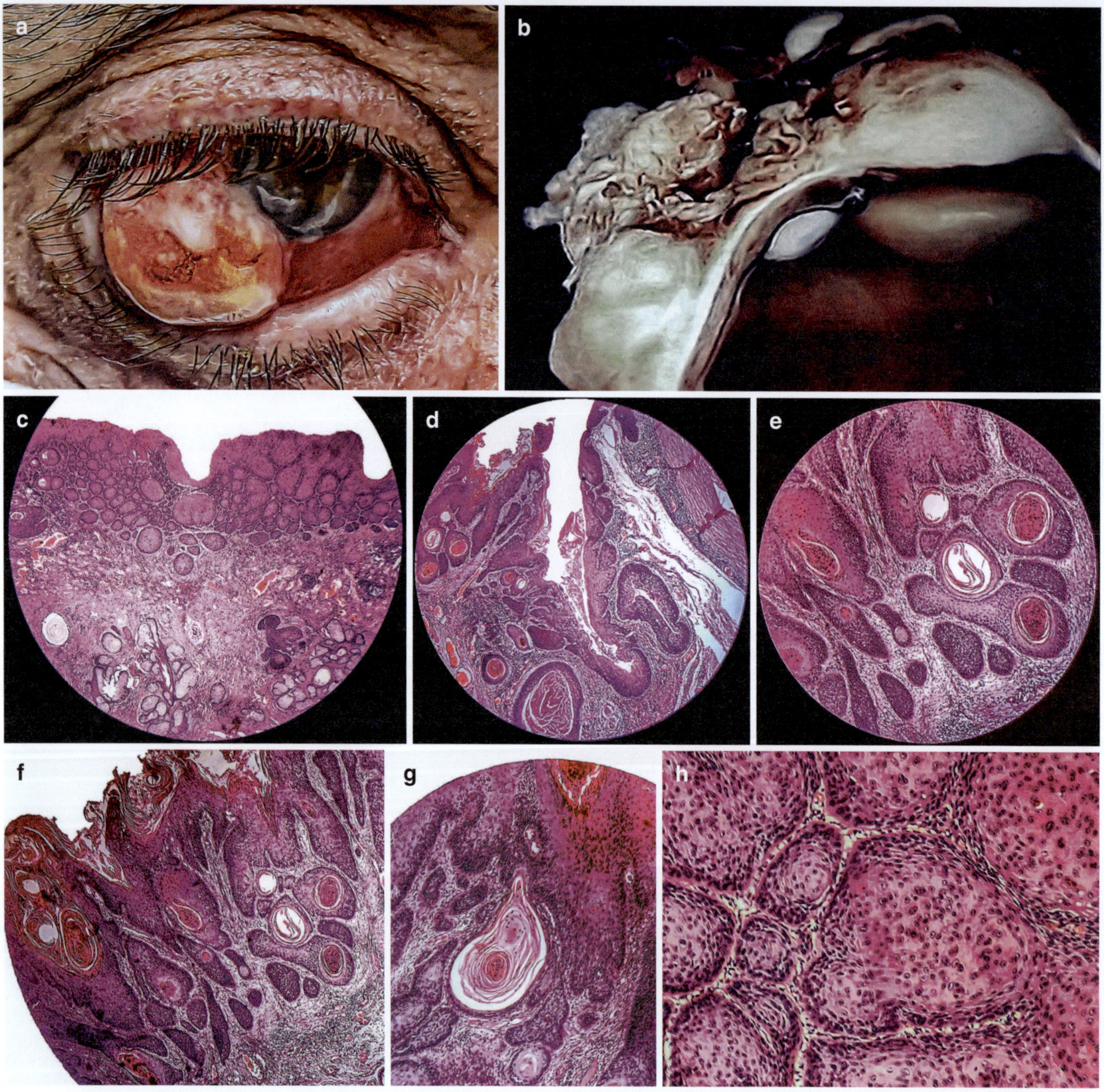

Clinically, there is an exophytic gray-white mass with surface ulceration at the limbus surrounded by inflamed conjunctiva. In (b), there is intraocular invasion by advanced conjunctival squamous cell carcinoma. The choroid and ciliary body are thickened by the tumor.

Sections show clusters of malignant squamous cells forming islands and nests with central parakeratin invading the subepithelial connective tissue and surrounded by chronic inflammatory cells. The overlying epithelium shows CIS.

Kaposi Sarcoma (a–d)

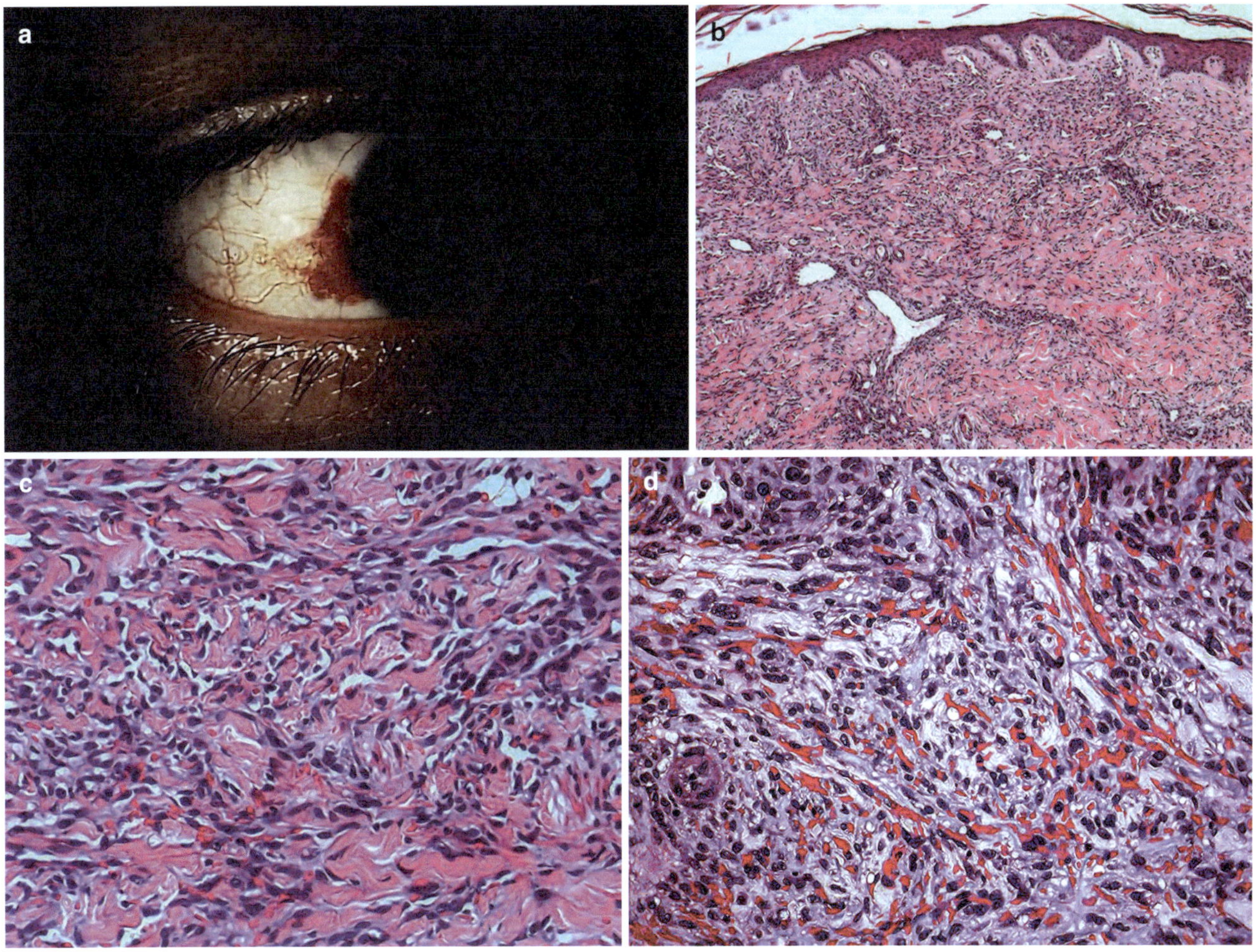

Clinically, the lesion is a subconjunctival hemorrhage in the bulbar conjunctiva.

Sections show dilated vascular channels dissecting through dermal collagen surrounded by larger, fusiform endothelial cells with hyperchromatic nuclei and thin, dilated vascular channels filled with erythrocytes and lined by flat endothelial cells with fusiform nuclei and scanty cytoplasm. Extravasated erythrocytes and hemosiderin deposits, together with lymphoplasmacytic infiltrate, surround the tumor areas.

Ancillary Tools

IHC [6]:

CD31, CD34, and podoplanin (D2–40) of the endothelial cells confirm the vascular origin of these tumors.

Factor VII, a clotting protein produced by endothelial cells.

HHV8 DNA in KS lesions can be detected by the reverse transcriptase polymerase chain reaction.

HHV8 latent-associated nuclear antigen-1 (LANA-1).

Primary Acquired Melanosis (PAM)/Conjunctival Melanocytic Intra-epithelial Lesions (C-MIL) (a–e)/ Invasive Melanoma (f, g)

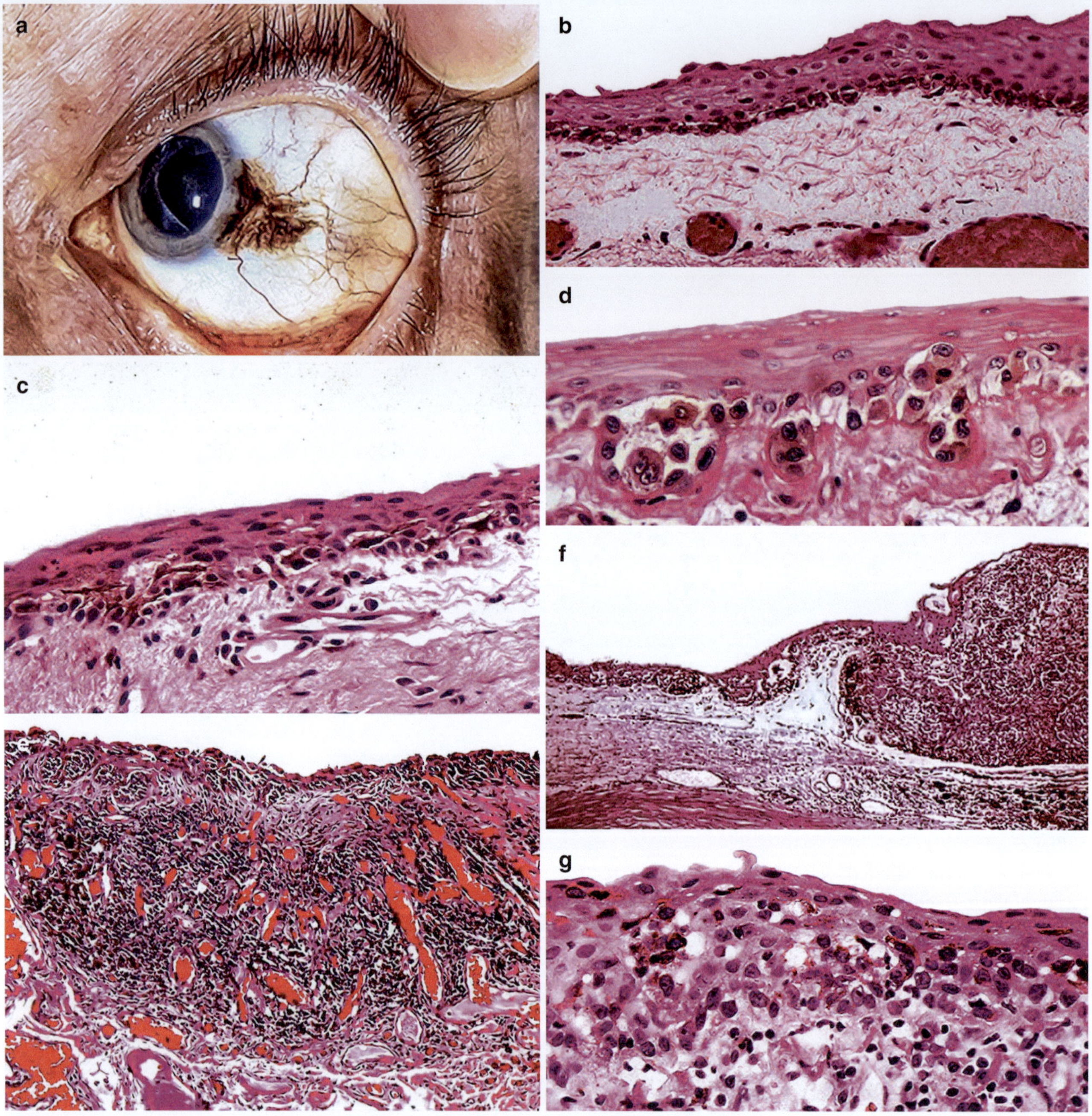

Clinically, the lesion is unilateral, flat, and develops in lightly complexioned persons.

Sections show C-MIL as follows [7]:

(b) **Benign melanosis: C-MIN grade (0–1)**: Conjunctiva! Hypermelanosis (increased pigment in epithelial cells without melanocytic hyperplasia or atypia). Slight or focal melanocytic hyperplasia without atypia (parabasal melanocytes with condensed round nuclei, smaller than basal epithelial cells, inconspicuous nucleoli, and inconspicuous cytoplasm) may be seen.

(c) **Low-grade C-MIL. PAM with mild atypia: C-MIN (grades 2–4)**: Predominantly basilar melanocytic proliferation with low-grade atypia (dendritic or small-to-moderate-size polyhedral, usually nonepithelioid melanocytes with round-to-irregular nuclear contours, often nuclear hyperchromasia, inconspicuous nucleoli, and inconspicuous or scant cytoplasm).

(d) **High-grade C-MIL. PAM with moderate to severe atypia: C-MIN (grade 5–10)**: More confluent basilar and significant nonbasilar proliferation of melanocytes with high-grade atypia (moderate to severe), evidence of intraepithelial nested and/or pagetoid growth, and epithelioid cell cytomorphology.

(e) **Melanoma in situ**: The term melanoma in situ may be used for (1) the most atypical high-grade C-MILs involving close-to-full thickness of the epithelium as in (e) and (2) histologically obvious melanomas without documented evidence of subepithelial invasion.

(f and g) **Invasive Melanoma**: Invasion of atypical melanocytes into epithelial and subepithelial connective tissue. Usually thin surface epithelium. Bizarre polygonal epithelioid cells with eosinophilic cytoplasm, large atypical nuclei, and prominent eosinophilic nuclei. Also, spindle cells are smaller cells. Often lymphocytes at the base or tumor margins

14.4 Lacrimal Gland and Duct

Dacryocystitis/Canaliculitis (a–d)

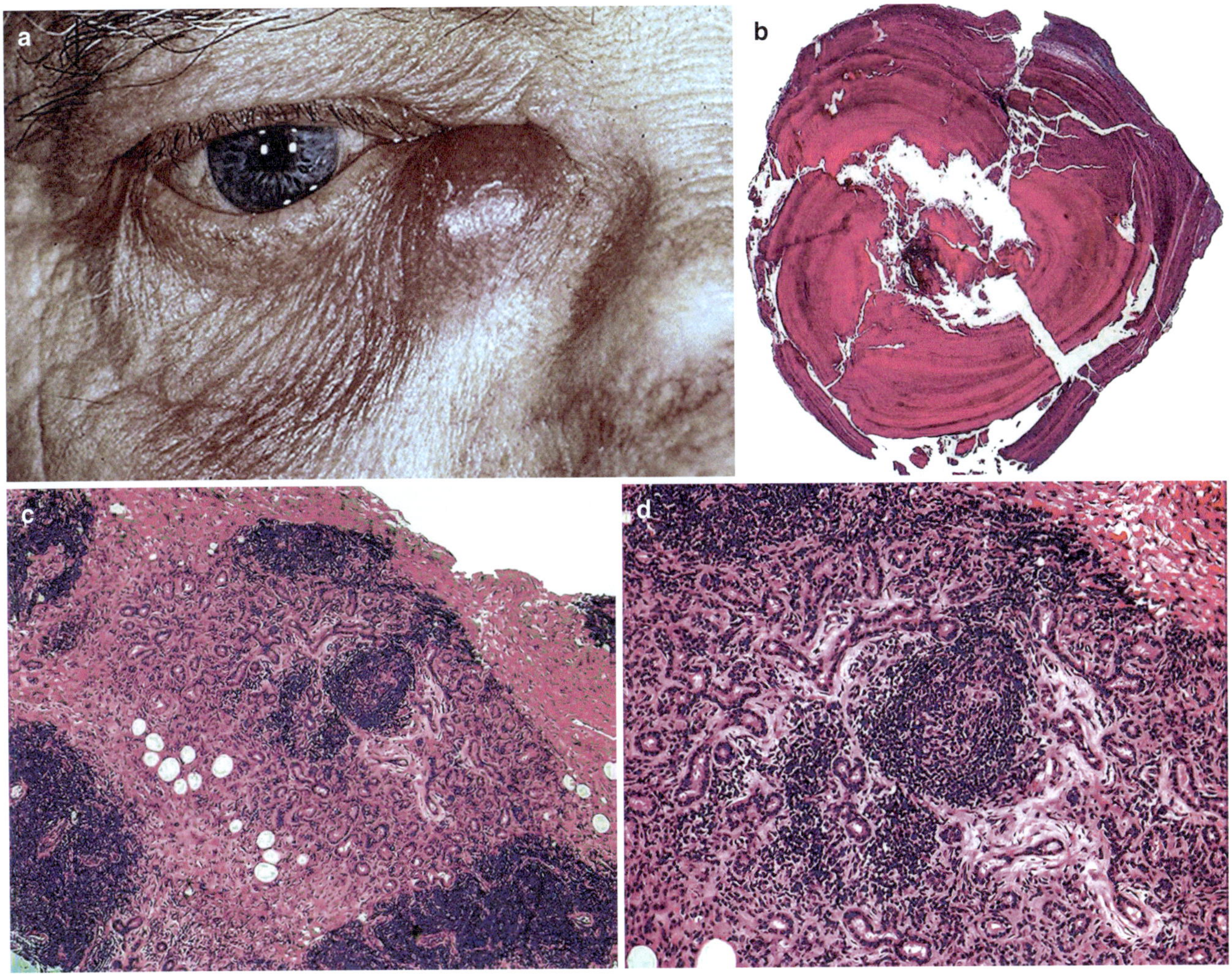

Clinically, the lesion is periorbital cellulitis, including erythema, warmth, and swelling around the eye, along with tenderness and purulent discharge from the tear duct. The swelling does not project above the medial canthal ligament.

Sections show

(b) Acute dacryocystitis, in which the lacrimal sac is dilated and filled with pus and acute inflammatory cells.

(c, d) Chronic dacryocystitis: showing diffuse stromal fibrosis infiltrated with chronic inflammatory cells with formation of lymphoid follicles and proliferation of capillaries and lacrimal ductules.

14.5 Uvea (Iris, Choroid, and Ciliary Body), Limbus, and Sclera

Lisch Nodule

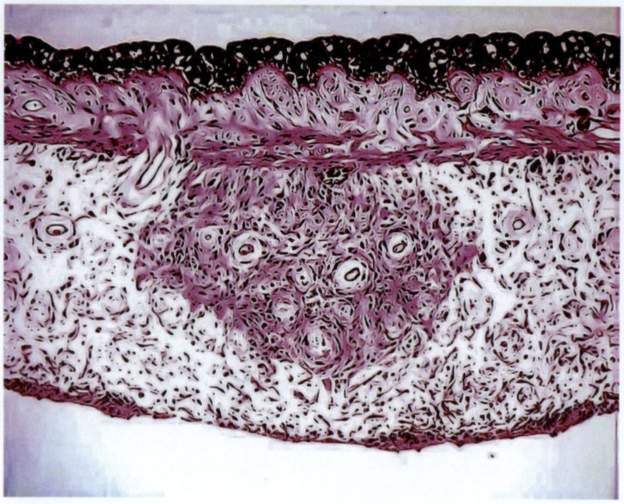

Sections show collections of spindle-shaped cells with oval nuclei and a pigmented cytoplasm arranged in dense, textured collagenous bundles. Fibroblast-like cells and mast cells were also observed.

Ancillary Tools

IHC [8]:

Vimentin, smooth muscle actin, neuron-specific enolase, and S100. These findings suggest that the spindle cells in Lisch nodules have characteristics of both Schwann cells and melanocytes.

Uveal Melanoma (Ciliary body and choroidal melanoma) (a)

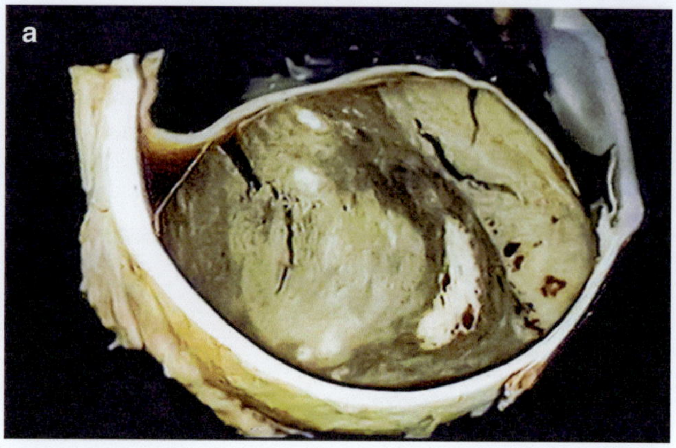

An enucleated eye showing a gray, solid, choroidal melanoma with a large basal diameter with retinal detachment and a focal area of necrosis that extends through the Bruch membrane into the retina and vitreous, producing retinal detachment, macular edema, and choroidal hemorrhage.

Microscopic Picture of Uveal Melanoma (b–i)

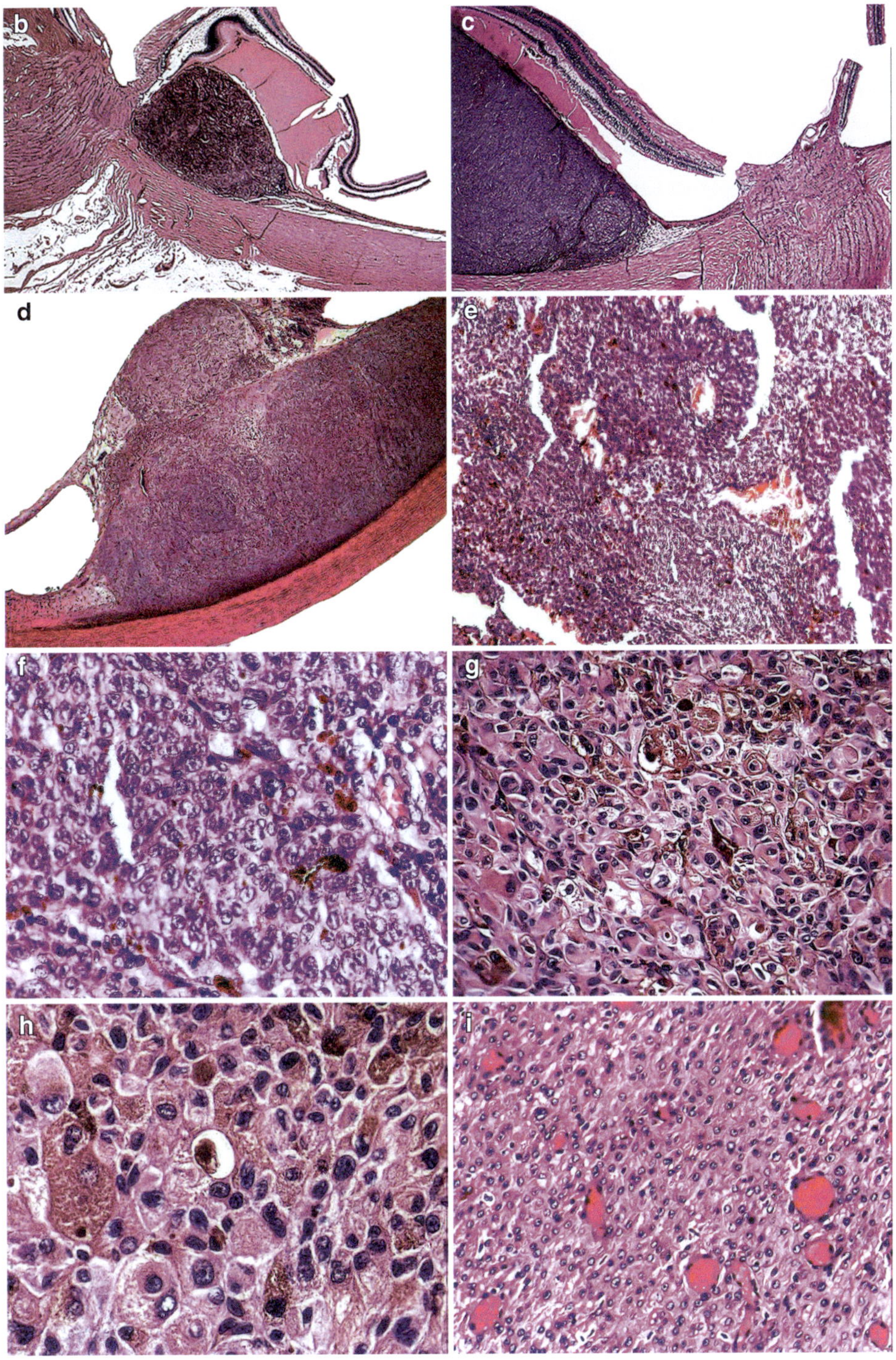

Sections show diffuse tumor mass not invading the optic nerve and causing a retinal break with the accumulation of subretinal fluid and fibrous metaplasia of the retinal pigment epithelium over the tumor apex. (d, e). The tumor is formed of 2 distinct cells, usually in combination: spindle-shaped cells with large oval nuclei and distinct nucleoli, and epithelioid cells: large polygonal cells with atypical nuclei and 1 or more prominent nucleoli. The tumor shows intra- and extracellular melanin pigment. Sometimes, the tumor may be amelanotic and need IHC evaluation of its cells (i).

Ancillary Tools

IHC [9]:

HMB45: specific and sensitive
S100: Sensitive
Vimentin, MelanA, MITF1Â
SOX10: highly sensitive to melanocytic proliferation
Ki67 and pHH3:Â
Molecular/cytogenetics description [10]:

- The most frequently mutated genes in UM are GNAQ and GNA11. Mutations in these genes occur in 71–93% of all UM tumors. They have no predictive value.
- The mutation status of secondary driver genes EIF1AX, SF3B1, and BAP1 is almost always mutually exclusive. Patients with a BAP1 mutation or absent BAP1 expression with immunohistochemistry (IHC) have a high metastatic risk, while patients with an EIF1AX mutation have a low risk of metastatic disease.
- Tumors with loss of chromosome 3 (monosomy 3) have decreased disease-free survival, which is associated with BAP1 mutations.

Necrotic Melanoma (a, b)

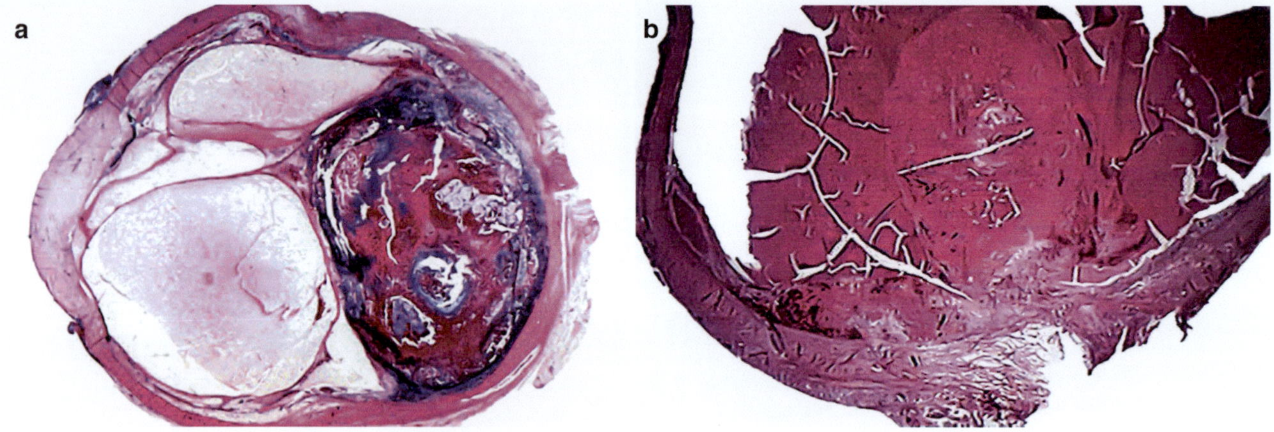

Sections show nearly 100% of the tumor is necrotic, with a thin rim of tumor cells present near the sclera. The necrotic tumor is formed of necrotic (ghost) melanoma cells with a scattering of melanin pigment and focal inflammatory cellular infiltrate (blue areas). In (b), the whole tumor is completely necrotic with the focal presence of melanin pigment near the sclera.

Metastatic Melanoma

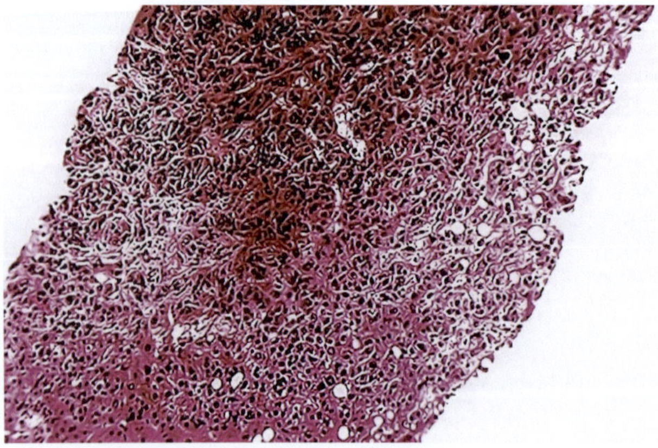

The section shows malignant pigmented melanoma cells in a non-destructive pattern around hepatocytes with perivascular (peritheliomatous) accentuation of tumor growth.

14.6 Retina

Retinal Astrocytoma (a, b)

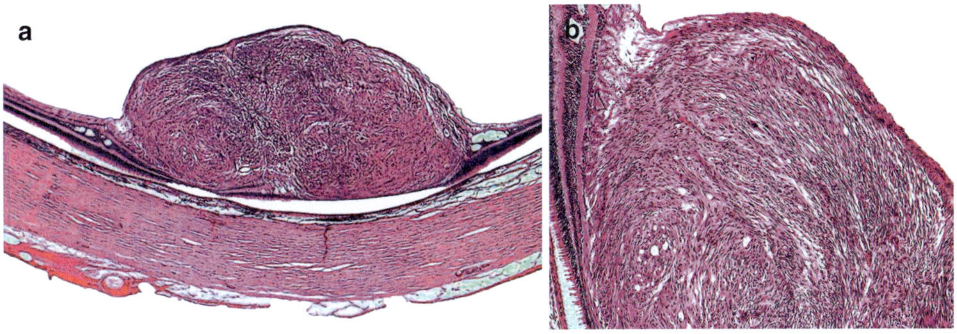

Sections show tumors composed of spindle-shaped cells that had short, spindle-shaped, densely stained nuclei and fibrillary eosinophilic cytoplasm. Cell borders were indistinct, with the cells forming vague fascicular patterns and small cystic cavities. No calcification, mitoses, or necrosis are noted.

Leukocoria

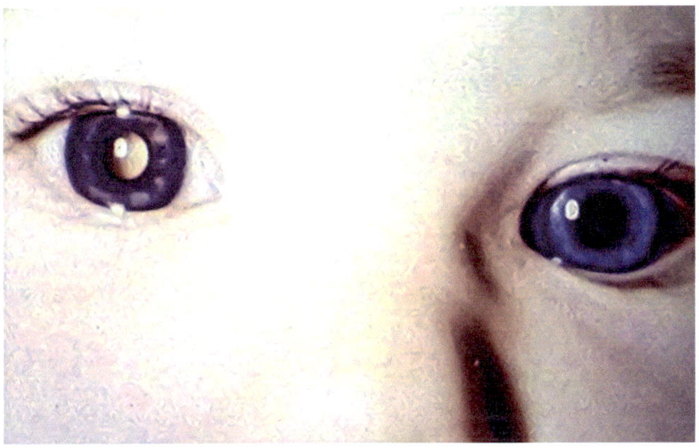

The term leukocoria means "white pupil." It is often used more broadly to encompass a spectrum of opacities and abnormalities. Leukocoria in an infant or older child may manifest the presence of retinoblastoma.

Retinoblastoma (a–c)

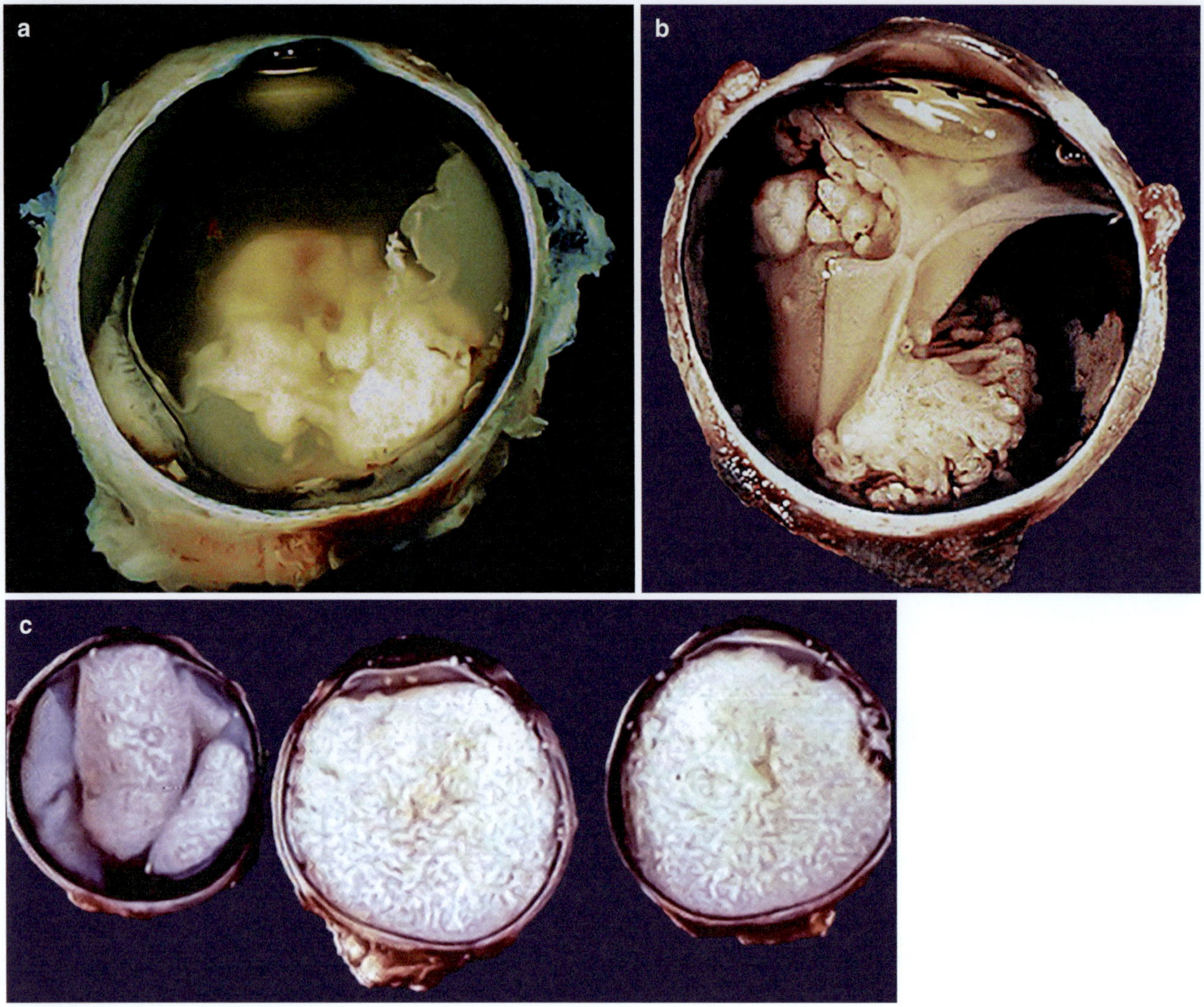

An enucleated eye showing a creamy white mass with chalky areas of calcification and yellow necrotic areas.

The tumor grows inward (endophytic growth).

The tumor may seed in remote parts of the eye (intraocular spread) (b) or fill the globe (c).

Microscopic Picture of Retinoblastoma (d–i)

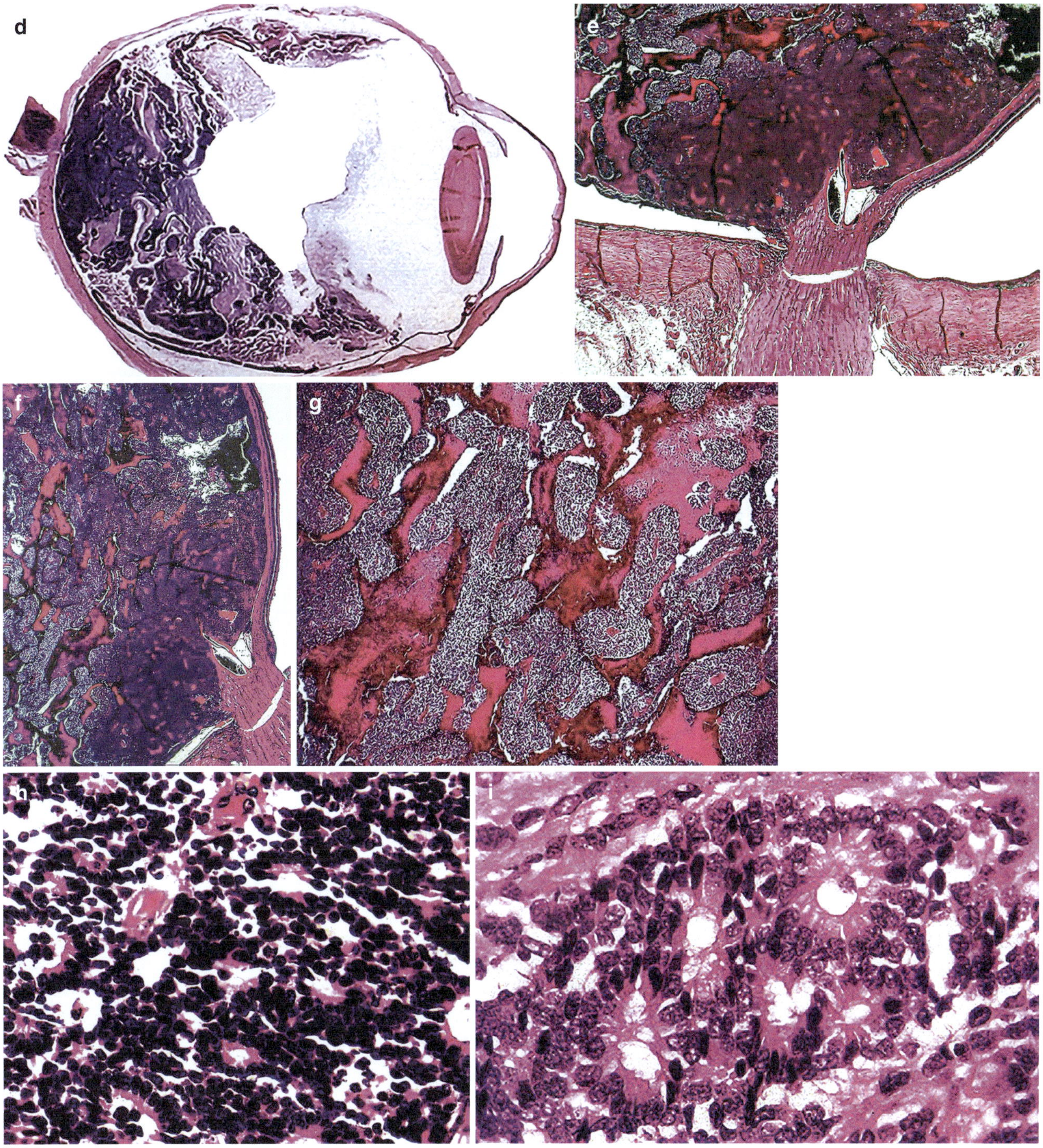

Sections show hyperchromatic small round blue cells with scant cytoplasm arranged in sheets, nests, and trabeculae. Flexner-Wintersteiner rosettes (most common): Central lumen with basally located nuclei analogous to the outer limiting membrane of the normal retina (Homer Wright rosettes are less common in retinoblastoma and lack of central lumen and tumor nuclei displaced away from the eosinophilic center).

Fleurettes (tumor cells arranged side by side with central lumen) may be seen. Areas of necrosis are observed.

Ancillary Tools

IHC [11]:

- SOX2
- MAP 2
- Neuron-specific enolase (NSE)
- Synaptophysin
- Retinoblastoma-associated protein (pRb)

14.7 Optic Nerve

Optic Nerve Melanocytoma (a–c)

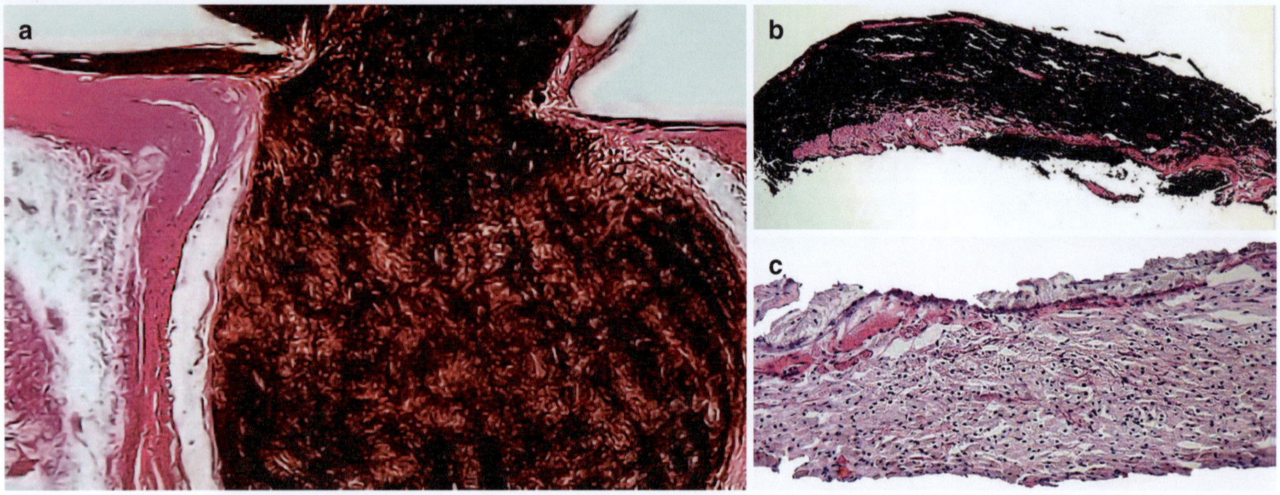

Sections show a heavily pigmented tumor involving the optic nerve head, optic nerve, and peripapillary choroid. Bleached preparation shows plump polyhedral melanocytes with small ovoid nuclei.

Optic Nerve Meningioma (a, b)

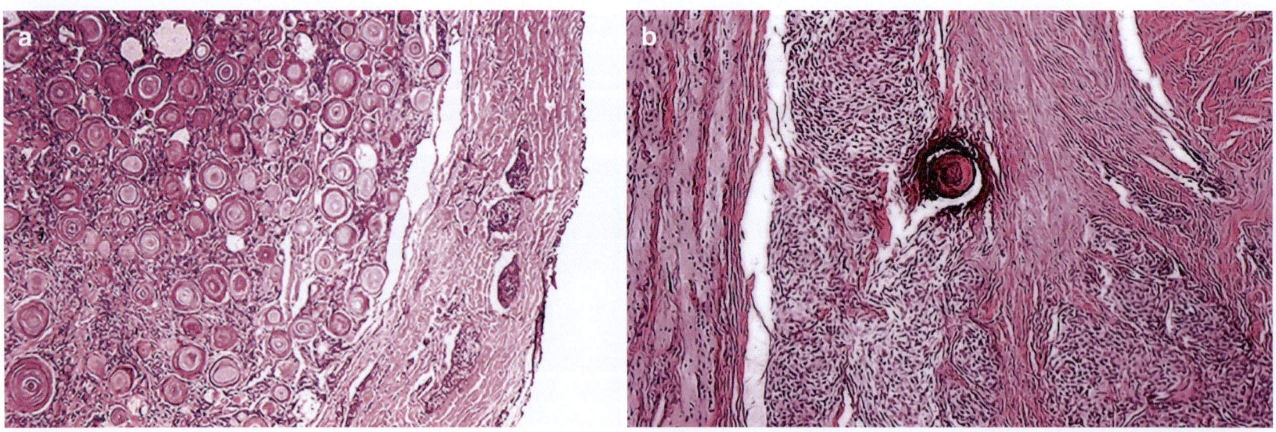

Sections show meningothelial cells arranged in small nests with a whorled pattern in the presence of psammoma bodies.

Optic Nerve Glioma (a, b)

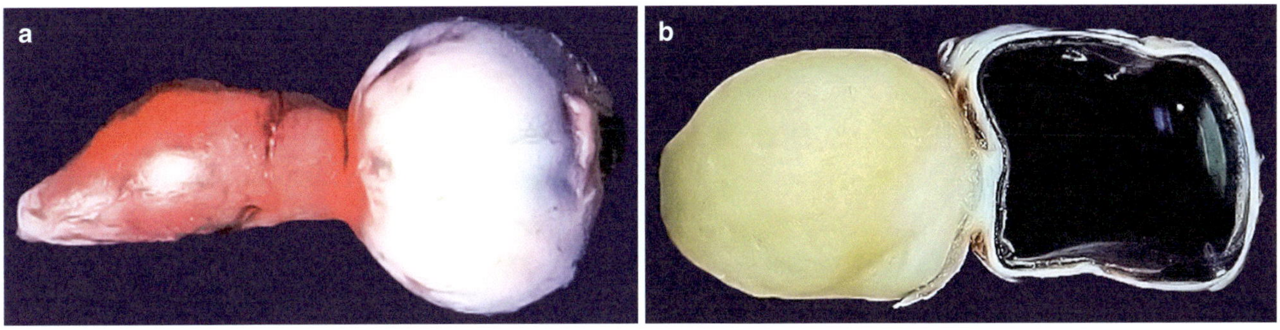

An enucleated eye showing a larger tumor-forming bulbous enlargement of the nerve often infiltrates the pia, causing arachnoid thickening. The cut section is solid and pale yellow.

Microscopic Picture of Optic Nerve Glioma (c, d)

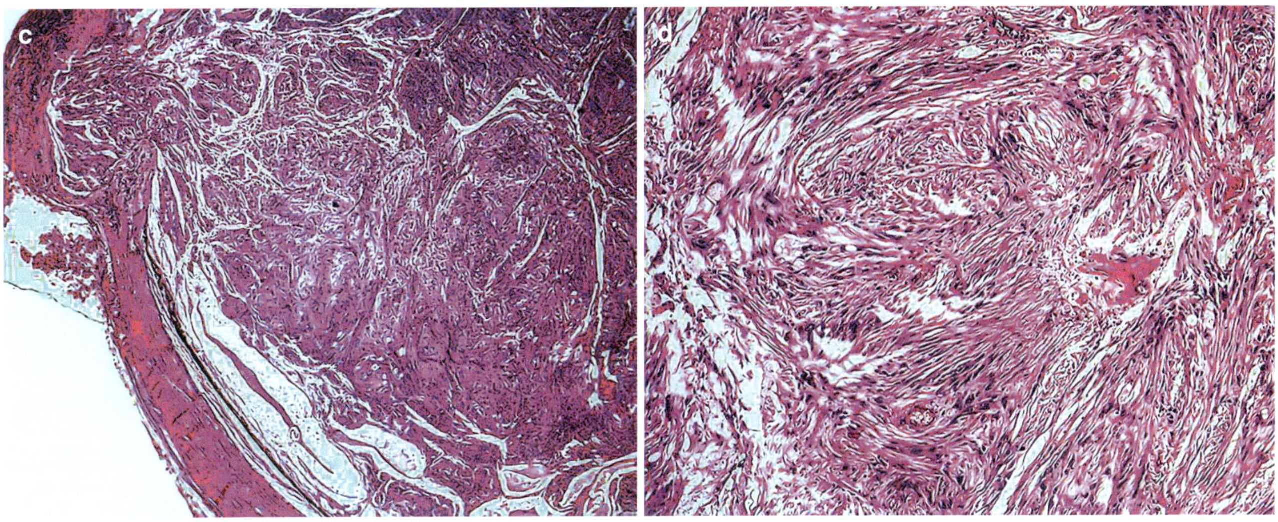

Sections show low-grade pilocytic astrocytoma, similar to cerebellar and third ventricle tumors, with round to spindled nuclei and dendrite-like cytoplasmic processes. Rosenthal fibers (fusiform, cigar-shaped eosinophilic structures within astrocyte cytoplasmic processes are a nonspecific degenerative change), hypercellularity with brisk mitotic activity are observed. Difficult to differentiate reactive vs. neoplastic resection margins

Optic nerve atrophy (a)

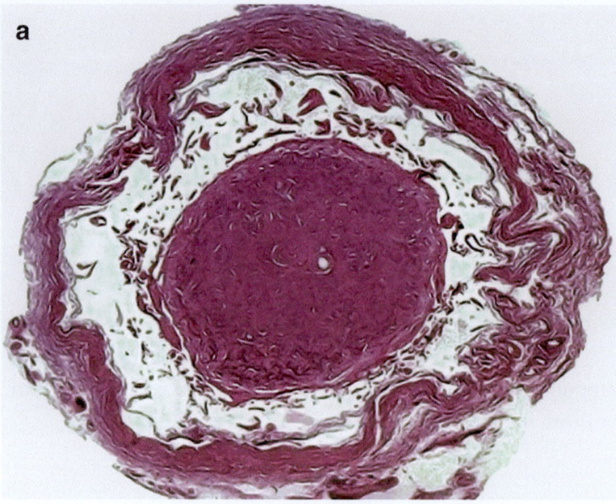

The section shows the loss of substance of the optic nerve due to degeneration of myelin sheaths and axons. Dura appears redundant due to loss of substance. Gliosis within nerve

14.8 Orbit

Orbital Dermoid Cyst (a, b)

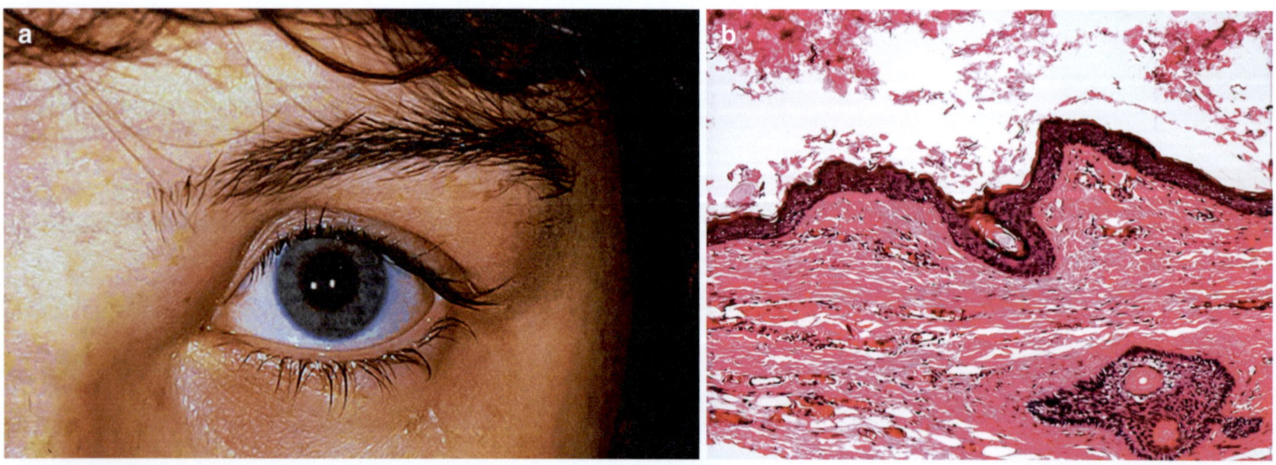

Clinically, the lesion is a soft, non-tender, round/oval cyst on the outer edge of the eyebrow.

The section shows an encapsulated cyst, lined by well-differentiated epidermis and dermis. The lumen is filled with keratinous debris, hair, and sebum.

Embryonal Rhabdomyosarcoma (a–j)

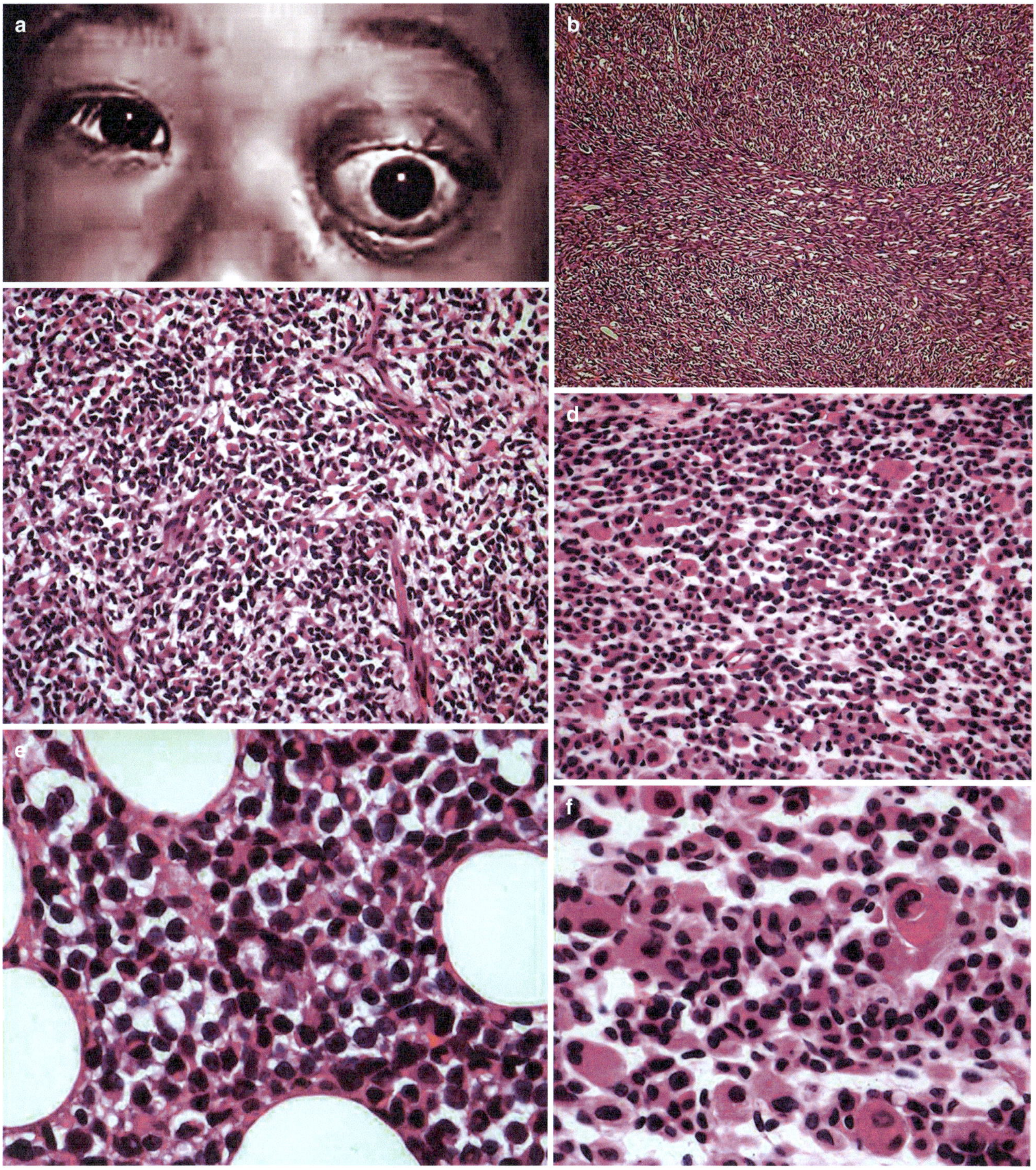

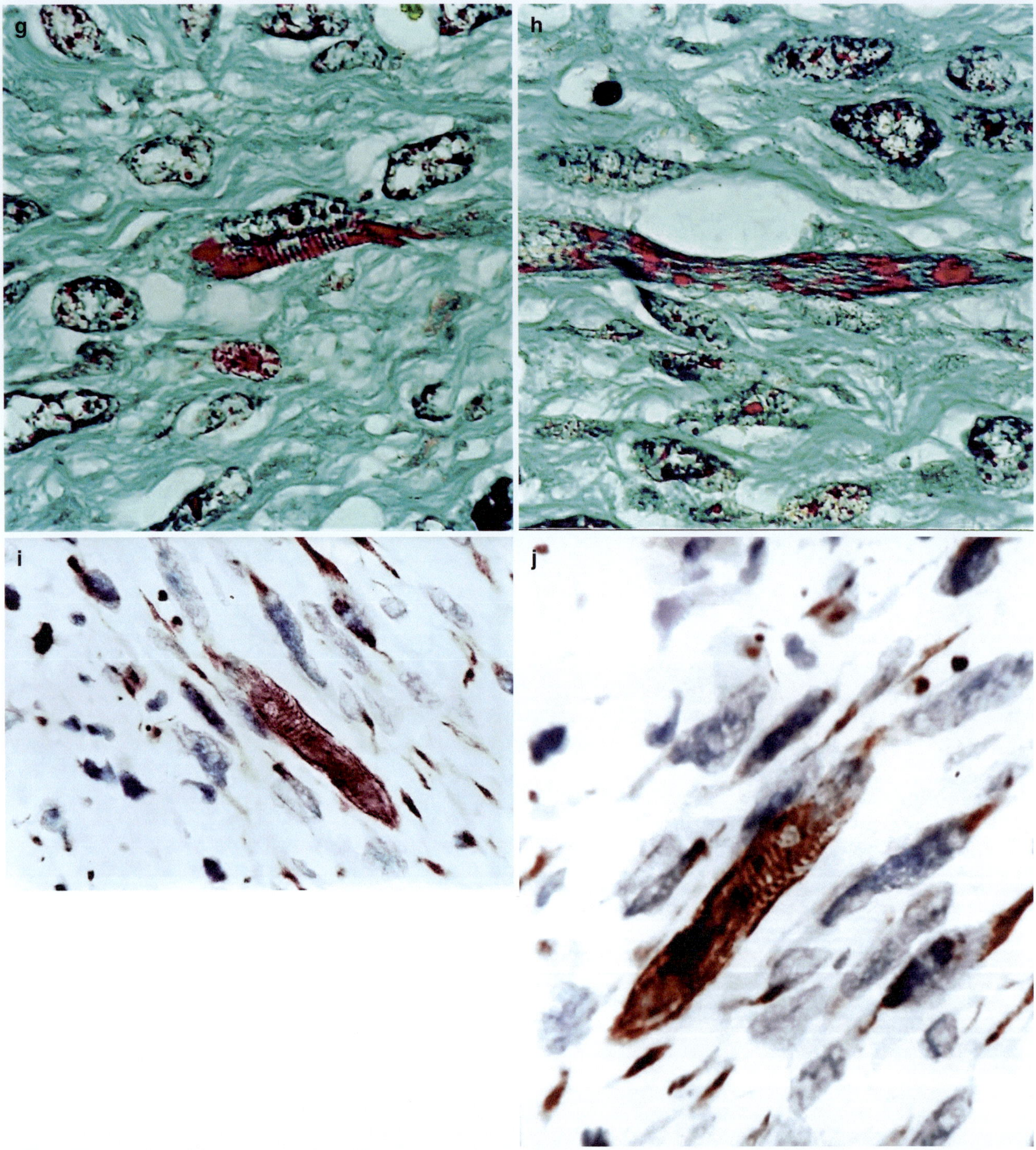

Clinically, the patient may present with a rapid onset of unilateral proptosis.

Sections show primitive mesenchymal rounded and spindle cells arranged in nests and sheets with prominent cytologic atypia, focal cleared cytoplasm, notable crush artifacts, and nuclear molding with variable degrees of skeletal muscle differentiation.

Ancillary Tools

IHC [12]:

Masson trichrome (g and h) may highlight the muscle differentiation.

Desmin (i), MyoD1, or myogenin are critical to document.

Vimentin (j) in all cells (even the most primitive).

Actin, myoglobin, myosin, and creatine kinase M staining in more differentiated cells.

There may be aberrant staining for several antigens: occasional immunoreactivity to cytokeratin, S100 protein, neurofilaments, and B cell markers such as CD20.

Molecular/cytogenetics description [13]:

11p15.5 Loss of heterozygosity or loss of imprinting is a frequent finding.

Chromosomal aneuploidies are very common, especially with gains of chromosome 8 (seen in 90% of patients).

- Additional gains frequently seen include chromosomes 2, 11, 12, 13, and 20.

Inactivating mutations of TP53 and CDKN2A and activating mutations of RAS family genes.

References

1. Helm K, Findeis-Hosey J. (2008). Immunohistochemistry of pigmented actinic keratoses, actinic keratoses, melanomas in situ, and solar lentigines with Melan-A. J Cutan Pathol. 35(10):931-4. doi: https://doi.org/10.1111/j.1600-0560.2007.00921.x. PMID: 18494818.
2. Inman GJ. et al. (2018). The genomic landscape of cutaneous SCC reveals drivers and a novel azathioprine-associated mutational signature. Nat Commun. 9(1):3667. doi: https://doi.org/10.1038/s41467-018-06027-1. PMID: 30202019; PMCID: PMC6131170.
3. Kim BC. et al. (2012). An immunohistochemical study of the origin of the solid strand in syringoma, using carcinoembryonic antigen, epithelial membrane antigen, and cytokeratin 5. Int J Dermatol. 51(7):817-22. doi: https://doi.org/10.1111/j.1365--4632.2011.05069.x. PMID: 22040364.
4. Wu WM, Lee YS. (2010). Autosomal dominant multiple syringomas linked to chromosome 16q22. Br J Dermatol.162(5):1083-7. doi: https://doi.org/10.1111/j.1365-2133.2010.09677.x. PMID: 20132207.
5. Orr CK, Yazdanie F, Shinder R. (2018). Current review of sebaceous cell carcinoma. Curr Opin. Ophthalmol. 29(5):445-450. doi: https://doi.org/10.1097/ICU.0000000000000505. PMID: 29985175.
6. Venkateswaran N. et al. (2021). Spotlight on ocular Kaposi's sarcoma: an update on the presentation, diagnosis, and management options. Expert Rev Ophthalmol. 16(6):477-489. doi: https://doi.org/10.1080/17469899.2021.1962294. PMID: 36325272; PMCID: PMC9624465.
7. Hardeep Singh Mudhar. et al. (2024). A Multicenter Study Validates the WHO 2022 Classification for Conjunctival Melanocytic Intraepithelial Lesions With Clinical and Prognostic Relevance, Laboratory Investigation, 104,(1). https://doi.org/10.1016/j.labinv.2023.100281.
8. Richetta A. et al. (2004). Lisch nodules of the iris in neurofibromatosis type 1 JEADV 18, 342–344. doi: https://doi.org/10.1111/j.1468-3083.2004.00915.x.
9. Rashid AB, Grossniklaus HE.(2014). Clinical, pathologic, and imaging features and biological markers of uveal melanoma. Methods Mol Biol.1102:397-425. doi: https://doi.org/10.1007/978-1-62703-727-3_21. PMID: 24258990.
10. Patrone S. et al. (2018). Prognostic value of chromosomal imbalances, gene mutations, and BAP1 expression in uveal melanoma. Genes Chromosomes Cancer. 57(8):387-400. doi: https://doi.org/10.1002/gcc.22541. PMID: 29689622.
11. Orellana ME. et al. (2016). Immunohistochemical analysis of retinoblastoma cell phenotype using neuronal and glial cell markers. Arq Bras Oftalmol.79(6):395-399. doi: https://doi.org/10.5935/0004-2749.20160111. PMID: 28076568.
12. Machado I, Mayordomo-Aranda E, Giner F, Llombart-Bosch A.(2015). The Role of Immunohistochemistry in Rhabdomyosarcoma Diagnosis Using Tissue Microarray Technology and a Xenograft Model. Fetal Pediatr Pathol. 34(5):271-81. doi: https://doi.org/10.3109/15513815.2015.1042604. PMID: 26125949.
13. Paulson V. et al. (2011). High-resolution array CGH identifies common mechanisms that drive embryonal rhabdomyosarcoma pathogenesis. Genes Chromosomes Cancer. 50(6):397-408. doi: https://doi.org/10.1002/gcc.20864. PMID: 21412928.

Index

G. Dawood, *Color Atlas of Human Gross and Microscopic Pathology*, https://doi.org/10.1007/978-3-031-76007-5

MIX
Papier aus verantwortungsvollen Quellen
Paper from responsible sources
FSC® C105338

If you have any concerns about our products,
you can contact us on
ProductSafety@springernature.com

In case Publisher is established outside the EU,
the EU authorized representative is:
Springer Nature Customer Service Center GmbH
Europaplatz 3, 69115 Heidelberg, Germany

Printed by Libri Plureos GmbH
in Hamburg, Germany